CHRONIC COMPLEX DISEASES OF

CHILDHOOD

A PRACTICAL GUIDE FOR CLINICIANS

CHRONIC COMPLEX DISEASES OF
CHILDHOOD

A PRACTICAL GUIDE FOR CLINICIANS

Edited by

Shahram Yazdani, MD
Associate Clinical Professor
Department of Pediatrics
David Geffen School of Medicine, UCLA
Mattel Children's Hospital
Los Angeles, California

Sean A. McGhee, MD
Assistant Clinical Professor
Department of Pediatrics
David Geffen School of Medicine, UCLA
Mattel Children's Hospital
Los Angeles, California

E. Richard Stiehm, MD
Professor of Pediatrics
Department of Pediatrics
David Geffen School of Medicine, UCLA
Mattel Children's Hospital
Los Angeles, California

BrownWalker Press
Boca Raton

Chronic Complex Diseases of Childhood:
A Practical Guide for Clinicians

BrownWalker Press
Boca Raton, Florida
USA • 2011

ISBN-10: 1-59942-535-1 *(paper)*
ISBN-13: 978-1-59942-535-1 *(paper)*

ISBN-13: 978-1-59942-536-8 *(Adobe PDF)*
ISBN-13: 978-1-59942-571-9 *(Mobi/Kindle)*
ISBN-13: 978-1-59942-572-6 *(ePub/iPad)*
ISBN-13: 978-1-59942-573-3 *(Google Editions)*

www.brownwalker.com

Publisher's Cataloging-in-Publication Data

Chronic complex diseases of childhood: a practical guide for clinicians/edited
by Shahram Yazdani, Sean A. McGhee, & E. Richard Stiehm.
p. cm.
ISBN: 1-59942-535-1
1. Chronic diseases in children. 2. Chronically ill children—Care. 3. Children—Diseases . 4. Chronic disease.   I. Stiehm, E. Richard, 1933- II. Yazdani,
Shahram. III. McGhee, Sean A. IV. Title.
RJ380 .C583 2010
618.92—dc22
                                                                                    2010924756

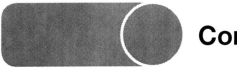

Contents

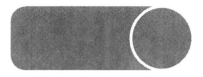

Tables & Figures

Tables

Figures

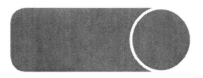

Acknowledgements

This book is dedicated to Marcy and Madison Smith who have inspired us, and the caring clinicians-educators who masterfully care for these children. We go forward with the notion that there is yet much to be done in understanding and caring for them.

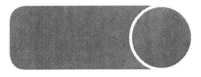

Contributors

Dafna Bababeygy, MD
Resident in Pediatrics
Department of Pediatrics and Medicine
Keck School of Medicine of the University of
    Southern California
Children's Hospital Los Angeles
Los Angeles, California

David E. Bronstein, MD, MS
Staff, Pediatric Infectious Diseases
Department of Pediatrics
Southern California Permanente Medical Group
Palmdale, California

Stephen Cederbaum, MD
Professor of Pediatrics and Human Genetics
Mental Retardation Research Center
Department of Pediatrics
David Geffen School of Medicine, UCLA
Mattel Children's Hospital at UCLA
Los Angeles, California

Randall Chan, MD
Resident in Medicine and Pediatrics
Department of Pediatrics and Medicine
Keck School of Medicine of the University of
    Southern California
Children's Hospital Los Angeles
Los Angeles, California

Jerry C. Cheng, MD
Staff, Pediatric Hematology Oncologist
Department of Pediatrics
Southern California Permanente Medical Group
Los Angeles, California

Natascha Ching, MD
Assistant Clinical Professor of Pediatrics
Pediatric Infectious Diseases
David Geffen School of Medicine, UCLA
Mattel Children's Hospital at UCLA
Los Angeles, California

Ronald W Cotliar, MD
Clinical Professor of Dermatology and Pediatrics
Department of Pediatrics
David Geffen School of Medicine, UCLA
Mattel Children's Hospital at UCLA
Los Angeles, California

Stephen A. Feig, M.D
Professor of Pediatrics, Emeritus
Pediatric Hematology and Oncology
David Geffen School of Medicine, UCLA
Mattel Children's Hospital at UCLA
Los Angeles, California

Mitchell E. Geffner, MD
Professor of Pediatrics
Keck School of Medicine of the University of
    Southern California
Acting Chief, Division of Endocrinology, Diabetes,
    and Metabolism
Fellowship Program Director
Children's Hospital Los Angeles
Los Angeles, California

Christopher C. Giza, MD
Associate Professor of Pediatric Neurology and
    Neurosurgery
Interdepartmental Program for Neuroscience and
    Biomedical Engineering
UCLA Department of Neurosurgery
David Geffen School of Medicine, UCLA
Mattel Children's Hospital at UCLA
Los Angeles, California

Leslie J. Hamilton, MD
Medical Director
Medical Home Project at UCLA
David Geffen School of Medicine, UCLA
Mattel Children's Hospital at UCLA
Los Angeles, California

Eba H. Hathout, MD
Professor of Pediatrics
Chief, Division of Pediatric Endocrinology
Director, Pediatric Diabetes Center and Islet Transplant Laboratory
Loma Linda University School of Medicine
Loma Linda, California

Shaun Hussain, MD
Fellow, Division of Pediatric Neurology
David Geffen School of Medicine, UCLA
Mattel Children's Hospital at UCLA
Los Angeles, California

James N. Jarvis, MD
Professor of Pediatrics
CMRI/Arthritis Foundation Oklahoma Chapter Research Chair
Chief, Pediatric Rheumatology
University of Oklahoma College of Medicine
Oklahoma City, Oklahoma

Roberta M. Kato, MD
Postdoctoral Fellow in Pediatric Pulmonology
Pediatric Pulmonology
Keck School of Medicine of the University of Southern California
Children's Hospital Los Angeles
Los Angeles, California

Thomas G. Keens, MD
Professor of Pediatrics, Physiology and Biophysics
Pediatric Pulmonology
Keck School of Medicine of the University of Southern California
Children's Hospital Los Angeles
Los Angeles, California

Pamela Kempert, MD
Assistant Clinical Professor of Pediatrics
Director of Hematology
Pediatric Hematology and Oncology
David Geffen School of Medicine, UCLA
Mattel Children's Hospital at UCLA
Los Angeles, California

Thomas S. Klitzner, MD, PhD
Jack H. Skirball Professor of Pediatrics
Chief, Division of Pediatric Cardiology
Vice-Chair for Academic Affairs
David Geffen School of Medicine, UCLA
Mattel Children's Hospital at UCLA
Los Angeles, California

Sheila Kun, RN, BSN, MS, CPN.
Nurse Care Manager
Pediatric Pulmonology
Keck School of Medicine of the University \of Southern California
Children's Hospital Los Angeles
Los Angeles, California

Delphine J. Lee, MD, PhD
Assistant Professor of Dermatology
Department of Medicine,
Division of Dermatology
David Geffen School of Medicine, UCLA
Los Angeles, California

Sean A. McGhee, MD
Assistant Clinical Professor
Division of Allergy and Immunology
David Geffen School of Medicine, UCLA
Mattel Children's Hospital at UCLA
Los Angeles, California

Theodore B. Moore, MD
Professor of Pediatrics
Clinical Director, Pediatric Hematology/Oncology
Director, Pediatric Blood and Marrow Transplant Program
David Geffen School of Medicine, UCLA
Mattel Children's Hospital at UCLA
Los Angeles, California

Kenji Morimoto, MD
Clinical Fellow
Division of Pediatric Hematology/Oncology
David Geffen School of Medicine, UCLA
Mattel Children's Hospital at UCLA
Los Angeles, California

Khiet D. Ngo, D.O.
Clinical Instructor of Pediatrics
Pediatric Gastroenterology &Transplantation
David Geffen School of Medicine, UCLA
Mattel Children's Hospital at UCLA
Los Angeles, California

Karin Nielsen, MD, MPH
Associate Clinical Professor of Pediatrics
Pediatric Infectious Diseases
David Geffen School of Medicine, UCLA
Mattel Children's Hospital at UCLA
Los Angeles, California

Katherine Wesseling Perry, MD
Assistant Clinical Professor of Pediatrics
Pediatric Nephrology
Department of Pediatrics
David Geffen School of Medicine, UCLA
Mattel Children's Hospital at UCLA
Los Angeles, California

Michelle Pietzak, MD
Assistant Clinical Professor of Pediatrics
Pediatric Gastroenterology and Nutrition
Keck School of Medicine of the University of
    Southern California
Children's Hospital Los Angeles
Los Angeles, California

Wendy H.P. Ren, MD
Assistant Clinical Professor of Anesthesiology
Department of Anesthesiology
David Geffen School of Medicine, UCLA
Ronald Reagan UCLA Medical Center
Los Angeles, California

Linda M. Roof, RN, MPH
Clinical Director
UCLA Health System
Department of Pediatrics
Pediatric Gastroenterology
David Geffen School of Medicine, UCLA
Mattel Children's Hospital at UCLA
Los Angeles, California

Raman Sankar, MD, PhD
Professor and Chief, Rubin Brown Distinguished
    Chair
Pediatric Neurology
David Geffen School of Medicine, UCLA
Mattel Children's Hospital at UCLA
Los Angeles, California

Gary M. Satou, MD
Associate Clinical Professor of Pediatrics
Director, Pediatric Echocardiography
Pediatric Cardiology
David Geffen School of Medicine, UCLA
Mattel Children's Hospital at UCLA
Los Angeles, California

George B. Segel, MD
Professor of Pediatrics and Medicine
Departments of Medicine and Pediatrics
Hematology and Oncology
University of Rochester School of Medicine
Rochester, New York

Kathryn Smith, RN, MN
Assistant Clinical Professor of Pediatrics
Associate Director for Administration
USC University Center of Excellence in Develop-
    mental Disabilities
Keck School of Medicine of the University of
    Southern California
Children's Hospital Los Angeles
Los Angeles, California

Robert S. Venick, MD
Assistant Clinical Professor of Pediatrics and Surgery
Pediatric Gastroenterology, Hepatology and Nutri-
    tion
Department of Pediatrics
David Geffen School of Medicine, UCLA
Mattel Children's Hospital at UCLA
Los Angeles, California

Samuel H. Wald, MD
Clinical Professor of Anesthesiology
Department of Anesthesiology
David Geffen School of Medicine, UCLA
Ronald Reagan UCLA Medical Center
Los Angeles, California

Derek Wong, MD, M.S.
Assistant Professor of Clinical Pediatrics
Clinical and Biochemical Geneticist
Medical Director of Newborn Screening
Division of Medical Genetics
Keck School of Medicine of the University of
    Southern California
Childrens Hospital Los Angeles
Los Angeles, California

Laura J. Wozniak, MD
Fellow in Pediatric Gastroenterology
Division of Pediatric Gastroenterology, Hepatology,
    and Nutrition
David Geffen School of Medicine, UCLA
Mattel Children's Hospital at UCLA
Los Angeles, California

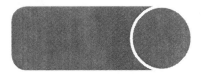

Preface

Recent advances in treatment of previously lethal pediatric illnesses has led to a growing population of children who require complex, chronic medical care. Most of this care is done at home or occasionally in chronic care facilities. Thus, the physicians including generalists, pediatricians and other health care personnel must provide acute and chronic care of these children in the office or emergency room setting.

This book was borne out of our own need for a concise, practical guide to assist in the care of children with complex diseases. This book focuses on the acute and long-term management of these children along with essential information regarding the pathogenesis, epidemiology, and prognosis of each disease. The diseases chosen for this book tend to be of a chronic, complex nature; require extensive specialized care; and lack readily accessible practice guidelines. Therefore, the authors have shared their knowledge and experience in order to assist primary care physicians better manage these illnesses. However, the more general chapters that focus on such issues as forming a medical home, management of medical devices, and disease drug interactions are relevant to the care of all children.

We thank all of our authors for their invaluable input and expertise and it is our hope that this guide book will assist physicians and other caretakers in improving the health and quality of life for these children and their families.

Shahram Yazdani
Sean A. McGhee
E. Richard Stiehm

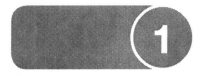

1 Creating the Medical Home

Introduction

Children with special health care needs interact with and receive services from a myriad of complex systems, and their parents must learn to access, navigate and coordinate services related to health care, developmental disabilities, special education, mental health, insurers and more. In addition, families may face challenges related to language, culture, socioeconomic status, and the ongoing daily burden of caring for a child with a chronic health condition. A medical home is a practice model that can serve to assist families by providing high quality care for children that is comprehensive, family-centered and coordinated in nature.

The American Academy of Pediatrics (AAP) defines a medical home as "a model of delivering primary care that is accessible, continuous, comprehensive, family-centered, coordinated, compassionate, and culturally effective care." In March 2007, the American Academy of Family Physicians (AAFP), the AAP, the American College of Physicians (ACP) and the American Osteopathic Association (AOA) published the Joint Principles of the Patient-Centered Medical Home, which defined the patient-centered medical home (PC-MH) as "an approach to providing comprehensive primary care for children, youth and adults. The PC-MH is a practice paradigm that facilitates partnerships between individual patients and their personal physicians, and when appropriate, the patient's family."

Most medical home definitions make reference to primary care, and for most children, this care will be delivered by a primary care provider in the child's community. But, for some—as is the case of children with rare or complex conditions—the specialist-, university-, or children's hospital-based special care center may serve as the medical home. For children with chronic conditions, the medical home provides linkages to needed services and coordination of care, a central repository of information about the child, and a place for families to seek information and support. In addition, because the medical home provider knows the child well, parents and providers can work together as partners to assure that the needs of the child are met in a timely and efficient way. Literature suggests that the medical home can have a positive impact on both the individual child and family, and on the health care system, as emergency department use may be reduced. The medical home concept, by definition, improves coordination between primary and specialty care providers, and community based agencies and programs serving the child and family.

What Constitutes a Medical Home?

The joint position paper of the AAFP, AAP, ACP and AOA, describes the basic elements of the medical home to include the following:

- A personal physician for first contact, continuous, and comprehensive care.
- A physician-directed medical practice with a team of individuals to provide ongoing care.
- A whole person orientation in which the physician takes responsibility for providing or arranging for all of the patient's acute, chronic, preventive or end of life care.
- Care that is coordinated and integrated across all components of the health care system.
- Assistance in transition to adult centered health care systems and supports.
- Quality and safety of care including advocacy, evidence based practices, continuous quality improvement, patient participation in decision making, the use of information technology, and participation in voluntary recognition processes.
- Enhanced access to care, expanded hours, and new options for communication with patients.
- Payment that appropriately recognizes the added value of the medical home.

Simply put, a medical home provides a base from which families can operate in caring for the child's special health care needs. In addition to providing primary, preventive and episodic illness care, the medical home provider

- assists families in identifying needed services and supports,
- refers families to care providers as appropriate,
- coordinates the care between multiple providers,
- consolidates medical records in one location, and
- facilitates transitions between in- and outpatient-care; and from pediatric- to adult-oriented providers.

While the child's care may be delivered in multiple locations by various types of providers, the medical home and the family work together to oversee the big picture, and understand how all the services and supports work together to provide comprehensive care for the child. This prevents gaps or duplications in services, and results in care that is comprehensive and cost effective. In short, optimal health care.

Benefits of Medical Home

Although serving as a medical home is a significant responsibility, there are several benefits to be derived both for the practice and the family. Foremost, families have one central and unifying health care environment for their child and an ongoing source of information and support. For providers, a medical home model encourages increased practice efficiencies and innovation, allows for easier patient follow up, and provides for shared patient care responsibility with specialists and community based services.

Families play an important role in the medical home and its members are considered full partners in their child's care. While the primary care provider or specialist may be the expert in the *health* care needed by the child, the family is the *overall* expert in their child as a whole. They are the constant in the child's life and provide the primary day-to-day care and support. In the medical home, families can be empowered to take a more proactive role in their child's care. For instance, they can be encouraged to create care notebooks that can be used to organize their child's records and facilitate communication among providers. The medical home is also a place where they can be provided with information about their child's condition, services, and supports so that they can advocate more effectively on behalf of their child.

What Are the Goals of the Medical Home?

The aim of the medical home is to provide high quality health care that is family-centered and coordinated, and is a place where parents and providers work together to set goals, seek services, monitor care and advocate to achieve the best possible outcomes for the child. Goal setting is carried out collaboratively by the parent, child if appropriate, and physician, as well as other members of the care team. Goals should be realistic and achievable and may change as the child's condition or family circumstances alter.

Several factors come into play in achieving those goals. First, comprehensive primary, preventive and episodic illness care is provided by a team led by a personal physician. Other team members may include nursing staff, care coordinators and/or administrative support staff within the practice setting. Next, the medical home is responsible for meeting the standards of basic pediatric health care for the child, and providing ongoing health education and support to the family. In addition, the medical home provides referrals to appropriate specialists as needed, and services in the community, such as special education and therapies. Third, families are given information about how and where to receive services, and what to expect. Lastly, the medical home provider maintains contact with the family to assure that referrals are successful and that the child ultimately receives needed services.

In a medical home, care is patient- and family-centered. Patient- and family-centered care is "grounded in mutually beneficial partnerships among health care patients, families, and providers. Patient- and family-centered care applies to patients of all ages, and it may be practiced in any health care setting." The core concepts of patient- and family-centered care include

1) *Dignity and respect*: In which the provider listens to and honors patient and family perspectives and choices and incorporates patient and family knowledge, values, beliefs and cultural backgrounds into the planning and delivery of care.
2) *Information sharing*: Where providers communicate and share complete and unbiased information with patients and families who receive timely, complete, and accurate information in order to effectively participate in care and decision-making.
3) *Participation*: Where patients and families are encouraged and supported in participating in care and decision-making at the level they choose.
4) *Collaboration*: In which patients and families are included in policy and program development, implementation, and evaluation, in health care facility design; and in professional education, as well as in the delivery of care (Institute for Family Centered Care, 2009). Providers and parents work as partners to identify child and family needs, and to locate and choose appropriate resources to meet those needs. This requires adequate time for communication with the family.

In order to optimize care and meet the family's goals, patient and family-centered care should be practiced by all members of the medical home.

A primary responsibility of the medical home is care coordination and chronic care management. This includes coordination among specialist physicians, community based resources, and service systems such as special education or the developmental disabilities system. Care coordination is more than making a referral. It includes ensuring that the family understands the reason for other needed services; assisting the family to access care; and periodically reassessing the effectiveness of the service and adjusting care accordingly. The medical home provides information to the referral on the one hand; while on the other obtains information from the service provider; incorporates it into the medical record; and shares and interprets the information for the family.

It is impossible for an individual physician to provide all elements of care in the medical home, and an understanding of resources in the community, as well as relationships with specialty care providers can assist in meeting the needs of children and their families. Certain core resources including the Medicaid or CHIP program, mental health services, the State title V program for Children with Special Needs, the developmental disabilities system, the early intervention system, special education, family resource centers, Head Start, and the Special Supplemental Food Program for Women, Infants and Children (WIC) are used by many families of children with special needs. Learning about these basic resources and how referrals are made to each can help the provider both meet the child and family's needs and share responsibility for care with other programs, many of whom offer some form of care coordination or case management. Oftentimes, responsibility for learning about these entities can be delegated to support staff in the office who can then learn more about each and establish relationships upon which referrals can be built. Many of these programs also have outreach materials that can be kept in the provider's office and shared with families when referrals are made.

Transforming a practice into a medical home takes time, with gradual and ongoing changes in practices, processes and shifts in philosophy of care. The transformation takes persistence and patience to achieve desired goals. Serving as a medical home requires regular self assessment to ensure that family needs are met, and that the practice setting is operating in a cost effective and efficient manner. There are a number of tools that exist to assist providers in self assessment, and to make simple changes to enhance the quality of care in a medical home practice. Likewise, there are now voluntary recognition programs to acknowledge the efforts of a medical home. It is likely that some of the current voluntary efforts will become mandatory as a means of assuring quality in compensating medical homes for care. Two examples of tools for self assessment include: (1) The Center for Medical Home Improvement's Medical Home Index; and (2) the National Committee on Quality Assurance (NCQA) Physician Practice Connections- Patient Centered Medical Home program. The Medical Home Index measures the medical "homeness" of a practice across six domains including:

- organizational capacity;
- chronic condition management;
- care coordination;
- community outreach;
- data management; and
- quality improvement.

The NCQA program assesses whether physician practices are functioning as medical homes across nine standards, including:

- access and communication;
- patient tracking and registry;
- care management;
- patient self management support;
- electronic prescribing;
- test tracking, referral tracking;
- performance improvement; and
- advanced electronic communications.

Accumulating data increasingly supports the notion that the patient centered medical home for children with special health care needs can improve patient satisfaction while reducing inpatient hospital utilization and emergency room visits. For example, the Medical Home Program for Children with Special Health Care Needs is a medical home program in the resident continuity clinic at UCLA with a strong chronic care management component. When patient data was compared for one year prior to- and after-enrollment in the program, analysis of encounter data for patients enrolled in this program demonstrates a significant decrease in emergency room use. This finding is consistent with reports of other programs focused on populations of children with chronic disease. Thus, it is likely that parents of children with chronic conditions who are enrolled in an active medical home are empowered to use telephone consultations or schedule outpatient appointments, and urgent care clinics to avoid emergency room visits. This hypothesis is supported by several parents reports in the UCLA Medical Home Program's parent advisory group who gave this explanation when they were shown data on emergency room use and asked to comment. In addition, when compared to normative data for medical homes, we have found that the UCLA program results in much higher parent satisfaction scores as measured by the Medical Home Family Index which is a module of the Medical Home Index. Of note, the use of Spanish speaking Family Liaisons has resulted in high parent satisfaction scores among Spanish speaking families that are not significantly different from those of English speaking families.

A medical home is only valuable to patients and families if it is accessible. Accessibility constitutes a variety of factors. One factor is physical and includes *structural accessibility* for families who need additional space, ramps and elevators to move wheelchairs, ventilators and other equipment when bringing their child for a visit, or a larger than usual exam room in order to accommodate their needs, or a height adjustable exam table to be able to transfer a child with mobility impairments. Another factor is more temporal: Accessibility to providers at times that are convenient to families—such as late in the day and Saturdays—and access to other means of advice when the office is closed. *Cultural and language accessibility* is important in providing a medical home so that families can speak in their native language to their providers and that their culture is respected as part of the medical home processes. Finally, *financial accessibility* is a consideration, with the goal of access to a medical home regardless of the payer source.

A significant challenge for medical home providers is appropriate compensation. The activities that define a medical home take time, resources and appropriately trained staff. Currently, third party payers do not typically reimburse for the care coordination component of the medical home, but recent health reform proposals have identified the medical home model as an important means of ensuring access, enhancing care, and improving cost effectiveness. With heightened attention to the model, the possibility exists for recognizing the necessity of appropriate reimbursement.

Establishing a Medical Home

A variety of roles need to be filled in order to carry out the activities associated with a medical home. Primary care, acute/episodic illness care, and chronic disease management are key elements. While typically the pediatrician or family practitioner carries out these activities, nurse practitioners or physician assistants may play a role as well. Care coordination is a critical piece of the services provided in the medical home. While the physician may serve as the care coordinator in a smaller practice, this role is often assumed by a nurse, social worker, medical assistants, lay case managers, or specially trained parents in larger practices. Adequate training must assure that the care coordinator is knowledgeable about community resources and public programs that families may need to utilize. In addition, the care coordinator must have interpersonal skills that facilitate partnerships with families as well as providers, agencies and programs to which families are referred. They should have experience with the care coordination process of assessing family strengths and needs, identifying appropriate resources, referrals, follow up and evaluation and revising the plan as needed. Finally, they should have the ability to communicate with families in the family's native language or through a medical translator.

Additional resources at the end of the chapter provide information and strategies for setting up a medical home, and practice management tools to enhance this effort. Some simple strategies; however, are virtually universal. It is helpful to identify the charts of those children with special health care needs. This allows the medical home practice to track the number of such children for purposes of resource allocation and arranging time-appropriate appointment setting allowing for additional time that these children often require.

Orienting families to the practice and making parents aware of office practices and procedures allows them to successfully interact with office staff. Providing commonly used materials, sometimes by means of a simple handout or booklet in different languages and appropriate literacy level saves time and improves care by reinforcing important information. Parents can also be encouraged to assume a more active role in serving as their child's advocate and can be encouraged to prepare for visits by writing down concerns ahead of time. Families can be referred to family resource centers for education and peer support, and be assisted in organizing their child's health and related information into a binder so that it can be shared with other providers.

All medical homes will refer children and families to community resources and specialized programs. This can be facilitated by using resource directories or development of a file with referral information. Simple handouts with common referral information such as the name, location and phone number of the nearby Head Start program, as well as how one applies for services, can assist in the referral process and help to ensure receipt of such services. While there may be an initial investment of time on the part of the practice, it will result in the accumulation of resource information that can be readily distributed to families, ultimately saving time and effort.

A Case Study of a Successful Medical Home

Baby boy "M" was first enrolled in the Medical Home program at UCLA when he was 8 months old. He was the first born son of two Spanish-speaking low-income parents and faced extreme medical challenges from the time of his birth. M was born with a condition called holoprosencephaly, a birth defect affecting the brain. His condition was complicated by hydrocephalus which required multiple brain surgeries to relieve the pressure on his brain. M was also dependent on a permanent feeding tube for nutrition, and, during his first few months of life, had multiple complications requiring two major abdominal surgeries. He was also diagnosed with profound developmental delay.

At the time of M's enrollment into the Medical Home Program, he was found to have very inconsistent medical care. Although the parents were trying their best to navigate the health care system, many things had fallen through the cracks. For example, there were multiple, months-old urgent subspecialty referrals still pending. M had not received adequate hearing or vision screening and, despite his increase in size, was on a diet that had not been adjusted for 3 months. Because his parents had never established a relationship with a primary pediatrician (they were unsure of the difference between subspecialty doctors and general physicians), M was behind on his preventative vaccinations. Despite his significant developmental delays, M was receiving very limited therapies at home. In addition, the parents also had never been given a clear prognosis for their son and were uncertain whether his development was age appropriate or not for someone with his multiply health challenges. They were also unaware of the community resources available to them.

M is now 2-and-a-half years old and despite his initial original poor prognosis, M has been progressing very well. He is still fed through a feeding tube but is able to eat half his diet by mouth thanks to excellent occupational therapy. M's hearing and vision were screened and he has hearing aids and glasses, which allow him to interact and enjoy his environment. He has an adaptive wheelchair and bath seat and because of intensive physical therapy, is able to sit unassisted on his own. He continues to progress in his mobility strength. His progress is monitored by 6 pediatric sub-specialists, who see M every 3–6 months and manage his extensive medical conditions. His vaccinations are up-to-date, and all of his routine health maintenance (i.e., dentistry, nutrition, growth, development, etc) are being appropriately monitored by his medical home general pediatrician. The family carries their "All About Me" binder, which contains a comprehensive care plan and a detailed medical history including his physician contact information in case of an emergency room visit. The notebook helps M's parents navigate his multiple medical appointments.

In summary, when applied to children with special health care needs, the medical home concept has the potential to greatly enhance most aspects of their care. While there is no current universal funding mechanism for compensating the time and effort required to deliver care in this manner, it is possible that widespread use of medical home concepts may bring significant savings to our health care system. In addition, the enhanced care for children with special health care needs who are enrolled in a robust medical home cannot be overlooked. These benefits suggest a prominent role for the medical home in the future design—or re-design—of our expensive health care systems.

References

Bethell, C.D., Read, D., Brockwood, K. American Academy of Pediatrics (2004). Using existing population-based data sets to measure the American Academy of Pediatrics definition of medical home for all children and children with special health care needs. Pediatrics. 113(5 suppl): 1529–37.

Klitzner T.S., Rabbitt, L.A., Chang, R.K.R. Benefits of care coordination for children with complex disease: A pilot medical home project in a resident teaching clinic. J Peds 156(6):1006-10, 2010.

McAllister, J.W., Pressler, E., and Cooley, W.C. (2007). Practice-based care coordination: a medical home essential. Pediatrics. 120(3); e723–33.

McAllister, J.W., Pressler, E., Turchi, R., and Antonelli, R.C. (2009). Achieving effective care coordination in the medical home. Pediatric Annals. 38(9): 491–7

Rosenthal, T.C. (2008). The medical home: growing evidence to support a new approach to primary care. Journal of the American Board of Family Practice. 21(5): 427–40.

Strickland, B.B., Singh, G.K., Kogan, M.D., Mann, M.Y., van Dyck, P.C., and Newacheck, P.W. (2009). Access to the medical home: new findings from the 2005-2006 National Survey of Children with Special Health Care Needs. Pediatrics. 123 (6): e996–e1044.

Additional Resources

www.brightfutures.org
www.familycenteredcare.org
www.medicalhomeimprovement.org
www.medicalhomeinfo.org
www.ncqa.org

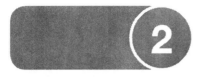

2 Cardiac Disorders

Table of Contents

Atrial Septal Defect (ASD)

Gary M. Satou, Thomas S. Klitzner

Atrial septal defect is a congenital heart disease whereby a defect or deficiency exists in a portion of the atrial septum which divides the right and left atrium of the heart. There are different atrial septal defect sub-types, but the general physiologic principles are the same: Oxygenated pulmonary venous blood "shunts" left to right through the defect, thus increasing the degree of pulmonary blood flow.

Etiology

In general, congenital heart disease is considered multifactorial in origin.

Clinical Presentation and Prognosis

Age of onset: Although the defect is present from birth, patients are often asymptomatic. Occasionally symptoms present in infancy or childhood.

Presenting signs and symptoms: Many children with ASD are asymptomatic. Often, they are referred to a pediatric cardiologist for evaluation of a heart murmur or with non-specific symptoms such as "chest pain" or intermittent shortness of breath. Infants with large defects may present with congestive symptoms, such as tachypnea, tachycardia or hepatomegaly. Insufficient growth or weight gain may be present. Adults, who will have long-standing left to right atrial level shunting, can present with pulmonary hypertension, including decreased saturations and respiratory symptoms/distress. There are rare occurrences where the first sign of an ASD is neurologic, particularly when a right to left embolic event and cerebrovascular insult occur.

Clinical course: The majority of patients remain asymptomatic and stable. The deleterious effects of an ASD can take decades to develop so there is usually not an acute need to close the defect. Although congestive circulatory symptoms and suboptimal growth occasionally occurs, these resolve with treatment. Left untreated into adulthood, the potential for pulmonary vascular disease and pulmonary hypertension is significant and likely irreversible leading to chronic symptoms and potentially shortened life span in children with large ASD's. This condition affects a very small subgroup of patients in the current era. However, it is the main reason that pediatric cardiologists recommend closure of ASDs despite the fact that most children are asymptomatic. Over time, children with smaller defects often show spontaneous diminution or closure. Thus, the cardiologist will choose to simply monitor these patients for a period of time. Occasionally, ASD's are closed to reduce the risk of paradoxical embolus which can occur in certain subgroups of patients, for example, pregnant females.

Prognosis: The overall prognosis for children with an ASD is excellent. Closure corrects the problem, alleviates symptoms and eliminates the potential for chronic pulmonary vascular disease. While there can be spontaneous closure in many children whose defects are small in general, there is less than 1% mortality associated with transcatheter-device or surgical closure. A very small subgroup of patients who undergo surgical or catheter directed closure of an ASD may develop heart block or atrial arrhythmias. For this reason, following ASD repair, pediatric cardiologists continue to monitor ASD patients in the long term. Adults with unrepaired ASD and secondary pulmonary vascular disease have suboptimal outcome and will remain symptomatic with an associated increase in morbidity and mortality.

Diagnosis

Echocardiography is the definitive diagnostic modality in the current era. Primary care providers should refer patients with a suspected ASD and symptoms of left to right shunting to a pediatric cardiologist who will guide the performance of the test so as to ensure optimal results. Initial findings may include tachypnea, tachycardia or venous congestion. Physical exam often reveals a split second heart sound on auscultation resulting from delayed closure of the pulmonary valve. If the clinician obtains a chest X-ray, there may be cardiomegaly and increased pulmonary vascular markings. If an electrocardiogram (ECG) is performed, findings may include right axis deviation, or an incomplete right bundle branch block pattern.

Management

When a child is diagnosed (by the pediatric cardiologist and echocardiography), the approach depends on the size of the lesion. Asymptomatic patients with small defects will be followed over time and given a chance to demonstrate spontaneous closure. Children with larger defects—with or without symptoms—will be referred for closure. At present, the majority of defects are closed in the catheterization laboratory by pediatric cardiac interventionalists who place special occlusion devices on the septum in a closed, non-surgical fashion. When the child is too small, or the defect not anatomically favorable for this approach, referral to a pediatric cardiac surgeon is appropriate.

Medication: Rarely, a small amount of diuretics (e.g., Lasix) or congestive heart failure (CHF) therapy may be prescribed for the patient who is symptomatic and awaiting repair. The same medications are utilized for a brief postoperative period, and then the patient is weaned off by the pediatric cardiologist. After a transcatheter device closure, patients are typically treated with Aspirin (3–5 mg/Kg/day) for 6 months.

Surgery: This is a relatively simple cardiac surgical procedure with primary or patch surgical closure of the ASD while on cardiopulmonary bypass. Some patients with ostium primum type ASD which is a hole located adjacent to the tricuspid and mitral valves (a form of AV Canal) will need suturing of an associated mitral valve cleft to alleviate mitral regurgitation.

Therapy: Physical therapy is generally not required following repair.

Social: Because of the simplicity of the defect and a relatively expeditious return to normal lifestyle after repair, the interest/need for social support groups is minimal. Websites and organizations considered reliable by pediatric cardiac specialists for parental education include those from the American Heart Association (AHA): www.americanheart.org and the Congenital Heart Information Network (CHIN): www.tchin.org.

Long-term monitoring: Most commonly, ASD closure is a one time intervention. Medications are usually not required after the postoperative period. The pediatric cardiologist may perform annual visits to monitor the very rare occurrence of heart block, arrhythmias or valvular/myocardial dysfunction. No exercise restrictions are imposed.

Pearls and Precautions

Incision: The incision should be kept clean and dry. Washing is achieved by using a damp cloth and soap. Do not completely soak incision in water or apply ointments or lotions until healed (usually 6 to 8 weeks). Itching is a normal sign of healing; scratching should be discouraged. Once healed, sunscreen should be applied prior to sun exposure. Parents should be instructed to call the cardiologist if redness, swelling, pain or drainage from the incision occurs.

Diet: Feedings may be more frequent, but smaller in quantity. Families should be educated that the infant/child may tire easily and require rest during feeding and that sweating may occur for a period of time. In general, if the feeding pattern is not slowly improving towards normalcy in the weeks following repair, the parents should contact the physician. Negative changes may be reflective of postoperative issues such as infection, effusions, or cardiac dysfunction.

Activities: Sternal precautions should be undertaken for the first 8 weeks after repair. This includes avoiding direct pressure or pulling on the sternum. Infants should not be lifted under the arms but rather scooped up under the back and bottom. Car seats should always be utilized when traveling. When possible, avoidance of ill friends and family or crowded public places is suggested for 2–4 weeks after discharge. As with feeding patterns, sleep patterns may be altered for a period of time after repair.

Endocarditis prophylaxis: Good dental hygiene is very important to reduce the risk of infective endocarditis and should be encouraged. If dental cleaning or care (or other non-cardiac procedures) are performed, the cardiologist should be contacted to discuss any postoperative patient issues. The most recent guidelines for endocarditis prophylaxis can be reviewed and are referenced below. Following ASD surgery, subacute bacterial endocarditis (SBE) prophylaxis is performed for 6 months (but not preoperatively).

Immunizations: Infants' vaccination should be delayed for approximately one month following surgery and should be discussed with the individual cardiologist.

Parental Education: Parents should be instructed to call the cardiologist or cardiac care team if any of the following occur:

- An incision demonstrates redness, swelling, pain or drainage.
- Increased work of breathing or shortness of breath occurs.
- Fussy behavior or poor feeding ensues. Swollen or puffy hands/feet are present.
- Vomiting or diarrhea occurs more than once.
- Fever develops (temperature 38.5 Centigrade or greater).

References

Atrial septal defect: spectrum of care. Kharouf R., Luxenberg D.M., Khalid, O., Abdulla R., Pediatr Cardiol. 2008 Mar;29(2):271–80.

Prevention of infective endocarditis: guidelines from the American Heart Association (multiple councils): Wilson W, Taubert KA, Gewitz M, Lockhart PB, Baddour LM, Levison M, Bolger A, Cabell CH, Takahashi M, Baltimore RS, Newburger JW, Strom BL, Tani LY, Gerber M, Bonow RO, Pallasch T, Shulman ST, Rowley AH, Burns JC, Ferrieri P, Gardner T, Goff D, Durack DT. Circulation. 2007 Oct 9; 116(15):1736–54.

Coarctation of the Aorta

Gary M. Satou, Thomas S. Klitzner

This is a congenital cardiovascular defect in which there is a narrowing or "waist" of the aorta and is usually located in the distal transverse aortic arch/proximal descending aorta in the thorax. Although often discrete in anatomy, coarctation can manifest as long segment hypoplasia or narrowing of the aorta. In neonates, there is often a patent ductus arteriosus which accompanies coarctation of the aorta. A large number of children with coarctation of the aorta also have a bicuspid aortic valve. This is a known association, the etiology of which is unclear. The complexity and severity of associated lesions, often several in number, can make the presentation of children with coarctation of the aorta quite variable. For the purpose of clarity in this section, we will limit the description to isolated coarctation of the aorta (with or without patent ductus arteriosus).

Etiology

The exact etiology of this anomaly is not clearly defined. However, some hypothesize that remnants of ductal tissue in the area of a "usual" coarctation leads to constriction of the ductus arteriosus (normal) and the adjacent aortic wall (abnormal), thus creating the aortic narrowing. This theory fails to explain the etiology of long segments of hypoplasia and stenosis seen in some patients. Others have postulated that the presence of left ventricular or aortic valve disease may diminish blood flow during fetal and postnatal life, leading to the more complex forms of coarctation.

Clinical Presentation and Prognosis

Age of onset: Children may present in the neonatal period, later in infancy or childhood, or occasionally during the adolescent years. In general, the "tightness" of the coarctation directly relates to the extent of its presenting symptoms and is inversely related to the age at diagnosis. Milder forms of narrowing are usually asymptomatic.

Presenting signs and symptoms: Children appearing to be healthy may be referred to the cardiology clinic for evaluation of a heart murmur or decreased femoral pulses. Symptomatic patients may present with varying degrees of upper extremity hypertension, poor lower extremity pulses, and a lower measured systolic blood pressure in the legs in comparison to the arms. If a large patent ductus arteriosus (PDA) is present (often neonates with a significant coarctation), there can be a "right to left" ductal shunting component present and thus a pulse oximetry differential noted between the arms and legs (demonstrating lower saturations in the legs). Spontaneous closure of the ductus arteriosis in infants with a PDA-dependent tight coarctation often can result in cardiac arrest or shock.

Clinical course: Coarctation of the aorta as a primary lesion can be mild and remain subclinical for a long period of time. Although the course may be relatively asymptomatic, at some point development of hypertension and its secondary effects are likely to occur. In prior eras, arterial collaterals might develop in longstanding coarctation in undiagnosed children. Given the wealth of knowledge of the ill effects of hypertension and its potential secondary end organ damage, patients in the current era with any significant degree of obstruction will be referred for intervention/repair. The same is recommended for the acutely ill infant or patient, where secondary cardiac and other organ dysfunction will occur. Heart failure and myocardial ischemia which are potential complications of significant narrowings in the aorta are untoward states to be avoided, especially in the neonate or infant with a closing ductus.

Prognosis: Timely surgical correction (or transcatheter intervention) of this lesion leads to an excellent prognosis. The procedure usually alleviates symptoms and opens the aorta either completely, or nearly so. The subgroup of patients who later develop re-narrowing of the aorta are primarily treated with transcatheter balloon dilation and possibly stent placement. Untreated coarctation is associated with variable degrees of morbidity and mortality risk.

Diagnosis

Although echocardiography is definitive, the astute clinician is aware of the diagnosis based on physical examination and bedside data. A combination of poor lower extremity pulses combined with heart murmur or upper extremity hypertension should provide clues to the clinician for diagnosis. If there is poor cardiac output and a shock-like state, coarctation should be suspected, but a murmur and a blood pressure differential may be absent. In the neonatal intensive care unit (NICU) or other hospital setting, any of these findings along with a pulse oximetry differential (desaturated lower extremities) or the "harlequin" appearance of isolated lower extremity cyanosis should suggest possible coarctation of the aorta with a right to left ductal shunt. Other scenarios such as Persistent Pulmonary Hypertension (PPHN) may create some overlapping findings.

Management

Especially in a symptomatic patient or in the asymptomatic child with hypertension at rest or during exercise, relief of the obstruction is generally indicated with coarctation. Mild degrees of narrowing and obstruction may be monitored by the pediatric cardiologist non-invasively until signs of secondary cardiac or systemic symptoms arise.

Medication: Medical management for coarctation of the aorta is primarily a temporizing maneuver in the ill patient. Preventive heart failure therapy such as diuretics and possibly mild inotropy, may be utilized until intervention is performed. In an effort to re-open or maintain patency to the ductus, prostaglandin (PGE) infusion is performed in all sick neonates and infants. This may be combined with congestive heart failure (CHF) therapy, but again, only while awaiting surgical repair.

Surgery: Currently, most centers prefer surgical repair consisting primarily of resection and end to end anastamosis, possibly including a tissue flap or patch for augmentation. In simple, isolated cases, coarctation surgery is performed through the side of the chest wall ("lateral thoracotomy") or centrally in cases where there is long segment arch hypoplasia or associated intracardiac disease, through a median sternotomy. Balloon angioplasty may be an effective intervention, but remains controversial in the patient with native coarctation, in part due to secondary aneurysm formation. Some centers will perform primary angioplasty and stent placement in older children when the necessary stent diameter is felt to approach the size of an adult aorta. For recurrent coarctation after surgical correction, angioplasty is often utilized and may include stent placement in the older patient.

Therapy: Physical therapy is generally not required following repair.

Social: Websites and organizations considered reliable by pediatric cardiac specialists for parental review include those from the American Heart Association (AHA): www.americanheart.org and the Congenital Heart Information Network (CHIN): www.tchin.org.

Pearls and Precautions

Pearls and Precautions

Incision: The incision should be kept clean and dry. Washing is achieved by using a damp cloth and soap. Do not completely soak incision in water or apply ointments or lotions until healed (usually 6 to 8 weeks). Itching is a normal sign of healing; scratching should be discouraged. Once healed, sunscreen should be applied prior to sun exposure. Parents should be instructed to call the cardiologist if redness, swelling, pain or drainage from the incision occurs.

Diet: Feedings may be more frequent, but smaller in quantity. Families should be educated that the infant/child may tire easily and require rest during feeding and that sweating may occur for a period of time. In general, if the feeding pattern is not slowly improving towards normalcy in the weeks following repair, the parents should contact the physician. Negative changes may be reflective of postoperative issues such as infection, effusions, or cardiac dysfunction.

Activities: Chest wall precautions should be undertaken for the first 8 weeks after repair. This includes avoiding direct pressure or pulling on the sternum. Infants should not be lifted under the arms but rather scooped up under the back and bottom. Car seats should always be utilized when traveling. When possible, avoidance of ill friends and family or crowded public places is suggested for 2–4 weeks after discharge. As with feeding patterns, sleep patterns may be altered for a period of time after repair.

Endocarditis prophylaxis: Good dental hygiene is very important to reduce the risk of infective endocarditis and should be encouraged. If dental cleaning or care (or other non-cardiac procedures) are performed, the cardiologist should be contacted to discuss any postoperative patient issues. The most recent guidelines for endocarditis prophylaxis can be reviewed and are referenced below. Systemic bacterial endocarditis prophylaxis is best discussed and determined by the pediatric cardiologist.

Immunizations: Infants vaccination should be delayed for approximately one month following surgery and should be discussed with the individual cardiologist.

Parental Education: Parents should be instructed to call the cardiologist or cardiac care team if any of the following occur:

- An incision demonstrates redness, swelling, pain or drainage.
- Increased work of breathing or shortness of breath occurs.
- Fussy behavior or poor feeding ensues.
- Swollen or puffy hands/feet are present.
- Vomiting or diarrhea occurs more than once
- Fever develops (temperature 38.5 Centigrade or greater)

References

Aortic coarctation: an overview. Abbruzzese, P.A., Aidala, E. J. Cardiovasc Med (Hagerstown). 2007 Feb;8(2): 123–8

Coarctation of the aorta: an update. Rothman, A. Curr Probl Pediatr. 1998 Feb;28(2):33–60.

Prevention of infective endocarditis: guidelines from the American Heart Association (multiple councils): Wilson W, Taubert KA, Gewitz M, Lockhart PB, Baddour LM, Levison M, Bolger A, Cabell CH, Takahashi M, Baltimore RS, Newburger JW, Strom BL, Tani LY, Gerber M, Bonow RO, Pallasch T, Shulman ST, Rowley AH, Burns JC, Ferrieri P, Gardner T, Goff D, Durack DT. Circulation. 2007 Oct 9; 116(15):1736–54.

Ebstein Anomaly

Gary M. Satou, Thomas S. Klitzner

This is a rare congenital cardiac malformation involving the tricuspid valve. The leaflets are abnormal in their position and are displaced apically, creating a larger sized functional right atrium and smaller functional right ventricle.

Etiology

The etiology of Ebstein's anomaly is uncertain at this time. In general, congenital heart disease is considered multifactorial in etiology. Environmental factors during pregnancy may play a role.

Clinical Presentation and Prognosis

Age of onset: Fetal echocardiography can diagnose this lesion in utero. Neonates with more severe forms of Ebstein's anomaly will be cyanotic and present in the newborn period. Milder forms may present later in childhood when a heart murmur is noted and referral to pediatric cardiology is made.

Presenting signs and symptoms: Symptomatic neonates will demonstrate cyanosis and possible acidosis and cardiac instability. The systolic murmur is created by the poorly functioning tricuspid valve which leaks and creates tricuspid valve regurgitation. Physical exam may demonstrate a gallop rhythm and tachycardia or, in older patients, distended neck veins and hepatomegaly. Older patients may be asymptomatic or present solely with the murmur of tricuspid regurgitation. Occasionally, supra ventricular tachycardia (SVT) may be the initial presentation occurring in patients with concurrent Wolf-Parkinson White syndrome (WPW) or distended atria.

Clinical course: Ebstein's anomaly may present with a spectrum of severity, consisting of varying tricuspid valve displacement and abnormalcy. Severe forms of this disorder will create an inadequate right heart and necessitate single ventricle palliation.

Symptomatic neonates can be very cyanotic, acidotic and require intensive care and medical/surgical management for survival. Children with milder tricuspid valve involvement are followed in the outpatient clinic, only needing intervention when progression ensues. Progression is variable and does not always occur. Despite intervention, chronic right heart failure can ensue in some patients, requiring consideration of heart transplantation.

Prognosis: Even with intervention, cyanotic neonates have a fairly high mortality. Children with mild forms of Ebstein's anomaly will be expected to live a full life, often without a need for intervention. Patients who have undergone right heart surgery will have some increased morbidity and mortality from chronic right heart issues and possible arrhythmias.

Diagnosis

Echocardiography is definitive and accurate in evaluating the degree of tricuspid valve involvement and regurgitation. Other cardiodiagnostic modalities do not eliminate the need for echocardiography. Chest radiograph may show mild to severe cardiomegaly or decreased pulmonary vascular markings. ECG may demonstrate right atrial enlargement and right bundle branch block. The physical exam may demonstrate distended neck veins, hepatomegaly and split first and second heart sounds. There may be a gallop rhythm and additional heart sounds.

Management

Medication: Cyanotic newborns require careful management while waiting for the pulmonary vascular resistance to drop. Prostaglandin infusion is used to maintain ductal patency while acid-base balance is important for myocardial and other tissue-protection. Inotropy and diuresis may be used for heart failure management. Occasionally, the degree of pulmonary blood flow will increase once the pulmonary vascular resistance (PVR) is lowered; this may eliminate the need for surgical intervention. If SVT presents, it is acutely treated as usual. However, if there is known WPW, one must be careful not to utilize digoxin as it can promote antegrade one-to-one atrial to ventricular pathway conduction which can create very fast ventricular tachycardia in which case various anti-arrhythmics are used in this setting.

Surgery: There are several types of tricuspid valve surgeries available for Ebstein's anomaly, but, it is a complex undertaking. The best approach for any given child can be controversial and may be based on institutional preference. In general, the goal is to improve tricuspid valve (TV) function and maintain a biventricular circulation which is not always achievable. Documented cases of tricuspid valve repairs have been performed with varying degrees of success. The procedure can be performed in older children but generally not in neonates or small infants. In cases of irreparable TV, the right heart is usually inadequate in size and/or function in which case a series of procedures are performed to create a single ventricular Fontan circulation (deoxygenated blood from the body bypasses the right heart and goes directly to the lungs while the left ventricle provides systemic circulation)

Therapy: Physical therapy is generally not required following repair.

Social: Websites and organizations considered reliable by pediatric cardiac specialists for parental education include those from the American Heart Association (AHA) at www.americanheart.org and the Congenital Heart Information Network (CHIN) at www.tchin.org.

Long-term monitoring: Generally, children who have not undergone surgery are not considered to be in heart failure. However, they may be managed on diuretic therapy and the frequency of their pediatric cardiology visits can vary. They are followed to ensure signs of CHF do not develop, such as fatigue, systemic venous distension, liver enlargement, and poor exercise tolerance. If the child has undergone TV repair or Fontan surgery, the visit frequency can vary as well, but is likely to be at least twice/year. Anticoagulation therapy may be utilized and this may include afterload reduction, often in the form of angiotensin converting enzyme (ACE) inhibitors. Depending on the drug types and amounts used, serum electrolytes are occasionally monitored. Although the pediatric cardiologist manages the chosen drug therapy, communication with the pediatrician is important. Exercise ability or restrictions are variable depending on the degree of TV regurgitation, residual cyanosis and level of myocardial function.

Pearls and Precautions:

Incision: The incision should be kept clean and dry. Washing is achieved by using a damp cloth and soap. Do not completely soak incision in water or apply ointments or lotions until healed (usually 6 to 8 weeks). Itching is a normal sign of healing; scratching should be discouraged. Once healed, sunscreen should be applied prior to sun exposure. Parents should be instructed to call the cardiologist if redness, swelling, pain or drainage from the incision occurs.

Diet: Feedings may be more frequent, but smaller in quantity. Families should be educated that the infant/child may tire easily and require rest during feeding and that sweating may occur for a period of time. In general, if the feeding pattern is not slowly improving towards normalcy in the weeks following repair, the parents should contact the physician. Negative changes may be reflective of postoperative issues such as infection, effusions, or cardiac dysfunction.

Activities: Sternal precautions should be undertaken for the first 8 weeks after repair. This includes avoiding direct pressure or pulling on the sternum. Infants should not be lifted under the arms but rather scooped up under the back and bottom. Car seats should always be utilized when traveling. When possible, avoidance of ill friends and family or crowded public places is suggested for 2–4 weeks after discharge. As with feeding patterns, sleep patterns may be altered for a period of time after repair.

Endocarditis prophylaxis: Good dental hygiene is very important to reduce the risk of infective endocarditis and should be encouraged. If dental cleaning or care (or other non-cardiac procedures) are performed, the cardiologist should be contacted. The most recent guidelines for endocarditis prophylaxis can be reviewed and are referenced below. Infective endocarditis prophylaxis is best discussed and determined by the pediatric cardiologist.

Immunizations: Infants vaccination should be delayed for approximately one month following surgery and should be discussed with the individual cardiologist.

Parental Education: Parents should be instructed to call the cardiologist or cardiac care team if any of the following occur:

- An incision demonstrates redness, swelling, pain or drainage.
- Increased work of breathing or shortness of breath occurs.
- Fussy behavior or poor feeding ensues. Swollen or puffy hands/feet are present.
- Vomiting or diarrhea occurs more than once
- Fever develops (temperature 38.5 Centigrade or greater)

References

How I manage neonatal Ebstein's anomaly. Bove EL, Hirsch JC, Ohye RG, Devaney EJ. Semin Thorac Cardiovasc Surg Pediatr Card Surg Annu. 2009:63–5

Ebstein's anomaly of the tricuspid valve: from fetus to adult: congenital heart disease. Paranon S, Acar P. Heart. 2008 Feb;94(2):237–43

Prevention of infective endocarditis: guidelines from the American Heart Association (multiple councils): Wilson W, Taubert KA, Gewitz M, Lockhart PB, Baddour LM, Levison M, Bolger A, Cabell CH, Takahashi M, Baltimore RS, Newburger JW, Strom BL, Tani LY, Gerber M, Bonow RO, Pallasch T, Shulman ST, Rowley AH, Burns JC, Ferrieri P, Gardner T, Goff D, Durack DT. Circulation. 2007 Oct 9; 116(15):1736–54.

Hypertrophic Cardiomyopathy (HCM)

Gary M. Satou, Thomas S. Klitzner

HCM is a primary heart muscle disorder in which the hypertrophied myocardium is both grossly and histologically abnormal leading to a myriad of cardiovascular issues including stiff heart muscle and poor filling, obstruction in the left ventricle (LV) outflow tract, ventricular arrhythmias and a risk of sudden death. Although there are other forms of cardiomyopathy, this description will be limited to HCM.

Etiology

HCM remains a fascinating heterogeneous spectrum of genetic disorders, few of which are presently fully elucidated. Overall, HCM is a collection of gene mutations which create abnormal sarcomere protein structure and function which is the underlying cause for abnormal myocardial performance and filling. The transmission of HCM is thought to be autosomal dominant, though approximately 50% are spontaneous mutations.

Clinical Presentation and Prognosis

Age of onset: This disease may present at all ages. However, children are often asymptomatic and may go undiagnosed, while adolescents may present with symptoms of heart failure, ischemia or sudden death. Both the onset of cardiac hypertrophy/dysfunction and the age at presentation is quite variable.

Presenting signs and symptoms and clinical course: Patients' first presentation may vary as well from asymptomatic to sudden death which makes early diagnosis of HCM difficult and its future clinical course unpredictable. When present, symptoms may include dyspnea, fatigue, chest pain and palpitations. Syncope (especially with exertion) is one of the most concerning presenting signs. Supra ventricular- or ventricular tachycardia may be the initial clinical presentation, leading to the subsequent diagnosis of the underlying HCM. Physical examination may reveal brisk carotid upstroke or a thrill; a systolic murmur of either outflow obstruction or mitral valve regurgitation may be present. There may be additional heart sounds consistent with filling a stiff LV.

Prognosis: Complex and not well-defined. The overall annual sudden death risk in patients may be estimated at 1%. Although uncommonly diagnosed in infancy, manifestation of the disease at this early stage is associated with increased mortality. General factors used to risk-stratify patients with HCM include positive family history of sudden death, syncope, exercise abnormalities and severe degrees of hypertrophy. These patients are considered for implantable cardiac defibrillator (ICD) implantation (in addition to drug therapy) and there is hope that this strategy may improve long term prognosis.

Diagnosis

Although there are different methods of diagnosing this disease, they are all limited by technical problems and may be of limited predictive value. At present, genetic screening is complex and limited by a number of factors including commercial availability of a small number of genetic subtypes and, if screened positive, a poorly predictable clinical course. Although if present, HCM can be diagnosed prenatal, it is extremely uncommon. Thus, screening in affected mothers of those with positive family history is usually negative. A small number of these normal fetuses will manifest HCM at some point in postnatal life. As with most cardiac abnormalities, echocardiography elucidates the diagnosis by showing the hypertrophied heart muscle. The distribution can be on the ventricular septum, concentric to the LV, or involve both ventricles. Experts in diagnosis and treatment of HCM are not in agreement on the risk factors that are best predictors of sudden death. However, the presence of a diastolic ventriculoseptal thickness of 15 mm in a child (or greater than 30 mm in an adult) is of great concern. The presence or absence of LV outflow obstruction generally plays a minimal role in diagnosis. The clinical history of syncope and/or positive family history, along with ventriculoseptal thickness and other echocardiographic measurements, are collectively considered in the possible diagnosis of HCM in a child or adolescent.

Management

Although remaining a difficult task, the goal of diagnosis and management is to alleviate any existing symptoms and to screen at-risk individuals for sudden death. Thus, irrespective of symptoms, many clinicians recommend medical management of all affected children and adolescents. Screening for exercise and rhythm abnormalities may be helpful in determining which patients may benefit from either ICD placement or LV outflow muscle resection (to reduce obstruction when present). If LV outflow obstruction or severe ventricular dyssynchrony is present, pacemaker placement and "synchronizing" of ventricular depolarization may be helpful. The goal of pacing in LV outflow obstruction is to create dyssynchrony and relieve the obstruction. Although it can work at times, the procedure has fallen out of favor because the initial study demonstrating efficacy has not been replicated.

Medication: Currently, irrespective of symptoms or outflow obstruction, a majority of clinicians are utilizing combination drug therapy (beta blockers and calcium-channel blockers) in most patients. Disopyramide has also been shown to reduce outflow obstruction in these patients. These drugs may help with facilitating relaxation and filling of the heart and, if initially present, possibly reducing the LV outflow gradient. They also have the additional function of serving as anti-arrhythmic agents. Direct inotropic agents or systemic vasodilators are generally avoided as they may aggravate the relative degree of obstruction, and systolic "pump" function is usually not compromised in HCM.

Surgery: Occasionally, children with HCM may have a degree of obstruction which is either creating additional symptoms or significantly worsening their myocardial perfomance. When the obstruction can not be relieved medicinally, operative intervention, while not perfect, generally will reduce the degree of obstruction. In most cases, a procedure entitled "myectomy" is performed whereby LV outflow muscle is resected through a median sternotomy while on cardiopulmonary bypass and the LV outflow can be accessed across the aortic valve. On rare occasions (and in combination with valve surgery), aortic- or mitral-valve surgery—or septal patching—is performed. There is a risk of heart block in this setting so a pacemaker system may be implanted at the time of the procedure. In addition, patients who are at risk of developing a malignant ventricular arrhythmia and sudden death receive an ICD implant as "back up".

Therapy: Physical therapy is generally not a part of patient care.

Social: Understandably, concern on the part of parents, the child and society at large that young healthy individuals may die suddenly creates significant anxiety.

Expeditious evaluation leading to diagnosis if the patient is at risk, or reassurance if the patient is not, can be extremely helpful. However, some families have a difficult time coping with the uncertainties that can exist during and after the evaluation process. Thorough, honest and thoughtful explanations often suffice to help alleviate these anxieties. Nonetheless, professional counseling may be indicated. General websites and organizations considered reliable by pediatric cardiac specialists for parental education include those from the American Heart Association (AHA): www.americanheart.org and the Congenital Heart Information Network (CHIN): www.tchin.org. A specific site found at www.sads.org, which although oriented towards arrhythmias and Long QT syndrome, may be helpful to families and friends involved with patients who carry the diagnosis of HCM. A cardiomyopathy site specifically related to children can be found at www.childrenscardiomyopathy.org.

Long-term monitoring: The frequency and timing of pediatric cardiology office follow-up for children with HCM is variable. It may be several times a year if there are levels of obstruction or valvular dysfunction to evaluate by echocardiography. If not, it may be on an annual basis. Exercise stress-testing may be performed along with 24 hour holter-monitoring, screening for EKG changes, arrhythmias, and LVOT gradients by echocardiography. Because beta blockers and calcium channel blockers are utilized, electrolytes are occasionally evaluated. For patients with ICD's or pacemakers, frequency of interrogation and prophylactic replacement for end of life batteries and/or lead issues are determined by the pediatric cardiologist.

Pearls and Precautions

Incision: This is applicable only to the subgroup of patients undergoing myectomy (see ASD chapter).

Medications and Endocarditis prophylaxis: Select categories of drugs including stimulants/sympathomimetics, nitrates, and inotropic agents should be avoided so as to reduce the risk of cardiac events. In general, patients with HCM do not need SBE prophylaxis, however, if cardiac surgery is undertaken, prophylaxis may be indicated for at least 6 months. Details should be reviewed with the pediatric cardiologist. The most recent guidelines for endocarditis prophylaxis materials can be reviewed and is referenced below.

Immunizations: Normal vaccination schedules can be followed. In the subgroup of patients who undergo cardiac surgery, delay of vaccinations for approximately one month following surgery is recommended. This should be discussed with the individual cardiologist as necessary.

Activity: Activity restriction is important in HCM in order to reduce the risk of sudden cardiovascular events. Patients are instructed to avoid high-level competitive and impact sports. Anaerobic activities (e.g., weight lifting) are discouraged. When HCM diagnosis is made in childhood, an altered lifestyle is often followed with relative ease as opposed to a new diagnosis being made in adolescence when an altered lifestyle may be more difficult to bear.

Parental Education and Screening

- First degree relatives of a child with HCM should undergo formal cardiovascular evaluation by a pediatric or adult cardiologist.
- CPR training should be obtained by family members and close friends. Some families may choose to purchase external defibrillators and keep them in the household.

- Parents should be instructed to call the cardiologist or cardiac care team if any of the following symptoms occur:
  - Increased work of breathing or shortness of breath
  - Dizziness/palpitations
  - Chest pain
  - Syncope
  - Fussy behavior or poor feeding in infants

References

Colan SD, Lipshultz SE, Lowe AM, et al. Epidemiology and cause-specific outcome of hypertrophic cardiomyopathy in children: findings from the Pediatric Cardiomyopathy Registry. Circulation. Feb 13 2007;115(6):773–81.

Maron BJ, Spirito P, Shen WK, et al. Implantable cardioverter-defibrillators and prevention of sudden cardiac death in hypertrophic cardiomyopathy. JAMA. Jul 25 2007;298(4):405–12.

Prevention of infective endocarditis: guidelines from the American Heart Association (multiple councils): Wilson W, Taubert KA, Gewitz M, Lockhart PB, Baddour LM, Levison M, Bolger A, Cabell CH, Takahashi M, Baltimore RS, Newburger JW, Strom BL, Tani LY, Gerber M, Bonow RO, Pallasch T, Shulman ST, Rowley AH, Burns JC, Ferrieri P, Gardner T, Goff D, Durack DT. Circulation. 2007 Oct 9;116(15):1736-54.

Yetman AT, McCrindle BW. Management of pediatric hypertrophic cardiomyopathy. Curr Opin Cardiol. Mar 2005;20(2):80–3.

Hypoplastic Left Heart Syndrome (HLHS)

Gary M. Satou, Thomas S. Klitzner

Hypoplastic left heart syndrome refers to a constellation of congenital cardiac anomalies with an underdeveloped left ventricle, in association with varying degrees of mitral stenosis/atresia and aortic valve stenosis or atresia. In addition, there is usually aortic arch hypoplasia and coarctation.

Etiology

Although the exact etiology of this anomaly is poorly understood, most theories revolve around the embryologic malformation of the aorta and mitral valve.

Clinical Presentation and Prognosis

Age of onset: This lesion is diagnosed in utero when fetal echocardiography is performed by properly trained clinicians. Otherwise, diagnosis is usually made in the first day or days of life (see below).

Presenting signs/symptom and clinical course: All HLHS neonates are symptomatic with congestive heart failure, low cardiac output (once the ductus arteriosis closes) and cyanosis. They require intensive care with medical and surgical management for survival.

Prognosis: Without medical and surgical care, HLHS is not compatible with life. Without intervention, the newborn will expire from acidosis, shock and myocardial failure. Conversely, with proper surgical and ICU management, these patients usually demonstrate an 85% early survival. Subsequent operations known as Stage 2 (Glenn shunt) and Stage 3 (Fontan Procedure) generally have an approximately 1% mortality (see below).

Diagnosis

Prenatal HLHS diagnosis is by fetal echocardiography. If not detected in utero, the newborn with acidosis, cyanosis and possibly poor systemic perfusion is quickly noticed right away by the NICU or nursery staff and cardiology consultation is requested. Echocardiography is performed and defines the anatomy as delineated above. Catheterization or other imaging modalities are rarely needed. Although rare in the modern era, sometimes patients' conditions are missed because an open ductus supports the systemic circulation so cyanosis is not immediately noticeable. These patients may be sent home, but invariably develop acidosis, cyanosis and poor systemic perfusion when the ductus arteriosis closes. This clinical presentation of extremis then draws attention to the infant and cardiac evaluation and diagnosis are usually made. However, in this scenario, the baby may have incurred irreparable injury or even death.

Management

Medication: In order to maintain ductal patency and systemic perfusion, prostaglandin infusion is necessary. Rapid treatment of acidosis is important for myocardial protection and inotropic support is usually initiated. Care must be taken not to administer supplemental oxygen as a response to cyanosis because this will enhance pulmonary blood flow at the expense of systemic perfusion.

Surgery: Currently, the majority of pediatric heart centers perform the Norwood (or Stage I) procedure or a modification of it. This usually includes removal of the atrial septum for improved mixing, a Stansel procedure connecting the main pulmonary artery with the ascending aorta, and aortic arch augmentation. A shunt or conduit is placed either from the aorta or the right ventricle (RV), to the branch pulmonary arteries, thus providing a source (the only source) of pulmonary blood flow. As the child later outgrows this connection, a second stage procedure is performed using the native superior vena cava. This is called a bidirectional Glenn shunt. A third stage called the Fontan procedure is then completed one or two years later. The procedure incorporates the IVC blood flow to the Glenn communication so that all systemic venous return is directed into the lungs, thereby bypassing the heart. This helps separate the systemic desaturated blood from the oxygenated pulmonary venous blood returning from the heart.

Therapy: In select cases of prolonged hospital stay, infants will be discharged with physical therapy, approximately three times/week. The goal of the therapy is to improve overall tone and range of motion after a prolonged period of supine positioning and deconditioning.

Social: Websites and organizations considered reliable by pediatric cardiac specialists for parental education include those from the American Heart Association (AHA): www.americanheart.org and the Congenital Heart Information Network (CHIN): www.tchin.org.

Long-term monitoring: After initial discharge following the Norwood procedure, careful and frequent follow up is given. Pediatric cardiologists may monitor the infant on a weekly to monthly basis. Many variables are monitored including oxygen saturation, blood pressure (note: not accurate when measured in the arm associated with the BT shunt, if performed), work of breathing, peripheral perfusion, nutritional status, and lower extremity pulses. Saturations will be in the general range of 75–85%. Medications used will include after load reduction (ace-inhibitors), and anticoagulation with either Aspirin or Coumadin. Occasionally, Lovenox is utilized. Diuretics and Digoxin may be used. Laboratory values are assessed to ensure adequate electrolyte balance and oxygen carrying capacity. Some institutions utilize home pulse oximetry to facilitate recognition of decreasing saturations. The Glenn shunt is performed at approximately 4 to 6 months of age and the discharge follow-up is less frequent and may be at 1 to 3 month intervals depending on both the cardiovascular status of the infant and physician style/preference. Medications and saturations are similar and may not change significantly, though diuretics are less-likely to be used after the early postoperative period. The Fontan procedure in the current era is performed on average at 2 to 4 years of age. It can be performed as early as one year of age if necessary. Generally, the oxygen saturations will increase into the 90%'s with this final procedure. For low risk patients, if a fenestration was created in the Fontan connection, it may be closed at 6 months to 1 year following surgery to further increase oxygen saturation. This is performed in a transcatheter fashion by placement of a septal occlusion device in the fenestration, eliminating the remaining right to left shunt and increasing the oxygen saturations, often into the 96–99% range. The afterload reduction and anticoagulation initiated pre-Fontan are usually continued indefinitely, so that most Fontan patients are taking at least two medications. The child with Fontan circulation and no significant cardiovascular residua are seen by the pediatric cardiologist 1–2 times/year. Outside of varsity level and contact sports, exercise is generally not discouraged. In most cases, it is usually a self-limiting scenario as the child/adolescent will have diminished exercise capacity at baseline. Long term issues for these patients can include a small risk of stroke or neurologic injury, arrhythmia, and cardiac dysfunction. A small subgroup of patients will have cardiac/single-ventricular failure not amenable to further medical or surgical care and require cardiac transplantion.

Pearls and Precautions

Incision: The incision should be kept clean and dry. Washing is achieved by using a damp cloth and soap. Do not completely soak incision in water until healed (usually 6 to 8 weeks). Do not apply ointments or lotions for 6–8 weeks. Itching is a normal sign of healing, and scratching should be discouraged. After healing occurs, sunscreen should be used when in direct sunlight. Parents should be instructed to call the cardiologist if redness, swelling, pain or drainage from the incision occurs.

Diet: Families should be educated that the infant/child may tire easily and require rest during feeding. Feedings may be more frequent but smaller in quantity. Sweating with feeds may occur for a period of time. In general, if the feeding pattern is not slowly improving towards normalcy in the weeks following repair, the parents should contact the physician. Negative changes may be reflective of postoperative issues such as infection, effusions, or cardiac dysfunction.

Activities: Sternal precautions are undertaken for the first 8 weeks after repair. This includes avoiding direct pressure or pulling on the sternum. Infants should not be lifted under the arms but rather cooped up under the back and bottom. Car seats should always be utilized when traveling. When possible, avoidance of ill friends and family or crowded public places is suggested for 2–4 weeks after discharge. Sleep patterns (similar to feeding patterns) may be altered for a period of time after repair.

Endocarditis prophylaxis: Good dental hygiene is very important to reduce the risk of infective endocarditis and should be encouraged. If dental cleaning or care is performed (or other non-cardiac procedures), the cardiologist should be contacted to discuss the patient's individual needs. The most recent guidelines for endocarditis prophylaxis can be reviewed and is referenced below. In general, these patients do require SBE prophylaxis.

Immunizations: Infants should delay vaccination for approximately one month following surgery. This should be discussed with the individual cardiologist.

Parental education: Parents should be instructed to call the cardiologist or cardiac care team upon the following findings after discharge:

- When an incision demonstrates redness, swelling, pain or drainage.
- If increased work of breathing or shortness of breath occurs.
- If oxygen saturations are decreased.
- When fussy behavior or poor feeding ensues.
- If swollen or puffy hands/feet are present.
- If vomiting or diarrhea occurs more than once.
- If fever develops (temperature 38.5 Centigrade or greater).

References

Hypoplastic left heart syndrome. Barron DJ, Kilby MD, Davies B, Wright JG, Jones TJ, Brawn WJ. Lancet. 2009 Aug 15;374(9689):551–64

New developments in the treatment of hypoplastic left heart syndrome. Alsoufi B, Bennetts J, Verma S, Caldarone CA. Pediatrics. 2007 Jan;119(1):109–17

Prevention of infective endocarditis: guidelines from the American Heart Association (multiple councils): Wilson W, Taubert KA, Gewitz M, Lockhart PB, Baddour LM, Levison M, Bolger A, Cabell CH, Takahashi M, Baltimore RS, Newburger JW, Strom BL, Tani LY, Gerber M, Bonow RO, Pallasch T, Shulman ST, Rowley AH, Burns JC, Ferrieri P, Gardner T, Goff D, Durack DT. Circulation. 2007 Oct 9; 116(15):1736–54.

Long QT Syndromes (LQTS)

Thomas S. Klitzner, Gary M. Satou

Long QT syndrome (LQTS) is a genetic syndrome resulting in risk of ventricular tachycardia and sudden death.

Etiology

The Long QT syndrome is the most common of the so called "repolarization abnormalities" that have genetic alterations in the proteins responsible for transport of ions across the cardiac muscle membrane. A variety of proteins and at least three ions (potassium, sodium and calcium) are known to alter the electrical activity of ventricular muscle in a manner which predisposes the individual to ventricular tachycardia and fibrillation. Genetic subtypes of the syndrome have been identified.

Clinical Presentation and Prognosis:

Age of onset: The Long QT syndromes are not a homogeneous group of conditions and thus the age at onset is variable. Cases of intractable ventricular tachycardia and second degree atrioventricular heart block due to extremely prolonged QT intervals have been reported in newborns, while in some cases, the condition is first discovered in adulthood. The majority of cases present after infancy with a predilection towards adolescence, likely secondary to the increased intensity of physical activity in this age group.

Presenting signs and symptoms: Unfortunately, many patients with Long QT syndrome present with an episode of cardiac arrest. However, as many as half have preceding symptoms of dizziness, chest pain, syncope, palpitations, and/or dyspnea. Occasionally, patients are discovered as the result of QT prolongation found on a screening EKG performed for unrelated reasons, and a small number experience ventricular tachycardia while undergoing general anesthesia. A growing number of patients are identified because of the premature, unexpected sudden death of a close relative. In addition it is recommended that a work-up for LQTS be conducted in patients with unexplained seizures, near drowning episodes and after un-witnessed accidents involving automobiles or heavy machinery. Congenital deafness may also be a presenting symptom of one particular subgroup of LQTS known as Jervelle-Lange-Neilson Syndrome, which includes all of the characteristics of LQTS along with congenital deafness. With the advent of genetic testing, it may be possible to make the diagnosis in an asymptomatic relative of an identified patient.

Prognosis: If left untreated, mortality from LQTS is thought to be between 0.15 and 20% per year depending on the LQTS subtype, the degree of QT prolongation and the age of onset. However, these estimates are based largely on speculation as true natural history studies are not possible. Many patients present with sudden cardiac death. Those who do not and are suspected of having the diagnosis are immediately placed on drug therapy.

Clinical diagnosis: Several factors contribute to the clinical diagnosis of LQTS. Patients who present with symptoms or history suggestive of LQTS should have an electrocardiogram on which the corrected QT interval is measured. The corrected QT interval is calculated by measuring the raw QT interval and dividing by the square root of the preceding RR interval. Normal values for this measurement are sex and age dependent, but a measurement of greater than 0.5 is almost always abnormal. Since many pharmacologic agents prolong the QT interval, it is important to ensure that the patient is not taking one of these medicines at the time of the EKG. In addition, QT prolongation may be evanescent, so several EKG's as well as EKG's on first degree family members is advisable. The second important feature of the diagnostic work-up of LQTS is a good family history. If the patient's history includes one or more first degree relatives who died suddenly at or before young adulthood, suspicions should be raised for the existence of the condition. Deaths of first degree relatives are particularly worrisome and consideration must be given to "accidents" that may have been preceded by cardiac arrhythmias such as single driver vehicle crashes, deaths while operating heavy machinery, un-witnessed skiing accidents and drowning. Other diagnostic features that may be helpful are the recording of the characteristic "Torsade de Pointes" tachycardia on event recorder, 24 hour holter monitor, hospital monitor or during anesthesia; ventricular tachycardia or Torsade de Pointe during stress exercise testing; or less commonly T-wave alternans on EKG.

Genetic testing: Under certain circumstances, genetic testing can be extremely valuable in making the diagnosis of Long QT Syndrome. At present, six genes have been identified. Five of these encode for subunits of cardiac ion channels and one extremely rare mutation has been found in the gene which encodes for cardiac ankyrin, a structural protein that anchors ion channels to the cell membrane. The clinical value of genetic testing lies in the ability to identify carriers of LQTS who themselves do not demonstrate QT interval prolongation and therefore may otherwise be missed. In addition, once the genetic determinant of the disease is identified in an individual patient, predictions of the likely clinical course and risk stratification may be facilitated. The most valuable aspect of genetic testing is identification of LQTS in relatives of a patient with a known gene mutation. Unfortunately, the value of genetic testing is greatly diminished when the etiologic mutation is unknown. Worse yet, in isolated patients suspected of having Long QT Syndrome, genetic testing can make the diagnosis only if a specific mutation is found. However, a negative test under these circumstances can mean that either the patient does not have the disease; or that the mutation affecting this individual patient is one that remains unidentified and therefore is absent from commercially available screening panels. The search for an as yet unidentified mutation is possible, but is extremely difficult and time consuming. Consequently, this analysis is currently the purview of research laboratories and, in general, is not helpful in the clinical setting.

Management

The mainstay of therapy in most cases of LQTS is the administration of beta blockers. This approach has been shown to reduce the risk of sudden death in approximately 70% of cases of LQTS.

Medication: All patients with Long QT syndrome should be on a beta-blocker. These medications are often used at maximal doses if tolerated. It may be helpful to use maximal treadmill or cycle stress to assess the effectiveness of this therapy. In general, an inability to raise the heart rate above 150/min in children indicates effective therapy. In some cases, adequate beta blocker effects may require higher than recommended doses of beta-blockers. However, in light of the protective effect of the medication, these supramaximal doses may be warranted in the absence of drug related symptoms. Propranolol and nadolol are the most commonly used beta-blockers, but atenolol and metoprolol are also prescribed in patients with LQTS. It is controversial as to whether different beta-blockers demonstrate differential effectiveness in preventing sudden cardiac death in patients with LQTS. In addition, all patients with LQTS should avoid drugs that prolong the QT interval or reduce serum potassium or magnesium levels. Any deficiencies in potassium or magnesium should be corrected.

Implantable devices: Therapy for LQTS has been significantly altered by the availability of Automatic Implantable Cardiac Defibrillators (AICD's) for children. The rate of sudden death can be reduced several fold by the implantation of a defibrillator. However, the risks of the procedure as well as the variance in data collected on these patients and the risk of sudden death must be evaluated by a trained pediatric electrophysiologist before a decision is made to place an AICD in a patient.

Social: The concern on the part of parents and society at large that young healthy individuals may die suddenly creates significant anxiety in many families. Expeditious evaluation leading to diagnosis, if the patient is at risk or reassurance if the patient is not, can be extremely helpful. Some families, however, do not seem capable of dealing with the uncertainties that can exist during and after the evaluation process. Thorough, honest and thoughtful explanations often suffice to relieve these anxieties. Nonetheless, professional counseling may be helpful in some cases.

Pearls and Precautions

Timothy Syndrome which manifests as LQTS plus syndactyly is caused by a calcium channel defect.

The original nomenclature for LQTS included the names Romano-Ward and Jervelle Lange Neilson Syndrome. Of interest, Romano Ward which consists of LQTS alone was thought to have a "dominant" pattern of inheritance while Jervelle Lange Neilson which includes both LQTS and congenital deafness was thought to be recessive. In fact, the defect in a potassium channel present in both the heart and ear is the same in both syndromes. When the gene is altered on one allele, sufficient potassium channels are produced in the ear to preserve hearing, while the arrhythmic effects on the heart are manifest. With a defective gene on both alleles, no functional potassium channels are produced, leading to both LQTS and hearing loss.

It is generally believed that patients who present with LQTS after age 40 do well. LQTS is often discovered for the first time when patients undergo general anesthesia.

Patients with LQTS should avoid taking medicines that prolong the QT interval. Common drugs to avoid are erythromycin, most pro-kinetics, most anti fungal agents and many anti-arrhythmic agents. A full and up to date list of medications that should not be taken by patients with LQTS can be found at http://www.sads.org/index.php/Drugs-to-Avoid/Drugs-to-Avoid.html.

References

Congenital long-QT syndromes: a clinical and genetic update from infancy through adulthood. Webster G, Berul CI. Trends Cardiovasc Med. 2008 Aug;18(6):216–24

Advances in congenital long QT syndrome. Collins KK, Van Hare GF. Curr Opin Pediatr. 2006 Oct;18(5):497–502.

Pulmonary Hypertension

Gary M. Satou, Thomas S. Klitzner

Disease: A variety of primary or secondary processes can alter pulmonary vascular physiology and create increased resistance and pulmonary arterial hypertension. This leads to chronic pulmonary hypertension, right heart failure and ultimately death. Thus, pulmonary hypertension as a "disease" category includes both primary and secondary pulmonary hypertension which can be idiopathic, familial, and/or associated with other systemic disorders including congenital heart disease.

Etiology

Despite being a heterogeneous disorder with multiple etiologic factors, some common physiologic components exist. In general, there is a triad of pulmonary vasoconstriction, thrombosis, and proliferation of smooth muscle or endothelial cells in the pulmonary arterial tree. An imbalance of multiple vasoactive factors creates this milieu, and pathologically, one sees "muscularization" of the pulmonary vessels with intimal and medial involvement, and subsequently, fibrosis.

Clinical Presentation and Prognosis

Age of onset: Because pulmonary hypertension is an endpoint with heterogeneous etiologies, there is no specific time at which patients present. Newborns, for example, can present with PPHN immediately at birth. Infants, children and adolescents all can present for the first time with the symptoms of pulmonary hypertension.

Presenting signs/symptom and clinical course: Neonates and infants may demonstrate desaturation, tachypnea, and irritability. Feeding may be poor. Common symptoms in older children include shortness of breath, a general sense of fatigue or tiredness, and poor exercise tolerance. There may be chronic cough, non-specific chest pain, or even syncope. Physical examination reveals tachypnea and possibly cyanosis. The older patient may have jugular venous distension. The precordium can be active with a right ventricular heave, and there may be a systolic murmur from tricuspid valve regurgitation. The second heart sound is single or narrowly split with a loud P2 component. With right heart failure, there may be hepatomegaly, ascites and lower extremity edema.

Prognosis: Historically, the treatment of pulmonary hypertension in children is poor. To date, even the results of children undergoing treatment have been relatively poor, though recent pharmacologic advancements demonstrate encouraging results in those patients who acutely demonstrate responsiveness to pulmonary vasodilator testing. Irrespective of etiology, the morbidity and mortality in pulmonary hypertension stems from the development of right heart failure. Once significant right ventricular (RV) failure ensues, secondary left ventricular dysfunction and failure can result. Sudden pulmonary, cardiac or neurologic events can occur with devastating consequences. The heterogeneity of pulmonary hypertension (i.e., idiopathic, familial, association with CHD) combined with the lack of research in pediatric patients makes exact outcome-statistics for any given age group difficult to determine in terms of treatment-success and survival. Adult survival data suggests approximately 15% mortality within one year on modern therapy. Outcomes in pediatric idiopathic pulmonary hypertension has been described as 97% survival at 5 years and 81% survival at 10 years. In CHD patients with fixed pulmonary vascular disease, long-term follow up reveals 80% untreated survival at 5 years and approximately 40% at 25 years out. Today, however, children with CHD usually undergo surgical repair at an early age thus preventing, for the most part, fixed pulmonary vascular disease. As a result, the population of untreated CHD patients has significantly decreased.

Diagnosis

Once the child with the above-described clinical presentation (history and physical examination) is identified, a number of tests are undertaken to diagnose pulmonary hypertension. Electrocardiogram (EKG) may demonstrate right heart enlargement and strain. Chest radiograph can show cardiomegaly and decreased peripheral vascular markings. Chest computerized tomography (CT) is utilized to rule-out other pulmonary disorders. Exercise and pulmonary function testing is performed. Echocardiography can rule-out associated congenital anatomic defects, and may show right heart enlargement (RV hypertrophy, dilation), tricuspid valve regurgitation, or ventricular dysfunction. Doppler techniques are employed to estimate the RV pressure. However, cardiac catheterization is the gold standard test, as it can directly and invasively measure intracardiac and pulmonary pressures and resistance. As well, one can perform acute pulmonary testing with pulmonary vasodilators such as oxygen and inhaled nitric oxide, and then re-calculate the pulmonary vascular resistance in an effort to determine the child's "responsiveness" to medical therapy.

Management

Current treatment strategies for children with pulmonary hypertension focus primarily on medical (as opposed to surgical) care. The duration of treatment is generally long-term/lifelong, and centers more on improving quality of life and reducing the risk of sudden pulmonary or cardiovascular events, rather than offering a "cure."

Medication: Several different categories of medications are currently used. Newer agents or categories are primarily selective pulmonary vasodilators and work in different ways with the common goal of reducing pulmonary vascular resistance.

- *Calcium channel blockers*: In children with acute responsiveness to pulmonary vasodilation in the catheterization laboratory, oral calcium channel blockade has been used with some success. Nifidipine is usually the oral agent utilized.
- *Prostacyclin Analogues*: Intravenous epoprostenal infusion has been shown to be effective in some children, including acute non-responders to testing. This requires reliable intravenous access and is continuously infused, making it somewhat cumbersome and placing children at risk of line complications, such as sepsis. Newer agents such as Treprostinil and Illoprost are being used, which allow for alternative subcutaneous or inhaled routes of administration, but still are suboptimal in that injections are generally not preferred by children and inhalations can be as frequent as every couple of hours.

- *Endothelin-Receptor Antagonists*: Endothelian is an endogenous peptide and potent vasoconstrictor that is found to be elevated in pulmonary hypertensive patients and inversely associated with survival. Thus, these agents work by reducing the concentration of endothelian. Bosentan, an oral non-receptor selective antagonist, is the most commonly used agent.

- *Nitric Oxide*: Used in the inhaled form, this is a selective pulmonary vasodilator with multiple beneficial effects on the pulmonary vasculature. It is most commonly used as a testing agent in the catheterization laboratory and in the postoperative care of the congenital heart surgical patient. Although it has been used in the chronic, ambulatory setting in the past, it is cumbersome and expensive.

- *Phosphodiesterase Inhibitors*: These agents work by selectively inhibiting the type of phosphodiesterase which breaks down cGMP, an important component in nitric oxide mediated vasodilation. Sildenafil is the main oral agent and at present, perhaps the most common drug utilized in pulmonary hypertension management. It can be used alone or in combination with other agents. It is often used to minimize rebound pulmonary hypertension found when weaning a child from inhaled nitric oxide.

- *Other*: Anticoagulation is an important part of management in patients with pulmonary hypertension. Patients may have a sedentary disposition due to physical limitations, and thus an increased risk of thromboembolism. As well, a pro-coagulable state can be found in some of these patients. Coumadin is the most common agent used, with a goal INR of usually 1.5 to 2.0. Oxygen by nasal cannula may be utilized at times when there is pulmonary parenchymal disease associated with the patient, or when severe alveolar hypoxemia exists. When right heart failure is present, heart-failure drugs such as Digoxin and diuretics are used at times.

Surgery: Although no surgical "cure" is available, atrial septostomy or lung transplantation is occasionally performed.

- *Atrial septostomy*: This is reserved for patients refractory to medical management and is a palliative maneuver to increase cardiac output by promoting right to left atrial level shunting/decompression and may serve as a bridge towards lung transplantation.

- *Lung transplantation*: Please refer to the lung transplantion section of Chapter 17 for details. Generally, morbidity and mortality remains significant with this approach, with continued issues of organ donor availability and a high incidence of subsequent bronchiolitis obliterans, transplant rejection, and infections. Also, the number of centers in the U.S. offering pediatric lung transplantation is small.

Pyscho-Social: When pulmonary hypertension is diagnosed, the needs of the child and family can be great. The concept of a debilitating, life-limiting disease, without a cure, is a tremendous and anxiety-provoking burden to have. Major centers offering care for these children usually provide support services such as social work, psychology and psychiatry.

Pearls and Precautions

Drugs: See below listing for adverse effects seen with the above described medications commonly used in pulmonary hypertension management. Because of chronic anticoagulation, one should avoid medications which will alter the metabolism of Coumadin. Stimulants and appetite suppressants can negatively affect cardiac or pulmonary function and should also be avoided.

- *Calcium channel blockers (Nifidipine)*: systemic hypotension, cardiovascular compromise.
- *Prostacyclin analogues (Epoprostenol IV, Trepostinil SQ, Iloprost: inhaled)*: headaches, nausea, flushing, diarrhea, rash, and jaw/leg pain. Potential complications of indwelling catheter.

- *Endothelian receptor antagonists (Bosentan):* liver function test (LFT) elevation, flushing, syncope, anemia. Teratogen.
- *Nitric Oxide:* Methoglobinemia. Rebound pulmonary hypertension when discontinued.
- *Phosphodiesterase inhibitors (Sildenafil):* headache, flushing, nasal congestion.

Immunizations/prophylaxis: Complete immunizations including influenza and pneumococcus are indicated. General avoidance of family, friends and settings where infectious exposure are present is wise. Incurred pulmonary infections should be aggressively treated so as to minimize any untoward, secondary effects.

Exercise: Low level physical activity is encouraged, but competitive sports and isometric exercises should be avoided.

Nutrition: Although a low fat, low salt diet is appropriate for all children, no specific diet is demanded.

Airplane travel: This should be discussed with the child's pediatric cardiologist. Depending on the circumstances, it may be allowed, but the pressurized cabin environment can induce alveolar hypoxia and pulmonary vasoconstriction. If allowed, supplemental oxygen therapy is likely to be recommended.

Pregnancy: This should be avoided at all costs, as the morbidity associated with pregnancy and the labor process are high. Oral contraception is problematic due to chronic coumadin therapy and potentially pro-coaguable state. Therefore, although it seems extreme, sterilization may be the recommended contraception of choice.

References

ACCF/AHA 2009 expert consensus document on pulmonary hypertension a report of the American College of Cardiology Foundation Task Force on Expert Consensus Documents and the American Heart Association developed in collaboration with the American College of Chest Physicians; American Thoracic Society, Inc.; and the Pulmonary Hypertension Association. McLaughlin VV, Archer SL, Badesch DB, Barst RJ, Farber HW, Lindner JR, Mathier MA, McGoon MD, Park MH, Rosenson RS, Rubin LJ, Tapson VF, Varga. J Am Coll Cardiol. 2009 Apr 28;53(17):1573–619.

Pulmonary arterial hypertension in children: a medical update. Rosenzweig EB, Barst RJ. Indian J Pediatr. 2009 Jan;76(1):77–81

Evaluation, risk stratification, and management of pulmonary hypertension in patients with congenital heart disease. Feinstein JA. Semin Thorac Cardiovasc Surg Pediatr Card Surg Annu. 2009:106–11

Supraventricular Tachycardia (SVT)/ Wolf-Parkinson-White Syndrome (WPW)

Thomas S. Klitzner, Gary M. Satou

Supraventricular tachycardia (SVT) and the related Wolf-Parkinson-White Syndrome (WPW) denote a rapid rhythm of the heart in which the origin of the electrical signal is either within the atria or the atrioventricular (AV) node.

Etiology

The most common forms of SVT result from the presence of two electrical pathways from the atria to the ventricles of the heart. These two pathways may reside entirely within the AV node, called AV Nodal Re-entrant Tachycardia (AVNRT). One pathway may be within the AV node, while the other forms are a bridge of tissue between the atrium and the ventricles. This connection is known as an "accessory pathway." Pathways can conduct from the ventricle to the atria (retrograde in direction), called a "concealed" pathway. These forms of tachycardia are also known as AV reciprocating tachycardia. When an accessory pathway can conduct in either direction, the electrocardiogram demonstrates a short PR interval with up-sloping of the initial portion of the QRS. This is the hallmark of the Wolf-Parkinson-White-Syndrome (WPW). In WPW, the tachycardia is retrograde or "concealed" and the EKG findings, which are due to anterograde pathway conduction, disappear during tachycardia. In the least common form of SVT in children, an ectopic focus in the atrium fires rapidly, creating a rapid ventricular response via conduction AV nodal conduction. The resulting rapid heart beat is known as Ectopic Atrial Tachycardia (EAT).

Clinical Presentation and Prognosis

Age of onset: The rapid heartbeat of SVT is most often recognized during one of three periods of life: Newborn (first 3 months of life), early school age (4–6 years) or early adolescence (12–15 years). This prevalence of presentations in these three time periods is well known, but not well understood.

Presenting signs and symptoms: The common presenting feature of SVT is sustained rapid heart beat which may be as fast as 300/beats/minute in the newborn, but is commonly above 200/beats/minute at all ages. In the newborn, the only symptoms may be poor feeding and lethargy, unless the parent notices rapid pumping of the ventricles while holding the infant or breastfeeding. In this early age group, patients do not develop signs of cardiac failure for 24 to 72 hours. Thus, many infants are diagnosed by pediatricians who are asked to evaluate for poor feeding. In older age groups, the most common presentation is a complaint that "my heart is beating fast" often during exercise, but occasionally at rest. Particularly in adolescents, the problem may manifest during strenuous exercise with the patient becoming tired or short of breath and stopping exercise only to find that their heart is beating rapidly and does not slow down.

Clinical course: When SVT presents in the newborn period, with or without WPW, there is a reasonable chance that the condition will disappear by one year of age. Typically, medical management is instituted in the first year of life and a majority of patients will not require further therapy. When the diagnosis is made at a later age or the condition persists after the first birthday, the clinical course is one of medical control or "cure" by catheter intervention (see below). Except for occasional breakthrough episodes and periodic visits to a pediatric cardiologist, the clinical course for the vast majority of patients with SVT is relatively benign. Some more difficult to treat patients may require hospitalization or early catheter intervention to gain control of the arrhythmia. The very occasional patient who presents with cardiomyopathy in addition to SVT may on rare occasions, require heart transplantation or possibly succumb to the cardiomyopathy.

Prognosis: Prognosis is excellent. Rates of the condition's disappearance in the first year of life combined with newer catheter techniques, promises a resolution of the condition in greater than 90% of patients once they have reached school age.

Diagnosis

Definitive diagnosis of SVT requires an electrocardiogram or rhythm strip demonstrating the arrhythmia. These are often obtained by pediatric cardiologists utilizing 24 hour holter monitoring or an event recorder. In cases where symptoms are associated with exercise, a treadmill exercise test with continuous EKG recording may yield a diagnosis. A presumptive diagnosis can be made by history in an older child who describes a rapid heart beat which has been counted to be faster than 200/beats/minute or reported by a credible observer to be "too fast to count" and which resolves by stopping abruptly (or skipping a beat and then stopping). Termination of tachycardia in this fashion is often seen in temporal association with vagal stimuli, such as valsalva maneuver or emesis. Patients with suspected SVT for which no documentation is available should be instructed to go to an Emergency Room if the tachycardia persists for more that a few minutes as this may allow for obtaining a full EKG during the tachycardia. The most definitive diagnostic information can be obtained by invasive electrophysiologic study which may be required in some cases. More often, a diagnostic electrophysiologic study is performed as part of catheter directed radio-frequency ablation and thus is more often reserved for treatment as opposed to diagnosis.

Management

Until 1990, the management of SVT was restricted to antiarrhythmic medicine. With the advent of radio-frequency ablation in children, the alternative of eliminating one of the electrical connections responsible for re-entrant tachycardias or abolishing an ectopic focus in the atrium began to replace pharmacologic therapy as the treatment of choice for SVT. Currently, drug therapy is utilized for all but the most refractory cases in the first years of life. Above the age of four years, radio-frequency ablation is becoming the standard of care.

Medication: Numerous anti-arrhythmic agents are used in the treatment of SVT. Since the AV node is almost always involved, agents that slow conduction or increase the refractory period of the AV node such as digoxin and beta-blockers are often used. Verapamil, which also affects the AV node, is not used in infancy due to the immature heart's dependence on calcium influx to support contraction, but may be used, with success, after age one year. When a lateral accessory pathway is involved in a re-entrant circuit, fleccainide may be useful. Amiodarone is reserved for the more difficult tachycardias because of concern for its side effect profile. In the presence of WPW, digoxin may increase conduction through the accessory pathway. This can enhance the chances of rapid conduction of atrial flutter or fibrillation to the ventricles resulting in ventricular tachycardia.

Radio-frequency ablation: Catheter directed radio-frequency ablation of one AV nodal pathway (AV node modification) or a lateral accessory pathway has become a mainstay of therapy in both children and adults. The procedure involves placing electrode catheters in the heart in a variety of positions to "map" the course of the tachycardia and identify and localize dual AV nodal pathways, a lateral accessory pathway or an ectopic focus. Use of a specialized "steerable" catheter allows positioning of the electrode tip with a high level of precision so that cauterizing energy can be transmitted to a localized area of the heart, ablating the extra pathway or ectopic focus. This procedure is commonly performed as an outpatient with a greater than 90% success rate for most types of SVT. Newer imaging techniques have reduced the use of fluoroscopy, and some ablations can be performed without the use of ionizing radiation.

Social: SVT is a prevalent condition, occurring in as many as 1/200 live births and 1/500 adolescents and adults. Thus, parents and patients may find comfort in knowing that amongst their relatives, friends and acquaintances are people who have or have had the condition. A simple mention of the problem in a social or work setting may elicit reassuring stories of others who have had SVT. Reliable web sites acceptable for review include www.americanheart.org and www.sads.org.

Pearls and Precautions

The airway, breathing, circulation (ABC's) of cardiopulmonary resuscitation/advanced cardiac life support (CPR/ACLS) are always pertinent in any age patient if tachycardia acutely develops while in the care of the primary care provider. Direct current (DC) cardioversion may be necessary in the acute care setting.

Neonates and infants are treated after an SVT diagnosis but may outgrow the condition and have anti-arrhythmic therapy discontinued at 6–12 months of age. Except for WPW, initial drug choice is usually beta blockers or digoxin. Breakthroughs can be treated with ice to the face (no more than 15 seconds to minimize injury) or vagal maneuvers. As the infant outgrows the per kilogram dosing of a drug, the cardiologist upsizes the dosing until the time of discontinuation. Pediatricians and families should notify the pediatric cardiologist if recurrent tachycardia ensues. Emergency room visits are likely in these scenarios, depending on the circumstances.

Older children and adolescents with SVT are educated regarding the various vagal maneuvers available (Valsalva, unilateral carotid message, having a patient hold his breath or place his thumb in his mouth and "blow"). Beta blockers are commonly used in this age group. Radio-frequency ablation is also widely performed with low risk and high success rates.

Pediatric cardiology visits will usually include history-taking, examination and EKG's as needed. Holter and event monitoring may be performed to record rhythms at various times and states. Exercise stress-testing may be used as well.

- Most patients will not have activity or exercise restrictions despite the diagnosis.
- Never use Digoxin with the diagnosis of WPW (as explained above).
- Sub-acute bacterial endocarditis (SBE) prophylaxis is not indicated.

Families should be educated that although the diagnosis/condition is serious, it is usually not fatal and often resolves over time. Treatment strategies are very effective and a full life style/life cycle is expected in most cases.

References

Supraventricular tachycardia in the pediatric primary care setting: Age-related presentation, diagnosis, and management. Schlechte EA, Boramanand N, Funk M. J Pediatr Health Care. 2008 Sep–Oct;22(5):289–99. Epub 2008 Mar 4.

The role of radiofrequency ablation for pediatric supraventricular tachycardia. Campbell RM, Strieper MJ, Frias PA. Minerva Pediatr. 2004 Feb;56(1):63–72

Diagnosis and treatment of arrhythmias. Perry JC, Garson A Jr. Adv Pediatr. 1989;36:177–99

Tetralogy of Fallot (TOF)

Gary M. Satou, Thomas S. Klitzner

In Tetralogy of Fallot, there are several intracardiac lesions. Most important is a large, unrestrictive VSD. Due to an arrest in conotruncal development, the aorta sits or "overrides" the septum and the VSD. In addition, there are varying degrees of RV to pulmonary artery obstruction. This obstruction can be sub-valvar and/or valvar and may have a supravalvar component. The degree of RV to PA obstruction dictates the degree of right to left shunting and desaturation.

Etiology

Congenital heart disease is considered multifactorial in origin. The major anatomic abnormality is anterior deviation of the cono-truncal septum resulting in four classic features of the condition: a ventricular septal defect (VSD), subpulmonary stenosis, aortic override and secondarily right ventricular hypertrophy.

Clinical Presentation and Prognosis

Age of onset: This lesion can be diagnosed in utero. Otherwise, diagnosis is often made in the first day or days of life as either desaturation or the usually loud murmur of the RV outflow/pulmonary valve obstruction results in a cardiology consultation and diagnosis.

Presenting signs/symptom and clinical course: This varies with the degree of RV outflow and pulmonary valve obstruction. Infants with tetralogy of Fallot can be classified as either "pink," meaning very little right to left intra-cardiac shunting and thus relatively normal oxygen saturations; or, "blue" meaning, desaturation which can be profound and is usually detected by clinical exam or pulse oximetry. These babies are susceptible to "spelling" or acute drops in pulmonary blood flow (by a "spasmodic" right ventricular outflow tract (RVOT)). If the RV outflow narrowing is very mild, there can be long term effects of pulmonary over-circulation. Most commonly, there will be increasing RVOT narrowing and this will result in desaturation and the long term effects of cyanosis.

Prognosis: Excellent with surgical intervention. Without surgical care, infants with tetralogy of Fallot are susceptible to "spelling" and acute decompensation, or the long-term sequelae of cyanosis (neurologic, hematologic, infectious).

Diagnosis

Prenatal diagnosis is by fetal echocardiography. When evaluated in the neonatal or infant period, a harsh murmur or cyanosis usually leads to the cardiology consultation. Echocardiography is performed as part of the evaluation. This confirms the diagnosis and is very good at demonstrating the level of RVOT obstruction and any associated lesions.

Management

Medication: Once the diagnosis is made, the approach to care depends on the degree of RV outflow obstruction and desaturation. For the "pink" tetralogy patient, watchful waiting and a surgical correction (see below) is performed. Medicine is rarely needed at this time. If the child is cyanotic, there may be an effort to maintain or re-open the patent ductus arteriosus (PDA) with PGE infusion to augment pulmonary blood flow, only as a temporizing maneuver prior to surgery. Some centers may attempt to stent the ductus via the transcatheter approach. For patients who are experiencing "Tet Spells" (see above), propranolol may lower the heart rate and decrease contractility to help avoid complications while awaiting surgery. By analogy, inotropic and chronotropic agents should be used with caution, or not at all, in unoperated patients with tetralogy of Fallot, as a spell may be precipitated.

Surgery: Corrective surgery entails repair of the defects while on cardiopulmonary bypass. This includes patch-closure of the VSD and varying degrees of RVOT surgery. Subvalvar obstruction usually includes muscle bundle resection and an outflow patch. When the valve is too small ("hypoplastic") to be preserved without leaving significant residual pulmonary valve stenosis, a "transanular patch" is performed. This is an extensive outflow patch which includes filleting open the valve. This adequately relieves narrowing and obstruction in most cases, but leaves the adverse effect of pulmonary regurgitation. This procedure is tolerated well in the short run, but long-term requires a follow-up procedure for pulmonary valve insertion. The details of the this procedure in terms of timing and type are still being determined. Newborns with severe cyanosis may be referred for a Blalock-Taussig shunt from the Aorta to the Pulmonary Artery to increase pulmonary blood flow to allow for growth before complete corrective surgery is undertaken. The Blalock-Taussig shunt is the first cardiac operation performed in children that resulted in its widespread use. An alternative approach that has gained some popularity in recent years is one that opens the RVOT to a limited degree without the use of cardiopulmonary bypass, while leaving the VSD for later surgery.

Therapy: Physical therapy is generally not required following repair.

Social: Websites and organizations considered reliable by pediatric cardiac specialists for parental education include those from the American Heart Association (AHA): www.americanheart.org and the Congenital Heart Information Network (CHIN): www.tchin.org.

Long-term monitoring: The frequency and timing of office follow-up for children with TOF is quite variable. Repaired patients without residual pulmonary valve dysfunction or other cardiac residua are often evaluated 1–2 times/year. The average patient will not require cardiac medication. No definite exercise restrictions are imposed though some high-impact sports are discouraged and each patient is evaluated individually with regards to clearance. In recent years, the sub-group of children and adolescents who underwent transannular patch repair are undergoing pulmonary valve insertion. The right ventricle in these patients becomes dilated after a number of years of pulmonary insufficiency and can be dysfunctional. It is hoped that insertion of a competent valve in this position will reverse the process. Careful surveillance of right heart size and function in these patients, particularly via cardiac magnetic resonance imaging (MRI) evaluations, is being performed with the idea that earlier re-intervention is warranted to avoid irreparable right heart abnormalities.

Pearls and Precautions

Incision: The incision should be kept clean and dry. Washing is achieved by using a damp cloth and soap. Do not completely soak incision in water until healed (usually 6 to 8 weeks). Do not apply ointments or lotions for 6–8 weeks. Itching is a normal sign of healing, and scratching should be discouraged. After healing occurs, sunscreen should be used when in direct sunlight. Parents should be instructed to call the cardiologist if redness, swelling, pain or drainage from the incision occurs.

Diet: Families should be educated that the infant/child may tire easily and require rest during feeding. Feedings may be more frequent but smaller in quantity. Sweating with feeds may occur for a period of time. In general, if the feeding pattern is not slowly improving towards normalcy in the weeks following repair, the parents should contact the physician. Negative changes may be reflective of postoperative issues such as infection, effusions, or cardiac dysfunction.

Activities: Sternal precautions are undertaken for the first 8 weeks after repair. This includes avoiding direct pressure or pulling on the sternum. Infants should not be lifted under the arms but rather cooped up under the back and bottom. Car seats should always be utilized when traveling. When possible, avoidance of ill friends and family or crowded public places is suggested for 2–4 weeks after discharge. Sleep patterns (similar to feeding patterns) may be altered for a period of time after repair.

Endocarditis prophylaxis: Good dental hygiene is very important to reduce the risk of infective endocarditis and should be encouraged. If dental cleaning or care is performed (or other non-cardiac procedures), the cardiologist should be contacted to discuss the patients individual needs. The most recent guidelines for endocarditis prophylaxis can be reviewed and is referenced below. After Tetralogy of Fallot surgery, SBE prophylaxis is recommended for at least 6 months and possibly longer in certain children with artificial material in situ and residual cardiac lesions and/or desaturation.

Immunizations: Infants should delay vaccination for approximately one month following surgery. This should be discussed with the individual cardiologist.

Parental Education: Parents should be instructed to call the cardiologist or cardiac care team upon the following findings after discharge:

- When an incision demonstrates redness, swelling, pain or drainage.
- If increased work of breathing or shortness of breath occurs.
- When fussy behavior or poor feeding ensues.
- If swollen or puffy hands/feet are present
- If vomiting or diarrhea occurs more than once
- If fever develops (temperature 38.5 Centigrade or greater)

References

Transatrial-transpulmonary repair of tetralogy of Fallot. Padalino MA, Vida VL, Stellin G. Semin Thorac Cardiovasc Surg Pediatr Card Surg Annu. 2009:48–53.

Early primary repair of tetralogy of Fallot. Jonas RA. Semin Thorac Cardiovasc Surg Pediatr Card Surg Annu. 2009:39–47

Indications and timing of pulmonary valve replacement after tetralogy of Fallot repair.

Geva T. Semin Thorac Cardiovasc Surg Pediatr Card Surg Annu. 2006:11–22.

Prevention of infective endocarditis: guidelines from the American Heart Association (multiple councils): Wilson W, Taubert KA, Gewitz M, Lockhart PB, Baddour LM, Levison M, Bolger A, Cabell CH, Takahashi M, Baltimore RS, Newburger JW, Strom BL, Tani LY, Gerber M, Bonow RO, Pallasch T, Shulman ST, Rowley AH, Burns JC, Ferrieri P, Gardner T, Goff D, Durack DT. Circulation. 2007 Oct 9; 116(15):1736–54.

Total Anomalous Pulmonary Venous Return (TAPVR)

Gary M. Satou, Thomas S. Klitzner

This is a congenital heart lesion in which all of the pulmonary veins, which normally bring oxygenated blood from the lungs to the left heart (via the left atrium), anomalously drain to a structure other than the left atrium. Usually, this is via a systemic vein which ultimately drains to the right-side of the heart. While this represents a left to right shunt, a right to left intracardiac shunt must also occur in order to ensure the pulmonary venous return makes it back to the left heart. There are subtypes based on the anatomic location of the pulmonary venous drainage, but the principle concept remains the same. When the anomalous flow connection has a narrowing or restrictive communication to it, this is referred to as an "obstructed" TAPVR.

Etiology

Congenital heart disease is considered multifactorial in origin. In general, the condition results from arrest in the embryologic development of the pulmonary veins and the left atrium.

Clinical Presentation and Prognosis

Age of onset: This lesion can be diagnosed prenatal by fetal echocardiography. It usually presents in the newborn period. Occasionally, the "unobstructed" type remains undiagnosed until early infancy.

Presenting signs/symptom and clinical course: Although most physicians exposed to this form of congenital heart disease during training will remember it as a cyanotic newborn emergency, this is not the only presentation. The clinical course is dictated by whether the anomalous pulmonary venous return is obstructed or not. The obstructed form, where flow though the pathway meets high resistance from anatomic narrowing at some point along the pathway, creates the classic picture of an ill neonate in the first day or so of life with cyanosis, tachypnea and hepatomegaly. The chest X-ray will show pulmonary edema, though not pulmonary overcirculation. Characteristically, the heart size on chest X-ray is normal. There often is not an impressive murmur. When there is unobstructed TAPVR, cyanosis is mild and may not be detected in the neonate. The physiology is similar to that of a large ASD with an accentuated pulmonary component and possibly fixed split second heart sound. In addition, there may be tachypnea and hepatomegaly.

Prognosis: Without surgical intervention, the majority of patients will die from pulmonary venous obstruction. Unobstructed TAPVR patients with ASD-like physiology have the longstanding risk of right heart and pulmonary arterial overcirculation. This can lead to irreversible pulmonary vascular disease.

Diagnosis

Prenatal diagnosis is by fetal echocardiography. Newborns are diagnosed by echocardiography and do not need other imaging modalities in most cases.

Management

Medication: Unlike many other cyanotic lesions in the newborn, ductal dependence is not part of the circulatory requirement and therefore prostaglandin infusion is not indicated. In fact, in certain scenarios, maintaining ductal patency can be detrimental. The majority of patients will present with cyanosis and quickly be diagnosed. Surgical correction is the first line of treatment and medical management is indicated only to ensure acid base balance and support cardiac output while arranging operation time. Diuretics may be utilized in the setting of pulmonary edema. Pulmonary vasodilators are generally not utilized as they may exacerbate pulmonary congestion. In a subgroup of postoperative patients, they may be used if there is abnormal pulmonary arteriolar architecture and elevated pulmonary vascular resistance. This may include nitric oxide or Sildenafil.

Surgery: Surgery is the mainstay of TAPVR treatment and is performed to redirect the pulmonary venous return to the left atrium. A communication is made from this common "confluence" to the back of the left atrium. This allows for the oxygenated pulmonary venous blood to return to the left atrium and then fill the left ventricle and aorta. Depending on the subtype, there is often a systemic vein that is ligated, in order to interrupt the communication responsible for the flow of blood from the lungs to the right heart.

Therapy: Following repair, physical therapy is generally not required. However, for the small subgroup of patients with a very prolonged hospital course, it may be indicated.

Social: Websites and organizations considered reliable by pediatric cardiac specialists for parental education include those from the American Heart Association (AHA): www.americanheart.org and the Congenital Heart Information Network (CHIN): www.tchin.org.

Long-term monitoring: The majority of infants undergoing TAPVR repair will have excellent results and will generally not be on medication. Pediatric cardiology visits are approximately annual. General well-being, oxygen saturations, and echocardiographic estimates of pulmonary artery pressure are included in the evaluation. Surveillance is to evaluate for the small incidence of recurrent pulmonary vein or anastomosis site obstruction occurring earlier rather than later in approximately 10% of the patients. Pediatricians should be apprised of any increased work of breathing, desaturation, or recurrent respiratory infections. Unfortunately, neither surgery nor trans-catheter balloon angioplasty (with or without stenting) has proved to be a perfect fix and there is an approximately 25–50% mortality in this subgroup. At present, pediatric lung transplantation remains fraught with limitations and is generally not a reliable treatment method despite the failure of other treatment modalities.

Pearls and Precautions

Incision: The incision should be kept clean and dry. Washing is achieved by using a damp cloth and soap. Do not completely soak incision in water until healed (usually 6–8 weeks). Do not apply ointments or lotions for 6–8 weeks. Itching is a normal sign of healing, and scratching should be discouraged. After healing occurs, sunscreen should be used when in direct sunlight. Parents should be instructed to call the cardiologist if redness, swelling, pain or drainage from the incision occurs.

Diet: Families should be educated that the infant/child may tire easily and require rest during feeding. Feedings may be more frequent but smaller in quantity. Sweating with feeds may occur for a period of time. In general, if the feeding pattern is not slowly improving towards normalcy in the weeks following repair, the parents should contact the physician. Negative changes may be reflective of postoperative issues such as infection, effusions, or cardiac dysfunction.

Activities: Sternal precautions are undertaken for the first 8 weeks after repair. This includes avoiding direct pressure or pulling on the sternum. Infants should not be lifted under the arms but rather cooped up under the back and bottom. Car seats should always be utilized when traveling. When possible, avoidance of ill friends and family or crowded public places is suggested for 2–4 weeks after discharge. Sleep patterns (similar to feeding patterns) may be altered for a period of time after repair.

Endocarditis prophylaxis: Good dental hygiene is very important to reduce the risk of infective endocarditis and should be encouraged. If dental cleaning or care is performed (or other non-cardiac procedures), the cardiologist should be contacted to discuss the patients individual needs. The most recent guidelines for endocarditis prophylaxis can be reviewed and is referenced below. After surgery for TAPVR, SBE prophylaxis is performed for at least 6 months and possibly longer in certain children with artificial material in situ and residual cardiac lesions and/or desaturation.

Immunizations: Infants should delay vaccination for approximately one month following surgery. This should be discussed with the individual cardiologist.

Parental education: Parents should be instructed to call the cardiologist or cardiac care team upon the following findings after discharge:

- When an incision demonstrates redness, swelling, pain or drainage.
- If increased work of breathing or shortness of breath occurs.
- When fussy behavior or poor feeding ensues.
- If swollen or puffy hands/feet are present
- If vomiting or diarrhea occurs more than once
- If fever develops (temperature 38.5 Centigrade or greater)

References

Surgical repair of total anomalous pulmonary venous connection. Kanter KR. Semin Thorac Cardiovasc Surg Pediatr Card Surg Annu. 2006:40–4.

Surgery for pulmonary venous obstruction after repair of total anomalous pulmonary venous return. Lacour-Gayet F. Semin Thorac Cardiovasc Surg Pediatr Card Surg Annu. 2006

Total anomalous pulmonary venous connection: surgical considerations. Norwood WI, Hougen TJ, Castaneda AR. Cardiovasc Clin. 1981;11(2):353–64.

Prevention of infective endocarditis: guidelines from the American Heart Association (multiple councils): Wilson W, Taubert KA, Gewitz M, Lockhart PB, Baddour LM, Levison M, Bolger A, Cabell CH, Takahashi M, Baltimore RS, Newburger JW, Strom BL, Tani LY, Gerber M, Bonow RO, Pallasch T, Shulman ST, Rowley AH, Burns JC, Ferrieri P, Gardner T, Goff D, Durack DT. Circulation. 2007 Oct 9; 116(15):1736–54.

Transposition of the Great Arteries

(D-TGA, complete transposition)

Gary M. Satou, Thomas S. Klitzner

Although there are different forms of transposition of the great arteries, the term usually refers to the most common type, in which the aorta is rightward or "dextroposed" in position, and is arising from the right ventricle. The pulmonary artery is relatively posterior and leftward and arises from the left ventricle.

Etiology

Congenital heart disease is considered multifactorial in origin.

Clinical Presentation and Prognosis

Age of onset: This lesion can be diagnosed in utero when fetal echocardiography is performed by properly trained clinicians. Otherwise the diagnosis is usually made in the immediate newborn period given the presence of significant cyanosis. Infants with transposition and a large ventricular septal defect (VSD) may have a later presentation/diagnosis given the increased degree of mixing afforded by the VSD.

Presenting signs/symptom and clinical course: TGA creates a circulation which is in parallel as opposed to series, requiring some level of mixing through an atrial septal defect, patent ductus arteriosis or ventriculoseptal defect. Otherwise, purely desaturated systemic venous blood will be ejected to the body and oxygenated, pulmonary venous blood will be re-circulated back to the lungs. This explains the cyanosis seen in transposition and the need for either an atrial communication or a patent ductus arteriosis (PDA) for mixing. Additional lesions can be seen with this defect, most commonly, a ventriculoseptal defect. All affected neonates are cyanotic to varying degrees. Those with a VSD or several levels of mixing will be less so. Typically these children are diagnosed by the cardiologist during their NICU stay.

Prognosis: With proper NICU and surgical care, these children have an excellent prognosis. The morbidity associated with surgical correction (see below) is approximately 1%. Without medical and surgical care, transposition is usually not compatible with life. If no intervention is performed, the newborn will develop myocardial dysfunction and ischemia, acidosis, and shock.

Diagnosis

This lesion can be diagnosed in utero when fetal echocardiography is performed by properly trained clinicians, or during the postnatal period in a cyanotic newborn. Occasionally, neonates with transposition and a large VSD may have a later presentation/diagnosis due to the increased mixing afforded by the VSD. Echocardiography defines the cardiac anatomy including the transposed great vessels.

Management

Corrective treatment for transposition of the great arteries is accomplished by neonatal cardiac surgery. The definitive procedure is called the arterial switch operation.

Medication: Prostaglandin infusion is utilized once the diagnosis is made, to enhance ductal patency and mixing at the great vessel level. However, if mixing is adequate by other means, administration of prostaglandin may not be necessary. Other uses of drug therapy are simply temporizing and may include gentle diuresis for pulmonary overcirculation and mild levels of inotropy to augment cardiac output. Oxygen carrying capacity should be optimized and occasionally blood transfusions are given.

Surgery: The treatment of choice for transposition of the great arteries is the arterial switch operation. It is performed through a median sternotomy, on cardiopulmonary bypass, and entails cutting the aorta and main pulmonary arteries in their proximal course, and "switching" them to the other root still arising from the heart. The coronary arteries must be resected from the old aortic root and re-implanted on the new, "neo" aortic root. If a VSD or other lesions are present, they are repaired. When performed in experienced centers, this procedure probably has an overall survival rate of 98–99% and seldom needs long-term re-intervention. This occurs in approximately 10–15% of patients with residual or progressive supra-valvular narrowing in the pulmonary artery or aorta.

Therapy: Physical therapy is generally not required following repair.

Social: Websites and organizations considered reliable by pediatric cardiac specialists for parental education include those from the American Heart Association (AHA): www.americanheart.org and the Congenital Heart Information Network (CHIN): www.tchin.org.

Long-term monitoring: Once the early postoperative period is over, pediatric cardiologists follow these patients approximately 1–2 times/year. The average patient will not require cardiac medication, though some institutions recommend long-term low-dose aspirin therapy (3–5 mg/Kg/day) due to coronary re-implantation at the time of the arterial switch operation. No exercise restrictions are imposed on the average, uncomplicated patient.

Pearls and Precautions

Post sternotomy care:

Incision: The incision should be kept clean and dry. Washing is achieved by using a damp cloth and soap. Do not completely soak incision in water until healed (usually 6 to 8 weeks). Do not apply ointments or lotions for 6–8 weeks. Itching is a normal sign of healing, and scratching should be discouraged. After healing occurs, sunscreen should be used when in direct sunlight. Parents should be instructed to call the cardiologist if redness, swelling, pain or drainage from the incision occurs.

Diet: Families should be educated that the infant/child may tire easily and require rest during feeding. Feedings may be more frequent but smaller in quantity. Sweating with feeds may occur for a period of time. In general, if the feeding pattern is not slowly improving towards normalcy in the weeks following repair, the parents should contact the physician. Negative changes may be reflective of postoperative issues such as infection, effusions, or cardiac dysfunction.

Activities: Sternal precautions are undertaken for the first 8 weeks after repair. This includes avoiding direct pressure or pulling on the sternum. Infants should not be lifted under the arms but rather scooped up under the back and bottom. Car seats should always be utilized when traveling. When possible, avoidance of ill friends and family or crowded public places is suggested for 2–4 weeks after discharge. Sleep patterns (similar to feeding patterns) may be altered for a period of time after repair.

Endocarditis prophylaxis: Good dental hygiene is very important to reduce the risk of infective endocarditis and should be encouraged. If dental cleaning or care is performed (or other non-cardiac procedures), the cardiologist should be contacted to discuss the patients individual needs. The most recent guidelines for endocarditis prophylaxis can be reviewed and is referenced below. After the arterial switch operation surgery, SBE prophylaxis is performed for at least 6 months and possibly longer in certain children with artificial material in situ and residual cardiac lesions and/or desaturation.

Immunizations: Infants should delay vaccination for approximately one month following surgery. This should be discussed with the individual cardiologist.

Parental education: Parents should be instructed to call the cardiologist or cardiac care team upon the following findings after discharge:

- When an incision demonstrates redness, swelling, pain or drainage.
- If increased work of breathing or shortness of breath occurs.
- When fussy behavior or poor feeding ensues.
- If swollen or puffy hands/feet are present
- If vomiting or diarrhea occurs more than once
- If fever develops (temperature 38.5 Centigrade or greater)

References

Transposition of the great arteries: from fetus to adult. Skinner J, Hornung T, Rumball E. Heart. 2008 Sep;94(9):1227–35.

Prevention of infective endocarditis: guidelines from the American Heart Association (multiple councils): Wilson W, Taubert KA, Gewitz M, Lockhart PB, Baddour LM, Levison M, Bolger A, Cabell CH, Takahashi M, Baltimore RS, Newburger JW, Strom BL, Tani LY, Gerber M, Bonow RO, Pallasch T, Shulman ST, Rowley AH, Burns JC, Ferrieri P, Gardner T, Goff D, Durack DT. Circulation. 2007 Oct 9; 116(15):1736–54.

Truncus Arteriosus

Gary M. Satou, Thomas S. Klitzner

Truncus arteriosus is a rare cyanotic heart disease whereby instead of the normal two arteries arising from the heart, only a single arterial trunk develops. A single, semilunar "truncal valve" exists. From this single arterial trunk, the pulmonary arteries arise. Although anatomic variations exist regarding where along the common trunk the branch pulmonary arteries originate, the most common type seen demonstrates confluent branch pulmonary arteries arising off a short common pulmonary trunk, which is located on the proximal portion of the main truncal artery. As well, truncus arteriosus always includes a large, outlet-type ventricular septal defect (VSD). Occasional additional findings include coronary artery and aortic arch abnormalities.

Etiology

Congenital heart disease is considered multifactorial in origin. Since truncus arteriosus, is one of the conotruncal cardiac malformations, there is an increased incidence of DiGeorge syndrome in these patients.

Clinical Presentation and Prognosis

Age of onset: Truncus arteriosus is present at birth as a result of abnormal cardiac development during embryogenesis. The diagnosis is often first made by fetal cardiac ultrasound. If no fetal ultrasound is performed, diagnosis is usually made in the newborn period, as high pulmonary blood flow (due to the pulmonary arteries arising from the systemic arterial trunk) and intracardiac mixing from the large VSD create varying degrees of cyanosis and pulmonary overcirculation, leading to cardiac consultation. In rare instances, newborns are discharged to home and come to attention due to the symptoms of heart failure in the first few weeks of life as pulmonary resistance falls (see below).

Presenting signs/symptom and clinical course: As stated above, the combination of increased pulmonary blood flow and a large VSD create a scenario in which congestive heart failure and respiratory distress will ensue. Thus, these babies are likely to be symptomatic in the first days or weeks of life. Clinical symptoms include desaturation, tachypnea, tachycardia and hepatomegaly. Poor feeding and growth are common. The clinical course, without treatment (see below) would include failure to thrive, recurrent respiratory illness and sustained heart failure. Physical exam findings can include, in addition to the above, systolic and possibly a diastolic murmur. The precordium may be active and the peripheral pulses bounding. The second heart sound is single (only one semilunar valve).

Prognosis: Without medical and surgical care, truncus arteriosus is usually not compatible with life. Due to congestive physiology and poor growth, the infant would ultimately develop pulmonary and myocardial failure.

However, these children have an excellent prognosis with proper NICU and surgical care. In the current era, early surgical mortality associated with truncus arteriosus is approximately 5%.

Diagnosis

Fetal or neonatal echocardiography is definitive in making the diagnosis. The common truncal valve and artery, the type of pulmonary artery branching pattern, and the VSD details should all be well seen by ultrasound. Thus, the use of cardiac catheterization or other imaging modalities is uncommon.

Management

Corrective treatment for truncus arteriosus is accomplished by neonatal cardiac surgery. This definitive procedure involves VSD closure and placement of a right ventricular to pulmonary artery conduit.

Medication: Except for the very rare case of truncus arteriosus with interrupted aortic arch, neonates do not require prostaglandin infusion. Preoperative pulmonary blood flow is plentiful and systemic perfusion adequate. Preoperative care may include diuresis for pulmonary over-circulation and mild levels of inotropy to augment cardiac output. Similar medications in the early postoperative period may be utilized, but are usually weaned off within a short period of time.

Surgery: Surgical correction of truncus arteriosus is performed through a median sternotomy, on cardiopulmonary bypass. The procedure includes patch closure of the VSD and a conduit or homograft insertion from the right ventricle (RV) to the pulmonary arteries. If the pulmonary arteries are not anatomically contiguous preoperative, then they are surgically "connected" so that the distal end of the conduit can communicate with both branch pulmonary arteries. This procedure is usually performed only in congenital heart centers with sufficient experience in neonatal heart surgery and has an overall survival rate of 95%. Re-intervention is necessary in all patients as the RV to pulmonary artery conduit placed during infancy does not grow and becomes inadequate over time. Timing of replacement is variable, but neonatally placed conduits may last up to 5 or 10 years after initial placement.

Therapy: Physical therapy is generally not required following repair.

Social: Websites and organizations considered reliable by pediatric cardiac specialists for parental education include those from the American Heart Association (AHA): www.americanheart.org and the Congenital Heart Information Network (CHIN): www.tchin.org.

Long-term monitoring: Once the early postoperative period is over, pediatric cardiologists follow these patients approximately 2 times/year. The average patient may not require cardiac medication, though some institutions recommend long-term low-dose (3–5 mg/Kg/day) aspirin therapy for the conduit. No exercise restrictions are imposed on the average, uncomplicated patient. Systemic bacterial endocarditis (SBE) prophylaxis is usually indicated, but should be reviewed with the pediatric cardiologist. All patients will develop increasing obstruction in their RV to pulmonary artery conduit. This is a function of somatic growth which "outgrows" the fixed-size conduit, and, progressive conduit calcification and stenosis. As the conduit becomes more obstructed, the RV pressure increases. Once RV pressure is elevated to approximately ¾ systemic blood pressure, intervention to reduce the conduit obstruction is usually undertaken. Transcatheter balloon dilation may be performed with or without stent placement and may delay the surgical upsizing of the conduit for up to two years. Ultimately, however, surgical conduit "upsizing" will be necessary. In a subgroup of patients, the truncal valve will have significant stenosis or regurgitation that requires intervention. Valvuloplasty is preferred to replacement, especially in small children.

Pearls and Precautions

Incision: The incision should be kept clean and dry. Washing is achieved by using a damp cloth and soap. Do not completely soak incision in water until healed (usually 6–8 weeks). Do not apply ointments or lotions for 6–8 weeks. Itching is a normal sign of healing, and scratching should be discouraged. After healing occurs, sunscreen should be used when in direct sunlight. Parents should be instructed to call the cardiologist if redness, swelling, pain or drainage from the incision occurs.

Diet: Families should be educated that the infant/child may tire easily and require rest during feeding. Feedings may be more frequent but smaller in quantity. Sweating with feeds may occur for a period of time. In general, if the feeding pattern is not slowly improving towards normalcy in the weeks following repair, the parents should contact the physician. Negative changes may be reflective of postoperative issues such as infection, effusions, or cardiac dysfunction.

Activities: Sternal precautions are undertaken for the first 8 weeks after repair. This includes avoiding direct pressure or pulling on the sternum. Infants should not be lifted under the arms but rather cooped up under the back and bottom. Car seats should always be utilized when traveling. When possible, avoidance of ill friends and family or crowded public places is suggested for 2–4 weeks after discharge. Sleep patterns (similar to feeding patterns) may be altered for a period of time after repair.

Endocarditis prophylaxis: Good dental hygiene is very important to reduce the risk of infective endocarditis and should be encouraged. If dental cleaning or care is performed (or other non-cardiac procedures), the cardiologist should be contacted to discuss the patients individual needs. The most recent guidelines for endocarditis prophylaxis can be reviewed and is referenced below. After truncus arteriosus surgery, SBE prophylaxis is performed for at least 6 months and possibly longer in certain children.

Immunizations: Infants should delay vaccination for approximately one month following surgery. This should be discussed with the individual cardiologist.

Parental education: Parents should be instructed to call the cardiologist or cardiac care team upon the following findings after discharge:

- When an incision demonstrates redness, swelling, pain or drainage.
- If increased work of breathing or shortness of breath occurs.
- When fussy behavior or poor feeding ensues.
- If swollen or puffy hands/feet are present
- If vomiting or diarrhea occurs more than once
- If fever develops (temperature 38.5 Centigrade or greater)

References

Neonatal truncus arteriosus repair: surgical techniques and clinical management. Rodefeld MD, Hanley FL. Semin Thorac Cardiovasc Surg Pediatr Card Surg Annu. 2002;5:212–7.

Prevention of infective endocarditis: guidelines from the American Heart Association (multiple councils): Wilson W, Taubert KA, Gewitz M, Lockhart PB, Baddour LM, Levison M, Bolger A, Cabell CH, Takahashi M, Baltimore RS, Newburger JW, Strom BL, Tani LY, Gerber M, Bonow RO, Pallasch T, Shulman ST, Rowley AH, Burns JC, Ferrieri P, Gardner T, Goff D, Durack DT. Circulation. 2007 Oct 9; 116(15):1736–54.

Ventricular Septal Defects (VSD)

Gary M. Satou, Thomas S. Klitzner

Ventricular septal defect is a congenital heart disease in which a portion of the ventricular septum, which divides the right and left ventricles, is deficient. There are several sub-types of ventricular septal defects, including membranous, muscular, inlet (AV canal type) and outlet (or mal-alignment) defects. In all forms, the pathophysiologic principle is that oxygenated pulmonary venous blood "shunts" left to right through the defect thus increasing the degree of pulmonary blood flow.

Etiology

Like most forms of congenital heart disease, VSD is considered multifactorial in origin.

Clinical Presentation and Prognosis

Age of onset: Although the defect is present from birth, patients can be asymptomatic, depending on the size and location of the defect. Symptoms may present in infancy when the defect is large. Small VSD's may be detected due to the loud murmur usually created by a restrictive communication.

Presenting signs and symptoms: Children are often referred to the pediatric cardiologist for evaluation of a heart murmur. Infants with large defects may present with congestive symptoms, such as tachypnea, tachycardia or hepatomegaly. Failure to thrive/poor growth may also be present. Older patients who have not had surgery to close the defect may develop irreversible pulmonary hypertension with chronic respiratory compromise and desaturation.

Clinical course: A large number of children are asymptomatic and are referred for evaluation of a heart murmur, which is created by blood-flow acceleration through the defect. If the defect is large and the flow significant, the effects of a left to right shunt through the VSD and pulmonary over-circulation can, over time, create irreversible pulmonary vascular changes by as early as 6 to 12 months of age. Thus, closure is undertaken in the first 6 months of life in children whose defects are felt to be large enough to create this scenario. Congestive circulatory symptoms and suboptimal growth resolves with treatment. If children with large VSDs are left untreated into later years, the potential for pulmonary vascular disease and pulmonary hypertension is significant and likely irreversible, leading to chronic symptoms and often a shortened life span. This affects a small subgroup of patients in the current era given the likelihood of referral when a heart murmur is identified. Children with small defects often show spontaneous diminution or closure over time. Cardiologists simply follow these patients, and treatment is rarely required.

Prognosis: The overall prognosis for these children is excellent. Closure corrects the problem, alleviates symptoms and eliminates the potential for chronic pulmonary vascular disease. Spontaneous closure or diminution in size occurs in many whose defect is rather small, especially if located in the muscular septum.

Diagnosis

Echocardiography is the definitive diagnostic modality in the current era. Primary care providers should refer patients suspected of having a VSD and/or symptoms of left to right shunting to a pediatric cardiologist to guide the performance of this test in order to assure optimal results and for the initiation of an appropriate treatment regimen.

The initial findings can include tachypnea, tachycardia or venous congestion, and poor growth. Physical exam reveals a systolic murmur. There may be a thrill palpable on the precordium. When the defect is large, there may be a diastolic rumble or even a gallop rhythm. The P2 component of the second heart sound may be loud in the presence of pulmonary hypertension. Chest radiograph may and increased pulmonary blood flow. Electrocardiogram may demonstrate left atrial and left ventricular enlargement or, in advanced cases, biventricular enlargement.

Management

The approach to the child with a ventricular septal defect depends on the size of the lesion. Asymptomatic patients with small defects will be followed over time and given a chance to demonstrate spontaneous closure. Based on revised American Heart Association (AHA) guidelines, endocarditis prophylaxis is no longer indicated. Children with larger defects (with or without symptoms) will usually be referred for closure. In infants, there may be a period of observation to plot the growth and watch for spontaneous restriction to develop. However, if this is not achieved by 6 months of age in infants with large defects and significant pulmonary blood flow, closure will be recommended. During this period, heart failure medication and an increased caloric diet may be prescribed.

Medication: Congestive heart failure (CHF) therapy may be prescribed for the child who is symptomatic and awaiting repair. Similar medications are utilized for a brief period postoperative, and then weaned off by the pediatric cardiologist. These can include diuretics (e.g., Lasix) often used to reduce preload and pulmonary overcirculation. Some cardiologists utilize Digoxin, or at times, afterload reduction (to reduce systemic vascular resistance). Increased calorie diets are used to optimize nutrition and offset the increased metabolic expenditure in the CHF state.

Surgery: This is a relatively simple cardiac surgical procedure with patch surgical closure of the VSD performed by the surgeon while on cardiopulmonary bypass. Though less-common, some patients are candidates for transcatheter VSD closure. These are typically mid-muscular VSDs, remote from valve structures. Not all pediatric heart centers offer or support this approach.

Therapy: Physical therapy is generally not required following repair.

Social: Websites and organizations considered reliable by pediatric cardiac specialists for parental education include those from the American Heart Association (AHA): www.americanheart.org and the Congenital Heart Information Network (CHIN): www.tchin.org.

Long-term monitoring: Most commonly, VSD closure is a one time intervention. Medications are usually not required after the postoperative period. The pediatric cardiologist performs annual visits to monitor the very rare occurrence of heart block, arrhythmias or valvular/myocardial dysfunction. No exercise restrictions are imposed.

Pearls and Precautions

Incision: The incision should be kept clean and dry. Washing is achieved by using a damp cloth and soap. Do not completely soak incision in water until healed (usually 6 to 8 weeks). Do not apply ointments or lotions for 6–8 weeks. Itching is a normal sign of healing, and scratching should be discouraged. After healing occurs, sunscreen should be used when in direct sunlight. Parents should be instructed to call the cardiologist if redness, swelling, pain or drainage from the incision occurs.

Diet: Families should be educated that the infant/child may tire easily and require rest during feeding. Feedings may be more frequent but smaller in quantity. Sweating with feeds may occur for a period of time. In general, if the feeding pattern is not slowly improving towards normalcy in the weeks following repair, the parents should contact the physician. Negative changes may be reflective of postoperative issues such as infection, effusions, or cardiac dysfunction.

Activities: Sternal precautions are undertaken for the first 8 weeks after repair. This includes avoiding direct pressure or pulling on the sternum. Infants should not be lifted under the arms but rather cooped up under the back and bottom. Car seats should always be utilized when traveling. When possible, avoidance of ill friends and family or crowded public places is suggested for 2–4 weeks after discharge. Sleep patterns (similar to feeding patterns) may be altered for a period of time after repair.

Endocarditis prophylaxis: Good dental hygiene is very important to reduce the risk of infective endocarditis and should be encouraged. If dental cleaning or care is performed (or other non-cardiac procedures), the cardiologist should be contacted to discuss the patients individual needs. The most recent guidelines for endocarditis prophylaxis can be reviewed and is referenced below. After ventriculoseptal defect surgery, SBE prophylaxis is performed for at least 6 months and possibly longer in certain children with artificial material in situ and residual cardiac lesions and/or desaturation.

Immunizations: Infants should delay vaccination for approximately one month following surgery. This should be discussed with the individual cardiologist.

Parental education: Parents should be instructed to call the cardiologist or cardiac care team upon the following findings after discharge:

- When an incision demonstrates redness, swelling, pain or drainage.
- If increased work of breathing or shortness of breath occurs.
- When fussy behavior or poor feeding ensues.
- If swollen or puffy hands/feet are present
- If vomiting or diarrhea occurs more than once
- If fever develops (temperature 38.5 Centigrade or greater)

References

Ventricular Septal Defects. Minette MS, Sahn MJ. Circulation 1996 114; (20):2190–7

Prevention of infective endocarditis: guidelines from the American Heart Association (multiple councils): Wilson W, Taubert KA, Gewitz M, Lockhart PB, Baddour LM, Levison M, Bolger A, Cabell CH, Takahashi M, Baltimore RS, Newburger JW, Strom BL, Tani LY, Gerber M, Bonow RO, Pallasch T, Shulman ST, Rowley AH, Burns JC, Ferrieri P, Gardner T, Goff D, Durack DT. Circulation. 2007 Oct 9; 116(15):1736–54.

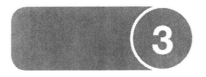 **Dermatologic Disorders**

Table of Contents

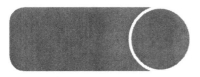

Ectodermal Dysplasias

Ronald W. Cotliar

Disease

Ectodermal Dysplasias (EDs) represent a group of inherited diseases in which there is a primary defect in hair, teeth, nails and sweat gland function. More than 170 different pathologic conditions have been identified and grouped under this banner. The various anomalies affecting both the epidermis and epidermal appendages are variable on a wide spectrum. Common features and clinical overlap are present in the majority of EDs. As clinicians we look for these so we can identify the syndromic forms of ED through the shared or common clinical findings.

- The skin is dry, fine and smooth, hypopigmented with areas of "eczema".
- Generally the hair is blonde and scanty. Hypotrichosis or varying degrees of partial or total alopecia is seen. Eyelashes and eyebrows may be absent. Body hair follicles may be absent or reduced.
- Oligodontia or anodontia are commonly seen. Enamel dysplasia along with rudimentary or conical teeth may be observed.
- The clinical appearance of the nails show a wide range of pathology including dystrophy, hypertrophy, abnormal keritinization, thickening, discoloration, splitting, fragmenting, or striations.
- While the apocrine glands are usually normally present, the eccrine sweat glands may be aplastic or hypoplastic, reduced in number or almost absent.
- The oral and nasal mucous glands, the salivary and mammary glands may be hypoplastic or absent. The mucous glands may be absent throughout the whole respiratory tract. The affected children may present with recurrent respiratory infections. The absence of the salivary glands can cause xerostomia.
- When gastrointestinal mucous glands are absent, the patient may present with dysphagia.

Hidrotic Ectodermal Dysplasia

(Synonym: Clouston's Syndrome)

Hidrotic ectodermal dysplasia (HED) is characterized by nail dystrophy and associated with defects of the hair and keratoderma of the palms and soles. Palmoplantar keratoderma (PPK) describes a diffuse or localized thickening of the palms and soles that can occur as a part of a genetic disorder, or as part of an inflammatory skin disorder.

Etiology

HED is an autosomal dominant disorder caused by a missense mutation in a gene that encodes for connexin 30. The connexins are gap-junction proteins that are important for cell communication. Connexin 30 is one of a family of connexins in which mutations cause other skin disorders. All cases have been linked to the *GJB6 locus.*

Clinical Presentation and Prognosis

Demographics: This is a rare condition; originally described in French-Canadian kindred and French populations, but now has been reported in individuals of varying racial and ethnic backgrounds.

Presenting signs and symptoms: HED may be present at birth or appear during the neonatal period. In affected individuals, hair and nails are affected while the teeth and sweating are normal. The hair is pale, brittle and often wiry. Patchy alopecia is common. Progressive hair loss and nail changes may occur during adulthood. In affected infants, the nails appear milky white, and thicken throughout childhood. In adults, the nail plates are noted to grow slowly, continue to thicken, and often separate from the nail-bed distally.

Clinical course: Hyperkeratosis (thickening) of the palms and soles may be progressive. Oral leukoplakia (white patches and plaques on the mucosa and tongue) has been reported in some cases. It is believed that sparse eyelashes can lead to conjunctivitis and blepharitis. Musculoskeletal changes may lead to tufting of the terminal phalanges and thickened skull bones. This is the most common type of ED. Their teeth are prone to caries although they are developmentally normal. Nail dystrophy with recurrent paronychia can lead to significant quality of life issues.

Prognosis: These individuals have a normal life span.

Diagnosis

In general, HED is a clinical diagnosis and laboratory testing is not of much use in diagnosing this disease. The diagnosis is straightforward. Clinical findings involve the nails, hair, and palmar/plantar thickening. In the absence of other findings of ED, these are very specific. Clinical molecular testing of GJB6 locus is available. Prenatal diagnosis is not currently available.

Management

The overall management of these individuals involves treatment of the skin and nails.

Medications: These patients greatly benefit from being followed by a dermatologist. Keratolytics such as Hydro40Foam® (contains urea in a new foam technology), Salvax® (6% salicylic acid in an emollient foam) are particularly useful. Additionally Kerol Emulsion® (urea and lactic acid in an ointment) can be both soothing and effective in reducing scaling. Occasional skin infections need to be treated with either bleach baths or compresses. An equivalent ratio of half a cup of regular Clorox added to a standard 40 gallon tub of water can be used in children one year of age and above. Appropriate dilutions are readily available. It is soothing and has had no bacterial resistance reported. To avoid systemic antibiotics, topical mupirocin as well as Altabax® (member of a new class of topical antibiotics) can be used for most infections.

Surgery: Debridement may be necessary for areas of anychia where hyperkeratosis and inflammation occur leading to pain. Ablation of the nail matrix may be required for pain from paronychia. The marked thickening of the nails itself can lead to inflammation and pain. In addition to use of keratolytics the child's parents can be taught to use a hand dremel or sand paper to afford pain relief. For cosmesis, nail sculpting/bonding, and wigs may be useful. Occasionally, mild syndactyly of toes 2 and 3 can occur.

Psych: It is extremely important that children are allowed to work around their physical limitations and not be defined or controlled by them. Due to their tendency to hyperthermia, sports and recreation must be chosen appropriately. Parents need to understand their role in strengthening both the child's ego and accepting the physical restrictions and minimizing them in the youngster's life.

Social: Patients and their families may find support at The National Foundation for Ectodermal Dysplasias (http://www.nfed.com).

Consultations: Oral surgery, ophthalmology.

Monitoring: Leukoplakia, blepharitis, conjunctivitis.

Pearls and Precautions

School/education: Schools need to be aware of the issue of nail disease and thickened palmar skin, and work with the family at ways to avoid and react if environmental circumstances cause difficulty.

Skin and dental care: Complete alopecia has been seen, and a wig is the only thing available for the hair loss. The nail findings are nondiagnostic, but common. In establishing the diagnosis of this syndrome, the swollen, tufted terminal phalanges may be more clinically helpful. The skin on the palms and soles can be very thickened and calloused, presenting as a keratoderma.

Miscellaneous: It is important to remember that this condition is not limited to French-Canadians and has been seen in other ethnic and racial groups.

Hypohidrotic Ectodermal Dysplasia

(Synonyms: Anchidrotic Ectodermal Dysplasia, Christ-Siements-Touraine Syndrome)

Hypohidrotic ectodermal dysplasia (HHED) is characterized by partial or complete absence of sweat glands, hypotrichosis and hypodontia.

Etiology

HHED is typically inherited as an X-linked recessive disorder. However, autosomal dominant, recessive and other x-linked (NEMO mutations) types have been rarely reported in the literature.

Mutation in ectodysplasin (EDA gene), a member of the tumor necrosis family, leads to abnormal development and regulation of ectodermal structures.

Clinical Presentation and Prognosis

Demographics: May present in infancy or early childhood with the incidence of 1:100,000 live births. Approximately 90% of the affected individuals are male, while female carriers are partially affected.

Presenting signs and symptoms: As noted above, there is absent or reduced sweating, hypotrichosis and partial or total anodontia. There is a clinical spectrum with more complete forms showing a distinctive appearance including prominent chin and frontal ridges, saddle nose, sunken cheeks, thick everted lips, large ears and sparse hair. The skin appears to be prematurely aged as it is smooth, soft, dry and finely wrinkled (especially around the eyes).

Alopecia may be the first feature to draw clinical attention. It is seldom total, and scalp hair is sparse, dry, fine and remains short. Eyebrows are sparse or absent, but the lashes are normal. The beard, pubic and axillary hair are sparse, and terminal hair on the trunk and limbs may be absent.

The nails are abnormal in about 50% of cases and may be thin, brittle or ridged, but are rarely grossly deformed. The temporary and permanent teeth may be entirely absent or a few teeth may be present. Even in complete anodontia the jaws develop normally, but the gums may be atrophic. The mouth may be dry from hypoplasia of the salivary glands and the lacrimal glands may be deficient.

Heat intolerance caused by absent or reduced sweating may present with unexplained fever in infancy or childhood.

Clinical course: General physical development may be stunted. Sexual development is usually normal, although a few cases of primary hypogonadism have been reported.

Prognosis: These patients usually have a normal life span. It is rarely fatal and improvement is seen in late childhood. Immunodeficiency may cause overwhelming sepsis and life-limiting complications.

Diagnosis

Affected neonates are often red and scaly at birth, and clinically can be confused with icthyosis. Over time the skin improves, but remains fragile. Affected infants have light-colored, sparse scalp and body hair. Hyperthermia due to decreased ineffective sweating is seen. Characteristic facies reveal periorbital wrinkling and hyperpigmentation, depressed nasal bridge (saddle-nose deformity), as well as everted lips. A raspy voice may be noted. Otolaryngologic findings can include thick nasal secretions, impaction, ozena, sinusitis, recurrent upper respiratory infections, pneumonias, decreased saliva production, and increased frequency of asthma. Reflux and feeding difficulties may be a problem in infancy. Late eruption of teeth with hypodontia with 5–6 teeth is common. The teeth may be conical or misshapen. Laboratory information that may confirm the suspected diagnosis of HHED include lack of eccrine glands on biopsy of palmar skin, and DNA analysis indicating mutation of the EDA gene. Prenatal diagnosis via DNA analysis and fetoscopy (20 weeks) skin biopsy looking for absent pilosebaceous units (eccrine sweat glands) is available.

Management

The most important consideration is to avoid overheating by the use of air conditioning, cool baths, light clothing, or simply moving to cool climates.

Medications: The underlying basis of treatment of these children is to bathe at least once or twice daily for 10–15 minutes. The goal is having the parents understand how to hydrate and lubricate the skin. Skin can only be hydrated through bathing and then trapping moisture with a proper emollient. It is strictly recommended that no towels be used, but have the parent gently wipe off excess water with their hands for a "squeegee" type effect. A wash such as Aveeno Baby Wash®, or Dove Body Wash® is effective. For lubrication, CeraVe®, an over-the-counter (OTC) moisturizer that contains ceramide is inexpensive and readily available, as well as Aveeno Baby Moisturizing Lotion®. A prescription moisturizer, EpiCeram® is another "medical device" that has a chemical composition that resembles the physiological balance of phospholipids in normal human skin. It is non-steroidal and in a study against Cutivate Cream® (fluticasone, a medium potency topical steroid approved for pediatric use on children 3 months of age and up), it was as effective for the treatment of "eczema." Since the underlying cause of atopic dermatitis (AD) and AD-like conditions is barrier dysfunction, the barrier repair capability of some of the new emollients is as effective as things we have used and continue to use that have side-effects, i.e., topical steroids and topical immunumodulators (Protopic® and Elidel®). Dermatologists call the protocol of hydration and lubrication, "wet and smear." Petrolatum based products like Vaseline® and Aquaphor® are often too occlusive and act as "sealers" leading to more difficult sweating and thermoregulation

The granulomatous dermatitis involving the scalp is often a major and most difficult problem to deal with. The involved clinicians must understand that this is an inflammatory condition and not infectious. Wound care consists of bleach compresses or sprays as well as barrier repair creams such as EpiCeram® (prescription mechanical device). Topical steroid lotions like 0.1 triamcinolone, or Cutivate Lotion® may be very effective.

Surgery: Maxillofacial surgery for cleft repair, lip abnormalities, as well as hypoplastic gum ridges may be necessary. Dental plates with implants need to be planned for from an early age. Improvement of everted lips as well as saddle nose deformity repair also need to be considered. Hand surgery may be required for syndactyly or ectrodactyly. Lacrimal duct aplasia or obstruction may need to be addressed. Malformed auricles can occur. Hypospadias has been described in several affected males.

Consultations: Taking care of these children requires a multi-disciplinary approach. The primary care provider needs to coordinate the involvement of geneticist, dentist, reconstructive (plastic) surgeon, immunologist, dermatologist and Ear-nose-throat (ENT) surgeons, as well as ophthalmologists.

Geneticists are helpful with the diagnosis of this disease and in future pregnancies, while dermatologists can help with the treatment of eczema and scalp lesions. Reconstructive surgery and ENT need to be involved in improving facial cosmesis and function. Early correction of these defects may improve patients' speech, and help the psychological well-being of the patient and family. ENT is also important in helping to manage recurrent sinopulmonary infections. It is important for the dentist to use plates early on, and implants as the child grows older. Ophthalmology needs to be involved if there are associated eye problems which most commonly are conjunctivitis and blepharitis. Immunology needs to be consulted to rule out and follow these children for possible immunodeficiency. These patients typically need wigs which is usually arranged by the plastic surgery staff; or can be obtained at cancer centers and clinics.

Therapy: These patients typically need speech therapy and it is best to offer adequate speech therapy (minimum of 3 hours/week) before the critical age of 3. Physical therapy is important for those with limited motion of their extremities and joints.

Psych: Family counseling and possibly ongoing therapy may be needed for some children and their families.

Social: Patients and their families may find support at The National Foundation for Ectodermal Dysplasias (http://www.nfed.com)

Monitoring: These patients should be monitored for skin infections, new lesions, feeding problems, and ophthalmologic issues.

Pearls and Precautions

These patients should avoid heat by all means.

Likely complications: These include skin, upper respiratory (mucous gland dysfunction) and systemic infections (in immunocompromised patients), blepharitis, feeling of isolation (particularly starting at adolescence), and depression.

School/education: The school needs to be made aware of exercise limitations and antipyretics to avoid hyperthermia. Speech difficulty in these children may interfere with their academic achievements and if needed, requires early and ongoing interventions.

Skin and dental care: Extraction of teeth should be avoided so that the alveolar ridge can be preserved. The presence of the typical fine wrinkles around the infant's eyes may lead an observant clinician to an HHED diagnosis in the nursery. If the mother is a carrier, she may have dry hair and skin, and be missing teeth.

Miscellaneous: ICD-9 Codes, 757.31-Ectodermal dysplasias.

References

Pinheiro M, Freire-Maia N. Ectodermal dysplasias: a clinical classification and a causal review. *Am J Med Genet* 1994; 53: 153–62.

Pinheiro M, Freire-Maia N. Ectodermal dysplasias. In: Harper J, ed. *Inherited Skin Disorders: the Genodermatoses.* Oxford: Butterworth-Heineemann, 1996: 126–44.

Epidermolysis Bullosa (EB)

Ronald W. Cotliar

Epidermolysis bullosa (EB) is composed of many clinically distinctive disorders that share three major features: genetic transmission, mechanical fragility of the skin, and blister formation.

There are three major types of inherited EB that are based on the level of the cleavage plane within the dermal-epidermal junction complex, or basement membrane zone (BMZ). These include:

1. Epidermolysis Bullosa Simplex (EBS)
2. Junctional Epidermolysis Bullosa (JEB)
3. Dystrophic Epidermolysis Bullosa (DEB)

Lesions in all types of EB clinically present as vesicles or bullae in response to frictional trauma.

Etiology

EB lesions arise secondary to defective attachment of the basal keratinocytes to the underlying dermis. These defects can arise from inside the keratinocyte plasma membrane or extracellularly in the BMZ. The same molecular defects which appear on the skin in each type of EB can be seen in other tissues that have an epithelial lining or surface such as the external surface of the eye, the oral cavity, the gastrointestinal tract (stomach excluded) and the genitourinary tract.

Epidermolysis Bullosa Simplex (EBS): is an autosomal dominant disorder. Mutations in genes for keratins 5 and 14 leads to production of a weakened basalar cytoskeleton that results in trauma, leading to intraepidermal bullae.

Junctional Epidermolysis Bullosa (JEB): is an autosomal recessive disorder. Heterogeneous mutations in the genes encoding hemidesmosomal proteins such as laminin 5 at the BMZ are responsible for the pathologic alteration of basal cell adhesion to the basement membrane.

Dystrophic Epidermolysis Bullosa (DEB): may be transmitted as autosomal dominant (Dominant DEB (DDEB)), or autosomal recessive (Recessive DEB (RDEB)). Mutations in the COL7A1 gene responsible for type VII collagen formation, the main structural protein in anchoring fibrils, lead to disruption of BMZ's integrity. The structurally defective and reduced numbers of anchoring fibrils contribute to this phenotype.

Clinical Presentation and Prognosis

Demographics: There is some variability in the incidence of different subtypes of EB. All subtypes have equal male to female prevalence.

- EBS is the most common form of EB with an incidence of 10–30 cases per million.
- JEB has an incidence of 2–3 cases per million live births.
- DEB has an incidence of 2.5 cases per million live births (dominant DEB is more common than recessive DEB, see below).

Presenting signs and symptoms: EBS has three different subtypes namely: Weber-Cockayne, Generalized (Koebner), and Dowling-Meara.

Weber-Cockayne typically presents during the 1st to 3rd decade of life, most commonly shows palmoplantar bullae, calluses, hyperhidrosis and may or may not be painful, or have superinfection. This subtype correlates with warmer temperatures and physical activity and is worse in summer months and tropical environments.

Generalized (Koebner) blisters appear at birth or early infancy, are most commonly generalized on the extremities, usually are not affected by warmer climates and have no superinfection. These patients may have mild oral mucosal involvement or nail dystrophy.

Dowling-Meara presents at birth or during the 1st month of life and may have widespread bullae in herpetiform grouping of lesions. Significant oral mucosa bullae with erosions may occur with esophageal involvement. Secondary hoarseness has been reported. These patients may have nail dystrophy with shedding but the lesions are usually nonscarring. This form of EBS may be severe, with increased morbidity, and sometimes mortality in infancy.

JEB has three subtypes including, *Herlitz JEB, Non-Herlitz JEB, and JEB-Pyloric Atresia.*

Herlitz JEB: Lesions appear at birth or shortly thereafter. Half of the affected infants die in infancy as a result of sepsis, dehydration, or respiratory complications. Generalized bullae may heal without scarring, or with milia and atrophy. Nonhealing granulation tissue occurs periorally, over the scalp, neck, upper trunk, nail folds, buttocks, and pinnae of the ears. Nail dystrophy or anonychia is also present. Head and neck lesions range from dysplastic teeth with hypoplasia of the enamel, and severe oral erosions, to hoarseness, croup, and edema secondary to laryngeal involvement. Malnutrition is common and leads to profound hypoproteinemia, anemia, infection, and eventually death by 3–4 years of age.

Non-Herlitz JEB: Is a milder form of Herlitz JEB. In this disease bullae tend to be more concentrated on the extremities and heal with atrophic scars. There is increased disease activity with increasing ambient temperature. Also, dystrophic nails and scarring alopecia is common while they have no granulation tissue, anemia, or growth retardation. These patients have normal life span and actually may improve with age.

JEB-Pyloric Atresia: Presents with severe congenital blistering and marked mucosal erosions, Pyloric stenosis or atresia, hydronephrosis, and renal failure secondary to stricture development. This form of JEB is fatal early on.

Dystrophic EB (DEB) has two forms, *Dominant dystrophic EB* (DDEB), and *Recessive dystrophic EB* (DDEB).

Dominant dystrophic EB presents at birth with bullae, which may either be widespread or localized to extremities. Bullae on dorsal aspect of extremities result in either hypertrophic or atrophic scars with milia. About 20% may have mucous membrane involvement while 80% have thickened nails. However, they typically have no hair or dental abnormalities. Following blisters at birth, random episodes of less severe blistering occur.

- Life span as well as growth and development are normal.
- The blistering episodes are worse than EBS, but milder than RDEB.

Recessive Dystrophic EB (RDEB) also presents at birth. In the more severe form (*Hallopeau-Siemens* variant) there is generalized dystrophic scarring with severe involvement of the mucous membranes, and severe nail dystrophy or anonychia. Bullae heal with atrophic scars and milia, resulting in "mitten" deformities of the hands and feet. Flexion contractures of the extremities may occur. In the more severe form, these lesions cause incapacitating deformity of the extremities. Eye involvement leads to blepharitis, symblepharon (adhesion of the eyelid to conjunctiva), conjunctivitis, keratitis, and corneal opacities. Hoarseness and aphonia are the result of laryngeal and pharyngeal involvement. If esophageal strictures occur, they can lead to failure to thrive.

- Teeth are malformed and susceptible to caries. Scalp and body hair is sparse or absent. Severe blistering may result in death due to sepsis, fluid loss or malnutrition. Surviving children become chronically susceptible to infection and repeated blistering leads to further disabilities. There are continued difficulties with laryngeal complications, esophageal strictures, and scarring of the anal and perianal areas. The scarred areas have a predisposition to develop basal cell and squamous cell carcinomas.

Prognosis: The prognosis of different types of EB vary from good to extremely poor. For details of each subtype please refer to the section above.

Diagnosis

It is of utmost importance to establish a diagnosis of EB and its subtype as soon as possible. This enables the clinician to discuss the prognosis and risk of recurrence in a family. The diagnosis of EB cannot be made in a neonate by casual exam.

There are multiple other disorders with confusing and overlapping phenotypes, which must be considered in a child with skin fragility.

A skin biopsy is performed to determine the cleavage plane and identify the affected protein components of the epidermis. The biopsy specimen is placed in specialized transport medium and is sent for indirect immunofluorescence to identify the presence, reduction, or absence of certain protein components such as type VII collagen, laminin 5, keratins 5 + 14, and plectin.

Electron microscopy is very helpful in mild cases by identifying the cleavage plane when this cannot be determined by routine microscopy.

Diagnosis of EB can now be made prenatally in order to provide far better genetic counseling. DNA-based testing utilizing chorionic villus samples are now routinely used in pregnancies at risk for a recurrence of EB. The problem presented by molecular based DNA testing is the need to know the precise genetic defect from an affected proband. In the absence of this info, a fetal skin biopsy remains the best diagnosis.

Management

Epidermolysis group of diseases are typically life long, affect many organ systems and require an intensive medical home approach. Presently, the management of EB is supportive and is aimed at ameliorating and relieving symptoms by providing infection control, wound healing, feeding, oral hygiene and rehabilitation therapy.

Medications and wound care: Bacterial colonization and infection delays or prevents would healing. While there are differences between the subtypes of EB, patients with EB have tendencies to develop chronic wounds that become colonized with bacteria that can lead to infections or delayed wound healing. Sepsis is one of the leading causes of infant mortality in these patients. Depending on the subtype, up to 24% of patients with JEB die from sepsis by 15 years of age. In one recent study, Staphylococcus species, streptococcus species, diphtheroids, pseudomonas aeruginosa, and candida species were the most commonly isolated microorganisms found in the wound cultures of EB subjects. It is also important to remember that both EB and Herpes Simplex virus can appear to be clinically similar. There are numerous reports that EB lesions can be supra-infected with HSV. Both topical and systemic antibiotics can be helpful and are necessary at times. Oral Cephalexin is often used. Topical Mupirocin (three times daily) and Retapamulin (twice daily) are effective. Both oral and topical antibiotics should be sued for short periods of time only, since bacterial resistance or sensitization to any topical medication can quickly occur. To decrease bacterial colonization, both acetic acid compresses or bleach baths and compresses are useful, but may cause stinging. Silver sulfadiazine cream or impregnated dressings have been used extensively for infected wounds. Although there are some theoretical concerns about its systemic absorption, there is inadequate data in EB patients to prohibit their use. Where available, 1% lipid-stabilized hydrogen peroxide cream has been used effectively. Ointments and dressings containing medical grade honey are also useful. Biafine®, a cream that is considered a "medical device" is a new and very effective agent in aiding wound healing and in caring for shave biopsy sites. Its effectiveness is thought to be due to its ability to attract macrophages into the wound and, by a yet unknown mechanism, stimulate fibroblasts.

Dressings: The perfect dressing for EB should maintain tissue moisture levels, be atraumatic and nonadherent, reduce pain, be available in a variety of sizes, hasten re-epithelialization, and be inexpensive.

Soft silicone dressings like Mepitel® and foams like Mepilex® are widely used. Mepitel® can be used as a primary dressing so that other therapeutic dressings which might adhere, can be used safely.

Dry wounds often do better with hydrogel dressings such as Vigilon® while for moist wounds, Mepilex® (a foam dressing) is effective. For very exudative wounds, a specialty absorptive dressing like Eclypse ® handles excessive fluid, and prevents the maceration and breakdown of surrounding skin. Barrier preparations such as Cavilon® can be used to protect normal skin from excessive exudates.

For EBS (Weber-Cockayne), silicon inserts in shoes that are well fit often keep the feet from blistering. Wearing two thin cotton socks with Vaseline® applied to the contact surface, often reduces friction. Drysol® applied to unbroken skin on a regular basis reduces hyperhidrosis and "toughens skin" and reduces blistering.

Oral tetracycline has been used to reduce the blistering with some efficacy. However, this needs to be further studied and cannot be used in children under 9–10 years old because of tooth discoloration.

Pain management is a major issue in caring for the more severe forms of EB (i.e., RDEB) and can be best administered by a pediatric pain management specialist. Withholding pain medications due to addiction concerns is unwarranted and at times (short life span) irrelevant. As with all chronic pains, adjunctive pain medications such as tricyclic antidepressants (Amitriptyline, nightly) along with anticonvulsants (gabapentine) and alpha-2 adrenergics (clinidine) can be useful. Although this is a chronic pain, opioids (i.e., Methadone) on an as needed or chronic basis may be used effectively.

Pruritus, particularly at night, can be controlled using hydroxyzine and other sedating antihistamines.

Surgery: In cases of failure to thrive due to difficulty with eating, a gastrostomy tube may be needed to provide adequate nutrition. Fusion of the fingers may also require surgical correction by plastic or hand surgery.

Consultations: A multidisciplinary medical team approach is needed to deal with the numerous secondary problems such as contractures, growth retardation, anemia, ocular, dental, pain, social and psychological problems that can overwhelm the affected children and their parents or other caretakers. We recommend involvement of genetics, dentistry, dermatology, gastroenterology, pain management, hand/plastic surgery, physical therapy, occupational therapy, ophthalmology, and infectious diseases on an as needed or ongoing basis to care for these children. For the milder subtypes, only one or a few specialty visits may be needed. EB clinics around the country (i.e., Stanford University) may also provide invaluable patient and physician support for the more severe or advanced cases.

Therapy: Physical and occupational therapy to help with walking, and prevention/treatment of oral aversion (mucosal blisters) is necessary. For those who need speech therapy, be aware that any instrumentation of the mouth may cause severe trauma in some subtypes.

Psych: The affected child, siblings, parents, and extended family have to deal with a heavy burden of personal, physical, and emotional issues. Therefore, we strongly urge clinicians to seek ongoing counseling for the entire or extended family.

Social: Patients and their families can find information at EB Medical Research Foundation: www.ebkids.org and the Dystrophic Epidermolysis Bullosa Research Association of America: www.debra.org

Monitoring: In cases of RDEB, be watchful of squamous cell carcinoma.

Pearls and Precautions:

Immunization: These patients should be fully vaccinated. Caution the nurse to not hold the thighs or arms too tight.

Nutrition/diet: For children with mouth blisters, mechanically soft diet may help with some oral intake, but is usually not adequate. These children need to have age and weight appropriate caloric intake. At times, this may only be achieved through a G-tube placement.

Tracheal toileting: If possible, avoid mouth or tracheal suctioning by all means.

Sleep: Amitryptiline may be useful in managing the pain and inducing sleep at night. Sedating antihistamines (see above) may be of some use. All sleep medications should be used cautiously.

Skin and dental care: Avoid the use of any brush for dental cleaning. Wiping the teeth with gauze and gloved fingers are most useful. All dental procedures and evaluations in noncompliant children need to be under sedation to avoid trauma and excessive pain. It is important to be aware that acquired melanocytic nevi in children with chronic blistering disorders may present as clinically atypical nevi. These can have very dark pigmentation and irregular borders. Although clinically worrisome they display normal histological patterns. The best way to approach these is for the pediatrician to follow along with the dermatologist who is providing the skin care.

Toilet: Even mild constipation may cause severe trauma to the perianal area. Therefore, oral or G-tube stool softeners (Docusate sodium, Polyethylen glycol) should be used liberally.

Likely complications: Secondary complications (arising from secondary involvement of other organs) involving the eye, mucous membranes of the orifices, gastrointestinal, respiratory, urogenital tracts and even muscles to some extent, is common. Blisters involving the oral mucosa and esophagus lead to difficulty in chewing and swallowing, leading to secondary malnutrition, anemia, growth retardation and delayed wound healing. Intestinal erosions can lead to chronic protein and blood loss, contributing to the development of multifactorial anemia, hypoalbuminemia, hypoproteinemia, malabsorption, and growth retardation. Rectal strictures may result in chronic constipation and sometimes megacolon.

Dental problems arise due to inadequate dental hygiene because of the fragile oral mucosa. Blistering in the eye can result in severe pain as well as visual reduction for days at a time. Scarring and contractures in the hands and feet leading to formation of mittens and socks, limits movement and can lead to severe deformities.

In these children, the skin grows over the digits enclosing them in translucent sheets. If necessary, hand surgeons will do a thumb release procedure to produce an opposable thumb. Operating on the other fingers has not been successful. If feet are functional, no surgery is attempted.

Importantly, the incidence of squamous cell carcinoma in young adults with generalized DEB is high, and many patients develop metastasizing skin cancer before age 40.

School/education: These children are neurologically intact and deserve to receive the same education as other normal children. However, schools need to be made aware of their physical limitations, and in the more severe cases (requiring intensive wound care) they may need to be home-schooled.

Medical devices: The more severe children may need a G-tube for feeding and special strollers for ambulation to avoid pressure points as they get older.

Other approaches: Presently, there are two prenatal diagnosis techniques under development.

Single-cell preimplantation diagnosis involving a single blastomere biopsy from the 6–10 cell stage of the fertilized embryo, followed by DNA mutation analysis will allow the treating physicians to implant the disease-free embryos into the uterus. This technique will prevent any pregnancy termination procedures. Currently, the extremely high level of technical expertise and its cost, make this prohibitive. However, this may be a technique widely available at low cost in the future.

Recent advances have enabled the isolation of nucleated fetal erythrocytes from maternal blood at between 8 and 11 weeks estimated gestational age (EGA). The cells are isolated and single-cell DNA analysis by polymerase chain reaction (PCR) can be done. The problem is that if the fetus is female and carries no Y chromosome, it becomes difficult to determine if the cell is of fetal or maternal origin. As this is a noninvasive procedure though, if the difficulties can be ironed out, it promises to be the most helpful and productive technique to date.

Reference

Brandling-Bennett HA, Morel KD. Common Wound Colonizers in Patients with Epidermolysis Bullosa. Pediatric Dermatology 2010 Jan 1;27 (1):25-8

Fine J-D, Eady RAJ. et al. The classification of inherited epidermolysis bullosa (EB): Report of the Third International Consensus Meeting on Diagnosis and Classification of EB. J of the American Academy of Dermatology June 2008 (Vol. 58, Issue 6, Pages 931–950).

Infantile Hemangiomas (IH)

Ronald W. Cotliar

Infantile hemangioma (IH) and hemangioma of infancy (HOI) are benign vascular tumors that are composed of proliferation of endothelial tissue. All congenital vascular lesions are categorized as vascular tumors or malformations.

Etiology

The exact etiology of this disease is unclear at this time. Most cases of IH are sporadic. The link between chorionic villus sampling (CVS) and IH formation is not as strong as once thought.

Clinical Presentation and Prognosis

Demographics: Infantile hemangiomas are present in 1% to 2% of healthy newborns and can be noted in 10–12% of infants by one year of age. Associated risk factors include being premature at birth and female; a product of multiple gestation; white, non-Hispanic ethnicity; exposed to pre-eclampsia and placenta previa; and having an older birth mother.

Presenting signs and symptoms: Most IHs present in the first 3 weeks to 3 months of life. Precursor or "premonitory marks" may be present at birth or within the first 48 hours of life. These lesions may appear as a small bruise, telangiectasia, area of skin pallor, or discoloration. They represent the area where the IH is forming.

IHs are categorized as superficial, deep, or combined (mixed). In addition, they can be focal, segmental, or indeterminate as described below:

- *Superficial:* IHs are bright red (strawberry) lobulated or smooth papules or plaques.
- *Deep:* IHs appear as compressible bluish subcutaneous nodules or plaques. The surface may show telangiectasias or a surrounding venous plexus. These lesions are usually noted in the first 3 months of life.
- *Combined*, or *mixed:* IHs clinically demonstrate features of the superficial and deep hemangiomas.
- *Localized*, or *focal:* IHs are well-defined papules, nodules or plaques that seem to arise from a central focus.
- *Segmental:* IHs are plaques that appear to involve a developmental or embryological area of the body. It is important to note that the lesion does not have to encompass the entire segment but only a portion.
- *Intermediate:* IHs are those lesions that cannot be diagnosed as either focal or segmental.

The majority of IHs are solitary, but multiple lesions occur in up to 20% of infants and are especially common among multiple births. IHs have a predilection for the head and neck, although they can occur anywhere on the skin, mucous membranes, or internal organs.

Clinical course: Infantile hemangiomas undergo a "proliferative" or growth phase that is often rapid for the first few months and is, at times, followed by 6–12 months of continued slow growth. However, deep IHs act differently and may continue growing up to 18 months, with some brief plateaus during this period. Generally, growth halts at one year of age and is followed by a gradual "Involution." The superficial involuting IH first shows a color change from a bright red to a violaceous hue, followed by a steel gray tone. The lesion softens and flattens. Deep lesions become less warm and blue as their subcutaneous size becomes smaller. Completed involution occurs at an estimated minimum rate of 10% per year, leading to a 50% resolution of IHs by age 5, 70% by age 7, and 90% by age 9.

Approximately 80% of IHs occur in isolation (a single lesion), while 20% involve multiple lesions. "Hemangiomatosis" is the term used to describe the clinical presentation of several to hundreds of small, generalized hemangiomas that are sometimes associated with visceral lesions (most commonly liver). Thus, two categories of this clinical picture have been created: Benign and Disseminated neonatal hemangiomatosis. Clearly not all affected infants will fall neatly into one category. It is now thought by most clinicians that hemangiomatosis represents a spectrum of diseases with varying degrees of cutaneous and visceral involvement. Doctors Ilona J. Frieden, and Anna L. Bruckner, have suggested the term "multifocal hemangiomas, with or without extracutaneous involvement," as a more descriptive clinical term. Each case should be assessed individually and there is no association between the number of cutaneous hemangiomas and possible visceral involvement. Visceral lesions can occur in the absence of skin lesions.

Prognosis: In general, children with smaller (up to about 1.5 cm) isolated hemangiomas have a good prognosis. However, female infants with segmental IHs are more likely to have complications. Premature infants with low, or very low birth weight are at risk of increased rate of complications. Segmental IHs are more likely to be associated with structural malformations. It is extremely important to let the parents know that after the resolution of the lesions, up to one-half of children have residual changes that include fibrofatty redundant skin (gray in color), atrophy, scarring, telangiectasias, and discoloration (e.g., hypopigmentation, etc.).

Diagnosis

The diagnosis of IH is typically prompted by its appearance on the skin. Imaging studies done by knowledgeable, experienced staff can be helpful in differentiating IHs from vascular malformations or other soft-tissue tumors. Doppler ultrasound has been the standard initial test of choice. It is the least invasive and most cost effective test to differentiate between vascular tumors and malformations. Recent introduction of color, 3D, high-resolution ultrasound machines that show real-time blood flow in even the smallest vessels, has eliminated the need for other imaging modalities. In many cases, computed tomography (CT) and resonance imaging (MRI) have been helpful in making a diagnosis at times. Magnetic resonance angiography (MRA) is generally only used in patients requiring embolization.

Although it is uncommon, occasionally a tissue biopsy of a lesion is necessary to correctly identify a vascular tumor. IH is the only neonatal/infant lesion in which the endothelial tissue on immunostaining is positive for glucose transformer isoform-1 (GLUT-1), a placenta-associated marker.

It is important not to confuse IHs with the other neonatal vascular tumors as below:

- *Rapidly involuting congenital hemangioma (RICH)* is fully formed at birth, does not proliferate during the neonatal period, but involutes later.
- *Non-involuting congenital hemangioma (NICH)* is fully formed at birth, but does not proliferate or involute in the neonate.
- *Tufted angioma* is a vascular tumor characterized by indolent growth. Typically they arise before 5 years of age and may be congenital and are located on the neck, upper torso, or shoulders.
- *Kaposiform hemangioendothelioma* is an aggressive vascular tumor that appears in children under 2 years of age and congenital cases have been reported. It is a deeper lesion.

- *The Kassabach Merritt Syndrome* is only seen in the tufted angioma and the kaposiform hemangioendothelioma. It is not seen in IHs.

Management

Hemangiomas should be treated only if the lesions interfere with function (feeding, vision, hearing, or breathing), or cause cosmetically deforming or disfiguring changes (lips, nasal tip, eyes, ears, and genitalia). Ulceration is by far the most common complication and reason for intervention in IHs. It has been shown in multiple studies to vary in incidence between 5–16%. Ulceration occurs during the proliferative phase and is not a sign of involution, as previously thought. Although the cause is unknown, mechanical trauma, and maceration, along with its anatomical location seems to play a role. Perioral, perineal, intertriginous, segmental, and posterior scalp lesions are more likely to undergo breakdown. Ulcerations are painful, can bleed, and may become secondarily infected. They heal with scarring, and depending on the size and site of the lesion may be disfiguring. If left alone, all other IH lesions have better cosmetic outcome than the ones that have undergone unnecessary procedures, often due to parental pressure.

The major goals of management as outlined in the "1997 Guidelines of Care of the American Academy of Dermatology" include:

- Preventing or reversing life or function-threatening complications.
- Preventing disfigurement.
- Minimizing psychosocial stress for the patient and family.
- Avoiding aggressive and potentially scarring procedures.
- Preventing or adequately treating ulceration to minimize scarring, infection, and pain.

Management of IH is complicated by its wide spectrum of clinical manifestations and the rapid biologic changes that occur during the neonatal period and infancy. Clinicians who are well trained and experienced in this discipline are often unable to predict which lesions are best left alone, and which ones present a threat. Thus, very close clinical observation of these patients by an experienced clinician is of utmost importance.

Medications: Intralesional steroids (usually triamcinolone) are the "gold standard" of treatment for localized lesions. All lesions above the neck need to be treated with extreme caution. Periocular IHs should be injected by an experienced clinician who is comfortable with this procedure. Parents need to be made aware of the risk of retinal artery embolization.

Superficial localized lesions may be treated nightly or twice daily with potent topical steroids. Ointments or the newer foam formulations seem to be effective. *Cordran Tape®* is a steroid impregnated tape that can be applied and left in place for several hours. We recommend that a medical staff experienced in using these tapes train the parents and monitor its use. Other Class I or II topical steroids can be used on the body. On the face, most clinicians use fluticasone cream 0.05%, or triamcinolone cream 0.1%, which are low to medium potency topical steroids.

Systemic corticosteroids are presently the mainstay of treatment for IHs that require intervention. While different physicians start treatment at 2–5 mg/kg/day, meta-analysis has led most centers to a starting dose of 3 mg/kg/day. We recommend "Ilona Frieden's protocol" that starts with 3 mg/kg/day of prednisolone as a single morning dose. Once the lesion is stabilized for 1–2 months, the dosage is then tapered at a rate that best suits the individual patient's response until a dosage of 1.5–2 mg/kg/day is reached. At that time, the patient's regimen is changed to an alternate day treatment while tapering over 8–10 weeks. In case of a rebound, taper can be slowed or stopped, but dosage should not be increased. This treatment is most effective if started during the growth or proliferative phase. We recommend some type of Histamine-2 blocker (i.e., Ranitidine 2–4 mg/kg/day divided twice daily) to prevent gastric upset or reflux. Some clinicians have recommended Pneumocystis Carinii Pneumonia prophylaxis in children over 6 months of age, using Trimethoprim Sulfamethoxazole at a dosage of 5–10 mg/kg/day divided twice daily on Monday, Wednesday and Friday, or on weekends. Avoid live vaccines while on high dose steroids (see below).

Nasal tip IHs can be treated with intralesional steroids, or sometimes a 3-week course of oral steroids. Visceral involvement requires higher doses over a longer period of time. It is unclear at this time whether the response of the cutaneous IHs parallel those of the visceral lesions, and thus can not be used as a surrogate marker for treatment monitoring.

Vincristine has been used in the treatment of the Kassabach-Merritt phenomenon (disseminated intravascular coagulopathy secondary to sequestration of platelets) which is not seen in IHs but only in the kaposiform hemangioendothelioma and tufted hemangioma (both vascular tumors). The use of Vincristine has been expanded to treat more aggressive IHs. It has replaced Interferon alpha and has been used by clinicians as a second-line therapy for IHs that have not responded to systemic steroids. It is administered by a central venous catheter and is best directed by a pediatric hematologist/oncologist.

Propranolol, a non-selective beta-blocker was serendipitously found to dramatically impact IHs and cause involution. In a letter to the editor, Leaute-Labreze C, et al. (Propranolol for severe hemangiomas of infancy. N Engl J Med. 2008;358:2649-2651.) reported their preliminary data on the use of Propranolol in 11 infants with severe hemangiomas. The authors suggest that this amazing therapeutic effect occurred as a result of vasoconstriction, decreased expression of VEGF and bFGF genes and the triggering of apoptosis of capillary endothelial cells. This new and exciting therapy awaits the results of placebo controlled studies to hopefully find a standardized protocol.

Blister care: Provide pain medications 20-30 minutes prior to the following steps to provide pain relief, if needed. Use clean techniques (not sterile) to drain each blister by inserting a sterile needle once or multiple times at its lower edge. This will allow the gravity to drain the blister without any need for pressure. Allow the overlying skin to stay intact. Avoid pressure dressing.

Dressing: Ulcerated IHs require local wound care using non-stick dressings (i.e., gel impregnated gauze), topical antibiotics (e.g., metronidazole), dilute bleach soaks, and frequent dressing changes. Pain control can be achieved with acetaminophen, ibuprofen, and topical lidocaine. Aggressive, persistent, large or deep lesions may necessitate the use of systemic or local steroids, pulsed dye laser, becaplermin gel, or excision.

Surgery: During the rapid growth phase of IHs, these vascular tumors can displace surrounding tissue in a way that tissue expanders do which can lead to the destruction of the dermal architecture resulting in cutaneous laxity. As the IH resolves (involution), it is not entirely absorbed but is replaced by a loose fibro-fatty stroma. This leads to residual tumor in the footprint of the "completely" regressed lesion. In addition, telangiectasias are often present. Therefore, after the natural involution of the IH, significant "scarring" or "disfigurement" is present in approximately 25% of IHs. Clinicians must be clear about this as to avoid false hope in the parents about results.

Surgery is indicated for certain lesions such as the nasal tip IH which is deeper and has great cosmetic significance. IHs of the perioral, periocular, and ear regions also need to be considered as possible surgical candidates. Interventional radiology is used when embolization is the treatment of choice.

Social: The cosmetic effect of IHs alone, in the absence of any associate anomalies, often creates a tremendous degree of anxiety and pressure on the parents. At times, this anxiety may lead to unnecessary treatment of self-resolving lesions. For the vast majority of children no therapy is indicated or warranted.

Parental education and guidance conferred through an honest and factual conversation may be all that is needed for many of these patients.

However, many parents turn to the Internet as their source of written information.

We recommend parents be referred to "Vascular Birthmarks Foundation" (http://www.birthmark.org) to obtain electronic information on this subject.

Table 3.1: Complications Associated with Certain Hemangiomas

Hemangioma	Complication(s)
Large segmental facial	PHACES syndrome.
Nasal tip, ear, large facial	Permanent scarring and disfigurement.
Periorbital and retrobulbar	Ocular axis occlusion, astigmatism, amblyopia, tear-duct occlusion.
Segmental "beard area" and central neck	Airway hemangioma (subglottal involvement), which may lead to stridor and respiratory difficulty.
Perioral, lips	Ulceration, disfigurement.
Lumbosacral spine	Tethered spinal cord, genitourinary anomalies.
Perineal, axilla, neck, perioral	Ulceration.
Multiple hemangiomas	Visceral involvement (liver, gastrointestinal tract are most likely) and can involve CNS or any other organ system including mucous membranes.
	Thyroid abnormalities have been reported in association with large hepatic hemangiomas. High levels of type 3 iodothyronine deiodinase activity has been found in hemangioma tissue. This enzyme is normally expressed in brain and placenta. It is involved in the inactivation of thyroxine. This can lead to hypothyroidism in the infant.

ICD-9 Codes, 228.01-Hemangioma, skin or subcutaneous (benign).

Monitoring: In an editorial opinion of the Journal Archives of Dermatology (vol 145 (No.3), authors pointed out that there is paucity of information supporting Hypothalamic Pituitary Adrenal (HPA) axis suppression induced by glucocorticosteroid (GC) treatment of IH. Supraphysiologic doses of systemic GCs can certainly cause HPA axis suppression, and thus parents and providers must remain "vigilant" of the need for stress dosing in the event of surgery, illness, or trauma. However, the data suggests that the risk of long-standing HPA axis suppression following a standard IH treatment protocol may be less common than previously thought, and should not militate against the appropriate use of the "gold-standard" treatment of IH.

Pearls and Precautions

Interferon alpha is a potent inhibitor of angiogenesis. In the past, it was used as a second-line agent in aggressive IHs that were unresponsive to corticosteroids. Due to its significant risk of neurotoxicity and permanent spastic diplegia, especially in preemies, this drug is no longer an acceptable treatment option.

Be aware of **PHACES syndrome** which is characterized by the association of **P**osterior fossa malformation (Dandy-Walker malformation is the most common structural brain abnormality) **H**emangiomas (large segmental facial lesions are the most common) **A**rterial anomalies, **C**oarctation of the aorta and other cardiac defects, **E**ye abnormalities, **S**ternal defects, and **S**upraumbilical raphe.

Table 3.1 shows the associated complications that should be kept in mind and monitored closely when certain hemangiomas are seen.

References

Leaute-Labreze C, et al. (Propranolol for severe hemangiomas of infancy. *N Engl J Med.* 2008;358:2649–2651.

Brucker Anna L, et al. Hemangiomas of Infancy. J Am Acad Dermatol 48(4):477–492, 2003.

Minzer-Conzetti K, Garzon MC, Haggstrom A, et al: Information about infantile hemangiomas on the Internet: How accurate is it? J Am Acad Dermatol 57(6):998–1004, 2007.

Sidbury Robert: Hypothalmic-Pituitary-Adrenal Axis Suppression is Systemic Glucocorticoid-Treated Infantile Hemangiomas. Arch Dermatol 145(3):319–320, 2009.

Childhood Vitiligo

Delphine J. Lee

Vitiligo is an acquired disorder of hypopigmentation that occurs in 1–2% of the general population.

Etiology

There are multiple hypotheses of its pathogenesis with the most popular including neural, oxidative stress, and autoimmune etiologies. Given the response to immunosuppressive treatment (e.g. topical corticosteroids), the association with other autoimmune diseases and laboratory abnormalities consistent with immune dysregulation, all etiologies may converge to a final autoimmune pathogenesis that result in the destruction of cutaneous melanocytes.

Pathology: The classic histopathology demonstrates absence of melanocytes with variable infiltration by leukocytes. Hematoxylin and eosin stain (H&E) of affected tissue may appear very similar to normal skin, while melanocyte-specific stains will reveal a loss of melanocytes. However, the diagnosis is usually based on the clinical exam.

Clinical Presentation and Prognosis

Age of onset: Half of all cases including adults develop before the age of 20 years, with the mean age in the pediatric age group being 4-5 years.

Presenting signs and symptoms: The majority of the pediatric vitiligo cases (78%) present as generalized symmetric patches, while up to 20% of the cases are "segmental," with localized lesions formed across the dermatomes. A much less common form of this disease in children is found in a focal distribution whereby the patches are localized in a single area, in a non-segmental distribution.

Clinical course: The course of this disease is typically slow and progressive, and somewhat unpredictable. While psychosocial stress can lead to flare-ups, approximately 10–20% of patients may experience spontaneous repigmentation, particularly with increased UV exposure during the summer months.

Prognosis: Vitiligo is a disease with no increased mortality or limitation of life-span. The affected children are generally otherwise healthy but have increased susceptibility to development of new lesions at the site of a new skin trauma (burns, cuts, etc.) known as the Koebner phenomenon. Children may be at increased risk of thyroiditis and (rarely) type 1 diabetes mellitus, pernicious anemia, or exacerbation of underlying endocrinopathy.

Diagnosis

Vitiligo is a clinical diagnosis based on the characteristic depigmented macules and patches that are enhanced with Wood's lamp. Skin biopsy is rarely required. Differential diagnoses of hypopigmented lesions include tinea versicolor, corticosteroid-induced hypopigmentation, post inflammatory hypopigmentation, idiopathic guttate hypomelanosis, hypopigmented/atrophic lichen planus, progressive macular hypomelanosis, lichen sclerosis-classic or generalized, hypopigmented mycosis fungoides, lupus and morphea.

Management

Early management may prevent cosmetic and psychological damage. However, given the non-life threatening nature of this disease, risks and benefits should be explained and discussed carefully. Studies have generally shown that combination therapy is superior to single agent therapy. Patients should be advised that repigmentation can wax and wane, though repigmentation efforts are often overall more successful in children than in adults and thus should be pursued.

Medications

Topical corticosteroids: Children under 12 can benefit from the use of low potency (class V) topical corticosteroids such as fluticasone propionate cream or desonide 0.05% cream once a day for four months. Patients should be monitored every four weeks. Rates of response vary from 15%–64%. Use of topicals can be impractical in generalized vitiligo. All topical steroids can cause striae, atrophy, and telangiectasias, but no large clinical trial has shown major side effects. These adverse effects are more common in higher potency topical corticosteroids and in fluorinated products, which if used, should be closely supervised by the prescribing physician. Unregulated use of high potency topical corticosteroids has been reported to cause hypothalamic-pituitary-adrenal axis suppression. Topical steroids should not be used near the eyes, given the potential risk for increased intraocular pressure.

Oral corticosteroids: This treatment is seldom recommended and only reserved for the rapidly progressive cases that are unresponsive to the more conventional methods. One study of 80 patients suggests that a low daily dose of oral prednisolone (0.3 mg/kg) can arrest progression of the disease, particularly in patients under 15 years of age.

Topical immunomodulators: For patients > 2 years of age in whom topical corticosteroid use is impractical or poses increased risk of adverse effects (e.g., near eyes), tacrolimus 0.1%, applied twice daily for 3 months is a useful alternative in management of face, eyelid, genital, and segmental vitiligo. Adverse effects include pruritis, stinging, and (very rarely) hypertrichosis. Patients and parents should be informed that the FDA has issued a black box warning for possible links between the use of topical calcineurin inhibitors and increased risk of lymphoma and skin cancer. However, no causal relationship of topical use (within the maximum recommended human dose) to skin cancer or lymphoma has been established. In general, patients using topical calcineurin inhibitors should use sun protection.

Vitamin D derivative: Calcipotriene (0.005% cream applied twice daily) is a vitamin D analog that can be used all over the body, including the eyelids and face. Topical calcipotriene is more effective in combination with steroids or phototherapy.

Phototherapy

NB-UVB (narrowband Ultraviolet B): 311 nm UV phototherapy has been shown to be equivalent in efficacy compared to PUVA (Psoralen-Ultraviolet A). Furthermore, NB-UVB results in a comparatively more cosmetically appealing repigmentation and carries a lower risk of photo contact allergenicity, phototoxic reactions, hyperkeratosis, and erythema. No protective eyewear is required. Twice weekly treatment has been shown to be equivalent to thrice weekly. Phototherapy is usually not the most practical method of treatment, and should be reserved for patients with generalized, symmetric involvement of >10% body surface area. Children should be old enough to be alone in the phototherapy unit. Home units should be monitored monthly after parents have been properly instructed on dosing. The most responsive areas, face and neck, followed by the trunk and non-acral surfaces, should demonstrate results by 6 months.

Excimer laser: 308 nm UV light has been shown to have a similar efficacy to NB-UVB in a small study that included children. This may be a useful modality for focal lesions.

The use of topical calcineurin inhibitors in combination with phototherapy should not be first line and the fact that risks are unknown should be carefully discussed.

Social: Attention should be paid to issues of self esteem, personal identity, and social conflicts, particularly when the disease manifests during puberty. Patients may seek support and information at the American Vitiligo Research Foundation (www.avrf.org).

Cosmetic: Though covering up lesions is not a therapy, patients may benefit psychologically by using cosmetic products to mask affected areas, such as Covermark® or Dermablend®, in addition to conventional cosmetics. Cinema secrets® (www.cinemasecrets.com) may also be effective in covering obvious lesions. Select patients may also benefit from skin dyes, such as Vitadye® (Elder) or quick-tan® preparations. Patients should always try test areas when applying a new product to be certain they do not develop a contact allergy.

Monitoring: Yearly thyroid function tests, complete blood count, and fasting plasma glucose are recommended for children with active vitiligo.

Pearls and Precautions

1. Provide parents and patients with ample support and education regarding the unpredictable prognosis and treatment response in this disease. Clinicians should emphasize the fact that repigmentation is possible. Parents and patients will have a more realistic expectation of the treatment outcome if they are made aware of the fact that facial and neck lesions are most responsive to treatment, while lesions over the bony prominences and acral areas are the most difficult to treat. Anecdotally, newer lesions are more responsive to treatment than older lesions.
2. The key to treating vitiligo involves immunosuppression by topical (usually) or systemic (rarely) therapy to inhibit the undesired immune response against melanocytes while stimulating melanocytes to encourage repigmentation of lesional skin.
3. Though stress as a triggering factor for rapid progression is observed/reported more often in adult patients, education of parents and the patient in the importance of adopting a life-long commitment to exercise and other stress management tools is good for the patient's overall health and may help prevent future flares.
4. Serial photography is the best way to document and assess the efficacy of treatments.

References

Halder RM. *Childhood vitiligo*. Clin Dermatol. 1997 Nov–Dec;15(6):899–906.

Huggins RH, Schwartz RA, Janniger CK. *Childhood vitiligo*. Cutis. 2007 Apr;79(4):277–80.

Sanfilippo AM, Barrio V, Kulp-Shorten C, Callen JP. *Common pediatric and adolescent skin conditions.* J Pediatr Adolesc Gynecol. 2003 Oct;16(5):269–83.

Sidbury R. *What's new in pediatric dermatology: update for the pediatrician.* Curr Opin Pediatr. 2004 Aug;16(4):410–4.

Silverberg NB, Travis L. *Childhood vitiligo*. Cutis. 2006 Jun;77(6):370–5.

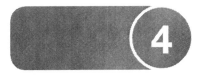 **Endocrinologic Disorders**

Table of Contents

Adrenal Hyperplasia

Mitchell E. Geffner

CAH refers to any of several autosomal recessive diseases resulting from mutations of genes for enzymes mediating the biochemical steps of cortisol synthesis, and, in some cases, aldosterone production by the adrenal glands. The more common forms of CAH are also associated with excessive production of androgens resulting in virilization of female fetuses, precocious adrenarche in children of both sexes, and abnormal menstruation, hirsutism, and acne in adolescent and adult women.

Etiology

Adrenal hyperplasia, formerly known as *congenital* adrenal hyperplasia, is now subdivided into two forms, *classical* adrenal hyperplasia (CAH) and *non-classical* adrenal hyperplasia (NCAH). The most common form of adrenal hyperplasia results from deficiency of the 21-hydroxylase enzyme [which catalyzes the conversion of 17-hydroxyprogesterone (17OHP) to 11-desoxycortisol (also known as Compound S)]. The classical form may be subdivided into salt-wasting (SWCAH) and simple-virilizing (SVCAH) subtypes which are associated with <1% and 1–2% of 21-hydroxylase enzyme activity, respectively. The milder non-classical variant has 20–60% of normal enzyme activity. The next most common form of adrenal hyperplasia is due to 11-hydroxylase deficiency (which catalyzes the conversion of Compound S to cortisol). As with most enzyme deficiencies, inheritance is autosomal recessive, with parents as obligate heterozygotes (carriers).

Clinical Presentation and Prognosis

Demographics: CAH secondary to 21-hydroxylase deficiency occurs in 1:15,000–16,000 births in most populations (the highest incidence of this disease being found in Yupik Eskimos). NCAH occurs in 0.2% of the general Caucasian population, but occurs much more frequently in certain other populations including 1–2% of Hispanics and Yugoslavs, and in 3–4% Ashkenazi Jews of Eastern European origin. Together CAH and NCAH account for 90% of all cases of adrenal hyperplasia. Since all other forms of adrenal hyperplasia are exceedingly rare, the discussion below will be limited to 21-hydroxylase deficiency, unless otherwise indicated.

Presenting signs and symptoms: Adrenal hyperplasia may be diagnosed at various ages. It can be detected by genetic testing during pregnancy via chorionic villous sampling (testing for which would be prompted by a prior affected sibling). In the past, development of salt-wasting and hyperkalemia along with male-looking genitals in females (fusion of labio-scrotal folds and enlargement of clitoris), would typically lead to the diagnosis of this disease in the first few days of life. However, newborn screening programs for 21-hydroxylase deficiency have made an earlier post-natal diagnosis possible. The genitalia of affected males are essentially normal, except for a mildly enlarged penis and hyperpigmented scrotum (with hyperpigmentation of the labio-scrotal folds evident in affected females). Without genetic screening, non-salt-losing males may not be diagnosed until later when they present with early development of pubic hair, with or without signs of virilization (including rapid linear growth and advanced bone age). NCAH patients without flagrant virilization may present with increased hair growth in females (60%), absence or loss of menstrual periods (54%), and acne (33%). Patients with NCAH never have salt loss or have been reported to have an adrenal crisis. Interestingly, there are patients with NCAH who never have any symptoms, but who are only detected as a result of screening because of an affected family member.

Note that the 11-hydroxylase form of this disease is typically associated with hypertension (and not salt loss except in the neonatal period). This is due to accumulation of salt-retaining aldosterone precursors, such as deoxycorticosterone (DOC).

Clinical course: Children with classical CAH will require lifelong glucocorticoid replacement while fludrocortisone is also required for salt-losers. Affected females will usually require frequent genital examinations and one or more surgeries. Patients with symptomatic NCAH will require glucocorticoid replacement at least throughout childhood. Those with CAH will always be at risk for adrenal crisis and all will require careful titration of medication doses to maximize height (an effect resulting from too much or too little glucocorticoid), to avoid weight excess and induction of cardiovascular risk factors (from too much glucocorticoid), and to maximize fertility rates (from too little glucocorticoid resulting in hyperandrogenism).

Prognosis: Meticulous medical care and proper use of replacement medications can significantly improve the prognosis of this disease and prevent progressive virilization and adrenal crises. Nonetheless, growth delay may occur with CAH or NCAH, and some degree of adult short stature is common. With increasing age, there is also a tendency toward obesity, which may be due to overdosing of glucocorticoids. Delayed onset of menses or symptoms of polycystic ovarian syndrome (PCOS)—including lack of ovulation and absent or irregular periods—may occur in adolescent girls. Of the women with SV CAH, 80% are fertile while 60% of those with severe SV CAH are fertile. New medical and surgical techniques have significantly improved the rate of successful pregnancies (usually requiring delivery by cesarean section).

Men with CAH have comparatively fewer problems with reproductive function and most have normal sperm counts and are able to father children. However, they are at risk for development of benign testicular adrenal rest tumors (or TARTS) that can nearly replace all normal tissue and decrease sperm production. These tumors are ACTH-sensitive and will usually shrink in response to pituitary suppression with dexamethasone (usually precluding the need for biopsy and/or surgery).

Diagnosis

Upon the suspicion of CAH, an immediate endocrine consultation is required. The best diagnostic test for 21-hydroxylase deficiency is an elevated serum level of 17OHP (which should be ordered immediately at an endocrine specialty laboratory). For children with either form of CAH, a random level will usually suffice. For select cases and most with NCAH secondary to 21-hydroxylase deficiency, measurements of 17OHP both before and after 250 μg of synthetic adrenocorticotropic hormone (ACTH) 1-24 (Cortrosyn® = Cosyntropin®) will likely be required to assure the correct diagnosis.

Other auxiliary diagnostic tests include serum concentrations of testosterone, androstenedione, renin, and electrolytes (in infants); a *stat* karyotype for sex determination [involving fluorescence in situ hybridization (FISH) testing for sex determining region on the Y chrosomoe (SRY)] in "virilized females," and occasionally other steroid precursors (*e.g.,* Compound S for 11-hydroxylase deficiency]. Note that when ordering the latter, the requested test should be a *specific* compound S. In virilized newborns with CAH, radiological studies, including pelvic ultrasound and genitogram (or possibly MRI), are required to confirm expected Müllerian duct-derived internal female anatomy (*i.e.,* fallopian tubes, uterus, and upper vagina).

Management

Medication: Oral hydrocortisone at 10–20 mg/m^2/day (or other glucocorticoid equivalent) in divided doses (usually 1/4 in AM, 1/4 in afternoon, and 1/2 at bedtime) is required to suppress the normal overnight rise in ACTH. Patients who need oral mineralocorticoid should receive 0.1 mg/day of generic fludrocortisone (Florinef® brand is no longer manufactured).

Although stress doses of glucocorticoids may not be necessary in patients with NCAH during a mild intercurrent illness, glucocorticoid doses must be increased 2- to 3-fold in CAH patients in this situation. All families should have parenteral glucocorticoid (Solucortef® Act-o-Vial) at home and know how and when to use it.

For more serious intercurrent illness or trauma requiring hospitalization, cortisol should be administered in the form of high-dose (~5–10X maintenance = ~50–100 mg/m^2/day) IV hydrocortisone in 4 divided doses or as a continuous infusion (these high doses also provide significant aldosterone effect which is fortunate since there is no pure IV mineralocorticoid available in the U.S.). Intravenous saline should also be empirically administered in these situations which are likely to be associated with dehydration and hyponatremia. Hyperkalemia may require its own specific emergency measures, but usually responds to hydrocortisone replacement. Intravenous glucose may also be required because of a predisposition to hypoglycemia secondary to the loss of counter-regulatory (anti-insulin) protection that is normally conferred by cortisol.

Surgery: Almost all females with CAH (but not NCAH) will require vaginoplasty, and frequently need surgery to recess the clitoris. The vaginoplasty is technically easiest to perform and psychologically least traumatic if done in the first 2 years of life. Males do not require surgery. Note that any surgical intervention during infancy or childhood is extremely controversial and should only be attempted after prudent consideration and extensive discussion with the parents (see below).

Psychological: The birth of a child with ambiguous genitalia creates a great deal of stress for parents and families. The optimal approach to such children involves a team of specialists with expertise in "disorders of sex development," the term now favored for all types of genital ambiguity. Inclusion of an experienced psychologist and ethicist is empiric in helping the families make decisions that will affect such long-term issues as sexual function, fertility, and gender identity/preference.

Social: All older children must wear Medic-Alert identification.

Laboratory tests and monitoring: In patients with any form of adrenal hyperplasia due to 21-hydroxylase deficiency, assessment of metabolic control should be undertaken by quantification of bone age (hemiskeletons prior to age 2 years and left hand and wrist radiographs thereafter) every 6 months. The bone age serves as an integrated quantification of control. Additionally, serum levels of 17OHP, testosterone, androstenedione, and, in salt-losers, plasma renin activity, should be checked every 3–6 months. Routine measurement of serum sodium and potassium is rarely helpful and urine testing for steroid metabolites should be discouraged. The aforementioned laboratory monitoring is best done prior to the morning medication dose ("trough" level), to assess the duration and effectiveness of the prior evening dosage of hydrocortisone. Note that there is no uniform consensus among the pediatric endocrinologists regarding the optimal protocol or frequency of testing to monitor this condition. Regardless, rapidly advancing bone age (often heralding an accelerated height velocity) in conjunction with elevated steroid intermediates indicates the need for greater glucocorticoid dosing, while the opposite findings (slowly advancing bone age, reduced height velocity, and suppressed intermediates) suggest overtreatment. The pattern of the plasma renin activity is used to modulate the fludrocortisone dosage.

Pearls and Precautions

Any infant, especially male infants, with hyponatremia and reciprocal hyperkalemia have CAH secondary to 21-hydroxlase deficiency until proven otherwise.

Any "male" infant with bilateral cryptorchidism and otherwise normal genitalia may be a "masquerading" female with severe virilization and should undergo immediate assessment for CAH (stat 17OHP and karyotype).

In the infant with SVCAH, elevated levels of 17OHP act as a mineralocorticoid antagonist and may cause electrolyte derangements similar to those seen in true salt-wasters.

Boys with CAH require careful testicular examinations at all visits. A careful sonographic screening should be scheduled at the onset of puberty and repeated every few years.

References

Lin-Su K, Nimkarn S, New MI. Congenital adrenal hyperplasia in adolescents: diagnosis and management. Ann NY Acad Sci 2008;1135:95–98.

Hughes IA. Congenital adrenal hyperplasia: a lifelong disorder. Horm Res 2007;68(Suppl 5):84–89.

Androgen Insensitivity Syndrome (AIS)

Mitchell E. Geffner

Androgen Insensitivity Syndrome (AIS) refers to a group of disorders of sex development caused by mutations of the gene encoding the *androgen receptor* which leads to a spectrum of undervirilization and/or infertility in affected XY males.

Etiology

AIS (formerly known as testicular feminization syndrome) is an X-linked recessive disorder in males (with little or no manifestations in 46,XX females) caused by mutations in the *androgen receptor (AR)* gene located on the proximal long arm of the X chromosome at Xq11-q12. 46,XX women with a single mutated copy of the *AR* gene are carriers of the condition and their 46,XY children (male) will have a 50% chance of being fully affected. Complete AIS results from total loss-of-function mutations of the *AR* gene, whereas partial AIS is due to mis-sense mutations that can be located in any domain of the *AR* gene. Over 300 gene mutations have been described in AIS.

Clinical Presentation and Prognosis:

Demographics: While the incidence of complete AIS is about 1 in 20,000, the incidence of milder degrees of androgen resistance is unknown. Evidence suggests that many cases of unexplained male infertility may be due to the mildest forms of androgen resistance. It has been estimated that 1–2% of "girls" with bilateral inguinal herniae have AIS.

Presenting signs and symptoms: The phenotype of the complete form of AIS is characterized by female external genitalia, absent uterus, lack of sexual hair, and labial gonads. The external genitalia in these individuals are identical to those of a normal female, except for the testes that are usually palpable beneath the labia majora. In the neonate, the external genitalia are fully female on inspection, although physical examination may reveal inguinal herniae or palpable testes. After puberty, the typical presentation includes full adult breast development, but no sexual hair. Spontaneous pubertal breast development typically occurs as a consequence of estrogen produced by peripheral aromatization from testicular androgens. Müllerian duct derivatives do not develop, similar to what occurs in normal males. The vas deferens, epididymis, and seminal vesicles, as well as the prostate, are absent. At puberty, lack of responsiveness to androgens leads to no or only sparse sexual hair development. Patients who have been reared as females may present with complaints of amenorrhea, lack of sexual hair, or short vagina.

Complete AIS (CAIS) should be suspected in infancy if inguinal or labial masses are recognized or, at puberty in the phenotypic female presenting with breast development and primary amenorrhea.

Partial AIS (PAIS) covers the spectrum ranging from the 46,XY infant presenting with a micropenis or genital ambiguity with perineo-scrotal hypospadias, bifid scrotum, and labial/inguinal masses (testes), to the 46,XY phenotypic adult male presenting with infertility and gynecomastia. Of note, carrier mothers may display some minor traits of the condition, including reduced amounts of axillary hair, pubic hair, and adolescent acne.

However a spectrum of partial varieties exist with a predominantly male phenotype, but small genitalia, gynecomastia, and decreased spermatogenesis.

Clinical course: Concerns related to the diagnosis of AIS will depend on the age of diagnosis, the presenting manifestations, and the severity of the phenotype. Early diagnosis via herniae appearance requires urgent medical attention. Detection of testicular tissue in the phenotypic female requires significant discussions between the family and a medical team well-versed in disorders of sex development in order to provide appropriate counseling with regard to the necessity for and timing of orchiectomy. Appropriately timed and staged introduction of estrogen therapy during the adolescent years is a key management issue in the setting of early orchiectomy. Appropriate screening strategies for testicular tumors must be considered for retained testes maintained in situ to allow natural feminization via aromatization of androgen to estrogen.

Prognosis: Due to the presence of a Y chromosome, the risk for gonadal tumors, particularly carcinoma in situ (CIS) and seminomas, is increased. Controversy exists regarding whether removal of the testes is necessary. For patients with CAIS, but not PAIS, delay of orchiectomy until after the completion of pubertal feminization may be beneficial. In males with PAIS, partially descended testicles could arguably provide some hope for fertility, function, and cosmesis in the future. If left intact, gonads should be carefully monitored for development of malignancy. One series reported that <5% of patients with CAIS who underwent gonadal biopsy had testicles with CIS.

Diagnosis

The receptor defect occurs not only in classical androgen-responsive tissues, but also in the hypothalamus and pituitary. Thus, lack of negative feedback inhibition during infancy and after puberty causes elevated serum testosterone and luteinizing hormone (LH) concentrations. Sequential LH and testosterone measurements in infants with androgen insensitivity show the normal post-natal LH and testosterone surge in infants with partial AIS, but not in those with complete AIS. By contrast, both in infancy and after 10 years of age, follicle-stimulating hormone (FSH) concentrations are normal or only mildly elevated.

Mothers (46,XX) of affected males have a single mutated copy of the *AR* gene, are carriers of AIS, and may display some minor clinical traits of the condition such as decreased secondary sexual hair and reduced adolescent acne.

Management

Medication: After orchiectomy, estrogen needs to be taken in order to support pubertal development, bone mineral density accrual, and completion of growth. This can be in the form of oral conjugated equine estrogens, oral ethinyl estradiol, or trans-dermal estradiol preparations (using dosage schedules as noted in the section on Kallmann syndrome). Since there is no uterus, progesterone may not be necessary.

Surgery: The overall necessity of testicular removal and its optimal timing (if any) remains the most controversial surgical management issue in these individuals. For women in whom a shallow vagina impedes normal sexual relations, self-dilation or surgical correction can be considered.

Psychological: Gender identity in patients with CAIS is almost always female. Counseling is a key element of CAIS management (see below). Many women with CAIS find value in making connections with others similarly affected. Internet support groups are available (http://www.indiana.edu/~ais/html/home.html; http://www.aissg.org/; and http://home.vicnet.net.au/~aissg/).

Social support: There are three ethical considerations regarding disclosure of the diagnosis of AIS. First, withholding information from these patients based on the assumption that physicians or parents are better able to determine what is in the patient's best interest, is ethically questionable. Second, the principle of informed consent asserts an ethical imperative to disclose such a diagnosis to the patient. For minors, participation in decision-making is guided by the concept of "assent" in line with a child's developmental capacity. Third, maintaining patient confidentiality is in direct conflict with the responsibility of informing other members of the family that they and their offspring may be at risk for the same condition.

Monitoring: Ongoing laboratory testing would be related only to monitoring for side effects of estrogen therapy (see section on Kallmann syndrome). For those individuals who opt to retain their testes, annual ultrasounds may help to detect early cancer.

Pearls and Precautions

- The diagnosis of AIS must be considered in an infant "female" who presents with bilateral inguinal herniae and in the adolescent "female" who presents with normal breast development, but little or no secondary sexual hair and primary amenorrhea.
- Each individual's phenotype generally correlates with the degree of androgen-action impairment, but phenotypic heterogeneity (*e.g.,* variation in clinical features) may occur in multiple affected individuals in one family.
- Since the risk of testicular cancer is relatively low, there is much controversy surrounding the necessity and timing of testicular removal.
- The diagnosis of AIS raises significant ethical issues with regard to if, when, and how disclosure should occur.

References

Galani A, Kitsiou-Tzeli S, Sofokleous C, Kanavakis E, Kalpini-Mavrou A. Androgen insensitivity syndrome: clinical features and molecular defects. Hormones (Athens) 2008 ;7:217–229.

Hughes IA, Deeb A. Androgen resistance. Best Pract Res Clin Endocrinol Metab 2006;20:577–598.

Craniopharyngioma

Mitchell E. Geffner

Craniopharyngiomas are congenital solid-cystic tumors of the hypothalamic-pituitary region, appearing most often in children and adolescents. The tumor and/or its surgical treatment may interfere with pituitary and hypothalamic function, damage the optic chiasm, and cause hydrocephalus.

Etiology

Craniopharyngiomas are unique tumors of embryological origin that typically develop in the suprasellar region. They are thought to arise from rests of pharyngeal epithelium deriving from remnants of Rathke cleft/pouch that subsequently form benign neoplastic cells. Most commonly, craniopharyngiomas are cystic with areas of focal solid components.

Clinical Presentation and Prognosis

Demographics: Craniopharyngiomas account for 80–90% of all childhood tumors originating in and around the pituitary region, and are the third most common cause of all intracranial tumors in children. In the U.S., the overall incidence of craniopharyngioma is 1.3 per 106 person-years, with ~28% of cases affecting children under 14 years of age. There are no differences in incidence by sex or race. There is a bimodal peak in incidence, with the first in childhood (ages 5–14 yrs.) and the second in adults >50 yr.

Presenting signs and symptoms: Craniopharyngiomas usually arise in the suprasellar region (and not in the pituitary gland itself) and may potentially involve many nearby critical structures, such as the optic chiasm and optic tracts, third ventricle, hypothalamus, thalamus, and pituitary stalk. Lateral extension of the tumor can impact major blood vessels such as the internal carotid arteries, as well as the medial temporal lobe. Posterior growth may involve the top of the basilar artery among other vascular connections to the brain, as well as impinge on and distort the rostral brainstem.

The most common presenting signs of craniopharyngiomas in children are headache, emesis, oculomotor abnormalities, papilledema, and other similar symptoms related to increased intracranial pressure. Optic chiasmatic compression and optic nerve atrophy may lead to visual field defects in some children.

Available data suggest that a significant number of patients (80–90%) have endocrine deficiencies at the time of tumor diagnosis. The details are described in the Table 4.1. It should be noted that much of these data preceded the era of CT/MRI imaging and, thus, the tumors were quite advanced at the time of diagnosis.

Table 4.1: Presenting Endocrine Deficiencies at Time of Tumor Diagnosis

Hormone	Percentage Abnormal	Comment
GH	• in 75%	52% present with growth deceleration
Gonadotropins	• in 40%	Rarely present with *precocious* puberty
TSH	• in 25%	—
ACTH	• in 25%	—
Prolactin	• in 20%	—
Anti-diuretic hormone	• in 9–17%	Causes diabetes insipidus

Clinical course: Once diagnosed, treatment planning for craniopharyngiomas consists of three areas: imaging, ophthalmological examination, and endocrinological work-up. Imaging is crucial to determine the full extent of the lesion (for details, see Diagnosis). In current practice, this often consists of both CT and MRI. CT scanning best delineates the presence of calcium which distinguishes these tumors from others. MRI best shows the full extent of the lesion, the ratio of cyst-to-solid tumor, and the involvement of local brain structures.

Prognosis: The prognosis of these patients greatly depends on the surgeon's ability to maximize tumor resection while minimizing damage to the critical adjacent brain structures. Some of the most common neurosurgical approaches used today include trans-callosal inter-hemispheric craniotomies along with sub-frontal, pterional, and trans-sphenoidal craniotomies that allow elevation of the brain and separation of the tumor from the optic apparatus. Even in the best hands, craniopharyngioma surgery has a mortality rate of 2–43%, and is associated with a high overall morbidity (12–61%), hypothalamic injury (40%), and visual deterioration (19%). The sequelae of the radiation treatment of this disease include visual deficits, endocrinopathies, neuro-cognitive and neuro-psychological disorders, and appetite and sleep abnormalities.

Post-operative endocrine dysfunction typically depends on the extent of the surgical intervention (*e.g.,* whether the infundibulum must be sacrificed) and radiation therapy.

Diagnosis

Detailed imaging with CT or MRI will reveal calcifications and cystic components, respectively. The differential diagnosis of tumors/lesions detected in the parasellar region includes chiasmatic/hypothalamic glioma, germinoma, Langerhans cell histiocytosis, and Rathke cleft cyst. Some patients are symptomatic and present with non-specific concerns, such as headache and visual disturbances, and some can even have specific endocrine abnormalities.

Management

Medication: High-dose intravenous dexamethasone (0.5–1.0 mg/kg pre-operatively followed by 0.25–0.5 mg/kg/d in four divided doses) is used to treat peri-tumoral edema in the peri-operative period (which will easily provide any stress-dose glucocorticoid coverage in case of known or unknown central adrenal insufficiency). Hormonal replacement is given pre-, intra-, and immediately post-operatively as needed [glucocorticoid (dexamethasone and later hydrocortisone), antidiuretic hormone (vasopressin or DDAVP), and/or thyroxine]. Subsequently, treatment with growth hormone and sex steroids is common.

Surgery: In almost all cases, surgery is the initial therapy. This also provides tissue to establish the diagnosis. Predominantly solid craniopharyngiomas require surgical approaches which maximize tumor resection while limiting damage to adjacent structures. In cases where large cysts are causing neurological dysfunction, the goal of surgery is to maximally resect the cyst(s), leaving the solid component for a second-stage surgery or for radiation. It should be noted that oftentimes the ability to separate the tumor from the optic apparatus and/ or hypothalamus can only be determined intra-operatively. Improved surgical techniques have resulted in a significant improvement in safety. Novel imaging techniques such as MR spectroscopy and high-definition MRI, allow better delineation of the tumor and sparing of critical brain structures. Surgical adjuvants, such as the cavitron ultrasonic aspirator, intra-operative ultrasound, and frameless stereotaxy, have made the surgery itself safer. Specific treatment of large residual cysts may be required in the form of direct administration of chemotherapy (bleomycin) and radiation therapy (phosphorus-32).

Radiation therapy: The role of radiation in the treatment of craniopharyngioma remains controversial. It is most efficacious for small solid tumors that do not directly contact the optic apparatus or hypothalamus. Some data suggest that subtotal tumor resection followed by radiation is an acceptable alternative to total surgical resection which has a high incidence of morbidity. Different groups have advocated different types of radiation therapy including conventional beam therapy, stereotactic radio-surgery (e.g., gamma knife), and proton beam therapy. With the development of some of these newer techniques, the morbidity of radiation may be further reduced. In recurrences and tumors that are not amenable to total resection, radiation should be considered as the next line of treatment. The conventional mode of radiotherapy has been fractionated external beam therapy with a recommended dose of 54–55 Gy at 1.8 Gy per fraction. While radiation dosage inversely correlates with the recurrence rate, it tends to directly relate to morbidity in these patients.

Psychological: Although the tumor itself is not associated with psychological/psychiatric manifestations, the presence of a brain tumor certainly can cause psychological trauma for the child and family. Additionally, resultant hypopituitarism may have direct (if untreated) or indirect psychological ramifications (e.g., depression). Hypothalamic obesity may also be associated with depression.

Social support: All older children with central adrenal insufficiency must wear Medic-Alert identification.

Monitoring: Hormone testing prior to surgical intervention can document the extent of pituitary damage caused by the tumor. Alternatively, this can be deferred until after surgery as panhypopituitarism, if not present pre-operatively, is likely to ensue from the surgical extirpation of the tumor. The hormonal abnormalities that require pre-operative vigilance are ACTH/cortisol and anti-diuretic hormone, as failure to diagnose and treat deficiencies could have catastrophic outcomes from the stress of surgery. However, high-dose dexamethasone is uniformly given for neurosurgical purposes and provides any required stress glucocorticoid coverage around the time of operation. In addition, the presence of pre-operative diabetes insipidus is quite unusual, but is usually readily apparent on simple clinical and biochemical grounds, and easily remediable with appropriate intravenous fluid regimens and desmopressin. Regardless of the results of pre-operative hormonal testing, repeat and more extensive hormone testing in the post-operative period is needed to evaluate pituitary function. As noted above, almost all children will have or develop growth hormone deficiency (GHD). The degree of other hormonal deficiencies will depend on the aggressiveness of the tumor and the surgery, with panhypopituitarism a very common sequel.

A pre-operative vision assessment to assess damage inflicted by the tumor itself should be performed by a pediatric ophthalmologist or neuro-ophthalmologist. This includes careful indirect ophthalmoscopy with dilatation and formal visual field testing (*e.g.,* by Goldman field examination or computerized perimetry). Repeat post-operative testing will document any worsening or improvement that ensues.

Pearls and Precautions

- Craniopharyngiomas are histologically benign tumors that are geographically malignant in terms of their ability to involve vital brain structures, making complete surgical removal problematic.
- Patients with craniopharyngioma more commonly present with irregular quadrianopsias rather than the classically described bitemporal hemianopsia (symmetrical bilateral loss of portions of the outer visual fields). Irregular quadrianopsias are due to the presence of uneven effects of these tumors impinging on the optic chiasm.
- There is a high incidence of permanent GHD in these children with frequent diabetes insipidus in the post-operative period which may remit. Other central hormone deficiencies may occur, but always in the setting of GHD, and must be replaced accordingly.
- Some children with documented GHD have normal growth in height throughout childhood.
- GH treatment has not been shown to increase the risk of craniopharyngioma growth or recurrence rates.
- Hypothalamic obesity tends to be the most frustrating complication of craniopharyngioma and its treatment. It is highly associated with all the typical complications of morbid obesity and, in almost all cases, remains refractory to standard and experimental therapies.
- Lateral skull X-ray can facilitate a diagnosis in 89% of cases. Presence of suprasellar or sellar calcifications and/or changes in the bony architecture of the sella (*e.g.,* thinning/erosion of the anterior and/or posterior clinoids and/or a double floor of the sella) are the diagnostic radiographic findings in craniopharyngiomas.

References

Keil MF, Stratakis CA. Pituitary tumors in childhood: update of diagnosis, treatment and molecular genetics. Expert Rev Neurother 2008;8:563–574.

May JA, Krieger MD, Bowen I, Geffner ME. Craniopharyngioma in childhood. Adv Pediatr 2006;53:183–209.

Diabetes (Type 1)

Eba H. Hathout

Type 1 Diabetes is caused by insulin deficiency due to genetic, environmental, autoimmune and idiopathic destruction of pancreatic β-cells, which tilts glucose homeostasis towards pathologic hyperglycemia.

Etiology

Although the precise cause of this disease is unknown, some of the possible contributory factors include:

- *Autoimmune* destruction of beta cells, evidenced by detected antibodies to islet cells, glutamic acid decarboxylase and insulin in newly diagnosed patients' sera, and association with other autoimmune disorders (thyroiditis 3–5%, celiac 2–5%, and Addison's <1%).
- *Genetic* factors are implied by the identification of numerous susceptibility loci several of which are located in the major histocompatibility complex (MHC) region on the short arm of chromosome 6 which contains genes that regulate the immune response. For example, higher risk is conferred by the presence of DR3 and DR4, and by the absence of an aspartate residue at position 57 of the DQB chain. The allele DQB1*0602 is considered protective.
- *Environmental* culprits include viral, chemical, nutritional, and stress etiologies.

Pathology

In view of insulin's pivotal anabolic role in directing glucose towards glycogen, lipid and protein synthesis, its deficiency halts a number of glucose homeostatic mechanisms. The result is a decrease in glucose uptake by muscle and fat, together with an increase in glycogenolysis and gluconeogenesis. Progressive hyperglycemia exceeds the renal threshold, leading to osmotic diuresis and dehydration. Lipolysis leads to excess fatty acids and ketone bodies, metabolic acidosis, and respiratory compensation. Increased stress hormones (glucagon, adrenaline, cortisol, and growth hormone) exacerbate hyperglycemia, dehydration, acidosis and hyperosmolality which together decrease consciousness and are fatal if untreated.

Clinical Presentation and Prognosis

Age of onset: The highest incidence of this disease has typically been during infancy to early adulthood, with peak incidences of 5 and 15 years of age. However, currently the largest increase in incidence worldwide is in children under five years of age.

Presenting signs and symptoms: Symptoms over 1 week to 6 months include polyuria, nocturnal enuresis, polydipsia, weight loss, anorexia, hyperphagia, lethargy, constipation, blurred vision and infection, especially cutaneous candidiasis. Rarely, symptoms of hypoglycemia reflect early islet cell instability. Patients presenting as diabetic ketoacidosis (DKA, 25%) may also have vomiting, abdominal pain and systemic infection. Other signs of DKA include dehydration, sweet-smelling breath, Kussmaul breathing (tachypnea with hyperventilation), decreased consciousness, coma, signs of sepsis, ileus, and signs of cerebral edema. DKA is a more likely presentation in children under 5 years of age in whom the symptoms of polyuria and polydipsia are harder to recognize.

Clinical course: Most symptoms and signs are reversible with appropriate insulin therapy.

Prognosis: With intensive glycemic control, children with type 1 diabetes have a favorable prognosis. Hypoglycemia and weight gain are chronic concerns. Long-term microvascular complications including retinopathy, autonomic and peripheral neuropathy, and nephropathy (starting with microalbuminuria) are less likely in patients with intensive basal/bolus insulin therapy (see Management).

Diagnosis

Blood glucose concentration >200 mg/dL or fasting blood glucose >126 mg/dL, or hemoglobin A1c > 6.5% in the presence of symptoms makes the diagnosis of diabetes straightforward. Type 1-diabetes is more likely in younger non-obese patients without a family history of type 2-diabetes or signs of insulin resistance, and its diagnosis is aided by the detection of diabetes autoantibodies (see Etiology). Transient hyperglycemia may occur in the context of concomitant illness. Borderline glucose levels warrant consultation with a pediatric endocrinologist and possibly a glucose tolerance test to confirm the diagnosis. Hyperglycemia in the presence of ketonuria—with or without acidosis—is the most frequent clue to the diagnosis. Initial management is dependent on the presence or absence of DKA.

Management

At onset, management of patients in diabetic ketoacidosis (DKA) mainly involves intravenous hydration and insulinization along with correction of electrolyte abnormalities and guarding against cerebral edema. For patients who are not in clinical and biochemical DKA (i.e., alert with stable vital signs, no postural hypotension, no Kussmaul breathing, bicarbonate level >15 mmol/L), subcutaneous insulin is given as basal/bolus therapy.

Insulin: Multiple Daily Injections

- Basal therapy (40% of total insulin dose) utilizes a long acting insulin such as Lantus every 24 hours or Levemir every 12 hours. Bolus therapy with rapid acting insulin (e.g., Apidra, Humalog, Novolog) is given with meals as a standard base dose of 0.1–0.15 units per kg or according to carbohydrate intake as 1 unit for 15 grams of Carbohydrate (this ratio changes individually and with age). Additional correction with rapid insulin is given at the same time if preprandial blood glucose is above 150 mg/dL (e.g., 1 unit for every 50 mg/dL above 100 mg/dL).

Continuous Subcutaneous Insulin Infusion:

- These devices are in the form of programmable pumps that contain rapid acting insulin, connected by an infusion line to a small plastic cannula inserted subcutaneously, and fixed by self-adhesive tape.

The goal is to deliver variable basal rates based on glycemic profiles in addition to bolus insulin coverage for carbohydrates and unanticipated hyperglycemia (please refer to "Insulin Pump" in the Medical Devices section). Total daily insulin (basal and bolus) by injection or pump ranges from 0.5 to 1.5 units per kg per day. Poor glycemic control on doses >1.5units/kg/day usually denotes non-compliance.

Diet: Carbohydrate counting is encouraged. A sugar-free (ADA) diet is instituted with age-adjusted calories of 1000+100 Kcals per year of age for a maximum 2600 Kcals. Carbohydrates as 50% of total meal calories are encouraged, but less if the patient is overweight.

Self blood glucose monitoring: Greater testing frequency improves metabolic control. Fingerprick checking is recommended daily before meals and at bedtime. Additional checks after meals and between 2 and 3 AM are recommended once or more per week particularly in cases of frequent hypoglycemia or significant physical exercise. Electronic meters with a memory to be downloaded for pattern detection and management are recommended in conjunction with patient/family documented logbooks. Target blood glucose levels are 70–140 mg/dL pre-meals, 120–180 mg/dL at bedtime and a maximum of 180 mg/dL after meals. Hypoglycemia (glucose <60 mg/dL) should be promptly treated with glucose orally (tablets or juice), and in the event of unconsciousness or seizures, with parenteral glucagon (0.5–1.0 mg SC/IM).

Urine Ketone Testing: This is recommended using special strips when blood glucose exceeds 250 mg/dL or during periods of illness. Ketonuria denotes fluid or insulin deficiency or imminent ketoacidosis.

Glycosylated hemoglobin measurement: HbA1c, which is formed by the binding of glucose to adult hemoglobin, best reflects a patient's glycemic control in the preceding 6–8 weeks. This should be measured quarterly on all patients with diabetes. Assays should compare to those used in the "Diabetes Control and Complications Trial" with a goal value of under 7.6%, and an ideal target range of 6 to 7%, to minimize future complications.

Other routine lab tests: At diagnosis: Diabetes autoimmune antibodies (glutamic acid, islet cell and GAD=diabetes autoimmune test group at Quest or Esoterix lab facilities), celiac panel, thyroid peroxidase and thyroglobulin antibodies, thyroid stimulating hormone (TSH). The following tests should be done in the fasting state (6 AM with the patient NPO since midnight): plasma glucose, C-peptide and lipid panel.

Annually, TSH fasting lipid profiles: If diabetes duration is >5 years, urine microalbumin to creatinine ratio should be measured and ophthalmologic evaluation be done.

Symptom-driven tests and referrals: Unexplained abdominal pain or pallor, or inadequate weight gain: CBC, ferritin, celiac panel. Unexplained hypoglycemia or inadequate weight gain: Cortisol and ACTH (8 AM). Referral to pediatric neurology, nephrology, psychiatry, dermatology, or podiatry is indicated for evidence of neuropathy, progressive nephropathy, psychopathology particularly depression, unusual skin manifestations or recurrent foot infections.

Pearls and Precautions

1. Diabetes presenting under one year of age, particularly under 6 months of age, may be monogenic and treatable with oral sulfonylureas. DNA testing is available in research laboratories.
2. Diabetes presenting at age 11 years or later in lean individuals with a similar picture in siblings, parents and grandparents may be maturity onset diabetes of the young (MODY), also treatable with sulfonylurea's and diagnosable by DNA testing in commercial laboratories.
3. The most common reason for frequent ketoacidosis (DKA) is noncompliance.

4. Failure of recovery from DKA despite careful fluid, electrolyte and insulin therapy may denote concomitant adrenal insufficiency or cerebral edema. Cerebral edema may result from rapid glucose and sodium decrease.

5. Frequent hypoglycemia may lead to hypoglycemic unawareness, which is potentially fatal.

Miscellaneous

Associated diseases include celiac disease, thyroiditis, and adrenalitis. Also see Type 2 Diabetes.

The following organizations' websites have useful information regarding childhood diabetes: International Society for Pediatric and Adolescent Diabetes (ISPAD.org), American Diabetes Association (Diabetes.org), Juvenile Diabetes Research Foundation (JDRF.org), International Diabetes Federation (IDF.org).

Social and school issues require the assistance of a pediatric diabetes team to facilitate compliance including self glucose monitoring and insulin administration during school, camp, and extracurricular activities.

Adolescence is the most challenging age-group to handle as the counter-insulin pubertal hormones rise, and compliance suffers due to depression, peer pressure, problems with self-image including body weight and eating disorders.

A pediatric diabetes team with social workers, psychologists, nurse educators and dietitian working together with the pediatric endocrinologist and the patient's family is highly recommended for the care of children with type 1 diabetes.

References

Raine JE, Donaldson MDC, Gregory JW, Savage MO and Hintz RL. *Practical Endocrinology and Diabetes in Children*. Oxford, Blackwell Publishing Ltd, 2006.

Steck AK, Klingensmith GJ, Fiallo-Scharer R. Recent advances in insulin treatment of children. Pediatr Diabetes. 2007 Oct;8 Suppl 6:49–56.

Diabetes (Type 2)

Eba H. Hathout

Type 2 Diabetes is due to relative insulin deficiency that is caused by insulin resistance or decreased insulin secretion.

Etiology

Genetic factors are implied by the strong familial incidence as well as prevalence in African American, Hispanic and Asian populations. Higher risk is conferred by obesity, sedentary lifestyle, female gender and being small for gestational age at birth. Environmental culprits also include ambient pollution and stress etiologies.

Pathology: In view of insulin's pivotal anabolic role in directing glucose towards glycogen, lipid and protein synthesis, its dysfunction halts a number of glucose homeostatic mechanisms. The result is a decrease in glucose uptake by muscle and fat, together with an increase in glycogenolysis and gluconeogenesis. Progressive hyperglycemia can exceed the renal threshold leading to osmotic diuresis. Lipolysis may lead to excess fatty acids and ketone bodies.

Clinical Presentation and Prognosis

Age of onset: This form of diabetes is most common over 40 years of age, with notable increasing incidence in children and adolescents. Up to 33% of newly diagnosed patients aged 10–19 years with diabetes in the U.S., have the type 2 form of this disease. Type 2 Diabetes has been detected in obese children as young as 4 years of age.

Presenting signs and symptoms: Many patients are asymptomatic. Therefore, screening of patients at risk by virtue of family history or obesity is indicated. Most are overweight at diagnosis, with absent or mild polyuria and polydipsia, and little or no weight loss. They may also have hyperglycemia and glycosuria without ketonuria. However, ketoacidosis is present in 5–25% of patients at diagnosis (see Type 1 Diabetes). Acanthosis nigricans (thickened darkened skin of neck or axillae), symptoms of ovarian hyperandrogenism (irregular menses or hirsutism), hypertension and hyperlipidemia may also be present.

Clinical course: Most symptoms and signs are reversible with appropriate diet, exercise, oral hypoglycemic agents and/or insulin therapy.

Prognosis: With intensive glycemic control, most patients have a favorable prognosis. Long-term microvascular complications including retinopathy, autonomic and peripheral neuropathy, and nephropathy (starting with microalbuminuria) are less likely in patients with good glycemic control. Macrovascular complications (ischemic heart disease and peripheral vascular disease) are more likely in adults with prolonged poor glycemic control.

Diagnosis

Blood glucose concentrations >200 mg/dL fasting blood glucose >126 mg/dL, and/or HbA1c > 6.5% make the diagnosis of diabetes straightforward Type 2 diabetes is more likely in older obese children with a family history of type 2 diabetes and/or signs of insulin resistance, and its diagnosis is aided by the detection of high endogenous insulin (C-peptide) levels concomitant with hyperglycemia. Transient hyperglycemia may occur in the context of concomitant illness or high-dose glucocorticoid use. Borderline high glucose levels warrant consultation with a pediatric endocrinologist and a glucose or mixed meal tolerance test to confirm the diagnosis. Initial management is dependant on the degree of hyperglycemia and the presence or absence of ketoacidosis.

Management

The aims of treatment are: (1) Maintenance of a normal glucose profile at all times (70–150 mg/dL pre-meals and maximum 180 mg/dL postprandially and at bedtime); and (2) Normalization of HbA1c to < 7%. See Type 1 Diabetes management for self-monitoring of blood glucose, urine ketone testing and HbA1c monitoring. The following stepwise approach can be used in type 2 diabetes if preprandial blood glucose is <250 mg/dL in the absence of DKA:

Medications

Metformin: This is an oral hypoglycemic agent (of the biguanide family) which, in the presence of endogenous insulin secretion, increases muscle glucose uptake and metabolism, and decreases hepatic gluconeogenesis. Starting doses are 250–500 mg b.i.d to t.i.d taken with food to minimize nausea, abdominal discomfort and diarrhea. Hypoglycemia is extremely rare compared to other hypoglycemic agents and lactic acidosis is unlikely in the presence of normal hepatic and renal function.

Other oral hypoglycemic agents: Acarbose, sulfonylureas, thiazolidinediones, and dipeptidyl peptidase inhibitors can be used in combination.

Insulin: If, despite diet, exercise and oral agents, glucose levels are poorly controlled and frequently exceed 250 mg/dL before meals, insulin is recommended using basal-bolus therapy (see Type 1 Diabetes).

Nutrition: Diet is the most pivotal component in the management of type 2 diabetes. Carbohydrate restriction and saturated fat minimization help reduce weight and maintain a healthy lipid and cardiovascular profile, all of which reduce long-term complications.

Miscellaneous: Physical exercise enhances glucose uptake by liver and muscle and aids weight reduction efforts.

Pearls and Precautions

1. Some patients have type 1 diabetes with obesity and clinical signs of insulin resistance. These can benefit from metformin therapy in addition to insulin.
2. Some patients have slowly progressive type 1 diabetes that may be mistaken for type 2 diabetes at onset. These patients are best maintained on low dose basal insulin to preserve long-term beta-cell function.

3. Some patients with type 2 diabetes have positive islet cell or thyroid antibodies.

4. Patients with type 2 diabetes can present in ketoacidosis.

5. If the type of diabetes is still questionable after 2 years of diagnosis, a mixed meal tolerance test using commercially available formulas (such as Boost, Carnation, Ensure) can be performed. Administration of 6 cc/kg (up to 300 cc) orally is done with plasma glucose and C-peptide levels drawn before and 90 minutes after administration. Normal or elevated C-peptide levels with concurrent high glucose values, and a rise of more than 50% in C-peptide following formula administration are suggestive of type 2 diabetes. The test is best done eliminating the preceding doses of basal and bolus insulin.

See Type 1 Diabetes for routine and symptom-based laboratory tests, referrals, organizational websites, and social and school issues particularly during adolescence.

Miscellaneous

Other types of diabetes include, cystic fibrosis-related diabetes [CFRD (best treated with insulin)], post-transplant diabetes, and secondary diabetes. Excess glucocorticoids (e.g., exogenous or Cushing syndrome), glucagon, or growth hormone can lead to hyperglycemia.

Post-transplant diabetes may not be permanent, has features of insulin deficiency and resistance, occasionally presents in DKA, and is very dependent on the immunosuppressive regimen. Treatment options include oral hypoglycemic agents and/or insulin.

Other associations with diabetes include Down syndrome, Turner syndrome, Klinefelter syndrome, asparaginase treatment, thalassemia, diabetes insipidus/optic atrophy/deafness (DIDMOAD) and the autoimmune polyendocrine syndromes.

References

Raine JE, Donaldson MDC, Gregory JW, Savage MO and Hintz RL. *Practical Endocrinology and Diabetes in Children*. Oxford, Blackwell Publishing Ltd, 2006.

Peterson K, Silverstein J, Kaufman F, Warren-Boulton E. Management of type 2 diabetes in youth. An update. *American Family Physician*. 2007 Sep 1;76(5):658–64. Review

Congenital Hyperinsulinism (CHI)

Mitchell E. Geffner

Congenital hyperinsulinism refers to a variety of genetic disorders in which early-onset hypoglycemia is caused by excessive insulin secretion due to one of several known mutations involving exuberant glucose-coupled insulin secretion by the pancreatic ß-cell.

Etiology

Hyperinsulinism is the most common etiology of hypoglycemia persisting beyond the immediate neonatal period (first hour of life). This condition has been referred to by a variety of names over the past 50 years: nesidioblastosis and islet cell adenomatosis were in the 1970's, islet cell dysmaturation syndrome in the 1980's, and persistent hyperinsulinemic hypoglycemia of infancy (PHHI) in the 1990s. Several inborn errors of pancreatic ß-cell function disrupt the normal linkage between insulin release and the ambient glucose concentration. These include mutations in the following genes: (1) *Sulfonylurea receptor* (*SUR1*) diffusely throughout the ß-cells of the pancreas (~50% of genetic CHI cases) which can be inherited either in an autosomal dominant or an autosomal recessive manner; (2) *SUR1* focally in the pancreas (one-third of the time localized to the head of the pancreas) resulting from uniparental disomy with loss of heterozygosity (~40% of genetic CHI cases); (3) *inward rectifying potassium channel* (*Kir6.2*) diffusely throughout the ß-cells of the pancreas which can be inherited either in an autosomal dominant or an autosomal recessive manner; (4) *glutamate dehydrogenase* (*GLUD1*) in ß-cells and hepatocytes causing gain-of-function and also associated with hyperammonemia which is inherited in an autosomal dominant fashion; and (5) *glucokinase,* gain-of-function of which is inherited in an autosomal dominant fashion and leads to constitutive activation of the first and rate-limiting step of glycolysis, thereby increasing the intracellular ATP/ADP ratio, sufficient to trigger insulin release at lower-than-normal blood glucose concentrations. Neonatal hyperinsulinemic hypoglycemia also occurs in ~50% of infants with Beckwith-Wiedemann syndrome and is typically a transient issue. Transient forms of congenital hyperinsulinism may occur secondary to maternal factors as seen in the infant of diabetic mothers, perinatal stress (*e.g.,* birth asphyxia, low birth weight, pre-eclampsia, toxemia, premature labor, and premature birth), intravenous glucose administered during labor and delivery, and maternal use of certain medications (*e.g.,* terbutaline, propranolol, oral sulfonylureas, and other hypoglycemic agents used to treat gestational or type 2 diabetes).

Clinical Presentation and Prognosis

Demographics: Permanent CHI occurs in 1 per 30,000–50,000 live births.

Presenting signs and symptoms: Hypoglycemic infants typically display jitteriness, hunger, cyanosis, hypothermia, and irritability, and may progress to having overt generalized seizures. Many of these presenting features are non-specific and may be a sign of sepsis.

Clinical course: The typically affected child presents with recurrent and often severe hypoglycemia in infancy and, on occasion, in later childhood. Careful confirmation of hyperinsulinemia as the etiology is mandatory, with molecular testing often pinpointing the specific genetic cause and directing the type of medical therapy and/or the need for surgical treatment. In order to avoid brain damage, strict avoidance of low blood sugars—especially prior to 3 years of age—is critical. Medical therapy may be used in preparation for surgery or, on occasion, as sole long-term treatment. In the latter case, careful monitoring and, where possible, treatment of drug side effects is required.

Prognosis: The most significant long-term concern in any infant with recurrent and/or severe hypoglycemia is permanent brain damage. Recent evidence supports the possibility of impaired visual cortex function with ongoing severe hypoglycemia in term neonates, especially in the youngest infants whose nervous systems are rapidly maturing. Early brain MRI abnormalities seen in full-term hypoglycemic infants appear to be more predictive of neurodevelopmental outcome than does the severity and/or duration of their hypoglycemia.

Diagnosis

Clinicians should suspect hypoglycemia in any newborn whose jitteriness, hunger, and irritability are promptly relieved by eating. A history of fetal macrosomia or onset of persistent hypoglycemia within the first 12 hours of life should raise suspicion for CHI. Another clinical factor supporting a diagnosis of hyperinsulinism is rapidly developing hypoglycemia for which IV glucose delivery at a rate of >12 mg/kg/min is necessary to maintain adequate serum glucose. Untreated progressive hypoglycemia may lead to neuroglycopenic symptoms, such as declining level of consciousness or seizure. Definitive evaluation begins with procurement of a "critical" sample at the time of confirmed hypoglycemia. Hyperinsulinism is diagnosed by the presence of any detectable serum insulin (usually >2 µU/mL) measured simultaneously with a low glucose concentration, preferably <50 mg/dL. Occasionally, measurement of c-peptide (the equimolar co-cleavage product, along with insulin, that is derived from proinsulin) or proinsulin itself in the critical sample is helpful to diagnose or confirm the presence of hyperinsulinemia. At the time of hypoglycemia, this diagnosis is further supported by the absence of blood and urine ketones, low serum ß-hydroxybutyrate (<2 mM), and low plasma free fatty acids (<1.5 mM). These all result from the action of insulin to prevent lipolysis. Detection of a low serum level of insulin-like growth factor binding protein-1 (IGFBP-1) in the critical sample also points toward the presence of hyperinsulinemia as this analyte is inversely regulated by insulin. An inappropriate glycemic rise of at least 30 mg/dL (from a basal glucose concentration of <50 mg/dL) following 1 mg of intravenous or intramuscular glucagon further supports this diagnosis. This increase in blood glucose (which fails to occur in nearly all other etiologies of hypoglycemia) is due to hyperinsulinemia leading to continuous replenishment of hepatic glycogen, that is in turn broken down by the administered glucagon, into glucose. An elevated ammonia level would suggest the hyperinsulinemic/hyperammonemic form of CHI.

Management

Medication: The primary medical therapy for CHI remains diazoxide (5–15 mg/kg orally divided into two daily doses) which, when given by the enteral route, suppresses pancreatic β-cell insulin secretion. If not completely successful, the parenteral insulin suppressant, octreotide, is administered next (5–20 μg/kg/day subcutaneously divided in 3–4 doses daily). The final medical adjunct is glucagon (1 mg/day as a continuous subcutaneous infusion).

Surgery: If maximal medical therapy fails, either subtotal (for diffuse lesions) or pancreatic lesionectomy (for focal abnormalities) is performed. The choice may be aided by results of PET scans and/or arterial stimulation of venous sampling.

Therapy: For infants and older children with developmental delay secondary to hypoglycemic brain damage, occupational, physical, and/or speech therapy may be of benefit.

Monitoring: Clearly, frequent daily home blood glucose monitoring is required in the affected child whether treated with medication and/or surgery. Once the glucose levels are stabilized with treatment, the frequency of testing will decrease. To assess glycemia in an integrated fashion, HbA1c levels may be helpful, as chronic hypoglycemia causes a lower than normal result. These approaches will also detect persistent or returning hypoglycemia which may occur when a surgical result is incomplete or hyperglycemia when excessive pancreatic tissue is extirpated. For those children treated medically with diazoxide, periodic complete blood counts can detect neutropenia. For those receiving somatostatin analogs, periodic monitoring for effects on growth (length/height measurements), thyroid function (free T4 and TSH), and gall bladder function (ultrasound) is required.

Pearls and Precautions

- Diagnosis of the specific etiology of CHI by biochemical, radiological, and/or molecular methods should be attempted to optimize the recommended treatment to improve long-term outcome and to provide appropriate genetic counseling.
- Both medical and surgical therapies for CHI are fraught with risks. Diazoxide causes acute fluid retention and chronic hypertrichosis that can be quite disfiguring. Adverse effects of octreotide include diarrhea, gallstones, and suppression of other hormones, including GH and thyroid hormones. Finally, resection of more than 85–90% of the pancreas may lead to insulin-dependent diabetes in the future.
- In the U.S., the most experienced center for the management of children with CHI is Children's Hospital of Philadelphia.

References

De Leon DD, Stanley CA. Mechanisms of disease: Advances in diagnosis and treatment of hyperinsulinism in neonates. Nat Clin Pract Endocrinol Metab 2007;3:57–68.

Ferry RJ, Allen D. Hypoglycemia. In: Kappy M, Geffner M, Allen D (eds). Pediatric Practice: Endocrinology. McGraw-Hill, 2009.

Kallmann Syndrome

Mitchell E. Geffner

Kallmann syndrome is defined as the presence of both hypogonadotropic hypogonadism and either hyposmia (reduced sense of smell) or anosmia (absent sense of smell).

Etiology

During embryological development, GnRH-producing and olfactory neurons migrate together. GnRH is released from neurons in the arcuate nucleus of the hypothalamus in a pulsatile fashion to stimulate pituitary synthesis and secretion of LH and FSH, which in turn, promote gonadal steroidogenesis and gametogenesis. Impairment of both GnRH function and olfactory neuronal migration results in Kallmann syndrome, defined as the presence of both hypogonadotropic hypogonadism and either hyposmia (reduced sense of smell) or anosmia (absent sense of smell), respectively. This condition was described in 1944 by Franz Josef Kallmann, a German-American geneticist. However, others, such as the Spanish doctor, Aureliano Maestre de San Juan, had previously noticed a correlation between anosmia and hypogonadism in 1856. Kallmann syndrome can occur in either partial or complete forms. It is thought to be either a monogenic or digenic disorder involving one or more of the following genes: *Kallmann syndrome 1 sequence (KAL1), FGF receptor 1 (FGFR1), prokineticin 2 (PROK2), prokineticin receptor 2 (PROKR2),* and *nasal embryonic LHRH factor (NELF).*

Clinical Presentation and Prognosis

Demographics: The disease occurs in 1 in 10,000 male births and 1 in 50,000 female births. The lower frequency of this disease observed in females is due to the fact that its most common form (due to a KAL1 mutation) is inherited in an X-linked recessive manner.

Presenting signs and symptoms: Most affected individuals present with absence of pubertal changes during adolescence or infertility during adulthood. Occasionally, cryptorchidism and/or micropenis in infant males, or hormonal testing in a child with a positive family history, leads to earlier diagnosis. All patients with Kallmann syndrome have either hyposmia or anosmia, and may also exhibit unilateral renal agenesis, atrial septal defect, colorblindness, and synkinesia (mirror movements).

Clinical course: Once diagnosed—either early because of a micropenis and/or undescended testes, or late because of failure to enter or advance in puberty—and possessing an abnormal sense of smell, there are no significant clinical issues until adolescence when testosterone replacement needs to commence. There is no treatment for disordered sense of smell and for most other co-morbidities. Patients with Kallmann syndrome are generally healthy and must deal mostly with issues surrounding sex steroid replacement and, in young adulthood, assisted reproductive strategies for achieving fertility.

Prognosis: The overall prognosis is good. Puberty induction and fertility are accomplished through different hormonal replacements (see below). Osteoporosis may also be a long-term, but manageable issue.

Diagnosis

The sense of smell can easily be confirmed by testing the recognition for common substances such as coffee or peppermint. Very low random serum LH and FSH measurements by ultrasensitive immunochemiluminescent (ICMA) methodology may aid in the diagnosis of hypogonadotropic hypogonadism. However, hypogonadotropic hypogonadism and simple delayed puberty are difficult to differentiate, since low gonadotropin levels are found in both conditions. The serum LH response following administration of synthetic GnRH or its analogs is no longer considered a reliable method of diagnosis and should only be interpreted in conjunction with the clinical presentation and genetic testing. GnRH is administered as leuprolide acetate [20 mcg/kg subcutaneously (maximum dose 500 mcg)], with LH, FSH, and either estradiol (females) or testosterone (males) responses measured at baseline and then at 60, 120, and 180 min., and 24 hrs. after the medication is administered. Any LH level >0.3 mIU/mL indicates normal pituitary reserve and, thus, helps to identify patients who likely have constitutional delay rather than true hypogonadotropic hypogonadism. The above testing strategy can be performed in suspected teenagers or adults, recognizing the fact that the pulsatile nature of gonadotropin secretion may require either multiple or pooled samples. This testing method can also be used in diagnosing at-risk infants (*i.e.,* those with positive family histories) between 6–8 weeks of age when the "mini-puberty of infancy" is most active and, therefore, low function of the hypothalamic-pituitary-gonadal axis may be demonstrated. Additionally, since testosterone production follows a diurnal secretory pattern, "random" serum measurements should be obtained between 8–9 AM, when levels are the highest. Genetic analysis for the *Kal1* and *FGFR1* gene mutations is commercially available. An MRI of the brain with contrast dye enhancement in a closed tube system should be obtained in all patients with hypogonadotropic hypogonadism. Abnormalities of the olfactory placode confirm Kallmann syndrome. A renal ultrasound should also be performed.

Management

Medication: Therapy for boys is aimed at a stepwise replacement of testosterone in order to mimic normal physiology. Historically, this has been accomplished with intramuscular testosterone, starting at 50 mg/mo with a gradual increase over 2-3 years so that most adult men will reach a maintenance dosage of 200–300 mg of depot testosterone every 2–4 weeks. These dosing regimens are based on the adult male testosterone production rate of 6 mg/d. Once at final adult height, older adolescent boys can take testosterone by patch or gel. Although trans-dermal approaches have not been studied for pubertal initiation in the past, availability of the testosterone gel using a pump actuator potentially offers an alternative method of pubertal induction. Therapy for girls with Kallmann syndrome is initiated with daily low-dose estrogen therapy alone for 1–2 years. Conjugated equine estrogens (e.g., Premarin) have traditionally been utilized at a dose of 0.3 mg daily for the first 6 months, 0.625 mg daily for the second 6 months, and then 0.625–1.2 mg daily starting in the second year. Ethinyl estradiol (e.g., Estrace) has also been utilized as oral replacement at a starting dose of 0.02 mg/day for the first 6 months, followed by 0.1 mg for the second 6 months, and 0.2 mg thereafter. Trans-dermal estradiol preparations (e.g., Vivelle patch) are also available and are initiated to provide 0.0625 mg daily, advancing slowly over the following 2 years to a total daily dose of 0.05 to 0.1 mg. Although it is not clear that patch-cutting to accomplish escalated dosing will reliably provide the expected amount of estradiol, this mode is currently being prescribed off-label. Administration of unopposed estrogen (without any added progesterone) using one of the aforementioned formulations and dosage schedules for 1–2 years does not appear to expose the uterus to any undue risk for endometrial hyperplasia and/or malignancy. At the end of the first few years, cyclic progesterone must be added. The two options include oral medroxyprogesterone at 10 mg/day (e.g., Provera) and micronized progesterone at 200 mg/day (e.g., Prometrium) on days 20–30 of each cycle. With this approach, withdrawal bleeding generally occurs in the following 3–10 days, although there can be some variability among patients. Another option is to provide continuous estrogen followed by progesterone on days 100–120 of the cycle to minimize menstruation, but provide uterine protection. Alternatively, at adult dosing, the aforementioned estrogen delivery methods are often abandoned in favor of a more conventional oral contraceptive or substituted with a weekly estrogen patch used in conjunction with oral progesterone. There are now available oral contraceptive agents (e.g., Seasonale and Quasense) that decrease the frequency of menstruation to every 3 months. Patients of either sex with hypogonadotropic hypogonadism are potentially fertile, but sex steroid therapy alone will not usually initiate gametogenesis. Thus, assuming an intact pituitary gland, the typical approach to fertility induction is pump-administered GnRH therapy or parenteral combination gonadotropin treatment (synthetic LH/hCG and recombinant FSH) that is supervised by a reproductive endocrinologist.

Psychological: Affected patients may have depressive and social withdrawal symptoms related to delayed puberty and/or infertility similar to other individuals with hypogonadism, but are not otherwise uniquely prone to psychological problems.

Social support: Patient support organizations for individuals with Kallmann syndrome include: The Pituitary Foundation (http://www.kallmanns.org/) and HYPOHH (http://www.hypohh.net/).

Laboratory tests and monitoring: In addition to the diagnostic tests described above, males receiving testosterone replacement should have annual assessment of liver function tests and hemoglobin, as exogenous androgens can rarely cause hepatotoxicity and erythrocytosis, respectively. For those treated with transdermal preparations, periodic serum testosterone levels help to establish dosing that yields physiological levels. For females treated with estrogen and/or progesterone, annual assessment of a comprehensive chemistry panel and complete blood count is advised to monitor for side effects.

Pearls and Precautions

School: Although there are sporadic cases of patients with Kallmann syndrome and mental retardation, intelligence is generally described as normal or borderline low.

Miscellaneous:

- When testing for sense of smell, do not inquire about whether skunks can be smelled or test the sense of smell with ammonia because these are irritants that stimulate the trigeminal nerve (cranial nerve #5) as opposed to smells that test the olfactory nerve (cranial nerve #1).
- As it is not part of a routine MRI, anatomical detail of the olfactory region on a head MRI must be specially requested.
- To test for synkinesia, have the patient simulate opening a jar lid with one hand and the other will also move involuntarily.

- Note that FSH responses cannot be used to differentiate hypogonadotropic hypogonadism and constitutional delay, but should still be performed to document biological potency of the exogenously administered GnRH.

References

Fechner A, Fong S, McGovern P. A review of Kallmann syndrome: genetics, pathophysiology, and clinical management. Obstet Gynecol Surv 2008;63:189–94.

Crowley WF Jr, Pitteloud N, Seminara S. New genes controlling human reproduction and how you find them. Trans Am Clin Climatol Assoc 2008;119:29–37.

Klinefelter Syndrome

Mitchell E. Geffner

Klinefelter syndrome is a genetic disorder of males, caused by the presence of an extra X chromosome, and characterized by small testicles, reduced testosterone production, and, in most cases, infertility.

Etiology

Klinefelter syndrome includes a group of chromosomal disorders in which there is at least one extra X chromosome added to the normal male karyotype of 46,XY. The extra X chromosome most frequently results from an error in meiosis (non-disjunction during parental gametogenesis) where a sperm or egg carries an extra X chromosome in addition to the normal single sex chromosome. Less often, it results from an error in cell division during mitosis of the zygote. This condition is named after Dr. Harry Klinefelter, an endocrinologist at Massachusetts General Hospital, who first described it in 1942.

Clinical Presentation and Prognosis

Demographics: Klinefelter syndrome is the most common cause of hypergonadotropic hypogonadism in males, occurring in about 1:500–1000 live-born males.

Presenting signs and symptoms: Klinefelter syndrome is most often diagnosed in pubertal or adult males. However, this syndrome may also be diagnosed on fetal amniocentesis or during infancy, or as a part of a chromosomal evaluation of hypospadias, small phallus, or cryptorchidism. The older boy or adolescent may be discovered during an evaluation for delayed or incomplete pubertal development with a eunuchoidal body habitus, gynecomastia, increased fat mass, and/or small testes. These patients may have relatively normal development of secondary sexual characteristics, such as pubic and axillary hair. Previously undiagnosed adult men may come to medical attention because of infertility or, rarely, breast malignancy. At all ages, decreased verbal intelligence, language learning, and problems with executive functioning are also a noteworthy feature.

Clinical course: In those diagnosed early because of unexpected detection on amniocentesis or by micropenis and/or undescended testes at birth or later in infancy, there are no significant clinical issues until school age when learning problems begin to surface. Patients with Klinefelter syndrome are generally healthy and, when they reach adolescence, must deal mostly with issues surrounding sex steroid replacement and, in young adulthood, assisted reproductive strategies for achieving fertility. Educational and psychosocial issues need attention by specialists versed in these aspects of the syndrome.

Prognosis: Adequate virilization and fertility can be achieved with testosterone supplementation and the new techniques mentioned below. Men with Klinefelter syndrome are at increased risk for certain cancers and osteoporosis. Additionally, there may be an increased risk of restrictive lung disease, insulin-resistant diabetes mellitus, and autoimmune disease (see below).

Diagnosis

In cases of suspected Klinefelter syndrome, a chromosomal karyotype must be performed (a buccal smear is unacceptable). The condition is suspected by the detection of low testosterone levels and elevated gonadotropins, follicle-stimulating hormone (FSH) and luteinizing hormone (LH). The aforementioned hormonal profile, along with a heightened negative feedback sensitivity of the pituitary gonadotroph cells, is most easily discernible in the first few months of life and after 10 years of age.

Management

Medication: See section on Kallmann syndrome for management strategies related to testosterone replacement. In contrast to patients with hypogonadotropic hypogonadism (e.g., Kallmann syndrome), patients with Klinefelter syndrome suffer from primary hypogonadism and severe intrinsic gonadal damage. As a result, almost all affected individuals are infertile.

Surgery: There are promising surgical techniques such as intra-cytoplasmic sperm extraction (ICSE) for males which may afford these patients new fertility options. The optimal age for this procedure is unknown.

Psychological: IQ is highly variable. Learning disabilities (affecting verbal greater than performance IQ) are common. Language delay is a fairly consistent finding. Psychological and educational testing is paramount so as to allow creation of individualized treatment strategies.

Social: Problems with executive functioning and social interaction are common among boys and men with Klinefelter syndrome.

Monitoring: As males with Klinefelter syndrome are at increased risk for diabetes and hypothyroidism, annual chemistry panels, HbA1c levels, and TSH measurements are recommended. In addition, the chemistry panels may help to detect rare androgen-induced hepatotoxicity in those receiving testosterone treatment. Furthermore, at that time, annual complete blood counts should be obtained to screen for erythrocytosis. For those treated with transdermal testosterone preparations, periodic serum testosterone levels help to establish dosing that yields physiological replacement. For symptoms suggestive of an anterior mediastinal germ tumor which is a rare cancer with heightened predilection in males with Klinefelter syndrome, a serum level of human chorionogonadotropin (hCG) should be obtained.

Pearls and Precautions

School: Boys with Klinefelter syndrome are generally well-behaved at school. Most are shy, quiet, and eager to please the teacher. However, when faced with concepts that are difficult, they tend to withdraw. Teachers sometimes fail to realize they have an inherent language problem and dismiss affected boys as lazy. As a result, they fall increasingly behind and, eventually, may be held back a grade. Individualized attention at school can be quite helpful.

Miscellaneous

- In patients with Klinefelter syndrome, there is an increased incidence of autoimmune disorders such as hypothyroidism, systemic lupus erythematosus, rheumatoid arthritis, and Sjögren syndrome. This may be due to their relatively higher estrogen and lower testosterone levels that respectively promote and protect against autoimmunity (as has been suggested in normal individuals). It is unclear at this time if early identification of Klinefelter syndrome and earlier initiation of androgen replacement will decrease the incidence of autoimmune conditions.

- There is a heightened risk of germ cell tumors involving the anterior mediastinum. Occasionally, such tumors are the presenting manifestation so that any male initially identified in this manner must have a karyotype performed. There is also a slightly higher risk of male breast cancer in men with Klinefelter syndrome.

References

Bojesen A, Gravholt CH. Klinefelter syndrome in clinical practice. Nat Clin Pract Urol 2007;4:192–204.

Visootsak J, Graham JM Jr. Klinefelter syndrome and other sex chromosomal aneuploidies. Orphanet J Rare Dis. 2006;1:42 http://www.OJRD.com/content/1/1/42)

Polycystic Ovarian Syndrome (PCOS)

Mitchell E. Geffner

PCOS is a condition typically characterized by obesity, menstrual abnormalities, hirsutism, a heightened risk of infertility, and enlarged ovaries. It is frequently associated with insulin resistance and hyperinsulinemia which are thought to play a key role in the condition's main biochemical abnormality, *i.e.,* excessive androgen secretion of ovarian origin.

Etiology

Also known historically as Stein-Leventhal syndrome, the etiology of PCOS remains unknown and is probably multi-factorial, resulting in excess androgen production from both ovarian and adrenal sources. A genetic component is suggested by autosomal dominant familial clustering. In fact, PCOS may actually begin *in utero* as a result of exposure to a maternal hyperandrogenic and/or insulin-resistant hormonal milieu. Known childhood risk factors for future PCOS include: congenital virilizing disorders, above average or low (small-for-gestational age) birth weight; early adrenarche; and severe obesity with acanthosis nigricans, metabolic syndrome, and glucose intolerance or type 2 diabetes mellitus (T2DM). It has long been known that women with PCOS manifest alterations in gonadotropin secretion, characterized by increased LH secretion and subnormal FSH induction of CYP19 aromatase activity in granulosa cells. These changes lead to elevated estrogen levels and a heightened androgen-to-estrogen ratio. Additionally, both obese and thin (more so the former) women with PCOS manifest *resistance* to the *gluco-regulatory* action of insulin, which results in compensatory hyperinsulinemia. Since insulin can stimulate *in vitro* androgen secretion by both normal and PCOS ovarian tissue, it is thought that the main clinical manifestations of this syndrome are due to retained *sensitivity* to the *growth-promoting* action of insulin that contributes to increased ovarian growth and androgen secretion. Elevated insulin levels also can decrease hepatic sex hormone binding globulin (SHBG) production (based on *in vitro* effects of insulin on liver protein secretion). This series of biochemical changes leads to increased free testosterone that, in turn, greatly contributes to the clinical manifestations of this syndrome.

Clinical Presentation and Prognosis

Demographics: PCOS is the most common endocrine disorder affecting females of reproductive age, occurring in 5–10% of women (including adolescent females) worldwide.

Presenting signs and symptoms: PCOS is typically associated with chronic menstrual abnormalities and slowly progressive manifestations of hyperandrogenism (e.g., hirsutism and acne). Abrupt changes in menstrual pattern and/or rapid onset and/or severe manifestations of hyperandrogenism should suggest alternate etiologies, such as adrenal hyperplasia, androgen-secreting tumors, or Cushing syndrome. Generalized obesity occurs in 85% of women with PCOS and may be associated with typical co-morbidities of hypertension, hyperlipidemia, and cutaneous manifestations of hyperinsulinemia/insulin resistance. The typical skin manifestations include acanthosis nigricans [thickening and darkening of skin in intertriginous regions, i.e., those where skin rubs on skin, such as the (nape of the) neck, axillae, and groin] and skin tags (acrochordons) that usually emanate from the acanthotic regions.

Clinical course: Adolescents and women with PCOS are at risk for menstrual irregularities or amenorrhea and permanent infertility unless the underlying abnormal hormonal milieu can be corrected. The key treatment for this is also the most difficult, i.e., weight loss. Thus, medical therapy is used to improve insulin sensitivity and to treat components of the syndrome. Specific fertility treatments sometimes overcome the abnormal biochemistry. With increasing age, the co-morbidities related to the medical syndrome, i.e., abnormal glucose metabolism, hyperlipidemia, and hypertension, become increasingly problematic with regard to early cardiovascular risk enhancement.

Prognosis: Significant long-term medical consequences of PCOS include infertility and other manifestations of hyperandrogenism, endometrial hyperplasia and cancer (due to the relative hyperestrogenism), along with the co-morbidities of obesity. Lifestyle modification is a key, but difficult element to invoke successfully. If medical therapy is unable to promote ovulation, assisted reproductive technologies may be required. Careful gynecological follow-up is vital with regard to monitoring for uterine abnormalities.

Diagnosis

In 2006, the Androgen Excess Society suggested that the definition of PCOS include hyperandrogenism (clinical hirsutism and/or biochemical hyperandrogenemia, *i.e.,* elevated free testosterone) and ovarian dysfunction (oligo-anovulation and/or polycystic ovaries). In addition, obesity, insulin resistance, and metabolic syndrome occur in at least 50% of females with PCOS. The diagnosis may be aided by an elevated LH:FSH ratio as well as laboratory evidence of insulin resistance. Ovarian ultrasonography is sometimes used adjunctively, but multiple ovarian cysts are not always present in women with PCOS who have clear-cut clinical and biochemical phenotype and may be present in completely normal women.

Management

Medication: Historically, administration of estrogen and progesterone (oral contraceptive) has been the mainstay of treatment for those not seeking pregnancy. Such an approach results in regular menses, reduced risk of endometrial hyperplasia and cancer (by avoiding unopposed estrogen exposure), and improves androgenic manifestations such as acne and hirsutism (in part by estrogenic stimulation of sex-hormone binding globulin production). However, it is critical that the estrogen dose not be excessive (averaging about 30 μg/day of ethinyl estradiol) and that the progesterone component has low androgenicity or even an anti-androgenic effect (e.g., dropirenone).

Anti-androgen drugs may be used adjunctively. The most commonly employed agent is spironolactone, which acts predominantly by binding to and blocking the androgen receptor. It may also interfere with (adrenal) steroidogenesis. This drug must be avoided during pregnancy because of teratogenic potential. Flutamide, which has similar mechanisms of action to spironolactone, is occasionally used. However, at high doses, it has potential serious hepatotoxicity.

Occasionally, adjunctive glucocorticoid therapy is employed for those who have associated significant adrenal hyperandrogenism.

Improvement of insulin sensitivity is well recognized as one of the most important components of the therapeutic approach to PCOS. Use of metformin by obese adolescents with PCOS appears to improve insulin sensitivity, lower serum insulin and androgen levels, and possibly increase the rate of ovulation. Insulin-sensitizing agents of the thiazolidinedione class (rosiglitazone and pioglitazone) have also proven helpful in the treatment of adult women with PCOS by improving their ovulatory function, hirsutism, hyperandrogenemia, and insulin resistance, while causing minimal adverse effects. Clinicians should note that the use of any insulin-sensitizer medications in non-type 2 diabetic females with PCOS represents an off-label use of these drugs.

Mechanical: As pharmacological approaches to excess hair prevent only new growth, mechanical hair removal remains a key approach to the removal of pre-existing hair or for progressive hirsutism that is poorly responsive to medications. Non-permanent hair removal methods include shaving, waxing, and use of topical depilatory creams. Though effective, permanent methods, such as electrolysis and laser therapy, are more costly and may be uncomfortable.

Psychological: The psychological ramifications of obesity, such as depression, are also issues in females with PCOS.

Social support: Since most affected females are overweight, basic therapy in this dominant subset should target lifestyle modification involving diet and exercise. Successful weight reduction and maintenance may well restore ovulatory cycles via reduction of insulin resistance.

Laboratory tests and monitoring: Semi-annual fasting laboratory monitoring of treated or untreated women with PCOS should include: Free and total testosterone, SHBG, comprehensive chemistry panel, lipids, and hemoglobin A1c. Sequential ultrasonography is not usually recommended.

Pearls and Precautions

- PCOS should not be confused with *idiopathic hirsutism* in which there are no other signs of significant hyperandrogenism, *i.e.,* clitoromegaly, cystic acne, increased muscle bulk, temporal hair recession, or voice-deepening.
- Furthermore, the term, hirsutism, should not be used interchangeably with *hypertrichosis*, the latter which refers to non-androgen-mediated, excessive growth of lanugo hair over the entire body. This may have an ethnic basis, occurring more often in individuals of Mediterranean and Northern Indian descent or be associated with chronic use of certain medications, *e.g.,* diphenylhydantoin, cyclosporine, minoxidil, and diazoxide.

References

Blank SK, Helm KD, McCartney CR, Marshall JC. Polycystic ovary syndrome in adolescence. Ann NY Acad Sci 2008;1135:76–84.

Diamanti-Kandarakis E, Christakou C, Palioura E, Kandaraki E, Livadas S. Does polycystic ovary syndrome start in childhood? Pediatr Endocrinol Rev 2008;5:904–911.

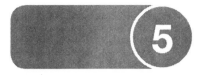

Gastroenterologic Disorders

Table of Contents

α_1-antitrypsin Deficiency

Michelle Pietzak

α_1-antitrypsin (α_1-AT) deficiency is the most common genetic liver disorder and the most common genetic cause for liver transplant in the pediatric population. It can present at any age, and α_1-AT deficiency needs to be in the differential of any age patient with unexplained liver disease. Diagnosis is based on measuring levels of the enzyme or detecting α_1-AT genetic mutations combined with characteristic histologic findings on liver biopsy.

Etiology

α_1-AT is a glycoprotein manufactured in the liver which belongs to the serpin family of serine protease inhibitors. The primary function of α_1-AT is to inhibit neutrophil proteases (elastase, cathepsin G and proteinase 3) which contribute to connective tissue remodeling and the proteolytic generation of antimicrobial peptides. This condition is inherited in an autosomal codominant pattern (two different versions of the α_1-AT gene may be expressed, and both contribute to the phenotype). A single amino acid substitution results in up to a 90% reduction in serum α_1-AT as the misfolded protein remains in the endoplasmic reticulum. In this sense, α_1-AT "deficiency" is really a disease of "accumulation" in the endoplasmic reticulum of hepatocytes.

Demographics: α_1-AT deficiency occurs worldwide, but its prevalence varies by population, being more common in people of northern European, Iberian and Saudi Arabian ancestry. In these populations, 4% are carriers and between 1 in 625 and 1 in 2000 are homozygous for the mutation. However, prospective population data from Sweden indicate that by 20 years of age, only up to 10% of those with the homozygous mutation develop clinical liver disease. The condition is less common in the Asian and black populations. In North America, α_1-AT deficiency is thought to affect up to 1 in 5,000 people. The American Lung Association estimates that 100,000 Americans currently have α_1-AT deficiency. Up to 25 million Americans, and 161 million people worldwide, are carriers for the disease.

Clinical Presentation and Prognosis

Presenting signs and symptoms: The hepatic presentation of α_1-AT deficiency can be varied, and can occur at any age. In the neonatal period, it can mimic biliary atresia or neonatal hepatitis, with jaundice, elevated transaminases and acholic stools. Presentations in school-aged children, adolescents and adults include isolated elevated transaminases, acute onset of liver synthetic dysfunction and chronic hepatitis. The disease may be subclinical until the development of portal hypertension, where the patient may present acutely with an upper GI bleed, splenomegaly and/or ascites (see separate chapter on portal hypertension). α_1-AT deficiency can present as cryptogenic cirrhosis in both the pediatric and adult population, with the gradual onset of pruritus, fatigue, anorexia, skin findings (telangiectasias, palmar erythema, xanthomas and caput medusa) and growth failure/protein-calorie malnutrition with evidence of fat-soluble vitamin deficiencies (A, D, E and K). Pulmonary manifestations of α_1-AT deficiency typically present during the fourth and fifth decade of life and are not typically seen in children.

Clinical course and Prognosis: Reported poor prognostic signs for the development of liver dysfunction include persistently elevated bilirubin, aminotransferases and PT as well as the physical signs of hard hepatomegaly and early splenomegaly. However, children with many of these "poor prognostic" signs, even portal hypertension, may have minimal disease progression for many years.

Diagnosis

Labs: Classic laboratory findings with chronic liver disease can include elevated transaminases, serum direct/conjugated bilirubin, serum alkaline phosphatase and γ-glutamyltransferase (GGT). In chronic liver disease with cholestasis and malnutrition due to fat malabsorption, low pre-albumin, total cholesterol, serum vitamins A, E, 25OH D and prolonged prothrombin time (from vitamin K deficiency) may be seen.

α_1-AT can be measured in several ways: Total serum α_1-AT, $\alpha1$-AT phenotype and α_1-AT genotype. A serum α_1-AT level can be measured by most laboratories. However, since α_1-AT is an acute phase reactant, it may be falsely elevated into the low normal range with cancer, stress, pregnancy, infections and other inflammatory disorders. Falsely low levels can be seen in protein deficient states (malnutrition) or protein losing states (protein-losing enteropathy or nephrotic syndrome) as well as in neonatal respiratory distress syndrome and in some cancers. Also, since α_1-AT is made by the liver, other liver diseases can give a falsely low level. Thus, a serum α_1-AT level is not as good a screening test as a genotype or a phenotype.

α_1-AT deficiency is caused by mutations in the SERPINA1 gene (serpin peptidase inhibitor, clade A [alpha-1 antiproteinase, antitrypsin], member 1), located on 14q32.1. More than 120 SERPINA1 mutations have been identified, with some associated with no disease, while others result in a moderate to severe deficiency of the enzyme. Most medical laboratories report α_1-AT blood levels and protease inhibitor (PI) phenotypes, while only specialized laboratories determine genotypes.

The most common allele of SERPINA1, called M, produces normal levels of the enzyme, and most people have two copies of the M allele (MM). Structural variants of α_1-AT can be divided into "normal allelic variants" (associated with no changes in α_1-AT concentration or activity), "null allelic variants" (no detectable serum α_1-AT), and "deficiency variants" (reduction in α_1-AT concentration and/or activity). Homozygosity for the null variant can result in premature emphysema, but no liver disease. The most common deficiency variants are S and Z. The S allele produces moderately low levels and the Z allele produces very little α_1-AT enzyme. ZZ individuals are likely to have α_1-AT deficiency. MZ individuals are thought to have negligible to a slightly increased risk of lung and liver disease. The MZ carriers may only develop chronic liver disease in the setting of other known etiologies for liver damage, such as obesity, alcohol, viruses (hepatitis B and C), medications and autoimmune liver disease. SZ individuals have increased risk of emphysema. MS carriers and SS individuals usually produce enough α_1-AT to protect the lungs and also do not develop liver disease.

Liver biopsy: With a positive phenotype or genotype screen, tissue confirmation of α_1-AT deficiency should be performed with a liver biopsy. This can be done percutaneously by a pediatric gastroenterologist or interventional radiologist under ultrasound guidance. Varying degrees of inflammation, fibrosis, cirrhosis and necrosis may also be seen.

Radiology: Cirrhosis and portal hypertension, which are serious complications of α_1-AT deficiency, may occur in childhood and can be imaged by ultrasound and CT of the abdomen. Please see separate chapter on portal hypertension for details of these studies.

Management

The treatment of α_1-AT deficiency-associated liver disease is primarily supportive. The primary goals of management are: Maintaining the quality of life, the prevention of life-threatening GI bleed (usually due to varices) and lifestyle modifications to decrease the risk of emphysema. Liver transplantation is an option to treat end-stage liver disease, and has an excellent survival rate. Agents which have shown promise for treating liver disease in *in vitro* and animal studies include PBA (4-phenylbutyric acid), iminosugar compounds, somatic gene therapy and hepatocyte transplantation.

Consultations: Referral to a pediatric liver transplant center should be considered early in the patient's course, especially if the child has portal hypertension and already has had an initial variceal bleed.

Social:

- Alpha-1 Foundation, www.alphaone.org: Funds research and provides resources, educational brochures and information on testing and diagnosis for physicians and patients.
- Alphanet, www.alphanet.org: Assists patients and families with support, education and strategies to manage their health.
- Alpha-1 Association, www.alpha1.org: Dedicated to improving the quality of lives of patients with α_1-AT deficiency through support, education and advocacy.
- The Alpha-1 Research Registry, www.alphaoneregistry.org: Confidential database which gives patients the opportunity to provide information to help advance research through questionnaires and clinical trials.
- Alpha-1 Kids, www.alpha1kids.org: Provides support and information for parents and children with α_1-AT deficiency.

Monitoring: Periodic assessment of growth, nutritional status, liver function and abdominal US with Doppler are sufficient to monitor uncomplicated liver disease. If evidence of protein-calorie malnutrition is present, or the patient has cholestasis, the fat-soluble vitamins should be measured. At present, it is not recommended that children with portal hypertension, who have not yet had bleeding esophageal varices, undergo periodic routine surveillance endoscopy.

Pearls and Precautions

Immunizations: All patients with α_1-AT deficiency should receive hepatitis A and B vaccinations. Polysaccharide pneumococcal and influenza vaccines should be given to those with risk for underlying lung disease. If the patient has received a liver transplant and is immune suppressed, live vaccines should not be given.

Family screening: Once the index case has been identified, other family members may be tested to establish risk for liver disease and/or emphysema. However, people with the same allelic variants may have very different clinical courses.

Lifestyle interventions: Those with liver disease should not drink alcohol or take medications which are known to be hepatotoxic (such as acetaminophen). In addition to not smoking, patients with α_1-AT deficiency should avoid lung irritants (such as second-hand smoke, dust, pollution and toxic fumes); seek prompt medical attention for respiratory infections; and exercise regularly to optimize lung function.

Complications

- *Emphysema:* While the liver disease of α_1-AT deficiency is considered an "accumulation disease," the chronic lung disease is thought to be due to "deficiency" or "lack of function" of the α_1-AT protein. Lack of α_1-AT in the lower respiratory tree allows for unchecked elastolytic attack on connective tissues, resulting in emphysema starting as early as the third decade of life. Cigarette smoking is thought to further inactivate α_1-AT via an oxidative mechanism, thereby accelerating the progression of the lung disease. Symptoms may include asthma, chronic bronchitis, emphysema, and/or bronchiectasis. Medications used to treat the lung disease include antibiotics, bronchodilators, corticosteroids, and supplemental oxygen. "Augmentation therapy" involves giving purified α_1-AT from human blood donors intravenously weekly, and may slow the progressive loss of lung function. Those with severe lung disease may be candidates for lung volume reduction surgery or lung transplantation.
- As with other chronic liver diseases which may result in portal hypertension, complications can include hepatopulmonary syndrome (pulmonary arterio-venous shunting), pulmonary hypertension, ascites, bacterial peritonitis, hepatorenal syndrome and liver failure with hepatic encephalopathy. Please see separate chapter on portal hypertension for more details about these specific complications.
- *Hepatocellular carcinoma:* Individuals over the age of 50 with worsening cirrhosis are at increased risk for hepatoma, and should have periodic CT imaging of the liver.
- *Panniculitis:* This is an inflammatory skin condition where subcutaneous areas of fat harden to cause painful lumps or patches. It can occur at all ages, has been linked to ZZ and MZ phenotypes, and is thought to be due to destruction of the skin by unrestrained neutrophils.

References

Perlmutter DH, Pierce JA. The alpha-1-antitrypsin gene and emphysema. Am J Physiol 1989;257(4 Pt 1):L147–162

Starzl TE, Porter KA, Busuttil RW, et al. Liver disease in alpha-1-antitrypsin deficiency: prognostic indicators. J Pediatr 1990;117:864–870.

Sveger T. Liver disease in α_1-antitrypsin deficiency detected by screening of 200,000 infants. N Engl J Med 1976;294:1216–1221.

Volpert D, Molleston JP, Perlmutter DH. Alpha1-antitrypsin deficiency-associated liver disease progresses slowly in some children. J Pediatr Gastro Nutr 2000;31:258–263.

Celiac Disease (CD)

Michelle Pietzak

Celiac disease is also known as celiac sprue or gluten sensitive enteropathy and is an immune-mediated condition which occurs in genetically predisposed individuals who ingest gluten.

Etiology

Gluten is a protein which occurs in wheat, rye and barley. CD is the only autoimmune disease for which there is such a narrowly defined trigger. Elimination of this offending agent from the diet results in clinical, serologic and histologic improvement in the patient. The majority (about 95%) of celiac patients possess human leukocyte antigen (HLA) DQ2, which also predisposes to many other autoimmune diseases, such as type 1 diabetes. The majority of other patients possess HLA DQ8. Serologic screens for this condition are excellent. However, biopsy-confirmed disease remains the gold standard for diagnosis, and is important to validate prior to the initiation of a lifelong gluten free diet (GFD).

Clinical Presentation and Prognosis:

Demographics: CD is thought to affect about 1% of the U.S. population. However, more than 90% of these patients are not yet diagnosed. CD used to be thought of as a disease of childhood, primarily affecting those of European descent (U.K., Scandinavia, Italy and other Mediterranean countries). It is now known that the disease can present at any age and can affect those of non-Caucasian heritage. CD has been described in Central and South America, the Middle East, Asia and Africa. At present, more women than men are diagnosed with CD. This most likely represents a reporting bias, as women are more likely to seek care from multiple practitioners for chronic, unexplained symptoms. Large serologic screening studies in several countries indicate that the male:female prevalence is identical. Many studies indicate that patients seek care from an average of 4–6 health care practitioners and spend an average of 11–12 years with symptoms before the correct diagnosis of CD is made.

Presenting signs and symptoms:

- *"Classic presentation"*: This occurs during the toddler years, after gluten has been introduced into the diet. These young children usually have chronic diarrhea with fat malabsorption, resulting in watery, gassy, floating and foul-smelling stools. However, some children exhibit severe constipation rather than diarrhea. Left untreated, this results in failure to thrive, anemia, short stature and fat-soluble vitamin deficiencies.

- *Late-onset gastrointestinal form*: GI symptoms occur after the toddler years, and can present in school age, adolescent, adult and even elderly patients. Symptoms include diarrhea, constipation, gastro-esophageal reflux, delayed gastric emptying, gaseousness and bloating. Left untreated, this can result in protein-calorie malnutrition, anemia, infertility, osteoporosis and fat-soluble vitamin deficiencies. These patients often get mislabeled as having irritable bowel syndrome or lactose intolerance. While these latter two conditions can present with gas and diarrhea, they do not cause the other chronic nutritional problems and are not associated with other autoimmune conditions as described below.
- Extra-intestinal forms:
  - *Skin:* Dermatitis herpetiformis (DH) is the skin rash of CD. The rash begins as erythematous macules, progresses to urticarial papules, and then tense vesicles. The two hallmarks of this rash are that it is symmetrical and pruritic. Because of the pruritus, patients often scratch open the vesicles, and the rash can mimic chronic eczema. Locations include face, elbows, buttocks, and knees. An office skin biopsy of normal appearing skin adjacent to affected skin, sent frozen and stained for granular IgA deposits in the dermis, can confirm the diagnosis. Patients with a positive skin biopsy for DH have CD, and do not require serologic or intestinal histologic confirmation. Dapsone, an anti-inflammatory antibiotic, may alleviate the pruritus, but a life-long GFD is required to maintain remission. Some DH patients have additional skin sensitivities, such as to latex and Betadine.
  - *Joints/bones*: Joint pain is the second most common complaint in celiac patients after GI symptoms. As in inflammatory bowel disease, joints affected are usually the large joints (wrist, elbow, hip, knee, and ankle). This can be differentiated from rheumatoid arthritis in that the patient is rheumatoid factor negative and there is no joint destruction. Joint pain often improves on the GFD. Osteopenia leading to osteoporosis and fractures is common in CD, and can occur even in childhood. Rickets due to vitamin D deficiency can be seen in toddlers. If CD is diagnosed and treated with a GFD prior to the attainment of peak bone mass in the early 20's, osteoporosis can be avoided.
  - *Mouth/dentition*: Recurrent oral aphthous ulcers can be seen in both CD and Crohn's disease. If CD is present during the toddler years, while the secondary dentition are developing, dental enamel defects may occur. Sealants are recommended for these defects, which are permanent.
  - *Endocrine/Reproductive system*: Infertility and delayed puberty are seen in both sexes who have undiagnosed CD. As in Crohn's disease, isolated short stature may be the only symptom. Women have more spontaneous abortions and fetuses with neural tube defects due to folic acid malabsorption. Type I diabetes and autoimmune thyroid diseases have increased risk for CD.
  - *Anemia*: Iron deficiency is one of the most common micronutrient deficiencies in undiagnosed children with CD. Deficiencies in vitamin E can lead to a hemolytic anemia. Advanced small bowel disease can lead to B12 malabsorption.
  - *Neurologic/psychiatric*: Patients with CD have higher rates of depression, schizophrenia and epilepsy. Vitamin deficiencies may lead to peripheral neuropathy, ataxia and neurologic symptoms. Young children with undiagnosed CD have been reported to have irritability and separation anxiety issues which improve on the GFD. Despite claims of improvement in autistic symptoms on a gluten free/casein free diet, there does not appear to be an increased incidence of CD in patients with autism, nor an increased rate of autism in celiac children.

Clinical course: Many children experience immediate relief of symptoms after initiation of the GFD. Diarrhea and gaseous distension may also be relieved with lactose restriction for several months after diagnosis. Weight gain is often immediate. Improvement in stature may not be seen for 6 months to a year after initiation of the GFD. There is a steep learning curve with the diet, as accidental or intentional ingestions of gluten may trigger immediate GI symptomatology which can last for several days.

Prognosis: The prognosis for a child diagnosed with CD who adheres to a GFD is excellent. A relapse in symptoms is usually due to inadvertent ingestion of gluten due to contaminated foods. A persistence of unexplained symptoms should prompt the practitioner to look for the presence of another autoimmune disease. Iron deficiency anemia and fat-soluble vitamin deficiencies can be corrected with supplementation after diagnosis. Once enteropathy has healed on the GFD, and absorption has normalized, routine vitamin supplementation can be used.

Diagnosis

The diagnostic approach to the child with CD is to first suspect the diagnosis. A thorough history and physical are essential, and should include serial plotting of weight, height, BMI, pubertal staging, and a bone age if there is growth delay. A family history for CD, GI cancers and autoimmune diseases are essential. On physical exam, the young child with undiagnosed CD may exhibit protein calorie malnutrition, with decreased subcutaneous fat stores and muscle bulk. Older children may have normal weight, height and BMI, or have shown a crossing of percentiles over the years on the pediatric height and weight curves. Isolated short stature can be seen. Abdominal distention with tympani can be appreciated due to gaseousness. Symptoms of iron deficiency anemia may include pica, decreased appetite, abdominal pain, generalized fatigue, sleep disturbances, frontal headache and shortness of breath with exercise. Signs of iron deficiency anemia may include clubbing, brittle hair and nails, and a sore, smooth, shiny and/or reddened tongue. Fat-soluble vitamin deficiencies may present with increased bruising and bleeding (vitamin K), rickets or osteopenia (vitamin D), hemolytic anemia, impaired balance and muscle weakness (vitamin E) or impaired night vision, dry eyes, rough skin, loss of taste and poor wound healing (vitamin A). Zinc and selenium deficiencies have also been described.

Routine laboratory testing may show some subtle findings for CD. A CBC may show microcytosis, with or without an anemia, due to iron deficiency. A chemistry panel may show low potassium due to chronic emesis, low bicarbonate with chronic diarrhea, low albumin and protein with protein-losing enteropathy, and slightly elevated transaminases due to a lymphocytic hepatitis. A very low alkaline phosphatase result may indicate a deficiency of this enzyme's co-factor, zinc, which can also be seen with chronic diarrhea.

There are excellent serologic screens for CD, even in young children. However, practitioners should be aware of the advantages and disadvantages of each one (see Table 5.1). Individuals need to be on a gluten containing diet for several months prior to testing, as these antibodies normalize on the GFD. Patients with IgA deficiency have an increased risk for CD, and will have negative anti-gliadin (AGA) IgA, tissue transglutaminase (TTG) IgA and anti-endomysial (EMA) IgA. However, AGA IgG and TTG IgG may be positive. Thus, a total IgA level should be measured concomitantly with serology.

Genetic testing for variants of HLA DQ2 and DQ8 can stratify risk for CD. One does not need to be on a gluten containing diet to have genetic testing. Therefore, infants not yet exposed to gluten, or patients who are already on a self-imposed GFD can have genetic testing. It would be rare for someone to not possess variants of either HLA DQ2 and/or DQ8 and have biopsy-confirmed disease. However, HLA DQ2 and DQ8 are found with high frequency in the general population, and therefore a positive test result does not confirm the condition.

Until proven otherwise, serology with a positive TTG IgA or EMA IgA in an otherwise healthy child indicates CD. Positive AGA IgG or TTG IgG in an IgA deficient patient is also suggestive of CD. A young child who has markedly elevated AGA IgG and IgA but normal EMA IgA and TTG IgA may still have CD. Regardless of serology, if a child has symptoms suggestive of CD, or a family history of CD, he should be referred for intestinal biopsy.

Small bowel biopsy is performed endoscopically either under conscious sedation or general anesthesia. Visually, the proximal duodenum and jejunum may appear normal; or there may be scalloping of the folds,

Table 5.1: Serologic Screens: Advantages and Disadvantages

Test	Advantages	Disadvantages
AGA IgG and IgA	• Inexpensive ELISA test • Positive in young patients • AGA IgG positive in IgA deficients • First to rise and fall with GFD	• Less sensitive and specific than TTG IgA and EMA IgA • Requires gluten ingestion • Positive with increased intestinal permeability (food allergy, viral infection, Down syndrome, cystic fibrosis)
TTG IgA	• Inexpensive ELISA test • High sensitivity and specificity	• May not be made by young children • Requires ingestion of gluten • Falsely negative in IgA deficients • Falsely positive in other autoimmune conditions (type 1 diabetes, autoimmune hepatitis, autoimmune thyroid disease, inflammatory bowel disease (IBD))
EMA IgA	• Highest sensitivity and specificity • Unlikely to be positive in other auto-immune conditions	• May not be made by young children • Requires ingestion of gluten • Falsely negative in IgA deficients • Expensive, subjective test run on primate tissue by specialized laboratory
HLA DQ2/DQ8	• Does not require ingestion of gluten in the diet for testing • Results do not change with GFD • Can be used on infants not exposed to gluten	• Expensive • Run by specialized laboratory • Presence of genes do not equal presence of active disease, only risk
Endoscopic biopsy	• Gold standard of diagnosis • Severity of disease can be graded • Diseases with similar presentations (Crohn's disease, GERD, eosinophilic diseases) can be ruled out	• Expensive, "invasive" • Requires ingestion of gluten • Requires sedation • Requires a gastroenterologist • Subjective interpretation of histology by pathologists with high interobserver variability

nodularity or aphthous ulcerations. Multiple small bowel biopsies should be taken from different levels, as the disease may be patchy.

Management

Nutrition/diet: The only current valid treatment for CD is the GFD. All sources of wheat, rye and barley need to be eliminated completely from the diet. In the U.S., oats are often milled with wheat, and can be contaminated. As of January 1, 2006, the Food Allergen Labeling and Consumer Protection Act of 2004 ensures that wheat is plainly stated on the labels of foods manufactured and sold in the U.S. Pre-2006, wheat could masquerade under many different names, including bulgar, couscous, emmer, einkorn, emmer, faro, filler, kamut, spelt or semolina. Rye is usually disclosed on a label as "rye." Triticale is a wheat/rye hybrid. Barley may appear as "malt" on a label. Unfortunately, the food allergen labeling does not apply to restaurants. Obvious sources of gluten include bread, cereal, cookies, pasta and pizza. Non-obvious sources include candies, communion wafers, soy sauce, gravies, soups and imitation meats and seafood. Food which are naturally gluten free, such as fruits, vegetables and meats (without gravy or breading) are considered safe. Any item which can be potentially ingested, such as play dough, lipstick, mouthwash and toothpaste, should be checked for gluten content.

Patients often don't receive enough fiber on the GFD, and may experience constipation. Alternative sources should be encouraged, such as amaranth, arrowroot, buckwheat, corn, flax, millet, potato, quinoa, rice, sorghum, tapioca, teff and flours made from nuts, beans and seeds. The GFD can be especially challenging for the patient with type 1 diabetes and CD, as foods derived from corn, potato and rice have a higher glycemic index than their gluten-containing counterparts. As with most chronic diseases, compliance during the teenage years can be especially challenging.

Medications: Wheat starch, which is used as filler in medications and vitamins, may be a potential source for gluten contamination, and is an issue that is currently being examined. If the Food and Drug Administration decides that 20 parts per million of gluten is an acceptable level for gluten-free foods, then medication in pill form is unlikely to surpass this cut-off. Until this issue is resolved, liquid medications are preferable for the pediatric patient with CD whenever possible.

Consultations: Successful management of the child with CD requires a team approach involving the patient, parents, other caretakers, school, gastroenterologist, primary care practitioner, and a dietician. After a biopsy-confirmed diagnosis, the child should be referred to a registered dietician knowledgeable about CD for a personalized nutritional assessment and education about the GFD. If poor growth, short stature or delayed sexual maturation remains present despite compliance with the GFD, referral to a pediatric endocrinologist should be considered. Children with CD may have co-morbid growth hormone deficiency, osteopenia or another concomitant autoimmune condition (such as type 1 diabetes, thyroid disease or hypoparathyroidism).

Therapy: Some malnourished children with CD and low muscle mass may benefit from physical and occupational therapy. However, most improve on GFD alone.

Psychological: In addition to the feelings of social isolation which can be seen on the GFD, CD patients have higher rates of depression and schizophrenia, and may require psychological or psychiatric interventions. Increased separation anxiety, reported in celiac toddlers, usually resolves with the GFD.

Social: Local, national and international support groups exist for both children and adults with CD. They can easily be found on the internet, and provide not only emotional support, but tips on shopping, eating out, education about resources and living a gluten-free lifestyle. Likewise, books about living with CD, children with CD, and GFD cookbooks are readily available through mainstream bookstores and internet sources. As awareness of CD, food allergies and food sensitivities increases, more supermarkets and restaurants are also catering to those with special dietary needs. There are also summer camps available in the U.S. which can maintain a kitchen which can prepare items for the GFD.

Monitoring: The child with CD should have frequent monitoring of growth and sexual maturation. Measurements of iron, fat-soluble vitamins, and liver and thyroid functions should be done. Screening of family members for CD should be offered. Measurement of bone density is often helpful in discovering occult osteopenia, and would suggest more aggressive supplementation of vitamin D and calcium, along with weight-bearing exercise and closer monitoring of linear growth. Monitoring for compliance can be achieved by serologic measurements on the GFD, repeat biopsy and/or interviews by a trained dietician. In general, unless the initial diagnosis of CD is in question, repeat biopsy is not recommended for a child with CD who is clinically doing well. In adults, repeat biopsy is being advocated by some to assess healing of enteropathy, to check for "refractory sprue" (non-response to the GFD) and to screen for enteropathy-associated small bowel T-cell lymphoma (EATL) which is seen in higher rates in CD patients. Refractory sprue is thought to occur in those who have had CD for decades, and the intestine has lost its ability to regenerate, and is therefore not considered an issue in pediatric CD. Most children with CD who continue to have symptoms despite the GFD have inadvertent or intentional gluten ingestion. Likewise, increased rates of GI cancers have not been reported in children with CD, although the youngest reported case of EATL thought to be due to CD was 15 years old. Some have advocated that TTG IgA combined with dietary interview is the most cost effective way to monitor for compliance.

Pearls and Precautions

Likely complications: Although the fear of GI cancer is often what keeps CD patients compliant, nutritional complications are far more common. These include iron and fat-soluble vitamin deficiencies, and osteoporosis and fractures. Patients with CD are often lactose intolerant. This is due to a decreased production of lactase, an enzyme that is found at the tip of the villous structure. With healing of enteropathy and regrowth of the villi, normal lactase production may resume, especially in younger patients. In those lactose intolerant, it is key that adequate vitamin D and calcium are incorporated into the diet from non-dairy sources such as fortified soymilk, orange juice, fatty fish and eggs. Alternatives include milk pre-digested with lactase and taking a lactase pill prior to dairy ingestion. Many will also tolerate yogurt and cheese, even if fresh whole milk and ice cream cause symptomatology.

Associated conditions: Because of the HLA which predispose to autoimmunity, many celiac patients may present with other autoimmune conditions. These include type 1 diabetes, Sjögren's syndrome, rheumatic diseases, autoimmune thyroid disease (Grave's disease, Hashimoto's thyroiditis), and autoimmune liver diseases (autoimmune hepatitis, sclerosing cholangitis, primary biliary cirrhosis). The symptoms of CD may be masked by the presence of these other conditions.

Associated syndromes: Patients with Down, Turner and Williams syndrome have increased risk for CD. Screening is strongly suggested in these patients, as they often exhibit short stature and gastrointestinal symptomatology as part of their syndrome. However, if initial serologic screening for CD is negative, it is not clear how often repeat testing should be performed.

Immunizations: There are no contraindications to vaccination in the child with CD. Some adult studies indicate hyposplenism with chronic CD, and advocate for additional vaccines for diseases due to encapsulated organisms. There are no data for this in the pediatric CD population.

Dental care: Children with CD should have regular 6 month dental checkups, with emphasis on examination for dental enamel defects in the secondary dentition. If present, sealants may be indicated.

Prevention: Some studies suggest that there is a critical window for the introduction of immunogenic proteins in the diet. Retrospective European studies suggest that the introduction of gluten too early (before 4 months) or too late (after one year) may increase the risk of CD. As with most autoimmune diseases, prolonged breastfeeding appears to diminish the lifetime risk for CD.

References

NIH Consensus Development Conference on Celiac Disease, National Institutes of Health Consensus Development Conference Statement, June 28–30, 2004, http://consensus.nih.gov/2004/2004CeliacD isease118html.htm

Fasano, A., Berti, I., Gerarduzzi, T., Not, T., Colletti, R.B., Drago, S., Elitsur, Y., Green, P.H.R., Guandalini, S., Hill, I., Pietzak, M., Ventura, A., Thorpe, M., Kryszak, D., Fornaroli, Wasserman, S.F., Murray, J.A., Horvath, K. Prevalence of celiac disease in at-risk and not at-risk groups in the United States: a large multicenter study. Archives of Internal Medicine 163: 286–292, 2003.

Pietzak, M.M. Follow-up of patients with celiac disease: achieving compliance with treatment. Gastroenterology 128:S135–S141, 2005.

Chronic Diarrhea in Children, Malabsorption Syndromes, Protein Losing Enteropathy

Randall Chan, Michelle Pietzak

Diarrhea can be defined as an increase in stool volume, water content, and/or frequency resulting in at least three daily liquid bowel movements. Diarrhea illnesses can be categorized into acute diarrhea (<14 days), persistent diarrhea (14–30 days), and chronic diarrhea (>30 days or having a recurrent pattern). Persistent and chronic diarrheas are often also delineated by etiology, with the term persistent diarrhea being reserved for infectious diarrhea alone.

Pathophysiology: Chronic diarrhea with malabsorption in childhood is usually the result of either infections or a malabsorption syndrome. During and after an acute diarrheal illness, persistent diarrhea can result from ongoing injury to the intestinal mucosa from bacteria, enterotoxin and/or dietary constituents (such as lactose). Debate continues as to whether proteins, bile salts and/or bacterial overgrowth can also continue to damage the exposed mucosa. Protein-calorie malnutrition may also delay the repair of the damaged intestine. Chronic malabsorption syndromes must be considered in any patient with chronic diarrhea, particularly if an acute inciting episode cannot be identified. Malabsorption syndromes can be separated into those caused by gastrointestinal mucosal surface injury (such as infectious diarrhea, enzyme defects, inflammatory bowel disease and celiac disease), liver diseases with chronic cholestasis, pancreatic disorders (such as cystic fibrosis) and defects in intestinal lymphatic drainage.

Etiologies

Infectious

Bacterial

The majority of bacterial diarrheas in the U.S. are caused by four organisms: Campylobacter, Shigella, Salmonella and enterohemorrhagic E. coli. Campylobacter and Salmonella can result in persistent or even chronic diarrhea.

Campylobacter: Campylobacter infection is primarily a food-borne illness. Infection results from the consumption of undercooked poultry, unpasteurized milk or improperly treated water. Campylobacter disease is generally self-limited, but 20% will have a prolonged or relapsing course. Symptoms can include fever, abdominal pain and diarrhea, which may be bloody. Acute Campylobacter infection can mimic appendicitis and IBD in its clinical presentation.

Salmonella: Salmonella species are primarily found in animals, including poultry, livestock, reptiles and other domesticated animals. Other foods, such as vegetables and breads, may also harbor the bacteria. Salmonella has a predilection for attacking the very young, the elderly and the immunosuppressed (in particular those with acquired immune deficiency syndrome (AIDS), cancer or hemoglobinopathies). Clinical presentation ranges from asymptomatic shedding to enteritis with watery diarrhea to colitis with bloody diarrhea, tenesmus and signs of systemic infection.

Clostridium difficile: C. difficile is a spore-forming bacterium that is ubiquitous in the environment and is thought to asymptomatically colonize in the intestinal tract of half of normal healthy infants. This colonization decreases to less than 5% of children older than 2 years of age. The disease is associated with an increased exposure to C. difficile organisms as well as a decrease in the normal intestinal flora due to antimicrobial agents. Clinical course can range from mild diarrhea with abdominal cramps to pseudomembranous colitis, toxic megacolon and death. The organism has been reportedly isolated from fomites (linens, curtains, floors, bookshelves) associated with infected patients for up to 5 months. Recurrent diarrhea occurs in approximately 10% of patients, although up to 40% of patients treated for C. difficile will experience at least one relapse. The disease may be self-limited upon stopping antimicrobials. For more severe forms, oral vancomycin or metronidazole is recommended. Probiotics, such as Lactobacillus GG and Saccharomyces boulardii can be used to treat colitis refractory to antibiotics, and to prevent relapse.

Infectious bacteria in immunocompromised children: Aeromonas and Plesiomonas can cause chronic diarrhea, especially in immunocompromised children. These organisms are associated with acute, secretory diarrhea, dysentery, and subacute or chronic diarrhea. One should suspect these infections with a history of exposure to shellfish or untreated water (including sea water). Plesiomonas diarrhea can last for months and Aeromonas diarrhea for more than a year. Treatment is mainly supportive with rehydration, but treatment with the appropriate agents may reduce the duration of the diarrhea. The organisms are usually sensitive to aminoglycosides, tetracycline, trimethoprim-sulfamethoxazole, quinolones and 3rd generation cephalosporins. However, most strains of both organisms are resistant to ampicillin.

Parasitic

Giardia: Giardia is a flagellated protozoan that infects the small intestine and biliary tract. It is the most common parasitic diarrhea in the U.S. Infection can be self-limited, or it can last for years without treatment. Epidemics are common in group homes and daycare centers. Most patients will have a chronic mild diarrhea, with emesis and abdominal pain. Foul-smelling stools and flatulence are common distinguishing symptoms. Weight loss due to chronic malabsorption in a young child should prompt an examination for Giardia. Cysts and trophozoites can be seen in the stool with routine light microscopy. However, fecal antigen ELISA is also sensitive and specific. Metronidazole is considered effective first line treatment.

Cryptosporidium: Cryptosporidium is a spore-forming protozoan that ordinarily causes a brief course of diarrhea. In immunodeficient patients, however, it can cause a severe chronic diarrhea lasting several months. This is most notably seen in AIDS patients. Severe dehydration and malnutrition can lead to death in patients with severe chronic cryptosporidiosis. Detection of Cryptosporidium is best done with an acid-fast stool smear, as standard ova and parasite examination may be unrevealing. Immunofluorescent monoclonal antibody and ELISA are also sensitive and specific stool tests. Cryptosporidium can be treated with nitazoxanide (Alinia) for 3 days, and intravenous immune globulin or bovine colostrum may be beneficial in immunocompromised children. Antiretroviral therapy with resultant increase in CD4 cell count of an HIV-infected patient can also improve diarrheal symptoms and the disease course.

Viral

Viral diarrheas rarely have a persistent course, although enteric adenoviruses are known to cause infections lasting weeks in duration. In addition, immunocompromised children, particularly those with T-cell deficiencies, may experience persistent infections of rotavirus, astrovirus, cytomegalovirus (CMV), Epstein-Barr virus (EBV), and herpes simplex virus (HSV), and these children may have diarrhea for many months.

Non-infectious diarrhea and malabsorption syndromes

Carbohydrate malabsorption: Carbohydrate malabsorption is a frequent cause of chronic diarrhea. Carbohydrates are enzymatically processed and absorbed at the intestinal brush border, and when they are not absorbed in an efficient manner, the resulting osmotic load will cause loose watery stools. Gas formation results from increased bacterial metabolism of the unabsorbed carbohydrates. Methane, carbon dioxide and hydrogen are increased and can be detectable with breath tests. In carbohydrate malabsorption, stools have a low pH and are positive for reducing substances. Diseases in this category include post-infectious diarrhea and congenital brush border enzyme and transporter deficiencies. Acquired or secondary lactase deficiency can be seen in diseases with mucosal injury, such as Crohn's disease, celiac disease and radiation enteritis.

Post-infectious diarrhea: Acute gastroenteritis, even severe episodes, typically last only 5–7 days in an otherwise healthy child. However, in cases where damage of the mucosal brush border results in lactase deficiency, diarrhea can persist beyond this. Those at risk for this "intractable diarrhea" include infants, the malnourished and those with preexisting digestive disorders. Severe damage to the mucosa can lead to generalized carbohydrate malabsorption, not just lactose intolerance.

Congenital intestinal enterocyte brush border enzyme deficiencies and epithelial dysplasias (neonatal diarrheas): The intestinal brush border is a complex system of enzymes and transporters, and malfunction in these leads to carbohydrate malabsorption and diarrhea. While the most common reason for disaccharidase intolerance is an acquired deficiency, congenital absence of enzymes and transporters do exist. Patients with these congenital disorders have profound dehydration with acidosis shortly after birth. Intake of infant formula or human milk is often not able to correct the dehydration and acidosis. Diseases in the category include glucose-galactose transporter deficiency, congenital lactase deficiency, sucrase-isomaltase deficiency, tufting enteropathy, microvillus inclusion disease and IPEX (immunodysregulation polyendocrinopathy enteropathy X-linked syndrome). Due to increasing exposure to sucrose, sucrase-isomaltase deficiency presents in childhood, rather than in infancy. Tufting enteropathy (intestinal epithelial dysplasia) presents with severe diarrhea after birth, which persists despite no enteral intake, similar to MVID. IPEX syndrome—associated with FOXP3 mutations—presents with chronic watery diarrhea, eczematous dermatitis, and endocrinopathy (usually insulin-dependent diabetes mellitus). IPEX syndrome is also associated with other autoimmune phenomena (Coombs positive anemia, autoimmune thrombocytopenia, autoimmune neutropenia, tubular nephropathy) with most affected males dying within the first year of life due to sepsis or metabolic derangements. Testing for these conditions requires the expertise of a pediatric gastroenterologist, and may require special genetic testing, endoscopy with biopsy for routine histopathology and electron microscopy, and samples of the mucosa for direct disaccharidase measurements.

Protein malabsorption: Unlike fat and carbohydrate malabsorption, significant protein malabsorption is rare outside of the CF setting. A more common reason for protein loss through the stool is protein-losing enteropathy (PLE), which is due to excessive protein secretion. PLE is usually due to mucosal damage or impediment of venous/lymphatic flow away from the small intestine. PLE is seen in IBD, celiac disease and lymphangiectasias. This condition can be screened for by an elevated fecal alpha-1-antitrypsin or fecal calprotectin.

Celiac Disease: Celiac disease is an immune-mediated reaction to gluten proteins in genetically susceptible individuals. Gluten is found in wheat, rye and barley, and elimination of the offending agent results in clinical and histologic remission. The inflammatory reaction to gluten occurs primarily in the proximal small bowel mucosa, leading to villous atrophy with malabsorption and secondary lactase deficiency. Chronic diarrhea often results, although patients can vary from asymptomatic or constipated to severe diarrhea with protein-calorie malnutrition. Young patients will commonly present with watery or bulky stools and a characteristically enlarged abdomen with wasted extremities. Short stature, delayed puberty, and musculoskeletal abnormalities (joint pain, osteopenia) are commonly associated. Please see the separate chapter on celiac disease for more details on the diagnosis and treatment of this disorder.

Crohn's Disease: Crohn's disease is a form of IBD that can cause multifactorial malabsorption and chronic diarrhea. Generalized small bowel mucosal injury can result in lactose intolerance, strictures can cause bacterial overgrowth, full-thickness bowel inflammation can lead to dysmotility (and bleeding), and rapid intestinal transit can also cause global malabsorption. In addition, PLE is common. Suspect Crohn's disease in a patient with chronic or bloody diarrhea associated with fever, weight loss, growth failure, stomatitis, and perianal disease. Please see the separate chapter on Crohn's disease for more details on the diagnosis and treatment of this disorder.

Fat malabsorption: Fat digestion requires both a functional exocrine pancreas and biliary tract. Fat is digested by pancreatic enzymes and emulsified by bile acids, both excreted through the ampulla of Vater into the duodenum. The resulting fatty acids are absorbed throughout the small bowel—short- and medium-chain fatty acids into the portal venous system and the long-chain fatty acids into the lymphatics. Interruption in any part of this complex physiologic process results in fat malabsorption with large, bulky, greasy stools that patients may interpret as chronic diarrhea.

Pancreatic disorders: Patients with pancreatic disorders such as CF, hereditary pancreatic insufficiency and chronic pancreatitis present with fat malabsorption. Destruction of pancreatic acini—or in the case of CF, obstruction of the ducts—occurs over time, leading to a loss of digestive enzyme secretion. Fat malabsorption can result in failure to thrive or weight loss. In addition, as with all fat malabsorption syndromes, fat-soluble vitamin deficiencies can occur, as well as deficiencies in essential fatty acids. Pancreatic enzyme supplementation can correct the fat malabsorption and appropriate multivitamins are recommended.

Bile acid malabsorption and chronic cholestasis: Bile acids are produced in the liver, secreted into the duodenum and actively resorbed in the terminal ileum to form an efficient enterohepatic circulation. Interruption of the resorption of bile acids in the ileum results in the passing of bile acids into the colon, where they act as a detergent, inducing chloride secretion and diarrhea. Conditions in which this may be seen include chronic cholestasis, ileal resection and radiation enteritis. Interestingly, post-cholecystectomy diarrhea may be due to increased enterohepatic circulation as well as increased passage of bile acids into the colon.

Intestinal lymphangiectasia: Long-chain fatty acids and fat-soluble vitamins are malabsorbed when lymphatic flow is obstructed as they cannot be absorbed via portal venous flow. The pressure from lymphatic obstruction can result in PLE. Intestinal lymphangiectasias can occur as a primary disease, or may be associated with celiac disease, mycobacterial infections, radiation enteritis or obstructive neoplasms. They can also be caused by distal lymphatic obstruction, such as with single-ventricle cardiac physiology after palliation (Fontan) surgery, as the thoracic duct may be obstructed. Generally, correcting the primary pathology will correct the disease, but in primary lymphangiectasia and in disease where the inciting disorders are not easily corrected, treatment should involve using short- and medium-chain fatty acids or parenteral nutrition.

Chronic secretory diarrhea

Congenital chloride diarrhea (Darrow-Gamble syndrome): Congenital chloride diarrhea is the most common of the congenital transport deficiencies. A chloride-rich stool causes profuse watery diarrhea, and this diarrhea begins prior to birth. It should be suspected if the intestines are dilated and fluid-filled on fetal ultrasonography.

Stool chloride will be elevated after the first few days of life. Electrolyte and water replacement therapy is essential to prevent growth retardation and renal involvement.

VIPoma (WDHA syndrome: watery diarrhea, hypokalemia, and achlorhydria): In patients with chronic watery diarrhea, hypokalemia, and alkalosis, a VIPoma should be suspected. Abdominal distension and growth arrest are frequently seen. Elevated levels of serum vasoactive intestinal peptide (VIP) are very suggestive of this disease, and imaging should be pursued of the adrenal glands and along the sympathetic nervous chain. VIPomas are most often ganglioneuromas, ganglioneuroblastomas and metastatic neuroblastomas. In adults, however, VIPomas are more often pancreatic islet cell tumors.

Zinc deficiency and acrodermatitis enteropathica: Zinc deficiency can occur due to chronic diarrhea, and it also can cause or exacerbate chronic diarrhea. Zinc exists in either a free state, or bound to metallothionein and stored in enterocytes. Free intraluminal zinc is absorbed into the portal circulation. Zinc is therefore lost in chronic diarrhea with increased enterocyte turnover. Wound healing is dependent upon zinc, and experimental models have shown that the intestinal mucosa recovers more slowly after a diarrheal episode in a zinc-deficient state. Deficiency leads to upregulation of cytokines and guanylate cyclase C, which produces cGMP. cGMP in turn alters the function of the cystic-fibrosis transmembrane regulator (CFTR), producing dysregulation of the sodium-chloride balance at the mucosal membrane and resulting in a secretory diarrhea. This may be seen in any zinc-deficient patient, but its effects are most dramatic in patients with acrodermatitis enteropathica (AE). AE is an autosomal recessive disorder due to a genetic mutation of SLC39A4 on 8q24.3, which encodes for a zinc uptake protein. Symptoms, which include profound diarrhea as well as dry, scaly, erythematous plaques of skin around the mouth and anus and on the scalp, hands and feet, occur within the first few months of life and appear shortly after discontinuation of breastfeeding (leading to the hypothesis that human milk has a beneficial ligand not found in cow's milk). Also seen in AE are vesicular and pustular lesions, alopecia, anorexia, paronychia, and superinfections with Staphylococcus and Candida.

Diagnosis:

History and physical exam: The first step in the diagnosis of a chronic diarrhea is to separate true chronic diarrhea—which generally is a result of intestinal malabsorption—from persistent diarrhea—which is usually infectious and secretory in nature. A careful history, including when and under what circumstances the diarrhea was first noted, is critical. Any clear history of a sudden starting point should suggest an infectious disease, and a suitable workup should include stool studies for bacterial culture and parasitic inspection. More indolent courses should point towards true chronic diarrhea and malabsorption. Most of these cases will present with failure to thrive or even frank weight loss, and a careful history including the construction of growth charts should be pursued. The characteristics of the stool should be illicited; greasy floating stools suggest fat malabsorption while watery stools associated with gas production may suggest carbohydrate malabsorption.

Physical exam may or may not be revealing. Growth failure with protein-calorie malnutrition will be present in many of the malabsorption syndromes. Jaundice and hepatomegaly may indicate cholestasis. A protuberant abdomen and wasted extremities can suggest celiac disease. Stomatitis and perianal lesions may indicate Crohn's disease.

Labs: Specific testing should be guided by the history and physical. Initial screening tests may include a CBC with differential, ESR or CRP for Crohn's disease, antibodies for celiac disease, hydrogen breath testing for carbohydrate malabsorption, and a sweat chloride test for CF. Stool tests may include alpha-1-antitrypsin or calprotectin for PLE, trypsin for pancreatic insufficiency (presence of trypsin indicates sufficiency), 3 day quantitative stool fat with corresponding diet history for fat malabsorption, and stool pH and reducing substances for carbohydrate malabsorption and postinfectious diarrhea. Low bicarbonate is generally seen with chronic diarrhea, particularly that of a secretory nature. Low albumin and protein can be seen in patients with PLE. In patients with chronic cholestasis or other diseases of the hepatobiliary system, elevated transaminases, bilirubin and alkaline phosphatase can be present. If the chronic diarrhea has resulted in a zinc deficiency, then a very low alkaline phosphatase may result, since zinc is a co-factor for the enzymatic reaction to detect this protein.

Radiographic studies: An abdominal plain film (KUB) is often unrevealing for causes of malabsorption. A calcified pancreas can indicate a hereditary pancreatitis. Upper GI series with oral radiocontrast may show enteritis due to infectious (Giardia, cryptosporidium) or inflammatory (Crohn's, celiac disease) conditions. Small bowel strictures, which can lead to bacterial overgrowth and malabsorption, can also be seen on UGI with Crohn's disease.

Endoscopy with biopsy: Endoscopic findings can be seen in infectious duodenitis, celiac disease and Crohn's disease in which there may be aphthous ulcers, bleeding, fissures and scalloping of the folds. Biopsies will be helpful in many of the diseases, such as celiac disease in which intestinal villous blunting will be seen. Special stains should be done for infections such as Giardia and mycobacteria. Light and electron microscopy can be revealing for the different causes of carbohydrate malabsorption. ERCP can be useful to diagnose (and potentially palliate) causes of biliary or pancreatic causes of malabsorption. Biopsy specimens can be also analyzed for enzyme deficiencies, such as lactase.

Management

Nutrition/diet: The American Academy of Pediatrics recommends that children with chronic diarrhea and malabsorption who are not dehydrated be fed age-appropriate diets, and those that are dehydrated should be fed shortly after rehydration. Bland diets—often lacking in protein—are no longer recommended. In those with malnutrition, a diet liberal in calories and protein should be provided to achieve catch-up growth. Some patients may require a calorically dense formula, either orally or via night-time nasogastric tube feeds. As shown via endoscopy in pediatric trials for diarrhea due to conditions such as inflammatory bowel disease, exclusive enteral nutrition using an elemental formula promotes healing and decreased inflammation. Intravenous nutrition may be required for those with very poor nutritional status associated with vomiting and diarrhea. However, for those who can tolerate enteral feeds complete "gut rest" with IV nutrition is not recommended.

Consultations: Successful management of the child with a chronic malabsorptive condition requires a team approach involving the patient, parents, other caretakers, school, gastroenterologist, primary care practitioner, and a dietician. After a diagnosis, the child should be referred to a registered dietician for a personalized nutritional assessment and education. If poor growth, short stature or delayed sexual maturation remain present despite compliance with medical therapy, referral to a pediatric endocrinologist should be considered. Children with autoimmune diseases, such as celiac disease and IBD, may have co-morbid growth hormone deficiency, osteopenia or another concomitant autoimmune condition.

Psychiatric: Children with chronic illnesses causing malabsorption have major concerns regarding their height, weight, use of chronic medications, and worrying about when their disease is going to flare up. Support must be given to the patient and family when dealing with a lifelong illness. Depression is common and may warrant a referral for individual or family counseling or to a psychiatrist.

Monitoring: The child with chronic malabsorption should have frequent monitoring of growth and sexual maturation. Measurements of iron, fat-soluble vitamins, and liver function should be done. Measurement of bone density is often helpful in discovering occult osteopenia, and would suggest more aggressive supplementation of vitamin D and calcium, along with weight-bearing exercise and closer monitoring of linear growth. Routine monitoring labs, such as CBC with differential, ESR, CRP, serum chemistries and vitamin levels should be tailored to the patient's disease location, medications, and clinical course. Repeat endoscopy should be considered for a child with celiac disease or IBD who is not doing well clinically in order to assess disease status. Capsule endoscopy is also starting to play a role in non-invasive monitoring of small bowel mucosal disease.

Pearls and Precautions

School/education: Urgency with chronic malabsorption may impact the child's ability to learn while in school. Because children with a chronic disease may not appear ill to the teacher, they are often denied restroom access during class. The patient's primary care physician or gastroenterologist may need to write letters for the patient to allow him or her to use the restroom when needed, or have the ability to use the school nurse's restroom if available. It is important for the hospitalized child to continue receiving school assignments, so as not to fall behind their classmates. Children with severe chronic diarrhea or recovering from bowel resection may require home schooling.

Medications to AVOID: Anti-diarrheal and antiemetic medications, such as Lomotil (diphenoxylate and atropine), Imodium (loperamide), Tigan (trimethobenzamide hydrochloride) and Reglan (metoclopramide) are contraindicated in children with acute and chronic infections and the majority of pediatric malabsorptive disorders. The side effects of these medications outweigh potential benefits in the pediatric population under these circumstances and should be prescribed with extreme caution.

Miscellaneous

- Autoimmunity does not exist in isolation. As such, a family history of type 1 diabetes, rheumatoid arthritis, Grave's disease, Hashimoto's thyroiditis, lupus, Sjögren's syndrome and other autoimmune diseases should cause the practitioner to investigate for these chronic malabsorptive conditions, such as IBD and celiac disease.
- Although historically CF, celiac disease and IBD have been described as common in the Caucasian population, other ethnicities can have these disorders.
- Iron is absorbed in the duodenum. As such, consider CF, celiac disease and Crohn's disease when investigating a child with chronic malabsorption and iron deficiency.
- Pathogens which usually cause a short, self-limited course of diarrhea in the normal host may lead to severe, protracted or relapsing disease in the immune-deficient host. The differential diagnosis of the causes of chronic diarrhea in immunocompromised children should broadly include bacteria (campylobacter, C. difficile, salmonella, shigella, yersinia, mycobacteria), fungi (candida, histoplasma, Paracoccidioides) as well as the above mentioned parasites and viruses.

References

Keating JP. "Chronic Diarrhea." Pediatrics in Review. Vol 26 No 1 (2005): 5–14.

Pietzak MM and Thomas DW. "Childhood Malabsorption." Pediatrics in Review. Vol 24 No 6 (2003): 195–206.

Hogdson HJF and Epstein O. "Malabsorption." Medicine. Vol 35 No 4 (2007): 220–225.

Crohn's Disease

Michelle Pietzak

Crohn's disease (CD) is a multi-system autoimmune disease which can affect the gastrointestinal tract anywhere from the oral cavity through the rectum. The diagnosis requires gastrointestinal endoscopy and biopsy. At present, there is no cure for Crohn's disease. Management primarily involves treating the symptoms while minimizing toxicity of chronic medications.

Etiology

As with most autoimmune conditions, Crohn's disease is thought to arise from a combination of genetic and environmental influences. Several genes have recently been associated with Crohn's disease, most of which involve the activation of Th1-related cells and cytokines. Multiple environmental factors have been studied. Increased risk for the development of Crohn's disease have been reported with diets high in refined sugars and omega-6 fatty acids and low in fruits and vegetables, lack of breastfeeding, diarrheal illness in infancy, cigarette smoking, and use of NSAIDS.

Clinical Presentation and Prognosis:

Demographics: It is thought that approximately one million people in the U.S. have Crohn's Disease. Of those, 50,000 children suffer from inflammatory bowel disease (IBD; Crohn's disease and ulcerative colitis combined). About 25% of them are diagnosed in the pediatric age range. IBD is a disease of the young, with the peak incidence occurring in the late teens and early twenties. Like most autoimmune diseases, IBD appears to occur more often in westernized—as opposed to developing—countries. Depending upon geographic location in the U.S., between 7 and 10 children per 100,000 will be diagnosed with IBD. It occurs with equal incidence among males and females, but has an increased incidence among Caucasians, especially Ashkenazi Jews. There tends to be a family predisposition to autoimmunity. As with most autoimmune diseases in westernized nations, the incidence appears to be increasing and the disease presenting at younger ages.

Presenting signs and symptoms: As opposed to acute infections which cause colitis, CD is insidious, not abrupt. Children with CD often have growth failure and protein-calorie malnutrition for years prior to the histologic diagnosis. CD can have presentations outside of the gastrointestinal tract. Patients may have extra-intestinal symptoms WITHOUT intestinal symptoms, and thus CD diagnosis is often missed.

(a) *Classic gastrointestinal symptoms:* Diarrhea, abdominal pain, fistulae and strictures, GI bleeding, stomatitis, nutritional deficiencies and perianal disease (skin tags, fissures, fistulae and abscesses) are classic findings.

(b) *Constitutional symptoms:* Fever, weight loss, fatigue and anorexia are common in CD.

(c) *Liver:* Active or autoimmune hepatitis, jaundice, pruritus, fatigue, cirrhosis, primary sclerosing cholangitis, bile duct carcinoma (late complication), steatosis, amyloid deposition and recurrent pancreatitis have all been associated with CD.

(d) *Rheumatologic:* Joint pain is the second most common complaint in CD patients after GI symptoms. Joints affected are usually the large joints (wrist, elbow, hip, knee, and ankle). This can be differentiated from rheumatoid arthritis in that the patient is rheumatoid factor negative and there is no joint destruction. Joint pain often improves with treatment of the IBD and flares when the GI tract flares. Osteopenia leading to osteoporosis and fractures is common in CD, and can occur even in childhood.

(e) *Endocrine:* Short stature, delayed growth and sexual maturation are presentations for CD and may present without concomitant GI symptoms.

(f) Skin:

    i. *Erythema nodosum:* tender red nodules usually near the anterior tibias which occur during IBD flares.

    ii. *Pyoderma gangrenosum:* skin ulcers which can occur on the extremities and around ostomies of patients with IBD.

    iii. *Vasculitis:* inflammation of peripheral vessels which blanch to the touch and may be tender.

(g) *Ocular:* Episcleritis (an inflammatory condition of the connective tissue between the conjunctiva and sclera) and uveitis may be ophthalmologic emergencies.

(h) *Renal:* Calculi are seen in about 5% of children with CD due to ileal dysfunction. Ureteric obstruction and hydronephrosis can result from chronically inflamed bowel adjacent to the kidneys.

(i) *Mouth:* Recurrent oral aphthous ulcers can be seen in both CD and celiac disease. Gingivitis can be due to granulomas within the gums. Pyostomatitis vegetans is a rare chronic inflammatory condition characterized by pustules and erosions on the gingival and labial or buccal mucosa.

(j) *Endocrine/Reproductive system*: Infertility and delayed puberty are seen in both sexes who have undiagnosed CD. Isolated short stature without overt GI involvement may be seen.

(k) *Anemia:* Fatigue, pallor and shortness of breath on exertion are common complaints. Anemia may be due to chronic disease or chronic GI blood loss. Iron deficiency is one of the most common micronutrient deficiencies in undiagnosed children with CD. Deficiencies in vitamin E can lead to a hemolytic anemia. Advanced small bowel disease can lead to B12 and folic acid malabsorption.

(l) *Neurologic/psychiatric*: Patients with CD have higher rates of depression than the general population. Vitamin deficiencies may lead to peripheral neuropathy, ataxia and neurologic symptoms.

Clinical course: Every child with CD has a unique presentation, clinical course and prognosis. It is thought that children who exhibit "fistulizing" (abnormal connections between gut and gut, gut and skin or gut and bladder) or "stenosing" (persistent narrowing of gut) disease have a progressively worse surgical outcome than those who exhibit simply "inflammatory" disease.

Prognosis: The prognosis for a child diagnosed with CD is guarded, as there is currently no cure for the condition. Overt GI symptomatology often waxes and wanes with flares, which may be idiopathic or due to stressors in the environment (diet, smoking, puberty, pregnancy, moving, going away to college, final exams, death in the family, etc.). Iron deficiency anemia and fat-soluble vitamin deficiencies can be corrected with supplementation after diagnosis. Growth failure may or may not improve with treatment, and may require supplemental calories via a special diet or formula, intravenous nutrition, or even growth hormone supplementation. Patients with structuring or fistulizing disease are thought to have the worst prognosis, as they often require multiple hospitalizations, strong immunosuppression and often bowel resection. The overall GI cancer risk for patients with long-standing CD is higher than for that of the general population, although rarely reported in the pediatric age range. The risk for colorectal cancer after 20 years of severe CD colitis has been reported to be about 8%.

Diagnosis

History and physical exam: The diagnostic approach to the child with CD is to first suspect the diagnosis. A thorough history and physical are key, and should include serial plotting of weight, height, BMI, pubertal staging, and a bone age if there is growth delay. A family history for IBD, GI cancers and autoimmune diseases are essential. On physical exam, the young child with undiagnosed CD may exhibit protein calorie malnutrition, with decreased subcutaneous fat stores and muscle bulk. Older children may have shown a gradual deceleration over years on the pediatric height and weight curves. Isolated short stature or delayed puberty can be seen without overt GI symptoms. Abdominal distention with tympani can be appreciated due to gaseousness. Overt upper or lower GI bleeding may be present. Symptoms of iron deficiency anemia may include pallor, decreased appetite, abdominal pain, generalized fatigue, sleep disturbances, frontal headache and shortness of breath with exercise. Signs of iron deficiency anemia may include clubbing, brittle hair and nails, and a sore, smooth, shiny and/or reddened tongue. Fat-soluble vitamin deficiencies may present with increased bruising and bleeding (vitamin K), osteopenia or osteoporosis (vitamin D), hemolytic anemia, impaired balance and muscle weakness (vitamin E) or impaired night vision, dry eyes, rough skin, loss of taste and poor wound healing (vitamin A). Zinc deficiency can occur with chronic diarrhea. Liver function tests should be routinely checked. Exams of the joints, skin and eye should be performed for the extra-intestinal manifestations as described above.

Routine laboratory testing: Elevations in white blood cell counts, platelet counts, C-reactive protein and sedimentation rate are often seen. A microcytic or macrocytic anemia may be present due to iron, B12 or folic acid deficiencies. A chemistry panel may show low potassium due to chronic emesis, low bicarbonate with chronic diarrhea, low albumin and protein due to protein-losing enteropathy, and elevated transaminases, bilirubin and alkaline phosphatase if the liver or biliary tree is involved. A very low alkaline phosphatase result may indicate a deficiency of this enzyme's co-factor, zinc, which can be seen with chronic diarrhea.

Tests for colitis and ileitis: If a child is presenting with colitis, tests for other more common infectious etiologies should include routine stool cultures for Salmonella, Shigella, Yersinia, Campylobacter, Aeromonas and E. coli 0157:H7, stool ova and parasites (for Amoebae), and Clostridium difficile toxins A and B. The patient should also have a PPD placed and chest X-ray taken to evaluate for Mycobacterium tuberculosis. If the disease appears to be located primarily in the terminal ileum (for example, when thickening of this area is seen on CT scan), infections with Yersinia and M. tuberculosis need to be ruled out. In patients with chronic diarrhea, growth failure, delayed sexual maturation, iron deficiency anemia and/or joint pain without overt GI bleeding, serologies should be sent to evaluate for celiac disease (see separate section on celiac disease for appropriate testing).

Stool tests: Alpha-1-antitrypsin is an enzyme made by hepatocytes, monocytes and macrophages. Elevations in fecal alpha-1-antitrypsin correlate with protein-losing enteropathy, IBD disease activity and response to therapy. Fecal calprotectin is a calcium- and zinc-binding protein which originates from neutrophils, monocytes, and macrophages, and can detect gastrointestinal inflammation and differentiate IBD from functional gastrointestinal disorders such as irritable bowel syndrome. Like alpha-1-antitrypsin, elevations correlate well to the endoscopic and microscopic disease activity in IBD, including in pediatric patients.

Serologic testing: Anti-Saccharomyces cerevisiae IgG and IgA are antibodies to Baker's and Brewer's yeast, and are elevated in 39% to 61% of patients with CD. pANCA are antibodies against cytoplasmic antigens which are most strongly associated with Crohn's colitis. OmpC is an antibody to outer membrane porin C on the cell wall of E. coli and is elevated in up to 55% of patients with CD. Anti-CBir1 is an antibody to flagellin on bacteria and is seen in about half of CD patients. Potential roles for IBD serology include categorizing a child with indeterminate colitis into either CD or ulcerative colitis, and to help identify patients at risk for aggressive disease behavior who may benefit from stronger medications. At present, these serologic screening tests are best utilized by gastroenterologists who are seeing patients at high risk for IBD, and not primary care practitioners who are screening for IBD in the general population.

Genetic testing: Although several key genetic mutations have been found to be associated with CD over the past decade (the best known, NOD2/CARD15, an intracellular pattern recognition receptor for a bacterial peptide coded located on chromosome 16), they are currently being utilized as research tools and not for screening the pediatric population.

Endoscopy with biopsy: Disease location should be determined by upper and lower endoscopy. Visually, the mucosa may range from slightly erythematous, edematous and nodular to having exudates, deep fissures, cobblestoning, and frank ulcerations with marked GI bleeding. Classically in CD, the terminal ileum is involved, and there may be "skip areas" (visually and histologically normal mucosa) within the colon. The mouth, esophagus and stomach may also be involved in CD. Colonic biopsies may show acute and chronic inflammation with mixed inflammatory cells. Ideally, surgical specimens should show transmural inflammation to all layers of the gut (as opposed to ulcerative colitis, which shows more superficial ulcerations). Histology may show granulomas, which are pathognomonic for either CD or infections such as those caused by Mycobacteria, fungi, Chlamydia, or Yersinia.

The small bowel may also be visualized by upper gastrointestinal imaging (UGI) with small bowel follow-through (to look for ulcerations and strictures), capsule endoscopy (to look for mucosal changes in the jejunum and ileum and occult GI cancers) or push enteroscopy.

Management

The goals of management in CD are to treat acute symptoms, induce and maintain remission, improve quality of life, avoid medication toxicity and prevent cancer.

Nutrition/diet: In those with malnutrition, a diet liberal in calories and protein should be provided to achieve catch-up growth. Some patients may require a calorically dense formula via night-time nasogastric tube feeds. Exclusive enteral nutrition using an elemental formula has demonstrated endoscopic healing and decreased inflammation in pediatric trials. However, compliance with this type of regimen in the U.S. has historically been poor, and relapse occurs in most patients within one year of resuming a normal diet. Intravenous nutrition may be required for those with severe nutritional status or anatomic disease (stricture or fistula). However, when compared to enteral nutrition, complete "gut rest" with IV nutrition has not proven to be superior to inducing remission. It is hypothesized that the Westernized diet, high in ω-6 PUFAs (polyunsaturated fatty acids), increases risk for IBD or contributes to flares. There may be a potential role for ω-3 PUFAs, found in fish oil, as anti-inflammatory agents in IBD.

Medications

Table 5.2 summarizes options for medical treatment of CD.

Surgery: Absolute indications for surgery include intestinal perforation, massive hemorrhage, chronic obstruction or evidence of dysplasia or cancer. Relative indications include perianal complications, complex fistulae or abscesses or refractory disease with growth failure.

Table 5.2: Options for Medical Treatment of Crohn's Disease

Medication	Indication	Adverse Effects
Antibiotics: metronidazole	• Mild active CD • Perianal disease • Prevention pouchitis	• Metallic taste, furry tongue, nausea, anorexia, candidiasis, peripheral neuropathy
Aminosalicylates: mesalamine, sulfasalazine	• Mild CD • May not be better than placebo in some studies	• Rash, fever, nausea, vomiting, headaches, hemolysis, agranulocytosis, alveolitis, hepatitis, pancreatitis, nephritis, male infertility
Oral corticosteroids: Prednisone	• Moderate CD • Rapidly active, inexpensive	• Aseptic necrosis, hyperglycemia, hypertension, diabetes, cataracts, osteoporosis, growth inhibition, striae, acne, cushingoid appearance
Immunomodulators: 6 MP, azathioprine	• Moderate CD	• Fever, myalgias, nausea, rash, pancreatitis, hepatitis, pancytopenia, increased risk of lymphoma
Methotrexate	• Moderate CD	• Nausea, hepatitis, hypersensitivity pneumonitis; little pediatric data
Intravenous corticosteroids: Solumedrol	• Severe CD	• As with oral steroids
Cyclosporin	• Severe CD	• Lack of pediatric data • Renal dysfunction, hirsutism, tremor, hypertension, gum hyperplasia, allergic reaction, hypomagnesemia, drug interactions, • PCP pneumonia, lymphoproliferative disease
Tacrolimus	• Severe CD	• Lack of pediatric data • Tremor, headache, diarrhea, hypertension, nausea, abnormal renal function, hyperkalemia, hypomagnesemia, hyperglycemia
Biologics: Infliximab (only one FDA approved for pediatrics)	• Severe CD	• Infusion reaction, reactivation TB, fungal infections, histoplasmosis, increased risk of lymphoma
Surgery	• Severe CD	• Risk for adhesions, strictures, fistulas

Consultations: Successful management of the child with CD requires a team approach involving the patient, parents, other caretakers, school, gastroenterologist, primary care practitioner, and a dietician. After a biopsy-confirmed diagnosis, the child should be referred to a registered dietician knowledgeable about CD for a personalized nutritional assessment and education. If poor growth, short stature or delayed sexual maturation remains present despite compliance with medical therapy, referral to a pediatric endocrinologist should be considered. Children with CD may have co-morbid growth hormone deficiency, osteopenia or another concomitant autoimmune condition.

Psychiatric: Children with CD have major concerns regarding their height, weight, use of chronic medications, and worrying about when their disease is going to flare up. Those on chronic steroids have self-esteem issues due to acne and cushingoid appearance. Support must be given to the patient and family when dealing with this lifelong, incurable illness. Depression is common and may warrant a referral for individual or family counseling.

Social: Local, national and international support groups exist for both children and adults with CD. They can easily be found on the internet, and provide not only emotional support, but tips on dealing with schools, eating out, traveling with IBD, and education about resources. These include Crohn's & Colitis Foundation of America, www.CCFA.org and IBD Support Foundation, www.ibdsf.com. There are also summer camps available in the U.S. which can maintain a kitchen which can prepare special meals for children with IBD, dispense medications, and have a physician and/or nurse on site for medical emergencies. It is often an eye-opening experience for the newly diagnosed child and family with IBD to meet others at camp dealing with the same physical and emotional issues.

Monitoring: The child with CD should have frequent monitoring of growth and sexual maturation. Measurements of iron, fat-soluble vitamins, and liver function should be done. Measurement of bone density is often helpful in discovering occult osteopenia, and would suggest more aggressive supplementation of vitamin D and calcium, along with weight-bearing exercise and closer monitoring of linear growth. Routine monitoring labs, such as CBC with differential, ESR, CRP, serum chemistries and urinalysis should be tailored to the patient's disease location, medications, and clinical course. In order to assess disease status, repeat endoscopy should be considered for a child with CD who is not doing well clinically. Imaging, such as UGI with small bowel follow-through to look for strictures, and CT scan to look for fistulas/stricture and intra-abdominal abscesses, may be required. However, the practitioner must take into account cumulative radiation exposure from these repeat radiographic studies in a child with CD. Capsule endoscopy is also starting to play a role in non-invasive monitoring of small bowel mucosal disease.

Pearls and Precautions

Likely complications: Nutritional complications of CD are common including protein-calorie malnutrition, iron and fat-soluble vitamin deficiencies, and osteoporosis and fractures. Patients with CD may be lactose intolerant with small bowel disease. Due to osteoporosis risk, adequate vitamin D and calcium may need to be incorporated into the diet from non-dairy sources such as fortified soymilk, orange juice, fatty fish and eggs. Alternatives include milk pre-digested with lactase and taking a lactase pill prior to dairy ingestion. Many will also tolerate yogurt and cheese, even if fresh whole milk and ice cream cause symptomatology.

Immunizations: There are no contraindications to vaccination in the child with CD unless they are receiving immune suppressing medications, in which case live viral vaccines should not be given.

School/education: Urgency with Crohn's colitis may impact the child's ability to learn while in school. Because children with CD may not appear ill to the teacher, they are often denied restroom access during class. The PCP or gastroenterologist may need to write letters for the patient to allow him or her to use the restroom when needed, or have the ability to use the school nurse's restroom if available. It is important for the hospitalized child with IBD flare to continue to receive school assignments, so as not to fall behind their classmates. Children with severe CD or recovering from bowel resection may require home schooling.

References

Ponsky T, Hindle A, and Sandler A. Inflammatory Bowel Disease in the Pediatric Patient. Surg Clin N Am 2007;87:643–658.

Kugathasan S, Judd R, Hoffmann R, Heikenen J, Telega G, Khan F, Weisdorf-Schindele S, San Pablo Jr W, Perroult J, Park R, Yaffe M, Brown C, Rivera-Bennett MT, Halabi I, Martinez A, Blank E, Werlin SL, Rudolph C, Binion DG for the Wisconsin Pediatric IBD Alliance. Epidemiologic and Clinical Characteristics of Children with Newly Diagnosed Pediatric Inflammatory Bowel Disease in Wisconsin: A Statewide Population-based Study. Journal of Pediatrics. 2003;143:525–31.

Griffiths AM, Nicholas D, Smith C. et al. Development of a paediatric IBD quality of life index: dealing with differences related to age and IBD type. J Pediatr Gatroenterol Nutr 1999;28:S46–52.

Cyclic Vomiting Syndrome

Dafna Bababeygy, Michelle Pietzak

Cyclic vomiting syndrome (CVS) is a disorder characterized by a distinct pattern of intense vomiting. By definition, this self-limited emesis cannot be attributed to a known organic cause.

Etiology

An organic cause to CVS has not been found. However it is thought that the dysfunction may originate in the central nervous system rather than the abdomen. Multiple mechanisms have been postulated for CVS including: migraine variant or equivalent, hypothalamic/adrenal dysfunction (Sato's syndrome), impaired neuro-immune interactions, fatty acid oxidation disorders, mitochondrial disorders, ion channelopathies and gastrointestinal motility disorders thought to be due to autonomic neuropathy.

Clinical Presentation and Prognosis

Demographics: The disorder is most commonly diagnosed in school-aged children, but the age of presentation can range from infancy through young adulthood. The disorder is more common in Caucasians, with a female predominance (3:2 female to male ratio).

Presenting signs and symptoms: The patient usually presents in the morning hours with incapacitating nausea which progresses to acute, intense and often bilious emesis. The forceful, constant emesis may lead to severe dehydration. Other symptoms may include fatigue, listlessness, pallor, anorexia, abdominal pain, headache, phonophobia and photophobia. The attacks may be triggered by both physical and emotional stressors such as infections, menstruation, sleep deprivation, birthdays, holidays and impending due dates for school projects or examinations. CVS is a diagnosis of exclusion. Acutely, it may mimic surgical and non-surgical disorders such as small bowel obstruction, hepatitis, pancreatitis, appendicitis, cholecystitis, ureteropelvic junction (UPJ) obstruction, metabolic syndromes, and neurological disorders such as a brain tumor, Chiari malformation, hydrochephalus or subdural hematoma.

Clinical course: CVS is composed of the "well phase" and the "episodic phase." During the well phase, the patient is asymptomatic. The episodic phase is divided into the prodrome, the emetic phase and the recovery phase. Abortive therapy, instituted in the prodromal or emetic phase, could potentially terminate the attack and/or reduce its severity. School age children may continue to have cyclic vomiting until adolescence at which point the vomiting abates and migraine headaches may commence. In a small percentage of patients, the vomiting continues through adulthood.

Prognosis: Mortality occurs when patients are misdiagnosed with CVS while there is an organic etiology for the vomiting (such as a malrotation with intermittent volvulus). In the emetic phase of CVS, patients may have intractable vomiting leading to dehydration, ketosis and possibly death. Unnecessary invasive procedures such as endoscopy, appendectomy, cholecystectomy, exploratory laparatomy and hysterectomy contribute to increased morbidity.

Diagnosis

History and physical exam: According to the NASPGHAN Consensus Statement on CVS (reference 1), all of the following six diagnostic criteria must be met to confirm the diagnosis:

- At least 5 attacks in any interval, or a minimum of 3 attacks during a 6 month period
- Episodic attacks of intense nausea and vomiting lasting 1 hour to 10 days and occurring at least 1 week apart
- Stereotypical pattern and symptoms in the individual patient
- Vomiting during attacks occurring at least 4 times/hour for at least 1 hour (although atypical CVS may exist with less frequent vomiting)
- Return to baseline health between episodes
- Emesis cannot be attributed to another disorder

According to the NASPGHAN Consensus Statement on CVS (reference 1), the following findings are "red flags" which warrant further workup for disorders other than CVS:

1. Bilious emesis, abdominal tenderness and/or severe abdominal pain
2. Attacks brought on by a defined trigger, such as illness, fasting, and/or a high protein meal
3. Abnormalities on neurologic exam including altered mental status, papilledema, abnormal eye movements, ataxia or motor asymmetry
4. Progressively worsening episodes or conversion to a continuous or chronic pattern of vomiting

Family history: There is often a family history of migraine headaches in children with CVS.

Labs: There are no specific laboratory markers used to diagnose CVS. In dehydrated patients, electrolytes, glucose, BUN and creatinine should be checked to help with IV fluid management. If all attacks are preceded by a defined trigger (such as fasting, high-protein meal or intercurrent illness), additional labs should include serum lactate, ammonia, carnitine, acylcarnitine and amino acids and urine for ketones and organic acids. In the presence of bilious emesis, amylase, lipase, AST, ALT, bilirubin, GGT and urinalysis should be obtained to evaluate for pancreatitis, hepatitis and urinary tract disorders.

Radiology: An upper gastrointestinal series with small bowel follow-through is mandatory to rule out malrotation with midgut volvulus in the acute setting, as this missed diagnosis is associated with high morbidity and mortality. Depending upon clinical symptoms, physical exam and screening labs, abdominal ultrasound or CT should be considered to evaluate the liver, pancreas and biliary tree (gallstones) and urinary tract system. Any abnormality on neurologic exam warrants a brain MRI, which is superior to CT for visualizing the posterior fossa.

Endoscopy: Endoscopic visualization of the upper GI tract should be considered if there is evidence to suspect a mucosal abnormality, such as esophagitis, gastritis, duodenitis, gastric or duodenal ulcer, celiac disease or Crohn's disease. These patients may present with hematemesis, anemia, short stature and/or protein-calorie malnutrition. Please see separate chapters on celiac disease and Crohn's disease.

Management

Medications: Prophylactic, abortive and supportive medications are used based on the patient's presentation and the phase of illness, as outlined below:

Acute attack management: Supportive measures, abortive therapies and treatment of coexisting complications should be addressed during the acute emetic phase of CVS. Supportive care includes placing the child in a dark and quiet environment, correcting dehydration and electrolyte abnormalities, using anti-emetics and providing pain relief. Dextrose-containing fluids help attenuate the metabolic derangements during this catabolic state. In general, the recommended intravenous fluid is D_{10} 0.45 NS with KCl at 1.5 times maintenance fluid rates (after correction of dehydration with normal saline boluses, if needed). If the patient has no enteral intake for 3–5 days, one should strongly consider parenteral nutrition with a minimum (depending upon the age of the patient) of 1.5g of amino acids/kg/day and total calories above the catabolic threshold (roughly 55–70 kcal/kg/day in the older child). Recommended anti-emetics include the serotonin 3 (5-HT3) receptor antagonist agents, including ondansetron (Zofran) or granisetron (Kytril), which may be administered orally, rectally or intravenously. Sedatives such as diphenhydramine and lorazepam are recommended when patients continue to vomit despite the use of anti-emetics. Ondansetron and lorazepam have been suggested to be the most effective combination therapy for symptomatic relief of nausea and vomiting. Severe abdominal pain can be treated initially with ketorolac (Toradol), morphine or hydromorphone. Ketorolac should be used with caution in the long-term management of these patients. As with other non-steroidal medications, GI ulcers, bleeding and perforation have been reported with ketorolac, as well as nephritis, hypersensitivity reactions and fluid retention with edema. If the pain is accompanied by dyspepsia, heartburn or esophagitis, oral or intravenous H_2 receptor antagonists or proton pump inhibitors can be added. A short acting angiotensin converting enzyme (ACE) inhibitor can be used for patients with transient hypertension. During the recovery period after the emetic phase, the child may be rapidly advanced to a normal diet. In patients with underlying dysmotility, a slow reintroduction of food may prevent further nausea.

Prophylactic care: Medications recommended for the prevention of emetic episodes are based upon expert opinion rather than evidence-based medicine. Most of these medications are also commonly used in migraine prophylaxis. Preventative medications should be considered when the patient has almost monthly episodes or the quality of life is being negatively affected by multiple hospitalizations and school absences. The medication used for prophylaxis depends upon several factors, including the child's age, side effects of the medications, dosage form, and medical and psychological comorbidities. Options to reduce the number and length of emetic episodes include cyproheptadine (Periactin, first choice), propanolol (second choice), amytriptyline, phenobarbital and pizotifen (also known as pizotyline, trade name Sandomigran). In children less than 5 years of age, it is recommended to start either cyproheptadine or propanolol. In children over 5 years of age, amytriptyline or propanolol can be used. Mitochondrial disorders have been reported in patients with CVS. Therefore, supplementing with nutrients involved in mitochondrial biology, such as carnitine and coenzyme Q, may be helpful in preventing future attacks. Acupuncture of the P6 (pericardial point) has also been reported to decrease the severity of attacks.

Psychological: The patient and family dealing with CVS may experience feelings of helplessness, despair, depression and anger. Anxiety and fear over future attacks may trigger CVS. Therefore, it is important that the clinician reassure the patient that the attacks are not self induced and will usually dissipate with age. Anxiolytic medications, guided imagery and/or deep breathing may help abort attacks brought on by anxiety. Psychotherapy utilizing age appropriate dramatic play and utilizing metaphors in stories and drawings have been reported to be beneficial.

Social: Families are often frustrated in dealing with CVS as there has often been a significant delay in obtaining the diagnosis. Also, once diagnosed, CVS is often unpredictable, and there is little long-term clinical data on effective therapies and prognosis. Patients and their families should seek the care of a physician familiar with the disorder and obtain information from support groups, such as the Cyclic Vomiting Syndrome Association: http://www.cvsaonline.org

Monitoring: A patient can maintain a vomiting diary to look for occult lifestyle and dietary triggers and to better tailor prophylactic therapy. If the patient is on prophylactic therapy, the appropriate drug monitoring should be obtained at regular intervals (i.e., checking EKG QTc interval before starting tricyclic antidepressants and 10 days after peak dose).

Pearls and Precautions

Lifestyle modifications implemented during the well phase such as avoidance of sleep deprivation, trigger-foods, motion sickness, high emotional states and fasting can reduce the recurrence of the emetic phase. Females with catemenial (menses-related) CVS have been successfully treated with low-dose estrogen oral contraceptives.

Nutrition/Diet: Fasting may precipitate an attack. As with migraines, trigger foods for CVS include chocolate, cheese, hot dog, aspartame, caffeine, alcohol and monosodium glutamate (MSG). Supplementing the diet with high-carbohydrate snacks between meals, prior to physical exertion and at bedtime, may prevent episodes.

Sleep: Regular sleep schedules may prevent further attacks.

Complications: With severe, prolonged emesis, chronic esophagitis, metabolic acidosis with hypokalemia and inappropriate secretion of antidiuretic hormone can be seen. Hematemesis can occur from a Mallory Weiss tear or prolapsed gastropathy.

Psychiatric: Due to lack of specific signs and symptoms, laboratories, radiographic findings and endoscopic abnormalities, the diagnosis of CVS is often missed for several years. As a result, CVS may dramatically impact the quality of life of the child and family, as well as lead to frustrations with the medical system and a high annual cost of care.

School/education: If untreated, children with CVS may miss school and experience a decline in their grades due to multiple hospitalizations.

Herbs that need to be avoided: Marijuana withdrawal can trigger the emetic phase of CVS. Marijuana used by adolescents to treat nausea and emesis may actually increase the frequency of CVS emetic episodes.

References

Li BUK, Lefevre F, Chelimsky GG, Boles RG, Nelson SP, Lewis DW, Linder SL, Issenman RM, and Rudoph CD. North American Society for Pediatric Gastroenterology, Hepatology and Nutrition consensus statement on the diagnosis and management of cyclic vomiting syndrome. Journal of Pediatric Gastroenterology and Nutrition. 2008;47: 379–393

Van Calcar SC, Harding CO, Wolff JA. L-carnitine administration reduces number of episodes in cyclic vomiting syndrome. Clin Pediatr 2002;41:171–174

Magagna J. Psychophysiologic treatment of cyclic vomiting. J Pediatr Gastroenterol Nutr 1995;21 (Suppl. 1):S31–36

Boles RG, Williams JC. Mitochondrial disease and cyclic vomiting syndrome. Dig Dis Sci 1999;44 (8 Suppl.):103S–107S

Polyposis Syndromes (Juvenile)

Dafna Bababeygy, Michelle Pietzak

The colonic polyposis syndromes which can occur in childhood are a heterogeneous group of rare hereditary disorders characterized by the development of polyps within the gastrointestinal tract that may have the presence of extraintestinal disease. The syndromes are classified histopathologically into hamartomatous or adenomatous type. Although adenomas are neoplastic in nature, hamartomas also carry a lifetime risk of cancer development.

Etiology

The syndromes are linked to genetic mutations within the loci of tumor suppressor genes. The **adenomatous syndromes** (also called neoplastic types) include familial adenomatous polyposis (FAP), attenuated FAP, Gardner's syndrome, Turcot syndrome type II and Peutz-Jeghers syndrome. Except for Peutz-Jeghers syndrome which is linked to a mutation in LKB1/STK11 (serine/threonine kinase), all involve mutations within the Adenomatous Polyposis Coli (APC) gene, a tumor suppressor involved in TP53-mediated apoptosis. The **hamartomatous syndromes** (also called inflammatory or juvenile types) include the juvenile polyposis syndromes (JPS). Among these syndromes are infantile JPS, generalized JPS, juvenile polyposis coli and JPS with hereditary hemorrhagic telangiectasia) and those which involve mutations in PTEN (Cowden syndrome, Bannayan-Riley-Ruvalcaba syndrome, Proteus syndrome, Bannayan-Zonana syndrome and macrocephaly/autism syndrome). PTEN is the gene for phosphatase and tensin analog, a tumor suppressor gene, located on 10q23.31. JPS are associated with mutations in SMAD, BPMPR1A and ENG, all of which are involved in TGF-β signal transduction.

Clinical Presentation and Prognosis

Demographics: **Adenomatous syndromes:** FAP is the most common polyposis syndrome in children. APC mutations are found in Ashkenazi Jews but also have a worldwide distribution. The age of presentation varies with each of the syndromes, and can occur from the neonatal period through adulthood. Both genders are affected equally. All of these syndromes are autosomal dominant except for Turcot syndrome, which is autosomal recessive.

Hamartomatous syndromes: JPS are rare conditions with an approximate incidence of 1 per 100,000 births. They are categorized based upon polyp location and age at presentation. Age of presentation ranges from infancy to adulthood and there is no gender prevalence. What separates JPS from the other hamartomatous syndromes is the absence of extraintestinal manifestations.

Presenting signs and symptoms and physical exam: Many of the pediatric patients with polyposis syndromes are asymptomatic and are detected because of screening due to an affected family member. If polyps are symptomatic, they may present with painless hematochezia, anemia, diarrhea, protein-calorie malnutrition, abdominal pain, intestinal obstruction, intussusception or rectal prolapse. Juvenile polyposis of infancy can be especially severe, presenting with anemia secondary to gastrointestinal bleeding, protein losing enteropathy, severe watery diarrhea, malnutrition and failure to thrive. Bleeding occurs as the polyps outgrow their blood supply, and also due to trauma from stool passage. Patients may even state that they have seen a flesh-colored or bloody polyp pass into the toilet. Children with FAP may have pigmented skin macules and ocular lesions, nasal polyps, gynecomastia, dental anomalies and lipomas.

Please see "Pearls and Precautions" section for physical findings associated with specific syndromes.

Clinical Course and prognosis: **Adenomatous syndromes:** Patients with FAP have progressive development of hundreds to thousands of adenomatous polyps in the colon, and therefore have a 100% lifetime risk of colorectal neoplasia. Size of the adenoma correlates with risk for malignancy, as those less than 1cm in diameter have <2% incidence of malignancy, while those >1cm have 2.7-fold increased risk of colorectal carcinoma over the general population. Mean ages for adenoma and colon cancer development in FAP are 16 and 39 years respectively. One-half of FAP gene carriers will have evidence of polyps on colonoscopy by the age of 15 years, and 1% will develop colorectal cancer between 15 and 20 years of age. Patients with FAP variants are at risk for developing benign and cancerous tumors of other organ systems such as duodenum (1–5%), pancreas (2%), periampulla, thyroid (2%), brain and liver (hepatoblastoma in 0.7% of children <5 years old). Compared to the general population, the risk of hepatoblastoma is 750–7,500 times higher in children predisposed to FAP, and the incidence of hepatoblastoma among children of FAP patients is 1 in 235, compared to 1 in 100,000 in the general population.

Hamartomatous syndromes: These patients also may develop colorectal cancer or cancers of other gastrointestinal organs including the stomach, duodenum or pancreas. There is a reported 17–22% chance of developing colorectal cancer in patients with JPS by age 35, and a cumulative lifetime risk of 68% by age 60 years.

Diagnosis

Adenomatous syndromes: These are characterized by:

1. Development of numerous adenomas in the colon and rectum.
2. Extraintestinal features involving cutaneous, endocrinologic, gonadal, head and neck, musculoskeletal, neurologic and other organ systems.

Hamartomatous syndromes: Criteria for JPS are:

1. More than three colonic hamartomatous polyps.
2. A patient with a family history who has any hamartomatous polyps.
3. The presence of hamartomatous polyps outside of the colon.

Labs: **Adenomatous and Hamartomatous:** A CBC and iron panel can show iron deficiency anemia due to chronic GI blood loss. Chemistry panel may show low albumin and total protein with protein-calorie malnutrition. Stools may be positive for occult blood and/or α_1 anti-trypsin or calprotectin (indicative of protein losing enteropathy. Please see separate chapter on chronic diarrhea).

Adenomatous: Transaminases, serum alpha-fetoprotein and liver ultrasound should be considered to screen for hepatoblastoma starting at age 7 years. Electrolytes, ACTH, plasma and urine cortisol should be checked in patients with Gardner syndrome to evaluate for Cushing's syndrome.

Please see Pearls and Precautions section for laboratory monitoring of specific syndromes.

Genetic testing: Many laboratories, both within the U.S. and internationally, are able to test for the genetic mutations associated with polyposis syndromes.

    Adenomatous: The APC gene mutation screening should be done in patients with >100 colorectal adenomas, first degree relatives of patients with FAP, and attenuated FAP with more than 20 cumulative colorectal adenomas.

    Hamartomatous: The following genes should be tested in symptomatic patients and first degree relatives of JPS patients: SMAD4, BMPR1A, ENG and PTEN.

Endoscopy with biopsy: Both symptomatic and asymptomatic patients with positive genetic testing should undergo a thorough esophagogastroduodenoscopy and colonoscopy with polypectomy. If a polyp is seen, a complete polypectomy is recommended, as grasp biopsies may miss histologic abnormalities. Capsule endoscopy can be used to visualize small bowel polyps distal to the duodenum.

    Adenomatous pathology: Colonic polyps can be classified into tubular, tubulovillous or villous types. In FAP, polyps can also be seen in the stomach, duodenum and small bowel. Most stomach polyps are benign fundic gland polyps and not adenomatous. Duodenal adenomas are usually asymptomatic and slow-growing.

    Hamartomatous pathology: These polyps should show a characteristic "branching" appearance of smooth muscle fibers mixed with collagen. JPS polyps are considered malignant if they have adenomatous characteristics.

Radiology:

    Adenomatous: It is recommended that a liver US be performed by age 7 to screen for hepatoblastoma. Upper GI with small bowel follow-through and air-contrast barium enema can further define small bowel and colonic polyps. Additional radiographic studies for particular syndromes are to be found in the "Pearls and Precautions" section below.

Management

Medication: The only available medications for adenomatous polyps are sulindac (Clinoril) and celecoxib (Celebrex), COX-2 inhibitors which have been reported to cause a modest reduction in the number and size of colonic and rectal adenomas in short and long term studies.

Surgery:

    Adenomatous: Given the large number of adenomas and 100% risk of the development of colon cancer, prophylactic colectomy is recommended. The recommended procedure is proctocolectomy with ileal-pouch-anal anastomosis, although other procedures, such as subtotal colectomy with ileorectal anastomosis (IRA), have been employed for patients with minimal rectal adenomas. Patients may initially require a diverting ileostomy if cancer is found. Ideally, the surgery should be performed by a colorectal surgeon who has experience in this area. If IRA is performed, which retains the last 10 to 15cm of rectum, the patient still requires monitoring endoscopy annually. For benign gastric polyps, no treatment is necessary and upper endoscopy should be repeated every 5 years. Since duodenal adenomas are generally small and slow-growing, surgery is not usually required, but side-viewing endoscopy should be repeated (every 6 months to 3 years depending upon size and location of adenoma). Treatment may include laser therapy, surgical resection, or only ongoing observation and biopsy.

Hamartomatous: If dysplastic changes occur or if there is a large polyp burden, resections of parts of the stomach, small bowel or colon may be necessary.

Consultations: Genetic counseling should be done prior to ordering genetic testing of family members. A pediatric gastroenterologist, pediatric surgeon and/or colorectal surgeon are necessary for long-term management. Depending upon the type of syndrome, a geneticist, developmental pediatrician, neurologist, gynecologist, urologist, otolaryngologist, oncologist, dermatologist, dentist, endocrinologist and psychologist or psychiatrist may be needed as part of the patient's medical care team.

Psychosocial: Patients and families affected by FAP may experience blame and guilt, and often benefit from support groups as listed below:

The American Society of Colon & Rectal Surgeons website lists patient and physician resources, including The Collaborative Group of the Americas on Inherited Colorectal Cancer and colorectal cancer registries: http://www.fascrs.org/patients/family_history_registries/

The Colon Cancer Alliance (CCA) is a national patient advocacy organization which provides patient support, education, research and advocacy across North America. http://www.ccalliance.org/C3: Colorectal Cancer Coalition is a nonprofit, nonpartisan advocacy organization that supports the work of research and grassroots advocates throughout the United States. http://fightcolorectalcancer.org/

Monitoring:

Adenomatous: For affected individuals, after colectomy, upper endoscopy is recommended roughly every three to four years; annually if an upper GI tract polyp is detected. Annual lower endoscopy should be performed on any residual rectum or pouch. For those asymptomatic with a family history and detected APC mutation, colonoscopy should be done annually starting at about the age of 10 years. For those with a family history but no detected APC mutation, flexible sigmoidoscopy is recommended starting at about the age of 25 years.

Hamartomatous: Endoscopic screening should be continued annually until no additional polyps are found, at which point screening every two years is thought to be sufficient. A patient with biopsy-proven JPS should have upper and lower endoscopy with polypectomy every two years. In patients with a family history of JPS, the absence of polyps does not exclude the presence of disease, and screening with upper and lower endoscopy every 2 years should continue. The patient's anemia and malnutrition should be corrected and asymptomatic first degree relatives should be screened with upper and lower endoscopy along with genetic testing starting in the second decade of life (roughly age 10–15 years).

Please see "Pearls and Precautions" section below for special recommended monitoring for specific syndromes.

Pearls and Precautions

Adenomatous

An adenomatous polyp in an individual younger than 30 years of age should prompt evaluation for a polyposis syndrome. The presence of more than three pigmented ocular fundic lesions on ophthalmologic examination confirms FAP.

Attenuated FAP is defined as oligopolyposis (<100 colorectal adenomas) which are predominantly right sided. This form of FAP has a delayed onset of presentation and cancer compared to classic FAP, and rarely has rectal involvement. Because of this, full colonoscopy (as opposed to sigmoidoscopy) should be used for screening, and the role of prophylactic colectomy is more controversial.

Peutz-Jeghers syndrome: Patients may have obvious hyperpigmentation of the oral mucosa, most commonly on the lower lip that may cross the vermilion border. Hyperpigmentation can also be seen on the gingiva, around the anus, genitalia, fingers and toes. The lesions may fade after puberty. Although colonic polyps are hamartomatous, almost half of patients with this syndrome die from cancer by age 57 years. The following organs are thought to have increased risk for cancer: Esophagus, stomach, small intestine, colon, pancreas, lung, breast, testes, uterus and ovary. Endoscopic ultrasound may help detect early pancreatic cancer.

Gardner syndrome is a form of FAP with cutaneous findings, osteomas, and skin and soft tissue tumors. The cutaneous findings can include epidermoid cysts, fibromas, lipomas, leiomyomas, neurofibromas and pigmented skin lesions. Osteomas are required to confirm this diagnosis, and are most often seen in the mandible, but can also occur in the skull and long bones. Osteomas often clinically precede GI polyps. Associated neoplasms involve the ampulla of Vater, CNS tumors, thyroid, bones and liver (hepatoblastoma). Screening should include radiographs of the skull, teeth and mandible; evaluation of the biliary tree by US, ERCP and/or MRCP; and abdominal US and/or CT to evaluate for masses.

Turcot's syndrome, which is autosomal recessive, is FAP associated with CNS malignancies, the two most common being glioblastoma and medulloblastoma. Cafe-au-lait spots, lipomas and multiple scalp basal cell carcinomas can also be seen.

Hamartomatous:

PTEN mutation: Recommended monthly self breast exam and annual clinical breast exam starting at age 12, and annual thyroid exam and baseline thyroid ultrasound starting in adolescence.

JPS: Routine surveillance for occult breast neoplasms recommended. CT or US of pelvis, or testicles, recommended in patients with precocious puberty or gynecomastia.

Cowden: The following are recommended: routine surveillance for occult breast neoplasm; thyroid imaging if suggestive of malignancy; ovarian imaging if suggestive of malignancy; head imaging if symptomatic; X-ray of spine to monitor for scoliosis.

Hereditary hemorrhagic telangiectasia *(Osler-Weber-Rendu syndrome):* May be a comorbid disease with JPS arterio-venous malformations, digital telangiectasia or digital clubbing.

Ruvalcaba-Myhre-Smith syndrome *(also known as Ruvalcaba's syndrome II):* Patients with this autosomal dominant syndrome have juvenile polyps in the stomach, small intestine, colon and tongue combined with elements of Sotos syndrome (cerebral gigantism). Findings include macrosomy, macrocephaly, abnormal facies, mental retardation, lipid storage myopathy, subcutaneous lipomas and pigmented macules on the penis.

Bannayan-Ruvalcaba-Riley syndrome: In this uncommon disorder, hamartomatous polyps are seen in the ileum and colon. Associations include macrosomia at birth (but normal adult size), macrocephaly, hemangiomas, lipomas, and penis freckles. Some patients have hypotonia, seizures and developmental delay. Patients with this syndrome need to be monitored for myopathy, scoliosis, and thyroid and breast malignancies.

School/education: Urgency with polyposis and colitis may impact the child's ability to learn while in school. Because children with a polyposis syndrome may not appear ill to the teacher, they are often denied restroom access during class. The PCP or gastroenterologist may need to write letters for the patient to allow him or her to use the restroom when needed, or have the ability to use the school nurse's restroom if available. Timing of colectomy for FAP children is an important concern, and summer months or school holidays are preferred to allow for a prolonged recovery time. Parents should discuss timing of prophylactic colectomy with the guidance counselor and home room teacher to plan accordingly. It is important for the hospitalized child to continue to receive school assignments, so as not to fall behind their classmates. Children recovering from bowel resection may require home schooling.

References

Schrieberman IR, Baker M, Amos C and McGarrity TJ. The Hamartomatous Polyposis Syndromes: A Clinical and Molecular Review. American Journal of Gastroenterology 2005; 100:476–490.

Huang SC, Erdman SH. Pediatric Juvenile Polyposis Syndromes: An Update. Current Gastroenterology Reports, 2009; 11:211–219.

Lofti AM et al. Colorectal polyps and the risk of subsequent carcinoma. Mayo Clin Proc 1986; 61:337–343.

Aretz S. Koch A. Uhlhaas S. Friedl W. Propping P. von Schweinitz D. Pietsch T. Should children at risk for familial adenomatous polyposis be screened for hepatoblastoma and children with apparently sporadic hepatoblastoma be screened for APC germline mutations? Pediatric Blood & Cancer 2006; 47:811–818.

Portal Hypertension

Michelle Pietzak

Portal hypertension is defined as an elevation of portal blood pressure greater than 5 mm Hg. Portal hypertension may be due to different etiologies, and is a common complication of many chronic liver diseases.

Etiology

Portal hypertension is due to increased portal resistance and/or increased portal blood flow. Diseases in the pediatric population associated with portal hypertension can be divided into intrahepatic and extrahepatic disorders. Extrahepatic causes include venous obstruction (portal vein, splenic vein or IVC thrombosis; Budd-Chiari syndrome); splenomegaly; arteriovenous fistulas; and chronic congestive heart failure. Intrahepatic diseases leading to portal hypertension include those primarily of the hepatocytes, biliary tract, and various miscellaneous conditions. Hepatocellular diseases include viral (hepatitis B and C); autoimmune (autoimmune hepatitis); metabolic/storage diseases (α_1-anti-trypsin deficiency [see separate chapter in this book], Wilson's disease, glycogen storage disease type IV, Gaucher's disease); toxins (drugs, alcohol, arsenic, vinyl chloride, vitamin A); and miscellaneous (histiocytosis X, venoocclusive disease). Biliary tract diseases include biliary atresia, cystic fibrosis, primary sclerosing cholangitis (see separate chapter is this book), schistosomiasis (of the intrahepatic portal venules and mesenteric veins) and diseases causing intrahepatic cholestasis (Alagille's syndrome, Byler's disease, Caroli's disease). The condition may also be idiopathic.

Clinical Presentation and Prognosis

Presenting signs and symptoms: The most common initial presentations of portal hypertension in the pediatric population are hemorrhage, splenomegaly and ascites. Gastrointestinal hemorrhage most often occurs from rupture of esophageal varices, but can also occur from gastric, duodenal or rectal varices, or from portal hypertensive gastropathy. Splenomegaly may be detected on routine physical exam, or the patient may have experienced left upper quadrant fullness, bruising or petechiae associated with thrombocytopenia.

Clinical course and prognosis: Because portal hypertension in the pediatric population is due to a wide array of both extrahepatic and intrahepatic diseases, it is difficult to generalize its natural history. In addition, most therapeutic interventions in pediatrics have been based upon adult data and applied in a non-controlled fashion. The two pediatric conditions which have adequate long-term follow-up are extrahepatic biliary atresia and extrahepatic portal vein thrombosis. In biliary atresia, success of the Kasai portoenterostomy is highly dependent upon the experience of the pediatric surgeon and medical center. Children with biliary atresia who experience progressive liver disease resulting in portal hypertension are those who either have poor post-operative biliary drainage, or suffer from recurrent bacterial cholangitis.

Prognosis: Poor prognostic signs in this group include total serum bilirubin above 4 mg/dL and variceal hemorrhage, which may occur even within the first year of life. Portal vein thrombosis (a fair number of which likely occurred in the neonatal period secondary to umbilical vein catheterization, omphalitis, hyper-coagulable state or congenital anomalies) can also be associated with life-threatening GI bleeds, but the time from obstruction to hemorrhage is more variable. Unlike biliary atresia, since there is no underlying hepatic disease, this type of portal hypertension has, in general, a more benign course, and some publications have suggested that these children may "outgrow" their disease as a result of developing collaterals or due to portal vein recanalization.

Diagnosis

A child presenting with GI hemorrhage and splenomegaly likely has portal hypertension and should be treated emergently as such, until proven otherwise. With chronic liver disease, there may be a long-standing history of growth failure, fatigue, intermittent jaundice, and/or anorexia. Physical findings with chronic disease may include pruritus, acholic stools, dark urine, palmar erythema, xanthomas, ascites and splenomegaly with or without hepatomegaly. Other physical findings may include splenomegaly with or without significant GI bleeding, caput medusa (prominent periumbilical collaterals through the umbilical vein which may demonstrate an audible venous hum [Cruveilhier-Baumgarten murmur]), rectal varices, peri-stomal varices, ascites, growth failure/protein-calorie malnutrition with evidence of fat-soluble vitamin deficiencies and protein-losing enteropathy. Patients may also have skin findings consistent with chronic liver disease such as telangiectasias, palmar erythema and xanthomas.

Labs: Classic laboratory findings in chronic liver disease include elevations in transaminases, serum direct/conjugated bilirubin, serum alkaline phosphatase and γ-glutamyltransferase (GGT). With advanced disease, low albumin and prolonged prothrombin time may be present. Pancytopenia may be seen due to hypersplenism. If acute cholangitis is present, there is often a leukocytosis with left shift, thrombocytosis, elevated bilirubin, and high sedimentation rate or C-reactive protein. Elevated amylase and/or lipase can be seen with pancreatitis. With chronic disease and malnutrition due to fat malabsorption, low serum vitamins A, E, 25OH D and prolonged prothrombin time may be seen.

Radiology: The diagnostic modality of choice to diagnose portal hypertension in childhood is an abdominal US with Doppler. Doppler US can determine portal vein patency and flow and can also detect thrombosis. Important information about the liver can be obtained in regards to size, nodularity, echogenicity and presence of intrahepatic or extrahepatic ductal dilatation with or without gallstones. The spleen size and patency of the splenic vein can also be assessed, although size of the spleen does not correlate with degree of portal hypertension. Collaterals, including esophageal varices, may also be visualized. Renal anomalies and ascites, which can be subclinical, can also be detected.

CT of the abdomen may reveal a coarse, nodular liver, large spleen, ascites and dilated intra-abdominal collaterals. However, since CT cannot directly measure portal flow, and involves radiation and often sedation of the pediatric patient, it is a suboptimal study to diagnose portal hypertension in this population.

In cases of acute portal vein thrombosis, selective angiography of the celiac axis, superior mesenteric artery and splenic vein may be useful to guide thrombectomy and/or shunt surgery.

Used in adults, the hepatic venous pressure gradient (HVPG) technique utilizes a balloon-tipped catheter inserted into an antecubital vein and advanced to the hepatic vein. HVPG is the difference between the free pressure and this wedged hepatic vein pressure. A gradient of >12 mm Hg increases risk for variceal hemorrhage, and this technique can be used to measure response to medications.

Endoscopy: Esophagogastroduodenoscopy (EGD) has the advantage of being diagnostic and therapeutic for acute GI bleeding in the setting of chronic liver disease. EGD can directly visualize esophageal, gastric and duodenal varices, portal hypertensive gastropathy, and also look for other etiologies of GI bleeding such as gastric and duodenal ulcers.

Management

The primary goal of management is the prevention of life-threatening GI bleed, usually due to varices. In adults, mortality during acute variceal hemorrhage may exceed 50%, and risk for re-bleeding is 50–75% within 2 years. Endoscopic and drug therapy lowers the risk for bleeding but do not significantly decrease long-term mortality. When possible, the underlying cause of the portal hypertension should be treated.

Medications and Surgery

Primary prophylaxis: The idea of primary prophylaxis is derived from adult data (cirrhosis due to chronic alcohol ingestion, primarily), and is intended to prevent the first episode of variceal hemorrhage. Given the unpredictability of the timing to the first episode of GI bleeding in a child with portal hypertension, primary prophylaxis should be cost-effective and be associated with a low morbidity and mortality. The primary drugs used are β-blockers which lower portal pressure primarily by diminishing portal flow. For adult patients with varices that have not yet bled, β-blockers lower the risk of bleeding. Doses may be titrated to lower heart rate by up to 25%. However, these drugs should not be used in children with underlying pulmonary disease such as in cystic fibrosis and asthma.

Treatment of acute variceal hemorrhage: Children with underlying liver disease and hematemesis should be brought to the immediate attention of the emergency room. Particular attention should be paid to temperature, respiratory rate, heart rate and blood pressure. A lack of a tachycardic response to acute GI bleeding in a patient on β-blockade may be seen, leading the clinician to underestimate the amount of blood being lost. Immediate aggressive fluid resuscitation should be initiated, first with crystalloid and then with packed red cells and perhaps fresh frozen plasma, vitamin K or recombinant factor VIIa, if there is evidence of coagulopathy. Thrombocytopenia is common with splenomegaly, but may worsen with disseminated intravascular coagulation (DIC). In adults in this scenario, it is thought that optimal hemoglobin levels are between 7 and 9g/dL, as overaggressive transfusion may increase the risk for variceal bleeding. A nasogastric tube may be of benefit with persistent hematemesis, but may also aggravate variceal hemorrhage with multiple attempts at placement. Because of the high risk of infectious complications, empiric antibiotics should be considered.

EGD should be performed urgently in the patient with ongoing hemorrhage who requires transfusion. If EGD cannot be performed in an expedient fashion, pharmacologic therapy with somatostatin or vasopressin can be initiated. Vasopressin decreases portal flow by increasing splanchnic vascular tone, but is associated with many side effects, including chest and abdominal pain which may be indicative of angina, left ventricular failure and/or bowel ischemia. Because of this, somatostatin (or its synthetic homologue octreotide) is being used more often in pediatrics. These drugs also decrease splanchnic blood flow, but their mechanism is thought to be due to the blockade of the effects of intestinal vasoactive peptides. Side-effects include a lowering of the seizure threshold and hyperglycemia due to inhibition of insulin secretion. However, this drug appears to be better tolerated than vasopressin in infants and small children. An initial bolus of 1–5 µg/kg/hour should be given, followed by an infusion of 1–5µg/kg/hour.

Long term: Combined long-term endoscopic and drug therapy may be slightly more effective than either modality alone. A variety of surgeries have been developed to decrease portal blood pressure. Patients not responding to medical and endoscopic therapy should be considered for a surgical shunt, transjugular intra-hepatic portal-systemic shunting (TIPS), or liver transplant, depending upon the underlying etiology for the portal hypertension. Types of portosystemic shunts include portacaval (portal vein to IVC), mesocaval (graft between SMV and IVC) and distal splenorenal (splenic vein to left renal vein). TIPS, done by an interventional radiologist, creates an artificial connection between the portal and hepatic venous circulation within the liver via a transjugular approach. Complications of shunts include hepatic encephalopathy, thrombosis of the shunt, recurrent bleeding and death. Pediatric patients with extrahepatic causes of portal hypertension have better results with shunts than those with intrinsic liver diseases. In the latter group, those with refractory portal hypertension are recommended to undergo liver transplantation.

Consultations: Referral to a pediatric liver transplant center should be considered early in the patient's course, especially if the child has an intrahepatic etiology for the portal hypertension and already has had an initial variceal bleed.

Monitoring: Periodic assessment of growth, nutritional status, liver function and abdominal US with Doppler are sufficient to monitor uncomplicated portal hypertension. At present, it is not recommended that children with portal hypertension, who have not yet had bleeding esophageal varices, undergo periodic routine surveillance endoscopy. For those who have bled, surveillance endoscopy roughly every few months for serial endoscopic banding or sclerotherapy to obliterate residual varices is recommended.

Pearls and Precautions

Ultrasound evidence of Budd-Chiari syndrome (hepatic vein thrombosis) warrants an evaluation for myeloproliferative diseases and a work-up for hypercoagulable state (such as low protein C, protein S or anti-thrombin III; factor V Leiden or prothrombin mutations).

Complications:

- *Hepatopulmonary syndrome (pulmonary arterio-venous shunting):* In this state, desaturations are seen due to intrapulmonic right to left shunting. It may present as shortness of breath on exertion. Patients may have digital clubbing. It is best imaged via agitated saline echocardiography and/or macroaggregated albumin scanning. It may be an indication for liver transplant, but may take months to improve post-transplant.
- *Pulmonary hypertension:* This entity is thought to occur as a result of obliteration of the pulmonary artery lumen. It is rare in children, but may be seen with cystic fibrosis. It does not typically reverse after isolated liver transplant. A pulmonary artery pressure >50 mm Hg is a contraindication to isolated liver transplant and may require combined liver/lung/heart transplant.
- *Ascites:* Thought to be due to a combination of sodium retention due to systemic vasodilatation, elevated portal pressure and impaired lymphatic drainage.
- *Bacterial peritonitis:* The child with ascites due to portal hypertension, who presents with fever, should have fluid aspirated for cell count and culture. Empiric antibiotics which cover enteric organisms should be initiated.

- *Hepatorenal syndrome:* This is functional renal failure with histologically normal kidneys in the setting of severe liver disease. It can occur acutely and is associated with a high mortality. The renal function returns to normal post-transplant.
- *Hepatic encephalopathy:* This occurs more as a complication of porto-systemic shunting, rather than as evidence of hepatic dysfunction. It can be difficult to diagnose in young children as Stage I may manifest with only irritability, behavioral changes and/or disturbed sleep-wake cycle.

References

Shneider B, Emre S, Groszmann R, et al. Portal hypertension in children: expert pediatric opinion on the report of the Baveno IV consensus workshop on the methodology of diagnosis and therapy in portal hypertension. Pediatr Transplant 2006;10:893–907.

Kasai M, Okamoto A, Ohi R, et al. Changes of portal vein pressure and intrahepatic blood vessels after surgery for biliary atresia. J Pediatr Surg 1986;16:152–159.

Mitra SK, Kumar V, Datta DV, et al. Extrahepatic portal hypertension: a review of 70 cases. J Pediatr Surg 1978;13:51–57.

Ozsoylu S, Kocak N, Yuce A. Propanolol therapy for portal hypertension in children. J Pediatr 1985;106: 317–321.

Primary Sclerosing Cholangitis (PSC)

Michelle Pietzak

Primary sclerosing cholangitis (PSC) is a chronic disease of the biliary tree. Inflammation of the intrahepatic and/or extrahepatic bile ducts can lead to strictures, dilatation, obliteration, and eventually biliary cirrhosis with end-stage liver disease. In children, it is often associated with inflammatory bowel disease (IBD) and may have significant overlap with autoimmune hepatitis (AIH).

Etiology

PSC is thought to be due to an immune-mediated process; however, the environmental triggers are not clear. PSC is likely triggered by infections, toxins or ischemia in genetically susceptible individuals who express abnormal HLA class II molecules on the surface of biliary epithelial cells. Other implicated genes involve mutations in CFTR, CLTA-4, ICAM, TNFα and metalloproteinase. PSC in IBD may occur due to increased intestinal permeability to gut flora, leading to portal bacteremia and an inflammatory cascade. In a rat model of PSC, intestinal bacterial overgrowth and endotoxin are hypothesized to cause intestinal and biliary injury.

Clinical Presentation and Prognosis

Demographics: While cases of pediatric PSC seem to be on the rise, the exact incidence is unknown, even in children with IBD. The highest reported prevalence is in Northern Europe and in Caucasians. The male:female ratio is approximately 2:1 in adults, and PSC can occur at any age, although men aged 25 to 40 years old seem to be most often affected. Approximately 2/3 of adults with PSC will eventually develop ulcerative colitis (UC) and roughly 5% of UC patients are affected by PSC. Patients with pancolitis (both from UC and Crohn's) are more likely to develop PSC. In pediatric studies, PSC may occur before, during or after the diagnosis of IBD.

Presenting signs and symptoms: In children, the disease usually has an insidious onset, often with vague symptoms for years prior to diagnosis. The exception to this is in the acute presentation of bacterial cholangitis, where children have fever, chills, right upper quadrant pain and jaundice. There is often a long-standing history of fatigue, intermittent jaundice, and anorexia. Some patients are asymptomatic when found to have abnormal laboratory findings on routine screening serum chemistries. Physical findings with chronic disease may include pruritus, acholic stools, dark urine, palmar erythema, xanthomas, ascites and hepatomegaly with or without splenomegaly. If portal hypertension exists, the child may present with variceal hemorrhage. Pancreatitis may occur, causing severe vomiting, dehydration, abdominal pain, anorexia and back pain.

If PSC is associated with IBD, the child may present with diarrhea, abdominal pain, GI bleeding, protein calorie malnutrition, oral aphthous ulcers, short stature, delayed puberty, skin rashes, joint pain and weight loss. However, PSC alone can also cause these symptoms. For more information on IBD in pediatrics, please see separate chapters on Crohn's disease and ulcerative colitis.

Clinical course and prognosis: As with other immune-mediated diseases, the heterogeneity of the patient population with PSC precludes making generalized statements about its clinical course and prognosis. Pediatric PSC may progress insidiously or rapidly to end-stage liver disease. Published independent prognostic factors include age at diagnosis, albumin, bilirubin, prothrombin time, splenomegaly, HLA haplotype and presence of high-grade strictures. It is difficult to predict which patients are at higher risk for cholangiocarcinoma.

Diagnosis

Labs: Classic laboratory findings in cholestatic liver disease include elevations in serum direct/conjugated bilirubin, serum alkaline phosphatase and γ-glutamyltransferase (GGT). With advanced disease, low albumin and prolonged prothrombin time may be present. If acute cholangitis is present, there is often a leukocytosis with left shift, thrombocytosis, elevated bilirubin, and high sedimentation rate or C-reactive protein. Elevated amylase and/or lipase can be seen with pancreatitis. With chronic disease and malnutrition due to fat malabsorption, low serum vitamins A, E, 25OH D and prolonged prothrombin time may be seen.

There is an overlap between PSC and AIH. Such patients may have an elevated globulin fraction seen on a routine chemistry panel (total protein − albumin = globulin fraction) due to the presence of autoantibodies such as antinuclear antibody (ANA), anti-smooth muscle antibody (ASMA) and anti-liver kidney microsome type I (anti-LKM 1). Isolated elevations of immunoglobulin G (IgG) have been reported.

Imaging of the biliary system: Abdominal ultrasound: In a child with acute abdominal pain and jaundice, this is the initial imaging modality of choice to look for gallstones, hepatitis, ductal dilatation, pancreatic disease and ascites. If there is evidence for portal hypertension, Doppler flow of the portal system can be interrogated.

Endoscopic retrograde cholangiopancreatography (ERCP): Characteristic findings of PSC can be visualized by looking at the biliary tree directly under fluoroscopy. ERCP is considered the "gold standard" for this purpose, best at evaluating chronic changes in the intrahepatic and/or extrahepatic biliary tree seen in PSC, such as strictures, dilatations, diverticula and a loss of peripheral functioning bile ducts (decreased "arborization" or a "pruned tree" appearance). An additional advantage of ERCP is that it can be therapeutic as well as diagnostic, allowing for interventions such as sphincterotomy, stent placement, balloon dilatation of a stricture and brushing for cholangiocarcinoma.

Magnetic resonance cholangiopancreatography (MRCP): As with ERCP, MRCP can visualize chronic changes to the intrahepatic and extrahepatic biliary tree seen in PSC. Its advantages are that it is non-invasive; is not limited by the age or size of the child; does not expose the child to radiation or contrast; does not require as much sedation (an older child may be able to lie still without medications); and may visualize ducts distal to an obstruction that ERCP contrast cannot.

Computed tomography (CT) cholangiography: As with ERCP and MRCP, this relatively new technique can detect biliary tract disease seen in PSC. Its advantages are that CT scanners are more readily available than MRI machines, and that an intravenous infusion of iotroxate (which mimics bilirubin) can be given to measure biliary excretion.

Percutaneous cholangiogram: This can be performed by an interventional radiologist under either ultrasound or CT guidance. However, this is a high-risk procedure and its use is limited to those children with markedly dilated biliary systems (such as seen with complications post-liver transplant). It has an advantage in that percutaneous drains can be placed at the time of visualization.

Biopsy: A fine needle liver biopsy may be obtained percutaneously by a gastroenterologist or radiologist with or without ultrasound guidance. The classic liver biopsy finding from a patient with PSC shows "onion skinning" fibrosis around the interlobular bile ducts. If AIH is present, swollen hepatocytes and a lymphocytic/plasma cell infiltrate may be seen in the portal and periportal areas.

Management

The goals of management are to treat symptoms (pruritus, protein-calorie malnutrition), improve biliary drainage and prevent progression of the disease, and to prevent complications.

Medications: Ursodeoxycholic acid, a choleretic bile acid based upon the chemical structure of bear bile, is commonly used to treat PSC at a dose of 20–40 mg/kg/day. This medication has been shown to improve bilirubin, alkaline phosphatase, AST and albumin levels in adult and pediatric patients. It may improve pruritus. The literature is conflicting as to whether its use slows the progression of PSC. It is commonly used because it is a relatively safe medication (its main side effect is diarrhea). Other medications used to alleviate pruritus include rifampicin, cholestyramine, phenobarbitol, carbamazepine and opioid antagonists (naloxone). If there is overlap with AIH, prednisone and azathioprine are commonly employed. The use of other immunosuppressants (in the absence of AIH), as well as chronic antibiotics (in the absence of cholangitis), chelation drugs and anti-fibrinogenics have been disappointing for the treatment of PSC.

Surgery: Indications for liver transplant surgery include cirrhosis, portal hypertension with variceal bleeding and refractory ascites, severe liver dysfunction with hepatic encephalopathy, refractory pruritus with markedly decreased quality of life, and recurrent bacterial cholangitis. Other biliary tract surgeries are to be avoided, as they may complicate the patient's anatomy for transplant. Endoscopic balloon dilatation of a dominant stricture, with or without stent placement during ERCP, may improve not only symptoms, but also transplant-free survival

Consultations: Referral to a pediatric liver transplant center should be considered early in the patient's course.

Psychological: Uncontrolled pruritus may lead to sleep deprivation, loss or normal activities of living, and may lead to suicidal ideation.

Pearls and Precautions

Children with IBD, especially those with ulcerative colitis, who have evidence of chronic liver disease, should be worked up for both PSC and AIH. Children with AIH which is not responding to medications should be evaluated for PSC. Some pediatric hepatologists advocate screening for PSC in all children with AIH.

Sleep: The pruritus associated with PSC may be severe enough to cause sleep deprivation. Medications containing diphenhydramine and hydroxyzine, while not treating the underlying cause of the itching, may allow the child to get some uninterrupted sleep.

Skin care: The pruritus in PSC is often the most debilitating symptom, and may be an indication for liver transplant. In addition to the above mentioned medications, some relief may be obtained from cool baths, moisturizers and topical steroid and anesthetic creams. Attention should be paid to keep the child's fingernails short, and breathable long-sleeved cotton shirts (as opposed to synthetics) should be worn.

Likely complications:

Bacterial cholangitis: If recurrent, may require patient to be on daily prophylactic antibiotics. Persistence of infection in a "bile lake" is an indication for liver transplant.

Cholelithiasis, with or without obstruction: Requires cholecystectomy.

Stricture of the bile duct: Dominant strictures as visualized by ERCP may improve with balloon dilatation. It is important that a benign stricture be differentiated from a cholangiocarcinoma, as their appearance on cholangiography can be similar.

Cirrhosis with portal hypertension: Please see separate chapter on portal hypertension for management.

Liver transplant: Although post-transplant survival in adults with PSC is good, they are at higher risk for complications such as rejection, thrombosis and biliary strictures. PSC may recur in the transplanted liver.

Cholangiocarcinoma: The majority of cases of this cancer occur in adults. However, the youngest reported case was in a 14 year old boy with ulcerative colitis. It is difficult to predict who is at higher risk for cholangiocarcinoma, as duration of PSC does not appear to be an independent risk factor. Those with strictures seen on cholangiography should be monitored aggressively.

Colonic adenocarcinoma: Children with ulcerative colitis are at high risk for this cancer. Duration and extent of colitis are known risk factors. The cumulative risk of colorectal cancer in ulcerative colitis patients is 2% after 10 years of active disease, 5% after 20 years, and 10% after 25 years. If the patient also has PSC, these risks increase to 9%, 31% and 50% respectively.

References

Roberts, EA. Primary sclerosing cholangitis in children. J Gastroenterol Hepatol 1999;14:588–593.

Worthington J, Cullen S, Chapman R. Immunopathogenesis of primary sclerosing cholangitis. Clin Rev Allergy Immunol 2005;28:93–103.

Balisteri WF. Bile acid therapy in pediatric hepatobiliary disease: the role of ursodeoxycholic acid. J Pediatr Gastroenterol Nutr 1997;24:573–589.

Feldstein AE, Perrault J, El-Youssif M et al. Primary sclerosing cholangitis in children: a long term follow-up study. Hepatology 2003;38:210–217.

Short Bowel Syndrome (SBS)

(Intestinal Failure)

Khiet D. Ngo

Intestinal failure (IF) is the inability to maintain appropriate growth, nutrition, and/or hydration using an individual's native gastrointestinal tract necessitating parenteral nutrition (PN) for >6 months. Short bowel syndrome (SBS) is one cause of intestinal failure characterized by a reduction in small bowel length. In the full term infant, small bowel length ranges from 200 to 250cm. There is no clear length of bowel that delineates a normal versus short bowel, but usually 2/3 of small bowel loss results in symptoms associated with SBS.

Etiology

Etiologies of intestinal failure are broadly divided into anatomical and functional causes with some overlap. Anatomical causes include necrotizing enterocolitis or gastroschisis with bowel resection, intestinal atresias, malrotation with volvulus, abdominal trauma, and vascular thrombosis. Functional etiologies include radiation enteritis, gastroschisis without significant bowel resection, dysmotility syndromes (such as chronic intestinal pseudo-obstruction syndrome, megacystic microcolon intestinal hypoperistalsis syndrome and total intestinal aganglionosis) and congenital malabsorptive syndromes (such as glucose galactose malabsorption, microvillous inclusion disease, immunodysregulation polyendocrinopathy enteropathy X-linked syndrome [IPEX], tufting enteropathy and enteroendocrine cell deficiencies).

Clinical Presentation and Prognosis:

Demographics: There is generally no gender, ethnic, or racial predominance in patients with intestinal failure.

Presenting signs & symptoms: The clinical presentation of children with short bowel syndrome is usually suspected in the context of one of the above etiologies. Clinical symptoms typically include voluminous diarrhea and/or steatorrhea resulting in significant weight loss or growth failure if untreated. Attempts at increasing oral or enteral nutrition result in increased stool output or other common symptoms such as nausea, vomiting, acute or chronic abdominal distension, and abdominal pain.

Clinical course: In general, the clinical outcomes of patients with IF can include: intestinal adaptation with complete independence from parenteral nutritional support, long term maintenance on parenteral nutrition with adequate growth and nutrition, development of intestinal failure associated complications and/or intestinal transplantation.

There are several good papers that have described the long-term outcomes of patients with IF and attempted to define the prognostic factors for adaptation. It is thought that having at least 20–30cm of small bowel length, the presence of an ilealcecal valve, a full or partial colon, and gastrointestinal continuity between all bowel segments are favorable predictors of adaptation. The ability to tolerate enteral feedings also serves to optimize the chances of adaptation. The underlying disease process can also help to define the chances for adaptation. For example, bowel resection from NEC has a better prognosis (compared to bowel resection from Crohn's disease), while gastroschisis, dysmotility syndromes and congenital malabsorptive syndromes have a less favorable prognosis for adaptation.

IF-associated complications that may impact a patient's clinical course include frequent central venous catheter infections, loss of vascular access sites, and chronic liver disease (persistent elevation in liver enzymes, elevation in direct and indirect bilirubin +/- coagulopathy). For patients who are unable to adapt and have persistent complications, intestinal transplantation is the standard of care.

Prognosis: Patients with IF who are not placed on parenteral nutrition have a poor prognosis including dehydration, malnutrition, growth failure, or death. The prognosis for patients who are appropriately managed with parenteral nutrition is generally excellent.

Diagnosis

Diagnostic criteria are as discussed above.

Management

The overall goal of managing patients with IF is to deliver the necessary amount of nutrition by a combination of parenteral, enteral, and oral routes to maintain normal growth and development. A prescription for parenteral, and enteral feeding should be individualized for every patient with the aim of maximizing absorption and reducing stool output.

Parenteral nutrition (PN): All patients with IF will usually require PN for varying lengths of time. A detailed discussion of the management of PN is beyond the scope of this text. A few of the underlying principals are as follows. PN is typically initiated in a hospital setting. Depending on the age and size of the patient, PN should be infused over 10 (older children and teens) to 18 (infants and toddlers) hours as blood sugars will tolerate to maximize the time available for normal daily activities. After initial discharge from the hospital, basic laboratory tests are closely monitored up to 1–2x/week, then monthly or with scheduled clinic visits thereafter. In general, pediatric patients are followed on a monthly basis. Older patients and patients who are on stable PN/EN programs can be seen less frequently.

Enteral Nutrition (EN): Enteral nutrition is essential in promoting intestinal adaptation, and reducing the likelihood of developing IF associated liver disease (IFALD). Patients who can consume an oral diet are encouraged to do so. For patients with intact colons, the proportion of carbohydrate, fat, and protein should approximate that of a normal diet 50–60%, 20–30%, and 20% respectively. Moreover, soluble fiber, oxalate restriction and oral rehydration solutions should be considered in patients who still possess an adequate amount of colon.

In order to reduce diarrhea, the following strategies can be considered: Complex oral nutrients such as complex carbohydrates, small frequent meals (5x/day), avoidance of simple and synthetic/artificial sugars, and the use of anti-diarrheal (loperamide, diphenoxylate/atropine sulfate, codeine) and anti-secretory agents (H2-blocker, proton pump inhibitors, octreotide). Antidiarrheal medications should be used with caution, and are contraindicated with acute GI infections and in patients at risk for toxic megacolon (such as in ulcerative colitis and Hirschsprung's disease). All fluid losses from emesis, enteral tubes, ostomies, or diarrhea should be closely monitored and replaced as needed.

Most pediatric patients with IF will require nasogastric (NG) or gastric tube (G-tube) feedings. Tube feedings should begin as early as possible via continuous feeding at a low rate (5-10cc/hr x 14–24hrs per day) and then slowly (1–5 mL per day initially) advanced as tolerated. The tolerated speed of EN advancement largely depends on the presence and severity of symptoms of feeding intolerance. These symptoms include increased stool output, increased abdominal distension/pain or discomfort, nausea/vomiting, and acute electrolyte disturbances. In the absence of these symptoms, feedings should be cautiously advanced. The choice of formula type has been controversial with regional practice differences. In the United States, protein hydrolysate and amino acid formulas have been favored, but intact protein formulas have also been successfully used in other countries.

Surgery: Patients with evidence of recurring bowel obstructions should be considered for surgical treatment. Intestinal lengthening procedures including the Bianchi and Serial Transverse Enteroplasty (STEP) procedures can be considered in select patients with dilated bowel segments. However, outcomes have not been consistent and generally have been a function of a center's surgical experience. If possible, gastrointestinal continuity should be restored as soon as possible. Early referral to a center of excellence for intestinal rehabilitation and transplantation is recommended for all patients who are high risk (see below).

Consultations & when to refer for intestinal transplant evaluation: Intestinal transplantation is a Medicaid-approved surgery that is no longer considered experimental and has become the standard of care in patients with IF who are unable to be maintained on PN. Patients with IF who are at high risk should be referred to an intestinal rehabilitation center with expertise in intestinal rehabilitation and intestinal/multivisceral transplantation. Consensus criteria for high risk patients include: Residual small bowel length <25cm, lack of an ilealcecal valve, early and persistent (total>3 or >1 per month) central venous catheter infections, difficult central venous catheter access, intractable diarrhea or inability to tolerate enteral feeds, significant liver dysfunction (persistent hyperbilirubinemia >3–6 mg/dL), preterm infants with massive bowel resection who are at high risk for liver disease, patients whose diagnosis and clinical course is uncertain, and the advisability of surgical intervention (e.g., Restoration of GI continuity, bowel lengthening procedures). Centers with intestinal rehabilitation services typically include a multidisciplinary team consisting of nurses specializing in PN/EN and central line care, pediatric gastroenterology, nutritionist, social worker, feedings specialists/occupational therapist, psychologist, general surgery, and transplant surgery. Although subspecialty care plays an essential role in the lives of these children, the importance of the general pediatrician's role cannot be overstated. The general pediatrician ensures that the routine acute and chronic childhood needs of these children are met and serves as a source of support for the family.

Therapy: Oral aversion is a common chronic challenge in a large number of patients with IF. Starting oral feedings as early as possible in infancy helps to reduce the chances and duration of long term oral aversion. Infants and children with oral aversion should be evaluated and treated by qualified occupational and speech therapists. Even in infants who take minimal oral feeds or are NPO, oral feeding/stimulation therapy should be considered so that they do not miss the critical window during infancy of learning how to suck and swallow (e.g., Non-nutritive sucking).

Psychosocial/development: As with many chronic childhood conditions, the burden on patients, care-providers, and families can be enormous. Many families are limited in both social and financial support. Involvement of an experienced social worker as part of a multidisciplinary team is important in supporting patient and family needs. The Oley Foundation (http://www.oley.org/) and American Society for Parenteral and Enteral Nutrition (ASPEN) (http://www.nutritioncare.org/) websites offer several resources to support families and clinicians.

Monitoring (labs, physical): Once a stable PN program has been established, patients are typically seen and labs monitored on a monthly basis. Accurate weight and height/length at each clinic visit is also essential. Routine laboratory tests should include: CBC, Na, K, Cl, CO2, BUN, Cr, Mg, Phos, iCa, AST, ALT, T/D bilirubin, protein, albumin, and prealbumin. Once or twice per year, extended nutrition parameters should be monitored. These extended parameters should include: Vitamin A/D-25-OH/E levels, INR, zinc, Se, Cu, Al, essential FA, Mn, B12, folate, parathyroid hormone, and iron studies (Fe, TIBC, ferritin, tranferrin) if anemia is

Table 5.3: Signs and Symptoms of Nutritional Problems

Vitamin or Trace Element Deficiency	Sign or Symptom
Biotin	dermatitis, alopecia, depression.
Essential fatty acids	xerosis (scaly, flaky dermatitis of the extremities), thrombocytopenia, follicular hyperkeratosis, dry, dull hair.
Folic Acid	pancytopenia, glossitis, stomatitis, diarrhea
Niacin	pellagra: scarlet, raw tongue, fissures of the tongue.
Pantothenic acid	abdominal pain, nausea and vomiting.
Vitamin A	xerophthalmia, keratomalacia, night blindness, sterility
Vitamin B1 (thiamine)	beriberi: cardiomyopathy, neuropathy, encephalopathy.
Vitamin B2 (Riboflavin)	stomatitis, glossitis, cheilosis.
Vitamin B6 (Pyridoxine)	peripheral neuropathy, convulsions, glossitis.
Vitamin B12 (Cobalamin)	megaloblastic anemia, neuropathy, glossitis
Vitamin C	scurvy, delayed wound healing, petechiae, perifollicular hyperkeratosis, hemorrhage.
Vitamin D	osteomalacia, rickets.
Vitamin E	hemolytic anemia, neuropathy, reticulocytois, thrombocytosis, edema.
Vitamin K	bleeding, increased pt
Chrominum	glucose intolerance, peripheral neuropathy, metabolic encephalopathy.
Cobalt	pernicious anemia
Copper	microcytic hypochromic anemia, leukopenia, neutropenia, menke's syndrome, bone changes, elevated cholesterol, hair and skin depigmentation.
Fluoride	dental caries
Iodine	thyroid disease (goiter, hypothyroidism, cretinism)
Iron	hypochromic microcytic anemia, apathy, weakness, cheilosis.
Magnesium	tetany, positive chvostek and trousseu signs, seizures, generalized weakness, anorexia, hypokalema, hypocalcemia, apathy, delirium.
Manganese	growth depression, bone deformities, retarded growth of hair and nails, changes in hair color, transient dermatitis.
Molybenum	growth retardation, impaired methionine and uric acid metabolism
Nickel	growth retardation, impaired lipid metabolism in animals.
Selenium	dilated cardiomyopathy, keshan's disease, white nails, idiopathic arrhythmias, myositis, growth retardation.
Zinc	apathy, anorexia, growth depression, dermatitis, alopecia, hair loss, impaired wound healing, dysgeusia.

present. Electrolyte components should be adjusted to correct any imbalances. Excess fluid loss (gastric, ostomy, rectum) replacement can be incorporated into the daily PN volume if it is small, or can be provided as a separate infusion in addition to PN. Vitamin and/or trace mineral deficiencies can be corrected by increasing the component via PN, separate IV infusions, or enterally if possible. For example, iron deficiency anemia is not uncommon in patients with IF and often requires separate infusions. Many centers also include periodic bone density measurements as part of a standard monitoring protocol.

Hearing exams should be considered every 2–5 years for children who are frequently treated with antibiotics such as aminoglycosides.

Signs and symptoms of nutritional problems listed in Table 5.3 should be elicited at every office visit.

Pearls and Precautions:

Immunization: All children with IF and an intact immune system should receive all preventative services similar to healthy children and routine vaccinations according to American Academy of Pediatrics (AAP) guidelines. According to the FDA website (contacted July 2009), there is not enough data to support the use of the existing rotavirus vaccine (RotaTeq ®) in these children.

Complications:

Potential complications of IF include: CVC-associated problems (infections, occlusion, breakage, vascular thrombosis, loss of vascular access), intestinal failure associated liver disease, malnutrition, micronutrient imbalance, essential fatty acid deficiency, fluid and electrolyte imbalance, small bowel bacterial overgrowth, D-lactic acidosis, oxalate nephropathy, renal dysfunction, metabolic bone disease, and peptic ulcer disease.

Central Venous Catheter (CVC) care: Frequent CVC infections can result in poor long term outcomes for patients with IF. Thus, optimizing CVC care to minimize infectious complications is crucial. CVC care guidelines are variable from institution to institution. At UCLA, patients and their care givers are educated to clean CVC access hubs 6 times with alcohol and 6 times with betadine or chloroprep prior to each access. Hub caps are recommended to be changed once a week and CVC site dressings are changed 1–3 times a week or as needed. Even in the best of hands, CVC-associated bacteremia can still occur.

Symptoms suggestive of infection include fever, chills, headaches, malaise, and blood sugar instability. Line clots can serve as a nidus for infection and should be suspected if there is difficulty with infusion of TPN or medications, or there are problems withdrawing blood back from the line. These symptoms should prompt urgent medical attention. Blood cultures from the CVC and peripheral sites should be obtained. A culture of the skin surrounding the line insertion site should also be done if pus or redness is seen at the entrance. Urinalysis and urine culture should also be considered. There should be a low threshold for hospitalization and initiation of antibiotic treatment. Given that there is a finite number of vascular sites in any patient, removal of a CVC should not be undertaken unless the infection is life threatening, recurrent/persistent despite adequate treatment, in the line tunnel under the skin, or fungal. Gram positive (S. aureus) and gram-negative organisms (klebsiella, E. coli, enterobacter, pseudomonas) are the most common etiologies.

Guidelines for treating and managing CVC-associated infections have been published by the Infectious Disease Society of America. Effective therapy should be documented with 2–3 negative blood cultures. The duration of therapy is from 10–14 days after the first negative blood culture. ID consultation should be considered in cases of resistant organisms or when there is any doubt regarding the source of infection or antibiotic treatment options. Patients with fungemia should have a renal ultrasound, a dilated ophthalmologic examination, and an echocardiogram to look for a potential nidus of infection. Frequent CVC infections leading to repeated catheter replacements can result in vascular thrombosis and ultimately loss of vascular access. Patients who have >1 CVC infection per year or who have had >3 CVC line replacements may be at risk for loss of vascular access and should be concomitantly followed by a center that performs intestinal transplantation.

IF Associated Liver Disease (IFALD): Is suggested by a chronic elevation in liver enzymes and/or hyperbilirubinemia. Patients with a gallbladder should have a hepatobiliary US to evaluate for gallstones. Evaluation for other causes of liver disease including viral hepatitis should be considered. Treatment involves maximizing enteral or oral nutrition and minimizing infectious complications. Ursodiol can be considered in patients with cholestasis, but its effectiveness can be variable. A small number of patients will have increased stool output with ursodiol. Omegaven® is an omega-3-fatty acid based lipid formulation that has recently become available in the research setting, and early results have shown some effectiveness in reversing IFALD.

Small Bowel Bacterial Overgrowth (SBBO): This condition can present similarly to feeding intolerance with diarrhea, abdominal distension, nausea/vomiting, D-lactic acidosis, malaise, or frequent CVC infections. D-lactic acidosis is suspected in patients presenting with a history of altered mental status with no obvious historical red flags or laboratory abnormalities. D-lactic acid levels are elevated in these patients. Treatment is with adequate re-hydration, observation, and treatment for SBBO. Some patients may require only one course of therapy while others may require a rotating schedule (e.g., 1 week on, 3 weeks off, a different antibiotic every other week, 3 weeks on and 1 week off). Many antibiotic regimens are available and will generally be center dependent (Table 5.4). There have been no large studies comparing the efficacy of each regimen. Probiotics and glutamine have been used on a limited basis for SBBO with no strong data to either support or discourage its usage.

Renal disease: Oxaluria associated nephrolithiasis is a known complication of chronic PN support. Oxalic acid stones develop as a consequence of lipid malabsorption; calcium then binds preferentially to lumen fatty acids compared to oxalate, leaving free oxalate available for uptake. This complication can be minimized by insuring adequate hydration and placing patients on a low oxalate containing diet.

Metabolic bone disease: Bone disease can develop in patients who have reduced bone mineral content. Serum calcium and phosphorous are monitored closely and replaced when necessary. vitamin 25OH D levels should also be checked and supplemented as needed. Baseline and annual bone density scans should be considered in patients with short bowel syndrome.

Peptic ulcer disease: Gastric hypersecretion is not uncommon after bowel resection and lasts up to 5 months or longer. Gastric hypersecretion can result in increased acid load, denaturing of pancreatic enzymes, and reduced pancreatic and bile salt function culminating in increased stool output. Patients should be treated for 6–12 months after resection with an acid suppressing agent.

School/education: Frequent hospitalizations and the intensity and volume of home health care needs contribute to developmental and educational delays for children with IF. For children <5 years, developmental/educational assessment should be performed by a qualified pediatrician or developmental specialist on an

Table 5.4: Antibiotics Used in Small Bowel Bacterial Overgrowth

Antibiotics Used in Small Bowel Bacterial Overgrowth	
Amoxicillin-Clauvulonate	Vancomycin
Ciprofloxacin	Rifaximine
Tetracycline	Gentamicin
Doxycycline	Fluconazole
Metronidazole	

annual basis. Identified physical, functional, or cognitive deficits should be addressed with appropriate resources. School aged children who lag in their academic achievement should have annual individual educational program (IEP) assessments.

References

Vanderhoof JA, Young RJ. Overview of Considerations for the Pediatric Patient Receiving Home Parenteral and Enteral Nutrition. Nutrition in Clinical Practice 2003;18:221–226.

Matarese LE, O'Keefe SJ, Kandil HM, et al. Short Bowel Syndrome: Clinical Guidelines for Nutrition Management. Nutrition in Clinical Practice 2005;20:493–502.

Gura KM, Duggan CP, Collier SB, et al. Reversal of Parenteral Nutrition–Associated Liver Disease in Two Infants With Short Bowel Syndrome Using Parenteral Fish Oil: Implications for Future Management. Pediatrics 2006; 118:e97–e201.

Parrish CR. The Clinician's Guide to Short Bowel Syndrome. Nutrition Issues in Gastroenterology September 2005;series 31.

Mermel LA, Allon M, Bouza E, et al. Clinical Practice Guidelines for the Diagnosis and Management of Intravascular Catheter-Related Infection: 2009 Update by the Infectious Diseases Society of America. Clinical Infectious Diseases 2009;49:1–45.

Ulcerative Colitis (UC)

Michelle Pietzak

Ulcerative colitis (UC) is a multi-system autoimmune disease which can affect the colon, liver and biliary tree, joints, skin and eyes. Confirmation of the diagnosis requires gastrointestinal endoscopy and biopsy. At present, there is no cure for UC except colectomy. Management primarily involves treating the symptoms while minimizing toxicity of chronic medications until the time a colectomy is appropriate.

Etiology

There is no clear etiology associated with UC, but like most autoimmune diseases, it is believed to be caused by a combination of genetic and environmental factors. Several genes have recently been associated with ulcerative colitis, most of which involve the pathways of apoptosis, epidermal growth factor or Th1-related cells and cytokines. Multiple environmental factors have been studied. Increased risk for the development of UC has been reported with the use of NSAIDS and oral contraceptives. Unlike Crohn's disease, cigarette smoking and appendectomy appear to decrease the risk of development of UC.

Clinical Presentation and Prognosis:

Demographics: The demographics of both forms of inflammatory bowel disease (UC and Crohn's disease) are very similar (please see Crohn's disease for details). There tends to be a family predisposition to autoimmunity, and 10–15% of children with UC have first-degree relatives with IBD.

Presenting signs and symptoms: The most common presenting symptoms for childhood UC are hematochezia, diarrhea and abdominal pain. As opposed to acute infections which cause colitis, UC is insidious, not abrupt. UC can have presentations outside of the gastrointestinal tract, as described below:

1. *Classic gastrointestinal symptoms*: Diarrhea, abdominal pain, lower GI bleeding, tenesmus, urgency, fever, weight loss, vomiting, fatigue and anorexia are common presentations of pediatric UC.
2. *Liver*: Active or autoimmune hepatitis, jaundice, pruritus, fatigue, cirrhosis, primary sclerosing cholangitis, bile duct carcinoma (late complication), steatosis, amyloid deposition and recurrent pancreatitis have all been associated with UC.
3. *Rheumatologic*: Approximately 1/3 of children with UC will complain of joint pain. Joints affected are usually the large joints (wrist, elbow, hip, knee, and ankle). This can be differentiated from rheumatoid arthritis in that the patient is rheumatoid factor negative and there is no joint destruction. Joint pain

often improves with treatment of the IBD and flares when the GI tract flares. Low bone density can be seen.

4. *Skin*:
   - *Erythema nodosum*: Tender red nodules usually near the anterior tibias which occur during IBD flares.
   - *Pyoderma gangrenosum*: Skin ulcers which can occur on the extremities and around ostomies of patients with IBD.
   - *Vasculitis*: Inflammation of peripheral vessels which may be tender and blanch to the touch.
5. *Ocular*: Episcleritis (an inflammatory condition of the connective tissue between the conjunctiva and sclera) and uveitis may be ophthalmologic emergencies.
6. *Thromboembolic disease*: Venous and arterial thrombosis of the lung, portal vein, hepatic vein, central nervous system and extremities have been reported in children with UC.
7. *Anemia*: Fatigue, pallor and shortness of breath on exertion are common complaints. Anemia may be due to chronic disease or chronic GI blood loss. Iron deficiency is one of the most common micronutrient deficiencies in undiagnosed children with IBD.

Clinical course: Every child with UC is unique in presentation, clinical course and prognosis. The majority of children enter remission within several months of diagnosis. However, predicting flares and relapse can prove difficult.

Prognosis: The prognosis for a child diagnosed with UC is guarded, as there is currently no cure for the condition other than colectomy. Overt GI symptomatology often waxes and wanes with flares, which may be idiopathic or due to stressors in the environment (diet, puberty, pregnancy, moving, going away to college, final exams, death in the family, etc.). Iron deficiency anemia can be corrected with supplementation after diagnosis. Growth failure may or may not improve with treatment, and may require supplemental calories via a special diet or formula, intravenous nutrition, or even growth hormone supplementation. Those with minimal disease limited to the rectum or rectosigmoid areas are thought to have a more benign course than those with pancolitis.

Diagnosis

History and physical exam: The diagnostic approach to the child with UC is to first suspect the diagnosis. A thorough history and physical are key, and should include serial plotting of weight, height, BMI, pubertal staging, and a bone age if there is growth delay. A family history for IBD, GI cancers and autoimmune diseases is essential. On physical exam, the young child with undiagnosed UC may exhibit protein-calorie malnutrition, with decreased subcutaneous fat stores and muscle bulk, or may have normal weight, height and BMI. Abdominal pain and distention with tympani can be appreciated due to gaseousness and colonic inflammation. Overt lower GI bleeding may be present on rectal exam, or only guaiac-positive stools. In fulminant, severe UC, the patient may have signs of acute blood loss, with fever, tachycardia, orthostatic hypotension, and more severe left lower quadrant abdominal pain and distension. Symptoms of iron deficiency anemia may include pallor, decreased appetite, abdominal pain, generalized fatigue, sleep disturbances, frontal headache and shortness of breath with exercise. Signs of iron deficiency anemia may include clubbing, brittle hair and nails, and a sore, smooth, shiny and/or reddened tongue. Zinc deficiency can occur with chronic diarrhea. Liver function tests should be routinely checked. Exams of the joints, skin and eye should be performed for the extra-intestinal manifestations as described above.

Routine laboratory testing: A CBC may show elevated white cell count with a left shift, an elevated platelet count and a microcytic anemia. ESR and CRP may be markedly elevated. Chemistries may reveal low potassium, bicarbonate, albumin, protein and zinc. Elevated transaminases, bilirubin and alkaline phosphatase can be seen if the liver or biliary tree is involved. Some children with mild UC at presentation may have entirely normal labs.

Tests for colitis: Common infectious etiologies should be ruled out, including Salmonella, Shigella, Yersinia, Campylobacter, Aeromonas, E. coli 0157:H7, ova and parasites (Amoebae) and Clostridium difficile. The patient should have a tuberculin test (PPD) and chest X-ray to evaluate for Mycobacterium tuberculosis. In patients with chronic diarrhea, growth failure, delayed sexual maturation, iron deficiency anemia and/or joint pain without overt GI bleeding, serologies should be sent to evaluate for celiac disease (see separate chapter).

Stool tests: Stool testing can be performed as non-invasive measures protein-losing enteropathy. Elevations in fecal alpha-1-antitrypsin correlate with protein-losing enteropathy, IBD disease activity and response to therapy. Elevations in fecal calprotectin suggest gastrointestinal inflammation and differentiate IBD from functional gastrointestinal disorders such as irritable bowel syndrome.

Serologic testing: pANCA are antibodies against cytoplasmic antigens detected by staining on the outer side of nuclear membrane of neutrophils, and are elevated in 50–67% of patients with UC. Anti-Saccharomyces cerevisiae IgG and IgA are antibodies to Baker's and Brewer's yeast, and are elevated in 5–14% of patients with UC. Potential roles for IBD serology include categorizing a child with indeterminate colitis into either UC or Crohn's disease, especially prior to colectomy. At present, these serologic screening tests are best utilized by gastroenterologists who are seeing patients at high risk for IBD, and not primary care practitioners who are screening for IBD in the general population.

Endoscopy with biopsy: UC may be localized to the rectum, left colon or involve the entire colon (pancolitis). Unlike Crohn's disease, the inflammatory response is confined to the colonic mucosa without transmural extension. These patients are thus much less likely to have strictures and fistulas. Visually, the mucosa may range from slightly erythematous, edematous and nodular, to having exudates and frank ulcerations with marked GI bleeding. As opposed to Crohn's disease, the small bowel should not be involved (although there can be "backwash ileitis" seen at the distal terminal ileum), and there should not be "skip areas" (visually and histologically normal mucosa) within the colon. Rectal sparing with pediatric UC is well described. Colonic biopsies may show acute and chronic inflammation with mixed inflammatory cells, neutrophilic crypt abscesses and depletion of goblet cells.

Management

The goals of management in UC are to treat acute symptoms, induce and maintain remission, improve quality of life, avoid medication toxicity and prevent cancer. The practitioner must bear in mind that unlike Crohn's disease, colectomy is curative. The risks of surgery must be balanced against medication toxicities in the pediatric UC patient.

Nutrition/diet: In those with malnutrition, a diet liberal in calories and protein should be provided to achieve catch-up growth. Some patients may require a calorically dense formula via night-time nasogastric tube feeds. Unlike Crohn's disease, exclusive enteral nutrition using an elemental formula has not demonstrated endoscopic healing and decreased inflammation in pediatric trials. Intravenous nutrition may be required for those with extremely poor nutritional status or toxic megacolon. It is hypothesized that the Westernized diet, high in ω-6 PUFAs (polyunsaturated fatty acids), increases risk for IBD or contributes to flares. There may be a potential role for omega-3 PUFAs, found in fish oil, and short chain fatty acids as anti-inflammatory agents in IBD.

Medications: Table 5.5 summarizes options for medical treatment of UC:

Table 5.5: Options for Medical Treatment of Ulcerative colitis

Medication	Indication	Adverse Effects
Antibiotics:	Mild UC	Lack of pediatric data
Metronidazole	Prevention of pouchitis	Metallic taste, furry tongue, nausea, anorexia, candidiasis,
Ciprofloxacin	post-colectomy	peripheral neuropathy, bacterial resistance
Aminosalicylates:	Mild to moderate UC	Lack of pediatric data
mesalamine,	Distal or left sided colitis	Rash, fever, nausea, vomiting, headaches, hemolysis, agranulocy-
sulfasalazine	(suppositories or enemas)	tosis, alveolitis, hepatitis, pancreatitis, nephritis, male infertility
Oral corticosteroids:	Moderate UC	Aseptic necrosis, hyperglycemia, hypertension, diabetes, cataracts,
Prednisone (rapidly	Distal or left sided colitis	osteoporosis, growth inhibition, striae, acne, Cushingoid
active, inexpensive)	(suppositories or enemas)	appearance
Immunomodulators:	Moderate UC	Fever, myalgias, nausea, rash, pancreatitis, hepatitis, pancytopenia,
6 MP, azathioprine		increased risk of lymphoma
Methotrexate	Moderate UC	Lack of pediatric data
		Nausea, hepatitis, hypersensitivity pneumonitis
Intravenous corticosteroids: Solumedrol	Severe UC	As with oral steroids
Cyclosporin	Severe UC	Mixed pediatric data
		Renal dysfunction, hirsutism, tremor, hypertension, gum hyperplasia, allergic reaction, hypomagnesemia, drug interactions, PCP pneumonia, lymphoproliferative disease
Tacrolimus	Severe UC	Lack of pediatric data
		Tremor, headache, diarrhea, hypertension, nausea, abnormal renal function, hyperkalemia, hypomagnesemia, hyperglycemia
Biologics:	Severe UC	Infusion reaction, reactivation TB, fungal infections,
Infliximab (only one FDA approved for pediatrics)		histoplasmosis, increased risk of lymphoma
Surgery	Severe UC	Small bowel obstruction, pouchitis, incontinence, high output
(curative)	Dysplasia Malignancy	ileostomy

Surgery: Absolute indications for surgery in pediatric UC include colonic perforation, exsanguinating hemorrhage or evidence of dysplasia or cancer. Relative indications include toxic megacolon or refractory disease with steroid dependency, growth failure or systemic complications. One of the more successful surgeries for pediatric UC is the ileal pouch anal anastomosis, using an ileal J-shaped pouch (a "neorectum") to preserve continence. Complications include small bowel obstruction and pouchitis, which can be treated with antibiotics, aminosalicylates or steroids.

Consultations: Successful management of the child with UC requires a team approach involving the patient, parents, other caretakers, school, gastroenterologist, primary care practitioner, a pediatric or colorectal surgeon, and a dietician. After a biopsy-confirmed diagnosis, if there is evidence of growth failure or protein-calorie malnutrition, the child should be referred to a registered dietician knowledgeable about UC for a personalized nutritional assessment and education. If poor growth, short stature or delayed sexual maturation remains present despite compliance with medical therapy, referral to a pediatric endocrinologist should be considered. Children with UC may have co-morbid growth hormone deficiency, osteopenia or another concomitant autoimmune condition.

Psychiatric: Children with UC have major concerns regarding their use of chronic medications, GI bleeding, and worrying about when their disease is going to flare up. Because of urgency and tenesmus, these children always have to know the location of the nearest bathroom. Sleep over parties and travel may not be feasible. Those on chronic steroids have self-esteem issues due to acne and Cushingoid appearance. Support must be given to the patient and family when dealing with this debilitating illness. Depression is common and may warrant a referral for individual or family counseling.

Social: Please see Crohn's disease chapter. Local, national and international support groups exist for both children and adults with IBD. They can easily be found on the internet, and provide not only emotional support, but tips on dealing with schools, eating out, traveling with IBD, and education about resources. These include Crohn's & Colitis Foundation of America (www.CCFA.org) and IBD Support Foundation (www.ibdsf.com). There are also summer camps available in the U.S. which can maintain a kitchen which can prepare special meals for children with IBD, dispense medications, and have a physician and/or nurse on site for medical emergencies. It is often an eye-opening experience for the newly diagnosed child and family with IBD to meet others at camp dealing with the same physical and emotional issues.

Monitoring: The child with UC should have frequent monitoring for anemia, liver disease and growth and sexual maturation. Measurement of bone density is often helpful in discovering occult osteopenia, and would suggest more aggressive supplementation of vitamin D and calcium, along with weight-bearing exercise and closer monitoring of linear growth. Routine monitoring labs, such as CBC with differential, ESR, CRP, serum chemistries and urinalysis should be tailored to the patient's disease location, medications, and clinical course. Repeat endoscopy should be considered for a child with UC who is not doing well clinically, to assess disease status. Because of the increased risk of colorectal cancer, bi-annual surveillance colonoscopy has been suggested to begin starting from 7–10 years from the initial diagnosis. There are no prospective studies to suggest optimal surveillance intervals in adolescent patients diagnosed at a young age.

Pearls and Precautions

Likely Complications:

- *Toxic megacolon:* Although rare, this is a medical and possibly surgical emergency, which can lead to sepsis, shock, hemorrhage and colonic perforation. Risk factors include use of anti-diarrheal medications (such as opiates or anticholinergics) and aggressive colonic distension with colonoscopy or barium enema.
- *Cancer:* Children with UC are at high risk for later development of colonic adenocarcinomas. Duration and extent of disease (for example, pancolitis is at greater risk than limited proctitis) are known risk factors. The cumulative risk of colorectal cancer in UC patients is 2% after 10 years of active disease, 5% after 20 years, and 10% after 25 years. If the patient also has primary sclerosing cholangitis, this risk increases to 9%, 31% and 50% respectively. Those with primary sclerosing cholangitis are also at higher risk for cholangiocarcinoma.

Immunizations: There are no contraindications to vaccination in the child with UC unless they are receiving immune suppressing medications, in which case live viral vaccines should not be administered.

School/Education: Please see Crohn's disease chapter. Children with severe UC or recovering from colectomy may require home schooling until they achieve continence.

References

Ponsky T, Hindle A, and Sandler A. Inflammatory Bowel Disease in the Pediatric Patient. Surg Clin N Am 2007;87:643–658.

Trudel JL, Lavery IC, Fazio VW, Jagelman DG, Weakley FL and Oakley JR. Surgery for ulcerative colitis in the pediatric population Indications, treatment, and follow-up. Diseases of the Colon and Rectum 1987;30:747–750.

Griffiths AM, Nicholas D, Smith C. et al. Development of a paediatric IBD quality of life index: dealing with differences related to age and IBD type. J Pediatr Gatroenterol Nutr 1999;28:S46–52.

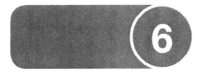

Genetic Disorders

Table of Contents

Introduction to Genetics and Inborn Errors of Metabolism

Stephen Cederbaum

In OMIM, the catalog of genetics diseases maintained by the National Library of Medicine, there are more than 10,000 conditions listed, all caused by mutations in a specific gene or genes (for example the number of genes involved in chromosome imbalance syndromes) or in some instances presumed mutations in a number of genes, (many unidentified) that cause a genetic predisposition to the disorder. In this presentation, we will discuss a select group of these disorders, but focus more attention on the inborn errors in which acute interventions may be life-saving.

Inborn errors of metabolism are a family of hundreds of genetic disorders that are caused by genetic mutations that cause enzyme deficiencies and prevent the conversion of substrate to product and result in one or more biochemical perturbations; deficiency of the product of the reaction, accumulation of one or more substrates proximal to the site of the block, accumulation of side products of one of the accumulated precursors of the reaction and often more widespread and less predictable changes in the enzyme content and physiologic dynamics of the patient. They generally are inherited in an autosomal recessive manner, but autosomal dominant, sex-linked recessive and mitochondrial inheritance is known. The majority of the genes involved in inborn errors have been cloned and DNA mutation analysis is available. There is considerable debate as to the value of mutation analysis in cases in which the diagnosis is unambiguous, but it is useful in all instances for prenatal diagnosis. The existence of a large number of inborn errors precludes discussion of each of them individually, but because many share common general characteristics for acute interventions and longer term symptomatic care, they can be grouped into general categories as we do in the chapters that follow.

Disorders of Small Molecules Circulating in the Blood

A. Disorders Presenting with an Acute Metabolic Crisis

Stephen Cederbaum

The majority of inborn errors that result in acute and sometimes life-threatening illness result from disorders in which the primary biochemical defect is manifest by elevated levels of the metabolites in the body fluids and not notably stored in the tissues themselves. Diagnosis is made initially by studying plasma and urine in particular, and sometimes cerebrospinal fluid for these disorders. Examples include: Amino acid disorders (maple syrup disease and non-ketotic hyperglycinemia, urea cycle disorders such as ornithine transcarbamylase deficiency (OTC)), organic acidemias (propionic, methylmalonic, isovaleric, glutaric acidemias), fatty acid oxidation disorders (medium-chain acyl CoA dehydrogenase deficiency (MCADD), long-chain hydroxyl-acyl CoA dehydrogenase deficiency (LCHADD)) and disorders of sugar metabolism such as galactosemia and fructosemia.

Etiology

With the exception of OTC which is X-linked recessive, Disorders presenting with an acute metabolic crisis are inherited in an autosomal recessive inheritance.

Clinical Presentation and Prognosis

Demographics: Autosomal recessive disorders are more common in consanguineous families and in patients from genetic isolates. Maple syrup disease is present in increased frequency in the Old Order Amish and Mennonite communities and glutaric acidemia in the Amish and in the Ojibway Indians of the Canadian plains.

Presenting signs and symptoms: Depending on the nature and severity of the mutations primarily, patients may present in the neonatal period after 24–48 hours of normalcy or may present later in life after a precipitating episode of catabolism due to infection, trauma or parturition. Other patients may present with a chronic course of poor feeding and weight gain, irritability and lethargy.

Presenting signs are generally those of an acute encephalopathy and may include cardiac failure, altered muscle tone (usually hypotonia), poor feeding, vomiting, coma (and of course death). Cerebral edema may be present in maple syrup disease and the urea cycle disorders. In the neonatal period particularly, these patients cannot be separated clinically from those with sepsis.

Prognosis: Prognosis in these conditions is guarded at best and is dependent on the severity of symptoms, the rapidity of diagnosis, the rapidity of response to treatment, and the severity of the triggering insult. Cerebral edema should raise a red flag in the disorders in which it occurs.

Diagnosis

The clinical features are not usually distinctive and offer no sure indication of the underlying condition. An exception is those conditions that may be accompanied by a distinctive odor such as the appropriately named maple syrup disease or isovaleric acidemia when the body and body fluids may smell like "sweaty feet." Routine laboratory studies offer the first clues: Acidemia with an anion gap, elevated ammonia, positive urinary ketones in the neonate with an organic acidemia may be important clues. Unfortunately, positive diagnosis is often dependent of highly specialized laboratory studies that are done in a few academic medical centers and commercial laboratories and the results will not be quickly available in the majority of clinical settings. Special studies include: Plasma amino acids, plasma acylcarnitine analysis, plasma carnitine and urinary organic acids. Once past the first week of life and often earlier, results of an expanded newborn screen should be available and may guide diagnostic thinking.

Management

This section will be divided into two broad and overlapping categories: (1) Management of an acute episode of encephalopathy; and (2) the longer term management of the chronically affected, but stable patient. The common feature of all of this class of disorders is that they can be modified by diminishing the load of substrate coming from either the diet or from the breakdown of body tissue. The latter poses a far greater hazard to the patient, but the former is the mainstay of chronic care, in particular. At the first acute episode, the diagnosis may not be known, either because the patient became ill before the result of newborn screening was known; newborn screening was not done; or, newborn screening is not sensitive for the diagnosis of a particular condition.

Acute: The patient must be stabilized and adequate intravenous access established. Respiration and hemodymics must be stable and should be secure before transfer to a tertiary care center is carried out. Care of the very sickest children is best carried out in a tertiary care facility where access to specialists, specialized procedures such as dialysis and specialized laboratory studies are more likely to be available. An inadequate supply of glucose is always a trigger to catabolism and 10% glucose, with insulin support (as is done for diabetic ketoacidosis) is always used as specific care is planned. Intravenous lipid as a second vital source of calories is critical in all but the fatty acid oxidation disorders, some of which may be amenable to medium chain triglyceride therapy. Electrolytes and blood volume should be maintained and bicarbonate supplementation is advisable if the bicarbonate falls below 10 meq/L or the pH becomes dangerously low. The offending metabolite can be removed effectively by dialysis in most instances. Extracorporeal membrane oxygenation (ECMO) gives the highest rate of exchange, but is often impractical and undesirable. Hemodialysis is the most commonly used effective method and is better by far than peritoneal dialysis and exchange transfusion which is useless. Any of these therapies can be used without knowledge of the diagnosis.

Having such a diagnosis may allow specific therapy to be used. The following specific therapies are recommended.

Maple syrup urine disease: These patients may be helped by nasogastric administration of the 17 amino acids that are metabolized normally.

Organic acidemias: Some clinicians use particularly high doses of carnitine, but rigorous proof for its efficacy has not been provided.

Isovaleric acidemia: Glycine is very helpful in the removal of isovaleric acid.

Urea cycle disorders: Sodium benzoate and sodium phenylacetate to divert ammonia from the dysfunctional pathway has been shown to mitigate the severity of the acute episodes.

Ultimately, metabolic stability cannot be fully attained without an adequate oral intake of calories and appropriate amounts of protein. In disorders with a known diagnosis, the normal diet is resumed as soon as the patient is stable enough to begin oral feedings (usually under the guidance of a metabolic specialist, even if at a distance).

Recurrent episodes of metabolic deterioration can often be managed locally with good glucose and appropriate electrolyte support serving to abort more severe deterioration in most cases.

Chronic treatment: Patients are maintained on a diet and regimen appropriate to their condition and degree of physical and cognitive disability. The diet must have adequate calories, adequate fluid, and an adequate amount of an appropriate mixture of proteins usually requiring specially formulated supplements, carnitine for a number of the organic acidemias and natural foods to provide calories and natural protein. Vitamins are usually found in the special products, but special note of this must be made. Constipation is undesirable as it may increase the production of offending metabolites by intestinal bacteria and mild inhibition of bacterial flora growth with metranidazole is part of the regimen. Ammonia diverting agents are used in urea cycle defects.

Patients should all carry an emergency letter, explaining to them and their families and to any emergency physician the nature of the condition and the most appropriate acute therapy. Most patients are provided with "sick day diets" which are modifications of their usual diet designed to mitigate the severity of the protein catabolism that occurs in conjunction with intercurrent illness. Prompt parentral response, first with these treatment modifications can often abort the need for hospitalization. In all cases, prompt and cautious parentral response improves the course of the illness.

Consultations: Management of these conditions must be undertaken under the supervision of a metabolic clinic in which medical, nursing, nutritional and social service support is available. Consultation with neurologists, developmental specialists and others is very often required.

Social support: National parent organizations exist for almost every disorder or family of disorders and can easily be found on the web. They are exceedingly helpful to and empower many families. Many children require special services which in California is provided by California Children's Services (CCS) and/or the Regional Centers.

Precautions and Miscellaneous Information:

Immunization: Children should be immunized in a normal fashion as dealing with an immunization reaction is easier than dealing with the acute illness that it can prevent.

Nutrition: The majority of these patients are on highly individualized diets that are limited in the quantity and type of natural protein. This is managed by the metabolic specialist and should not be modified without consultation. In most instances parents can be taught to read labels for protein content and introduce commercial products independently. Most alternative medicines deemed safe for unaffected children and which are protein free can be taken by patients with inborn errors of metabolism.

Routine medication: Medications used to treat ordinary pediatric conditions can be used if they do not contain a prohibited nutrient, for example lactose as a sweetener or carrier in an antibiotic as in the case of galactosemia. The pharmacist will usually have access to this information.

Likely complications: Patients with these disorders are at risk for acute episodes of deterioration at any time in their lives, although with age these episodes usually diminish in frequency and severity. Routine infections of childhood, trauma, or medical and dental procedures may pose a risk and have to be handled more carefully. Overnight fasting for a procedure may be contraindicated in some patients and may require overnight admission prior to the procedure and a hospital stay for observation of adequate nutrient and fluid intake afterward. In general, these patients are treated normally, but with a higher degree of awareness.

Many patients will be mentally retarded and/or physically handicapped and will require special services to optimize their function. These should be individualized.

School/Education: It is now customary to educate all children up to their ability to learn. Many patients with these conditions will require some form of special education and comprehensive testing to determine their needs. In addition they may need special services for administration of medication and feeding at school and may require assistance with toileting. Each school district has its own rules in this regard.

Reference:

Fernandes, J., Saudubray, J-M., van den Berghe, G., Walter, J.H. (eds.) Inborn Metabolic Diseases (4th ed.), Springer Verlag, Heidelberg, 2006.

B. Disorders Presenting with Chronic Metabolic Intoxication

Stephen Cederbaum

Examples include: Amino acid disorders like phenylketonuria (PKU) and homocystinemia, organic acidemias, cobalamin processing defects (cobalamin C), and fatty acid oxidation disorders such as carnitine transporter defect and carnitine palmityl transferase deficiencies.

Etiology

Autosomal recessive inheritance.

Clinical Presentation and Prognosis

Demographics: Autosomal recessive disorders are more common in consanguineous families and from patients from genetic isolates. For example, partial carnitine palmityl transferase I deficiency (CPTI) is more common in aboriginal Inuit populations of Canada and Alaska.

Presenting signs and symptoms: Depending on the nature and severity of the mutations, primarily, patients may present at different times of life, some never showing any but biochemical abnormalities. Some patients with cobalamin defects or some with CPT I may never present with a recognizable acute episode. Others, such as PKU and homocystinemia virtually never have an acute metabolic episode, except in the case of the latter where complications of the condition, such as a vascular accident may present acutely. Patients with carnitine transporter deficiency of severe degree have been found by chance when women gave birth to normal infants who were found to be carnitine deficient during the expanded newborn screening procedure. CPT2 deficiency may go undiagnosed if the patient never subjects him- or herself to the exercise conditions that provoke rhabdomyolysis or cramping.

Prognosis: The prognosis of these disorders is variable. In PKU in which both mutations in the phenylalanine hydroxylase gene are severe, mental retardation, microcephaly with variable symptoms of seizures or autistic like behavior occur. In mutations of lesser severity, symptoms of mild developmental delay and diminished school performance may go undetected. In homocystinemia some patients are mentally retarded, whereas others are ascertained through an ophthalmologist who discovers dislocated lenses. Many patients with homocytinemia have a distinct body habitus which is only recognized after the diagnosis is made. Those with the pyridoxine responsive form of the disorder may have lesser elevations of homocyteine in the blood at diagnosis and a milder clinical course.

Diagnosis

Patients with untreated PKU or with homocystinemia have distinctive clinical symptoms, but most of these disorders are now diagnosed preemptively by expanded newborn screening. The biochemical marker for homocystinemia, elevated methionine levels, may be absent in the first days of life and lead to this disorder being overlooked. Milder forms of other disorders may be missed as well. Under these circumstances, clinical description unique to one or another disorder is not relevant. Standard references (see bibliography) would contain the description of these conditions.

In case the diagnosis is missed in newborn screening, the conditions are usually uncovered by studies of plasma amino acids, urine organic acids, plasma acylcarnitine profiles or plasma carnitine determination.

Management

Management is dependent on the diagnosis. Chronic treatment for all patients consists of a special metabolic diet, often vitamin supplements in those conditions that are proven to be vitamin responsive, and specific symptomatic support. The overall management often requires a team of physicians, but the aspects specific to the inborn error should be managed in a metabolic center where expertise in the conditions is abetted by nursing and nutritional expertise. Infrequently, common intercurrent illnesses (such as diarrhea or flu) and environmental stressors may cause acute episodes not unlike those described in the previous chapter. Intervention can usually occur locally with glucose and fluid support. The episodes in these disorders are usually shorter and easier to treat.

Phenylketonuria is managed by a strict low protein diet with a supplement of an amino acid mixture containing no phenylalanine. The most familiar name is phenyl-free, but, in fact, there are more than 10 different formulas on the market with variations in composition appropriate to the patient's age whose names are constantly changing to distinguish them in the marketplace. More recently, a proportion of patients with PKU, increasing in frequency in those with a more mild form, have responded to high doses of the normal co-factor in this reaction, tetrahydrobiopterin (Kuvan®) with lowering or elimination of the need to limit dietary phenylalanine.

Homocystinemia is likewise treated with a diet except with those in whom there is a response to its natural co-factor, vitamin B6 given orally in doses from 100–500 mg/per day depending on the patient age. Excessive doses of B6 can cause neurotoxicity so that it cannot be increased with reckless abandon. Because folic acid wasting may occur, patients are supplemented with 1–5 mg of folate a day and are given a baby aspirin and sometimes other medications that diminish the tendency to arterial thrombosis.

Cobalamin deficiencies are treated with diet and in particular the administration of one or another form of vitamin B12 in high concentrations. Most commonly 1 mg of hydroxycobalamin is given by injection daily, but variations on dose and route of administration reflect individual patient variation and the limitations of our knowledge.

Fatty acid oxidation defects are treated with a higher carbohydrate intake and with care to avoid fasting. In the case of partial CPT2 deficiency, similar measures should be taken before exercise.

Carnitine transported deficiency responds readily to carnitine administration.

The more distant long term effectiveness of any of these therapies has not been determined, although in the case of PKU, in particular, the picture appears to be quite bright.

With the exception of those conditions that may react adversely to an exercise program, schooling with other children at the appropriate level of their ability is desirable.

Special Services: Some of these children and adults require special services, which in California is provided by California Children's Services (CCS) and/or the Regional Centers (RC).

Social support: National Parent organizations exist for almost every disorder or family of disorders and can easily be found on the web. They are exceedingly helpful to and empower many families.

Precautions and Miscellaneous Information

Immunizations: None of these conditions should influence the normal pattern of immunization.

Nutrition: Many of these patients are in highly individualized and quite limited diets. They should be managed by the metabolic specialist and the diet should not be modified without consultation. In most instances, parents can be taught to read labels for protein and other nutrient content and can be empowered to introduce commercial products independently. Most alternative medicines deemed safe for unaffected children and which are proven to be protein-free can be taken by patients with these inborn errors of metabolism.

Routine Medication: Medications used to treat ordinary pediatric conditions can be used if they do not contain a prohibitive nutrient, for example, lactose as a sweetener or carrier in an antibiotic in the case of galactosemia, or products sweetened with aspartame (NutraSweet®) in the case of PKU. The pharmacist will usually have access to this information.

Likely complications: Some patients with these disorders, as previously noted, may be subject to acute episodes of deterioration in response to severe intercurrent illness. Routine infections of childhood, trauma, or medical and dental procedures may pose a risk if they are particularly severe. Overnight fasting for a procedure may be contraindicated in some patients, although this need be less stringent than in the disorders which more routinely present with acute episodes.

School/Education: These children should be educated in a normal school with programs individualized to meet special needs. Patients with PKU may need dietary supervision while in the cafeteria. Patients with other disorders may require administration of medication during the day. With the exception of those conditions that may react adversely to an exercise program, activities with other children at the appropriate level of their ability is desirable.

Reference

Fernandes, J., Saudubray, J-M., van den Berghe, G., Walter, J.H. (eds.) Inborn Metabolic Diseases (4th ed.), Springer Verlag, Heidelberg, 2006.

Lysosomal Storage Disorders

(consists of mucopolysaccharidoses, gangliosidoses, mucolipidoses, oligosaccharidoses and Pompe Disease)

Stephen Cederbaum

Etiology

The majority of these conditions are inherited in an autosomal recessive manner. Two exceptions are Hunter Disease or mucopolysaccharidosis, type II (MPS II); and, Fabry Disease, both of which are inherited in an X-linked manner. As is the case with most autosomal recessive disorders, isolated or inbred populations are at greater risk of having an increased frequency of one or another of these disorders. The Ashkenazi Jewish population has a particularly high frequency of non-neuronopathic Gaucher Disease, referred to as type I, infantile-onset GM-2 gangliosidosis or Tay-Sachs disease and the severe form of sphingomyelinase deficiency also known as Neimann-Pick disease, type A. A form of Sanfilippo disease is particularly prevalent in the Caiman Islands. A mild form of Fabry disease is said to be prevalent in the Northern Italian mountains, quite possibly in an X-linked disorder of later onset that does not affect fertility.

Clinical Presentation and Prognosis

Demographics: Onset occurs from birth to middle age, depending on the disorder and the severity of the enzyme deficiency.

Presenting signs and symptoms: Excluding the rare instances when the disorder presents at birth, the children are often quite normal in the first weeks or months of life. Depending on the disorder, the patient development tends to plateau and then gradually regress. The children with sphingolipid storage disorders stop smiling, lose visual focus, may develop hyperacusis (over-sensitivity to certain sound frequencies), seizures or obvious neurologic findings. The head is likely to enlarge rather than be small. The mucopolysaccharide storage disorder patients begin to develop skin thickening, joint deformities, coarsening facial features, hirsuitism and organomegaly, a complex referred to unflatteringly as gargoylism. The presentation of later onset disease is more highly variable, but involves the same types of symptoms, loss of attainments, inattention, visual difficulties, etc. They may not resemble the infantile onset presentation. Fabry disease usually presents in the first decade of life with burning sensations beginning in the hands and feet which can be excruciating. Unlike most sex-linked disorders, manifestations occur quite early in the majority of females, albeit later and less severe than in their brethren.

Clinical course: This is inevitably progressive. Those with severe infantile onset lipid storage disorders often die within two to five years, depending on the intensity of intervention. Most children enter a vegetative state as the disease progresses. Later onset disease may progress more slowly. In non-neuronopathic Gaucher disease, patients may go through life without symptoms and may be diagnosed incidentally at autopsy. This is emphasized by the disparity between the carrier frequency and the recognized disease frequency among Ashkenazi Jews. Fabry disease may begin in the first decade as noted above, but may require 40 or 50 years before the more serious cardiac and renal manifestations become symptomatic.

Prognosis: That for the infantile onset disorders is dismal, with a relentless downhill course, a large part of which is spent with irritability and no meaningful interaction with family members. That for the other disorders has been already described.

Diagnosis

The first step leading to the diagnosis is clinical suspicion. Until recently specialized urine studies for mucopolysaccharide was the first line method available, followed by enzymatic studies on plasma, leukocytes or skin fibroblasts. Currently, it is more common to take advantage of the more readily available enzymatic methods as the first step in diagnosis for many of the disorders. Diagnostic confirmation can now be accomplished by mutation analysis for most of these disorders. Mucopolysaccharide storage disorders also have radiological features of dysostosis multiplex or multiple and often characteristic boney abnormalities. When a disorder is suspected and cannot be demonstrated, a skin or conjunctival biopsy examined by electron microscopy may be the only clue that you are on the correct diagnostic track.

Management

This is best carried out in specialized centers for the care of people with these disorders. The organ systems that are at risk and the therapeutic approach taken towards these patients depends on the specific disorder, the tissues which normally express the enzyme and the rate of progression. These would include the central nervous system, the spinal column independently of neurologic damage, viscera, the heart, skeletal muscle (Pompe disease) the lungs, the skin, and joints. The majority of interventions for all of them are symptomatic. Some may require stabilization of the cervical spine on the one extreme and physical therapy on the other. Care generally involves multiple specialties and consultations and must be coordinated. Difficulty in removing an endothecial tube because of thickening of the bronchial epithelium requires the special expertise of a highly trained pediatric anesthesiologist during surgery.

Medications: For a limited number of these disorders such as Gaucher, Fabry, Hurler, Hunter, Pompe and Maretaux-Lamy Diseases, enzyme replacement therapies are available. Because enzymes do not enter the central nervous system, the beneficial effects are limited to the visceral organs and those tissues accessible to the enzyme. In disorders that do not involve the central nervous system such as Gaucher and Fabry, the results have been excellent. The efficacy is more limited in other disorders because of the progression of the neurological problems. Intrathecal approaches to enzyme delivery for several of these disorders are being explored. All enzyme therapy is terribly inconvenient and terribly expensive. Therapy using small molecular weight biosynthetic inhibitors and enzyme chaperones are being studied and some seem quite promising. They have the potential of crossing the blood-brain barrier and thus treating and mitigating the neurologic deterioration. They offer little benefit in terms of cost. As of this writing, one such medication, miglustat (zavesca®) is approved by the FDA for the treatment of Gaucher disease.

Surgery: For some disorders involving central nervous system deposition of storage material and deterioration, stem cell therapy (previously referred to as bone marrow transplantation) has been tried and may be successful when used early. Other surgical interventions such as gastrostomy tube placement, tracheotomy, VP shunts and other symptomatic approaches are often required. Anesthesiology presents a particular risk to patients with moderate to advanced storage disorders as noted above.

Consultations: The care of patients with these highly specialized disorders requires specialized care centers with experience in these conditions. Consultations with such a center and an ongoing relationship is mandatory, even when enzyme replacement therapy and many of the symptomatic interventions can be carried out locally. Patients may have to be seen by neurologists, cardiologists, physical therapists, gastroenterologists, surgeons of various types, ophthalmologists, audiologists and others.

Social: The psychological impact of a progressive degenerative disorder which until recently had no potentially successful interventions is not a problem unique to this group of conditions and requires particular attention. The involvement of a social worker and if necessary, of a psychiatrist or a psychologist may be required. Disease specific and more generic support groups exist and can be found on the web. For the lipidoses, the United Leukodystrophy Foundation is an excellent resource (http://www.ulf.org). For mucopolysaccharidoses the MPS society provides excellent advocacy and support (http://www.mpssociety.org).

Special Considerations

Immunizations: It is recommended that these patients receive all of the usual immunizations including seasonal flu vaccine as the disorders are generally perceived to be much worse than the potential impact of the immunizations themselves. Exceptions to this rule would be patients in the advanced stages of the disorders in which the risk of an otherwise trivial immunization reaction may pose a particular hazard.

Nutrition/diet: This family of conditions does not require any specific dietary therapy, but dysfunction of the swallowing mechanism, GI tract problems and diarrhea may require special intervention such as placement of gastrostomy tubes or alteration of the diet specific to the problem. Because the complex molecules that are stored in these conditions are broken down in the GI tract, there is no need to limit their intake.

Tracheal toileting: As these disorders advance, a number of them cause respiratory difficulties and they require suctioning on a continual basis, and eventually tracheotomies.

Sleep: A number of patients who develop psychiatric symptoms as part of their neurological deterioration may have trouble sleeping in addition to their behavioral problems during the day. Interventions appropriate to the behaviors and the problems should be carried out with the advice of mental health professionals. There is no consensus as to the optimal treatment of these rare disorders.

Likely complications: Each disorder included in this group may differ from others and in addition they may differ from one another in severity. In the more severe cases of conditions involving the central nervous system, the end point is often death and in the process the patients may deteriorate toward this end slowly, require respiratory support, cardiotonic agents and other supportive measures. Other disorders may have disease specific complications such as joint and skeletal deformity, respiratory issues, problems with vision and hearing, or others. Reference to issues with specific diseases need to be sought.

School/education: Depending on the disorder, patients can be intellectually normal or handicapped. Within this variation, there are special challenges imposed by physical conditions that may accompany the disorder. There are exercise limitations, risk of physical contact, inability to manipulate the fingers and hands requiring assistive devices and special feeding regimens. Close contact between the parent, the school, and the school district is often necessary in order to obtain timely Individualized Educational Plan (IEP) and physical nursing support.

Medications/herbs: There are no specific medications that must be avoided by patients with these conditions. Any anesthetic should be used with caution and a literature search for complications with the particular disorder would be important. Recently genistin, a soy-derived natural product has had miraculous improvements attributed to it. Systematic controlled studies are underway to assess the true efficacy, if any, of this product.

Reference

Fernandes, J., Saudubray, J-M., van den Berghe, G., Walter, J.H. (eds.) Inborn Metabolic Diseases (4th ed.), Springer Verlag, Heidelberg, 2006.

Disorders of Energy Metabolism

A. Glycogen Storage Disorders (Glycogenoses, von Gierke disease)

Stephen Cederbaum

Etiology

The disorders of glycogen metabolism with or without glycogen storage are largely inherited in an autosomal recessive manner. The exception to this is an abnormality in the gene responsible for activation of liver phosphorylase, which is inherited in a sex linked recessive manner. Disorders of glucose metabolism such as in some patients with diabetes mellitus, may accumulate substantial amounts of glycogen in the liver and at first pass be confused with glycogen storage diseases. Intensive glucose therapy may also lead to substantial glycogen accumulation in the liver and if not factored in, may have a liver biopsy that is confused with glycogen storage disease.

Clinical Presentation and Prognosis

Demographics: As recessive disorders they are present in both genders with equal frequency and have no significant ethnic or geographic prevalence.

Presenting signs and symptoms: Glycogenoses usually present early in life with those causing hypoglycemia almost always presenting in the first year. Most patients present with hypoglycemic episodes not otherwise explained, usually, but not invariably accompanied by hepatomegaly. Hepatomegaly alone may be the presenting sign in those particular patients who have phosphorylase-activating defects or genetic deficiencies in phosphorylase itself. Less frequently, acidosis with elevated lactate may be the first clue found in the course of evaluation. In some instances of glycogen storage disease type 1B, neutropenia and a predisposition to infection may call attention to the diagnosis, leading to ascertainment of hepatomegaly, and finding abnormalities of blood sugars.

Clinical course: In the most severe form of glycogen storage disease, symptoms infrequently appear in the first months of life when feeding is very frequent and the hypoglycemia is not distinguishable from the normal infants' impulse to feed. As the child ages, the inability to stretch the period between feedings becomes more apparent and the hepatomegaly, which may have been present for awhile, is noted and the diagnosis may be made. A rigorous feeding regimen may mitigate the symptoms of hypoglycemia and the hepatomegaly would be the most common ongoing abnormality seen. Intercurrent illness and stress may precipitate a crisis which requires extraordinary intervention such as intravenous glucose maintenance. Over time, in glycogen storage disease Type IA, slow growth, renal enlargement, hypertension and liver adenomas may be a developing problem.

In Type IB, recurrent infections and GI problems may become particularly prevalent. Other forms of the condition may have more indirect and less traumatic manifestations. However, the hallmark of all is hepatomegaly and the risk, at least, for hypoglycemia. Exceptions to this rule would be glycogen storage disease, idiosyncratically labeled as Type 0 and Type IV or branching enzyme deficiency. With excellent care, quite long and normal lives, outside of the rigorous feeding schedule, may be anticipated. This contrasts with some doomsday scenarios found in the older literature.

Prognosis: With control of the blood glucose, growth, intellectual function and overall prognosis may be good. Severe and unsuccessfully treated episodes of hypoglycemia may cause brain damage. Complications of the disorder such as hypertension, the development of liver adenomas and gout may complicate long term care. Women with more severe forms of glycogen storage disease can undertake pregnancy, but may have periods of great instability of glucose homeostasis. In glycogen storage disease Type IB, control of infections and the GI problems which resemble inflammatory bowel disease can prove to be difficult and in some instances—even with modern therapy—may cause death. Patients with glycogen storage disease Type III may develop muscle weakness and cramping and cardiomyopathy, the latter in the 3rd decade of life or later. In the various phosphorylase deficiencies where activator deficiencies are the cause, patients may in fact improve with age, see reversion of liver size to normal, and not suffer from hypoglycemia.

Diagnosis

The diagnosis of disorders of glycogen metabolism is suspected from the physical examination, the presence of hypoglycemia and the X-rays, and is confirmed by enzymatic studies in liver, blood and fibroblasts, and patterns of metabolite excretion in the urine. The histolytic and urinary analytical procedures are carried out in multiple venues, but biochemical confirmation is carried out in a limited number of places in the U.S. and is best preceded by telephone consultation if ordered by physicians not experienced in caring for these disorders. In glycogen storage disease type IA, but increasingly in all cases, mutation analysis may replace liver biopsy and enzymology as the simpler, less invasive and preferred method of confirmation.

Management

Nutrition: The key to the care of these patients is maintenance of blood glucose in a normal range. With this, growth can be maintained, lactate acidemia controlled, plasma lipid levels kept down, and the need for allopurinol to control hyperuricemia diminished. Glucose control is most challenging in the type I forms with diminished glucose-1-phosphatase activity and sometimes in severe forms of type III or debrancher enzyme deficiency. Small, frequent feedings, the use of uncooked cornstarch (which slowly releases glucose in the GI tract), and in the first year of life especially, continuous overnight gastrostomy feeding with cornstarch and a soy-based formula, can prevent hypoglycemia. Needs will differ by the individual and by the form of glycogen storage disease. Patients with glycogen storage disease are advised to eat a moderate fat diet at most, and to avoid sucrose and fructose.

Surgery: The risk of hypoglycemia associated with fasting has been noted and must be addressed when surgery is planned. Intra-operative or post-operative blood glucose instability is a risk in these patients.

Pregnancy: Blood glucose instability is a risk during pregnancy, but with careful monitoring and the realization that hospitalization may be required, can be undertaken.

Social: There is an active support group for patients and families with glycogen storage diseases (http://www.agsdus.org). Patients are often short, have a cherubic face and may have a protuberant abdomen causing them to be shy and self-conscious. The abdomen becomes less obvious as the patients age and have good care and the problem tends to recede. Because some patients are in fragile glucose balance, an unhealthy and overly controlling relationship between parent and child may develop and inhibit the normal achievement of independence by the affected individual.

Consultations: Patients with glycogen storage diseases require management by a specialist team with a dietitian experienced in these disorders. Most often, this is a metabolic or endocrine clinic, but sometimes gastroenterologists care for these patients. Input from nephrologists, neurologists, psychiatrists and surgeons is sometimes needed.

Monitoring: Liver adenoma with a potential for malignant transformation occurs in a minority of patients with Type IA, and yearly ultrasounds beginning at age 6 and alternating with MRI exams after age 10–15 are indicated.

Miscellaneous precautions

Immunizations: Immunizations should be carried out in a routine fashion. There is no evidence that live vaccines are contraindicated in patients with type IB glycogen storage disease.

Likely complications: Complications may appear despite the most meticulous care. In type I, intercurrent illness may cause a rapid increase in glucose utilization and hypoglycemia. Nausea and vomiting requires intravenous glucose support and is a true medical emergency. The kidneys in this condition enlarge and hypertension occurs in a significant minority of affected patients, sometimes in the first decade. Patients with type III or IV (branching or debranching enzyme) are more prone to cirrhosis.

School/education: Unless the patient has had severe and late treated hypoglycemia causing brain damage, their intelligence is normal and school should present no special intellectual problems. Provision for school meals, snacks and corn starch ingestion during school hours needs to be made.

Reference

Fernandes, J., Saudubray, J-M., van den Berghe, G., Walter, J.H. (eds.) Inborn Metabolic Diseases (4th ed), Springer Verlag, Heidelberg, 2006.

B. Disorders of Pyruvate Metabolism
Pyruvate Dehydrogenase Deficiency, Pyruvate Carboxylase Deficiency, Pyruvate Decarboxylase Deficiency (PDH, PC, PDC)

Stephen Cederbaum

Etiology

The pyruvate dehydrogenase complex is a giant multimeric complex to which at least five genes contribute multiple subunits. It is the most common cause of elevated pyruvate and lactate and symptomatic disease seen in the clinic. Of the five enzymes involved, defects in E1α, encoded on the X-chromosome is by far more frequent. The others are inherited in an autosomal recessive manner. The third enzymatic subunit the dihydrolipoamide dehydrogenase is shared by two other complexes and mutations in it are found infrequently, but also affect metabolism of branch chain amino acids and glycine metabolism.

Clinical Presentation and Prognosis

Demographics: The most common form of this disorder, deficiency of the E1α subunit of the pyruvate dehydrogenase complex has no ethnic predilection which is quite typical for an X-linked gene. The most severe form of pyruvate carboxylase deficiency, a gene critical in gluconeogenesis and also presenting with lactate and pyruvate acidemia, has a higher prevalence in the aboriginal Canadian population.

Presenting signs and symptoms: The severe forms of this disorder may present in the newborn period with metabolic acidosis, seizures and neurologic problems. More mild forms of the condition may present later with varying symptoms that include intermittently exacerbating ataxia and developmental delay. Patients with intermittent ataxia, some athetosis and normal intelligence are known in cases of PDH deficiency.

Clinical course: The disease appears to be progressive in a majority of patients. They may succumb to increasing neurologic damage, the complications of skeletal deformity that results from inactivity, pneumonia, an intercurrent illness or exacerbation of the seizures. This deterioration may be extremely slow and indolent. However, a patient who presented in the first decade of life with intermittent bouts of ataxia lasting as long as six or eight weeks, continued to have these episodes, but was otherwise well and vigorous and was able to graduate college and was employed when last seen at age 28. Athetosis had progressed minimally, but he was otherwise asymptomatic between episodes.

Prognosis: These patients continue to confound their physicians. Some respond better than others to therapy and may continue to progress developmentally albeit slowly. These patients do, however, have severe debilitating episodes often triggered by intercurrent infection. In general, the more severe and earlier the presentation, the worse the prognosis.

Diagnosis

The physical examination is usually nonspecific but often includes athetosis, variable neurological abnormalities, developmental delay and in testing an elevated level of pyruvate and less frequently lactate and alanine. A distinguishing feature of PDH deficiency in particular is a normal lactate/pyruvate ratio. In PC deficiency, the ratio may be elevated, but seldom as high as in the disorders of the respiratory chain. The diagnosis may be confirmed enzymatically using lymphocytes, but cultured skin fibroblasts are more often used and are deemed more reliable because the assay can be repeated a number of times. A muscle specimen would be best of all, but there is generally no need for such an invasive procedure with no therapeutic gain.

Mutation analysis is readily available for the EIa subunit and is available with greater difficulty for the other genes. Please note that the availability of mutation screening for many disease genes is increasing apace and no anthology is likely to be up to date with this information. The most comprehensive survey of available tests is listed on GeneTests which can be accessed on the web (http://www.ncbi.nlm.nih.gov/sites/GeneTests/?db=GeneTests).

Management

Medications: The usual anticonvulstants are used to control seizures that may occur and are best managed by a neurologist. The biochemical abnormalities in pyruvate dehydrogenase deficiency are quite easily addressed with a high fat (ketogenic) diet with lactate and pyruvate levels often becoming normal. The clinical response may be dramatic, but can be quite limited. Indications from comparisons of younger siblings to their older brethren, suggests that on the whole the diet may make a difference in outcome and life span.

Therapy: Physical, occupational and speech therapy are appropriate in many patients.

Consultants: As indicated above, care of patients with these complex metabolic disorders "takes a village." Metabolic specialists, nutritionists, neurologists, intensivists and the educational assessment teams are all required.

Pearls and Precautions

Nutrition: This has been discussed above and consists of high fat natural foods, added fats, and medium chain triglycerides. This would be not too dissimilar to a ketogenic diet and sometimes have proportions of fat that are equivalent. Because of the metabolic block in these patients, they may be prone to the development of ketoacidosis and because of the metabolic block, do not rapidly get glucose into the mainstream of metabolism and so may respond much more slowly to correction of the acidosis.

Supportive care: A majority of these patients are neurologically and intellectually handicapped and the usual interventions, appropriate to the disability, should be used.

Reference

Fernandes, J., Saudubray, J-M., van den Berghe, G., Walter, J.H. (eds.) Inborn Metabolic Diseases (4th ed), Springer Verlag, Heidelberg, 2006.

C. Disorders of the Mitochondrial Respiratory Chain (MELAS, MERRF, Leigh disease)

Stephen Cederbaum

Etiology

The mitochondrial respiratory chain consists of at least 100 separate proteins encoded in at least as many genes and an equal number or more that are responsible for their proper assembly and function. It has the unique characteristic of having some of the subunits encoded in non-nuclear DNA located in the mito-chondrion, the so called mtDNA. Inheritance of these conditions has been described as autosomal dominant, autosomal recessive, sex-linked recessive and mitochondrial, a unique pattern of inheritance in which the disorder is passed down from the mother to offspring of either sex, but cannot be passed on by a male since only maternal mitochondrial DNA survives in the fertilized embryo. In the case of mitochondrial inheri-tance, there may be two different species of mtDNA, the normal one and the mutated one. This is referred to as heteroplasmy. Moreover, the proportion of mutated DNA may vary from organ to organ in a single individual and from sibling to sibling and thus lead to bewildering variation in clinical presentation. Finally, since mitochondrial respiratory chain activity diminishes in efficiency as an individual ages, the disease tends to worsen as the patient gets older and in a number of instances, no symptoms occur until the third or fourth decade of life, or later. Even in the disorders inherited in the mendelian fashion, there may be organ to organ variability for reasons that are not known, but may simply be due to the complement of other genes present in the individual.

Clinical Presentation and Prognosis

Demographics: With the genetic variety of this family of conditions, it is not surprising that some of the recessively inherited disorders are going to be found selectively in population isolates. Because of its rapid mutation rate, disorders due to mutations in the mitochondrial genome mutations are far more frequent than would ordinarily be inferred from its size of far less than one percent of that in the nuclear genome. It is estimated that the frequency of mitochondrial disorders due to mutations in the mitochondrial genome constitute fewer than five percent than those patients presenting in infancy and childhood, but may represent 20% or more of those presenting in later life. Thus, a normal result from one or another of the readily available mitochondrial mutation panels hardly rules out a disorder in this system in children, especially.

Presenting signs and symptoms: As one might expect of a function required in virtually all cells in the body, respiratory chain disorders are usually multisystem, although the time of onset in different organs may differ one from the other. The organs most frequently involved include the brain, skeletal muscle, heart, the liver, the kidney, endocrine organs, manifested more frequently by diabetes mellitus, and the sense organs including vision and hearing. Peripheral neuropathy and MRI abnormalities often occur. Included in the latter, are atypical basal ganglion lesions recognized by most neuroradiologists.

The most severe deficiencies may present at birth with evidence that damage began *in utero*. Unlike disorders of amino and organic acids in which the maternal circulation and organ function may cleanse the fetus of abnormal metabolites, the mother cannot compensate for poor ATP production in the fetus. Many other patients have a delayed onset varying to months or years of life, some with acute presentations and others with more indolent ones. Acute intercurrent illness and the attendant stress can precipitate episodes of decompensation.

Clinical course: The clinical course is almost always slowly progressive, although the rate may vary from individual to individual. The most severe early onset cases may progress to death in hours, days or weeks. Later onset cases might have a progressive course of 20–30 years or more. With time, more organ systems and more severe symptoms in these systems become apparent. The usual outcome is death, neurologic damage, cardiorespiratory failure, or less frequently, failure of another organ. Although the conditions are almost always multisystem, the onset of symptoms in different organs is unpredictable having cases when a single organ is severely affected and amenable to transplantation. This variability must be taken into account when such decisions are made.

Prognosis: The end point for most patients, eventually, is death. In some, the rate of progression is so slow that a normal life span with reasonably normal functionality can occur.

Diagnosis

Mitochondrial disorders have been described at one and the same time as the most under diagnosed and the most over diagnosed of all the metabolic diseases. This dismal state of affairs has been due to the relative nonspecificity of the symptoms and the very limited and invasive nature of the tests required to make the diagnosis. Because of this complexity, a number of schemes to increase diagnostic accuracy have been developed, most commonly that of Walker for adults and of Thoburn specifically tailored to children. The most important criteria for making a diagnosis include: Persistently elevated plasma lactate levels, elevation of lactate in the cerebral spinal fluid, elevation of lactate in the brain detected by magnetic resonance spectroscopy, the multisystem nature of the disorder with emphasis on visual and hearing deficits, muscle biopsy, analyzed histologically and biochemically and MRI. Family history is often helpful and can be critical. More recently, DNA technology has been brought to bear, and as these methods become increasingly less expensive and more widely available, the range of diagnostic methods will expand. It is a field that is currently deficient in the ease of making a definitive diagnosis and fortunately in a state of flux. At the present time, diagnosis should be made by a metabolic specialist and should be viewed with a critical eye by the primary pediatrician.

Management

This is perhaps the most controversial area in mitochondrial disorders. With the exception of replacement of coenzyme Q10 in a small minority of patients who have a defect in the biosynthesis of this critical electron transport chain component, no therapy can be considered to be proven or indeed even considered to be probably effective. Despite this, a large proportion—and perhaps even a majority of individuals who work in this field—use a variable cocktail of vitamins empirically, beginning with coenzyme Q10, and having other components such as carnitine, riboflavin specifically, other B vitamins, creatine and other types of antioxidants. The levels of reactive oxygen species may be somewhat diminished by these interventions, but their efficacy in clinical practice, and especially in a double masked trials have not been demonstrated. Other therapies are symptomatic and not specific to this family of disorders. Intercurrent illness can be dangerous for patients with mitochondrial disorders and they should be monitored carefully at these times and hospital admission for more vigorous symptomatic support considered.

Social support: There is a strong network of support groups for this family of disorders headed by the United Mitochondrial Disease Foundation (UMDF http://www.umdf.org).

Miscellaneous Precautions

Nutrition: A good balanced diet is recommended for patients with these disorders. Some practitioners in the field believe that a diet higher in fats may be more effective than a normal one, but the theoretical basis for this approach is poor and has not been formally tested in a randomized study.

Exercise: Exercise has been shown in at least one carefully controlled trial to increase endurance and functional capacity, but whether this is due to anything other than a training phenomenon is not known.

Other: All other treatments for these conditions are symptomatic and don't require specification at this time.

Reference

Fernandes, J., Saudubray, J-M., van den Berghe, G., Walter, J.H. (eds.) Inborn Metabolic Diseases (4th ed), Springer Verlag, Heidelberg, 2006.

D. Disorders of Fatty Acids Oxidation and Carnitine Metabolism (FAOD)

Stephen Cederbaum

Etiology

The disorders of fatty acid oxidation are comprised of defects in at least 20 of the 31 genes known to encode proteins involved in fatty acid oxidation. These functions include the uptake of fatty acids into the cell, the formation of the fatty acid CoA preparatory to its conversion to the carnitine ester for transport into the mitochondrion, and then the various steps of oxidation within the mitochondria to form the acetyl CoA products and the reducing equivalents that are converted to ATP. They are all inherited in an autosomal recessive manner.

Clinical Presentation and Prognosis

Demographics: With so many disorders involved, some are seen with increased frequencies in different genetic isolates.

Presenting signs and symptoms: Depending on the nature and severity of the disorder, the condition may present with cardio-respiratory collapse or liver failure in the newborn period. Acute symptoms in an otherwise healthy patient—particularly during intercurrent illness with fasting—could present with sudden death, or more frequently with indolent symptoms of lethargy, muscle stiffness, or rhabdomyolysis with exercise. A number of these disorders present at birth with the mother showing signs of acute fatty liver of pregnancy or the HELLP syndrome.

Clinical course: This is highly variable. A number of the disorders, even with complete loss of enzymatic activity, may never be symptomatic and only now are these patients being picked up with expanded newborn screening using tandem mass spectrometry. Whether or not some are entirely benign or represent predisposing conditions in which illness is triggered by other genetic or intercurrent causes is a matter of debate. Other patients present with recurrent episodes of cardiac or liver failure and some may have chronic cardiac problems and biochemical abnormalities in the blood. Many are treatable, the underlying principle being either to replace carnitine in those who are carnitine deficient or limit fat intake and fasting requiring fatty acid oxidation in others. Many of the conditions are compatible with long survival, some asymptomatic, some with subacute symptoms and others with intermittent difficulties.

Prognosis: The prognosis is dependent on the nature of the defect, the severity of the defect, the effectiveness of treatment and other unknown genetic and/or environmental modifiers. The patients should be handled and treated by specialists in the field of metabolic disorders, although the majority of their care can be carried out locally. In the worst case scenario, the patients are quite fragile and the smallest intercurrent event can tip them into acute decompensation and even death.

Diagnosis

These patients are usually physically normal unless they are in congestive heart or liver failure. The majority of these patients are now ascertained with expanded newborn screening using tandem mass spectrometry. Abnormalities in the acylcarnitine metabolite profile lead to follow-up studies of either DNA or enzymatic activity in lymphocytes and fibroblasts with the application then of appropriate therapeutic modalities. These procedures are carried out in specialized laboratories and are best ordered by or with the advice of a metabolic specialist. Examination of the acylcarnitine profile and urinary organic acids may be sufficient for an unambiguous diagnosis in many instances. The non-fasting analytical profiles may be normal in patients in whom the prognosis may be guarded and cannot be used as an unambiguous prognostic indicator.

Management

Medications: Patients with systemic carnitine deficiency due to a transporter defect require quite high doses of carnitine to maintain blood and tissue levels in the normal or near normal range. Patients with defects in the carnitine transporter system which is required for the ingress of long chain fatty acids into the mitochondrion, or defects in these enzymes themselves, are often treated with supplementation of medium chain triglycerides. There is some experimental work using benzfibrates in patients with longer chain defects that are partial and who may do better with the augmentation of the general fatty acid oxidation machinery brought about by this FDA-approved drug. Symptomatic therapy for cardiac failure and arrhythmias is often necessary as well.

Surgery: If the patient is to be fasted for any prolonged period of time, admission to the hospital and maintenance of intravenous glucose is mandatory. Resumption of feeding with the appropriate diet as soon as possible after surgery is recommended.

Social support: There is a fatty acid oxidation disorders patient support group which can be found on the web (http://www.fodsupport.org). Many families find this an important source of information and social support.

Consultants: These disorders are best managed in a metabolic center with a team consisting of a dietician, nurse and social worker. Consultation with cardiologists, gastroenterologists and neurologists is often necessary.

Pearls and Precautions

Nutrition: As noted previously, a diet relatively low in long chain fats and higher in carbohydrates, and the avoidance of fasting, particularly in times of intercurrent illness is critical to the care of these disorders. For some of the longer chain defects, augmentation of the diet with medium chain triglycerides bypasses the site of the block and provides a ready source of acetoacetate and β-hydroxybutyrate for immediate energy needs. This energy cannot be stored. In some instances of long chain disorders in which accumulation of the elevated levels of long-chain carnitine esters in the circulation cannot be completely suppressed, the use of uncooked cornstarch at bedtime as in the case of the glycogen storage disorders is an important element in care.

Sleep: Although long periods of fasting is contraindicated in these patients, it is generally unnecessary to interrupt sleep for a feeding when they are not otherwise ill with an infection except in the most severe instances.

Likely complications: In some of the long chain fatty acid oxidation disorders, optic nerve degeneration may occur. The cause of this is unknown and no specific therapy can be recommended. Patients are vulnerable during intercurrent infections and should be particularly vigilant during these times, making sure that there is adequate fluid and caloric intake. Prolonged vomiting may be reason for intravenous fluid support until a normal eating pattern has been re-established. Many specialists have found home glucose monitoring to be counter-productive since normal readings may lull families into a false sense of security in the face of impending disaster.

Reference

Fernandes, J., Saudubray, J-M., van den Berghe, G., Walter, J.H. (eds.) Inborn Metabolic Diseases (4th ed), Springer Verlag, Heidelberg, 2006.

Disorders of Folate and Neurotransmitter Metabolism

(includes disorders of pyridoxine metabolism, folate transport, tetrahydrobiopterin (BH4) synthesis and neurotransmitter synthesis, Segawa disease)

Stephen Cederbaum

Etiology

All members of this larger and somewhat disparate group of disorders are inherited in an autosomal recessive manner.

Clinical Presentation and Prognosis

Demographics: As is the case with all autosomal recessive disorders, isolated populations or those originating from a small founder population will have a higher incidence of some of these disorders. Among these disorders, there is no ethnic or geographic group that has a notably higher incidence of these unrelated conditions.

Presenting signs and symptoms: In their most severe form, these disorders all present with severe seizures in the neonatal period that may respond to the particular metabolite that is in genetically short supply. All can present more indolently with neurological symptoms and later onset seizures. The biopterin deficiencies may present with symptoms and signs of autonomic dysfunction such as temperature and blood pressure instability, oculogyric crises and changes in muscle tone. Disorders of biopterin metabolism often present with elevations in blood phenylalanine and can be confused with phenylketonuria, and is often referred to as "malignant hyperphenylalaninemia." Deficiencies of L-Dopa may present later in childhood with neurologic symptoms that increase in intensity as the day wears on.

Clinical course: These conditions share a remarkable responsiveness to therapy, but without intervention can be fatal or neurologically devastating. Thus, making the diagnosis is very important and as a result, is one instance when too much testing is preferable to too little.

Prognosis: Without treatment these disorders can be devastating, debilitating to the patient and the family and ultimately fatal. With appropriate therapeutic intervention, as described below, life can in many instances proceed relatively normally. Every specialist has witnessed what can only be called therapeutic miracles.

Diagnosis

Disorders of pyridoxine and pyridoxal phosphate-dependent seizures must be suspected and then the compounds administered empirically while the EEG is monitored. Pyridoxine is readily available for administration, but pyridoxal phosphate is not and cases of this new disorder may be overlooked because of this. Diagnosis can be confirmed with DNA studies demonstrating mutations in the genes known to cause these disorders.

The other disorders can be suspected from the clinical presentation, but are confirmed through study of neurotransmitter metabolites in the cerebrospinal fluid, which are done in one or two specialized laboratories in the U.S. and several overseas in Europe and Japan. Laboratories that do these specialized procedures can be found on a website sponsored by the National Library of Medicine named GeneTests, which has as one of its functions maintaining a list of all laboratories who inform them of the tests that they do (http://www.ncbi. nlm.nih.gov/sites/GeneTests/?db=GeneTests). Increasingly, neurologists are performing lumbar punctures in children with unknown disorders and are routinely measuring these metabolites as part of the evaluation. In any event, no elective lumbar puncture in a child without a neurological diagnosis should be done without performing these specialized studies. Folate levels are measured at the same time. Here too final confirmation is obtained from enzyme or mutation studies that can be done using peripheral blood samples.

Management

This has been hinted at previously and has been spelled out in the case of the pyridoxine disorders. In the case of BH4 deficiency, the basic treatment is replacement of the neurotransmitters, Dopamine and serotonin. This is accomplished by giving sinemet®, a commercially available product for the treatment of Parkinson disease that contains L-Dopa and an inhibitor of the enzyme that breaks it down and 5-OH-tryptophan which is converted to serotonin. OH-tryptophan is obtained from compounding pharmacies at relatively modest cost. BH4 is quite expensive, but is very useful in some BH4 biosynthetic deficiencies; less so in others, but is always useful when these deficiencies result in hyperphenylalaninemia. High dose folinic acid is useful in mitigating CSF folate deficiency which we now know is usually caused by a genetic deficiency of the appropriate folate transporter. Adequacy of treatment is assessed through periodic lumbar punctures and the response to therapy.

Nutrition: With the exception of those disorders accompanied by hyperphenylalaninemia, these patients can enjoy a normal diet to the limit of their ability to eat.

Surgery: This is always a risk in patients with autonomic instability and surgery, even for routine matters, is best carried out in a tertiary care center with pediatric trained anesthesiologists.

Social: A parent support group exists for persons afflicted with BH4 deficiency and can be found at http://www.bh4.org/BH4_deficiency_ParentSupport_Montgomery.asp. Other support groups will likely be formed as some of these other disorders become better known and their existence may be found through the National Organization for Rare Disorders (NORD) (http://www.rarediseases,org).

Consultations: These are complex disorders to manage and while most metabolic specialists will feel comfortable leading the team effort, some pediatric neurologists may feel comfortable as well. In any event, both specialties should be members of a team that may include physical therapists, dieticians, social workers and orthopedists.

Monitoring: It is critical that these patients be followed closely. A lapse in pharmacologic care can result in recurrence of symptoms or the occurrence of new ones developing in response to the diminution or withdrawal of pharmacologic support.

Other precautions:

Immunizations: These should be carried out according to the normal schedule. Immunization reactions are deemed far less serious than the occurrence of the diseases themselves. Seasonal flu vaccines are recommended as well.

School and Education: Schooling and the educational program should be tailored the individual needs of the students and cannot be specified.

Reference

Fernandes, J., Saudubray, J-M., van den Berghe, G., Walter, J.H. (eds.) Inborn Metabolic Diseases (4th ed), Springer Verlag, Heidelberg, 2006.

Disorders of Peroxisomal Metabolism

(includes Adrenoleukodystrophy, adrenomyeloneuropathy and Zellweger Syndrome)

Stephen Cederbaum

Disorders that involve a sub-cellular organelle that carries out specialized metabolic functions.

Etiology

This family of disorders is due to mutations in one of the many genes that make up the structure of a small sub-cellular organelle called the peroxisome. The best known and most frequently encountered disorder in the group, adrenoleukodystrophy, is inherited in an X-linked manner with a substantial minority of female carriers showing some clinical manifestation during their lifetimes. The remaining members of this family of disorders are inherited in an autosomal recessive manner. As with all recessive disorders, inbred groups and population isolates may have an increased frequency of these conditions.

Clinical Presentation and Prognosis

Presenting signs and symptoms: Adrenoleukodystrophy (ALD) generally appears in males at about age 7 to 8 years and begins with a subtle loss of neurological and cognitive function that may progress rapidly to a vegetative state and then to death. Another significant fraction of affected males escape this rapid onset and rapacious fate and present in their teens or later with a disorder of the spinal cord termed adrenomyeloneuropathy which may be indolent in onset and manifest primarily with problems with gait and balance and with abnormal lower extremity deep tendon reflexes. These two differing forms may present in the same family with the same mutation illustrating the involvement of other genetic or environmental causes for the disparity. Variations and mixed pictures occur as well.

The recessive forms often present in the newborn period with hypotonia, eye and visual abnormalities, hepatic enlargement with cystic changes, MRI abnormalities and dysmorphic facies given the eponym, "Zellweger facies" after the physician who first described this appearance. Epiphyseal stippling is common. Later onset forms present with ataxia, nystagmus, visual impairment, and increasing deafness.

Prognosis: The prognosis of juvenile onset adrenoleukodystrophy is grim and the progression is rapid, often running its course in a year or two. On the other hand, the adrenomyeloneuropathy may have a far more indolent course and be compatible with excellent functional health for many years. Complications may include some cognitive decline, gait difficulties and problems with bowel and bladder control. Prognosis in the early onset forms of the other peroxisomal disorders is grim and those that present later are slowly progressive.

Diagnosis

A major function of the peroxisome is to metabolize very long chain fatty acids and virtually all common forms of these disorders are amenable to screening by looking for elevated levels of these fatty acids in the blood. Abnormalities in plasmalogens, fatty acid ethers found in red cell membranes particularly may be abnormal in some. Phytanic acid found in green leafy vegetables accumulates in a single gene disorder as well as the more general membrane assembly disorders and is bundled together with very long chain fatty acid analysis for clinical biochemical analysis at a modest cost. All known genes are cloned and diagnosis can be confirmed by these means, although the same autosomal recessive syndromes can be caused by mutations in more than 10 genes, making mutation analysis outside of the research setting prohibitive.

Management

Specific therapeutic recommendations are available only for adrenoleukodystrophies. As the name implies, adrenal insufficiency is quite characteristic and when treated appropriately can make an important functional difference in affected patients. It may precede the onset of neurological symptoms and therefore should be investigated in family members at risk who are well neurologically. Conversely, patients with isolated adrenal insufficiency should have a very long chain fatty acid study done.

Medications: The major "buzz" in adrenoleukodystrophy is Lorenzo's oil, a combination of long chain fatty acids, used under experimental protocol, that appears to delay the onset of symptoms in boys who are gene carriers, but who are well. In combination with a lower fat diet, it will lower the 26 carbon chain length fatty acids to normal or near normal. Less clear is the effect on the onset of symptoms in those destined to develop adrenomyeloneuroapthy. This too is being addressed experimentally. Mustard seed oil is similar in composition to Lorenzo's oil and there is an underground among families ineligible for the trials of Lorenzo's oil to use mustard seed in an analogous manner. It carries a similar risk of platelet depression, but its use does not contravene any FDA guideline.

Surgery: Bone marrow transplantation at the very outset of symptoms of ALD has been shown to be effective in preventing progression to full blown disease in the majority of instances. Accordingly, males known to be at risk by virtue of being gene carriers should be followed semiannually with MRI studies of the brain, adrenal hormone studies and psychometric batteries to detect the earliest signs of the inflammatory presentation of the disease so that bone marrow transplantation can be planned as soon as possible. Since at least half of the carriers do not develop the juvenile inflammatory manifestations, marrow transplantation is too dangerous to carry out preventively.

Consultations: Care is best managed by a metabolic specialist familiar with the condition, but consultation with endocrinologists, neurologists, neuroradiologists, physical therapists and psychologists is required.

Social: The United Leukodystrophy Foundation is a very active support and advocacy group. They can be found at http://www.ulf.org.

Miscellaneous precautions

Immunizations: There is no reason to limit normal immunizations in these children.

Diet: The diet should be a normal one except in those patients being treated with Lorenzo's oil. A diet lower in fat can do no harm.

Advanced disease: Those patients with advanced disease present a myriad of management problems that require symptomatic intervention. No special techniques are available.

School/education: Schooling and participation in physical education should be appropriate to the level of functioning of the individual. Patients with adrenomyeloneuropathy are generally free of brain disease and are intellectually normal. Visual, hearing and physical aids may be required.

Reference

Fernandes, J., Saudubray, J-M., van den Berghe, G., Walter, J.H. (eds.) Inborn Metabolic Diseases (4th ed), Springer Verlag, Heidelberg, 2006.

Down Syndrome (Trisomy 21 Syndrome)

Derek Wong

Etiology

Down syndrome is a recognizable condition caused by an additional chromosome 21, which results in a 50% increase in the expression of approximately 300–400 genes. This genetic excess results in increased rates of malformations, developmental and growth delays, and increased susceptibility to a variety of medical problems.

Approximately 94% of Down syndrome patients have classic trisomy 21, 2% have mosaic trisomy 21, and 3% have a translocation. Mosaic patients have a variable phenotype that may be less severe than classic patients. Translocation patients are usually indistinguishable from classic patients, but this diagnosis is very important for recurrence risks.

Clinical Presentation and Prognosis

Demographics: Down syndrome had an overall incidence at birth of approximately 1 in 660 in the era prior to prenatal screening, but is undoubtedly less frequent today. The extra chromosome may arise from meotic nondisjunction in either parent, but in practice the largest majority are maternal in origin. The incidence of live born Down syndrome babies is closely tied to maternal age, with risks rising from less than 1 in 1000 at age <30, to 1 in 200 at age 37, and 1 in 30 by age 45. A mother who has had one classic trisomy 21 child has a slightly increased risk of recurrence. Recurrence risks in other cases depend on parental karyotypes, and can range from the maternal age-related risk to 100%.

Presenting signs and symptoms: In most patients with Down syndrome the diagnosis is obvious at birth with characteristic facies, including upslanting palpebral fissures, epicanthal folds, protruding tongue, and an excess of skin folds in the neck. Single transverse palmar creases are present in less than half of patients with Down syndrome, and are a common finding in normal patients. Other frequent signs in the neonate that may be helpful include hypotonia with poor Moro, hyperflexibility of joints, a wide gap between the first and second toes, and clinodactyly due to shortened or absent middle phalanges of the 5th fingers.

Gastrointestinal obstruction is a more frequent occurrence in Down syndrome. Cardiac anomalies may cause feeding difficulties, tachypnea, and cyanosis. Other common features include spinal anomalies, seizures, and congenital cataract. Although anomalies such as diaphragmatic hernias and tracheoesophageal fistulae are uncommon in Down syndrome patients, their incidence is much higher than in the general population.

Clinical course: The course of Down syndrome is quite variable, and depends upon the exact malformations. Down syndrome patients experience reduced linear and head growth compared with normal children. Infant feeding difficulties due to hypotonia are common, and are exacerbated by underlying cardiac disease. Respiratory infections cause an increased incidence of otitis media and sinusitis.

All Down syndrome children have some degree of developmental delay; however, the degree of mental retardation varies from mild to severe. Although most Down syndrome children have good social skills, their IQ declines with age. They require physical and occupational therapy as well as special education.

Prognosis: The average life span of a Down syndrome patient is 50 years, but varies greatly between individuals. Cardiac malformations and leukemia are more serious prognostic factors that may shorten the lifespan of Down syndrome patients. Most Down syndrome adults require some sort of assisted living. A few can hold jobs, but may require a full-time care facility. The incidence of precocious dementia, including Alzheimer disease, is markedly increased in adults.

Diagnosis

Although Down syndrome may be suspected on the basis of the clinical exam, a standard karyotype is the "gold standard" for the diagnosis. If a more rapid diagnosis is critical, a FISH study for trisomy 21 is available. If the karyotype is normal but the diagnosis is still suspected, referral to a geneticist for evaluation is indicated because some complex translocations involving small pieces of chromosome 21 may require comparative genomic hybridization (CGH) or similar tests to make the diagnosis.

Management

Growth: Growth charts for Down syndrome are widely available from the American Academy of Pediatrics and the National Down Syndrome Society. Down syndrome patients are shorter than their normal counterparts, and are at risk for obesity. Growth may be maximized by optimal management of concomitant cardiac, endocrine, gastrointestinal, and other disorders. Growth hormone is rarely used unless a true deficiency is present.

Thyroid disease: Hypothyroidism is common, and T4 and TSH should be obtained at birth, 6 months, 1 year, and annually thereafter. Thyroxine supplementation is similar to that used in other children, although some practitioners supplement patients with mildly elevated TSH and normal T4 because of potentially improved development. In older children, hyperthyroidism may occur.

Cardiac Disease: All patients should receive an echocardiogram after birth due to the increased risk of congenital heart disease. Endocardial cushion defects, ventricular septal defects, patent ductus arteriosus, and atrial septal defects are common. Medical and surgical management is similar to other children with these disorders. Older children need to be monitored for the development of mitral valve prolapse and valvular regurgitation.

Gastrointestinal disease: Gastrointestinal malformations, including duodenal atresia (double bubble sign on X-ray) and imperforate anus are common malformations. Hirschsprung disease and gastroesophageal reflux are also more frequent in Down syndrome children. There is an increased risk of celiac disease, and asymptomatic children should be screened with tissue transglutaminase (TTG) antibodies after the age of 3 years. Antibody positive patients should be referred to a gastroenterologist for endoscopic confirmation of the diagnosis.

Otolaryngologic disease: Middle ear effusion and hearing loss are common, and Down syndrome children should receive formal hearing screens at birth and at 1 year. Further testing and/or otolaryngologic referral should be done if the parents express concerns about hearing or if the tympanic membrane cannot be visualized.

Ophthalmologic disease: Cataracts should be screened at birth. Strabismus and nystagmus are common and warrant ophthalmologic referral.

Orthopedic: Flexion and extension X-rays for atlantoaxial instability continue to be recommended for Down syndrome children prior to sports participation. However, their clinical value is the subject of intense debate. Patients with signs of spinal cord impingement such as gait problems or loss of bowel/bladder control should be immediately referred to an orthopedist. High risk activities should be avoided in patients with radiographic or clinical evidence of instability.

Hematologic: Leukemoid reactions and polycythemia are common in the newborn period, and are detected with a complete blood count (CBC). Down syndrome children have an increased risk of leukemia, but periodic CBC testing is not indicated.

Consultations: The care of these patients may require multiple subspecialty consults. Often a genetics consultant may help with confirming the diagnosis and planning of future pregnancies, while a cardiology consultant at birth is necessary to look for congenital heart disease. All other consultants such as child development, endocrinology, gastroenterology, neurology, orthopedics, and otolaryngology depend on the patient's clinical presentation and needs at different stages of growth. Routine dental evaluations are essential to prevent periodontal disease and orthodontic issues are universally seen. However, cooperation and tolerance of corrective bracing may not be always possible.

Therapy: Most Down syndrome children benefit from physical therapy for both gross and fine motor development and speech therapy to help with language delay. A hearing test should precede speech therapy. Physical therapy can be implemented as early as 2–3 months of age while speech therapy should be implemented no later than one year of age.

Psychological: Depression, anxiety and disruptive behaviors have been frequently reported in children with Down syndrome and require prompt attention by a mental health care worker. Additionally, treatment and care of a child with Down syndrome is often burdensome and causes significant stress on the parents and the siblings of these children. Individual and family therapy to screen for depression and anxiety along with ongoing treatment of the distressed family members is essential to the care of these children.

Social: Parents of these children may qualify for social security supplemental income benefit. Explore other medical and income benefits that may be available to these children and their families in your community and state.

Parents can find internet support at:
National Down Syndrome Society
NDSS 666 Broadway, 8th floor, New York, New York 10012.
1-800-221-4602.
http://www.ndss.org

Monitoring: In addition to what is mentioned above, anticipate and monitor for the following: Duodenal atresia, constipation—that may indicate hypothryroidism or Hirschsprung disease—leukemoid reactions and polycythemia in the neonatal period, snoring and sleep apnea, and poor growth indicating neglect, poor nutrition or medical problems. As these patients enter puberty, as with all teenagers, sexual health, and fertility need to be discussed with the patients and their families to prevent sexual abuse, disease, or unwanted pregnancies.

Pearls and Precautions

Immunization: Down syndrome patients have more severe RSV infection than other patients, and RSV prophylaxis is especially important in those patients with additional risk factors such as prematurity and congenital heart disease. Down syndrome patients have reduced immunity that increases their risk of infection. It is especially important that they receive the recommended immunizations on time. When available, they should also receive an annual influenza vaccine.

Nutrition/diet: Those who are not affected by celiac disease do not need to follow any special diets. Herbal and vitamin supplements are widely advertised for Down syndrome patients, but have not been proven beneficial.

Sleep: Sleep apnea occurs frequently in older children and adults. Proper sleep study and possible use of night-time CPAP may be indicated.

School/education: These children need to receive socially integrated special education that is tailored to their cognitive potential and socialization skills. Those who have severe physical limitations may need to receive home schooling.

References

American Academy of Pediatrics. Committee on Genetics. American Academy of Pediatrics: Health supervision for children with Down syndrome. Pediatrics. 2001 Feb;107(2):442–9.

Davidson MA. Primary care for children and adolescents with Down syndrome. Pediatr Clin North Am. 2008 Oct;55(5):1099–111, xi. Review

22Q11.2 Deletion Syndrome

(DiGeorge Syndrome, Velocardiofacial Syndrome)

Derek Wong

Etiology

22q11.2 deletion syndrome is a condition that is caused by a large deletion in the long arm of chromosome 22, resulting in haploinsufficiency for a large segment of DNA. The deletion, combined with the patient's genetic background and environmental influences, causes a wide variety of malformations.

Clinical Presentation and Prognosis

Demographics: 22q11.2 deletion syndrome is thought to occur in at minimum 1 in 4000 births, making it the most common contiguous gene deletion syndrome. The syndrome is present in a substantial minority of patients with cleft lip and/or palate and a larger proportion of patients with conotruncal heart lesions.

Presenting signs and symptoms: Many infants with 22q11.2 deletions have aberrant development of the 3rd and 4th pharyngeal pouches, also known as "DiGeorge sequence." Patients may have absent thymus and parathyroid glands, and present with immunodeficiency and hypocalcemia as well as a wide variety of congenital heart disease including VSD, ASD, and Tetralogy of Fallot.

Older children may present with "Velocardiofacial" features such as cleft palate with or without cleft lip, hypernasal speech, congenital heart disease, short stature, and developmental delay. Characteristic facies include a long face, hooded eyebrows and tubular nose.

It has been increasingly recognized that some patients with 22q11.2 deletions present with isolated congenital heart disease or cleft palate. Behavior problems and schizophrenia may also be presenting symptoms.

Clinical course and prognosis: Because 22q11.2 deletion syndrome has such a wide range of presentations, the clinical course is remarkably variable. In the first few years, the severity of the congenital heart disease and immunodeficiency are the most important factors in the clinical course. In addition, infant feeding problems with vomiting are common.

During childhood, issues such as hearing loss and speech problems become more important. Developmental delay and learning disabilities are extremely common and may be exacerbated by attention deficit disorder. Psychiatric issues become more important as the patient approaches adulthood.

The average life span of a 22q11.2 deletion syndrome patient is unknown. However, there are many adults with the condition, and at least a few reports of several 60–70 year old patients.

Diagnosis

Although 22q11.2 deletion syndrome may be suspected on the basis of the clinical exam, a FISH test or an array comparative genome hybridization (αCGH) for the chromosomal deletion is essential for the diagnosis. Most patients with velocardiofacial features have the deletion, but some patients with DiGeorge sequence have a chromosome 10p13 deletion or an environmental cause such as prenatal alcohol exposure.

Management

Growth: Growth charts for 22q11.2 deletion syndrome were not widely available as of 2008. However, they have been published in "Velo-Cardio-Facial Syndrome, Volume 1" by Shprintzen and Golding-Kushner. Some studies suggest that approximately half of 22q11.2 deletion syndrome patients have short stature during childhood. The majority of these patients have constitutional delay and will have normal adult heights.

Endocrine disease: Hypocalcemia due to hypoparathyroidism may present at any age. Calcium levels should be checked annually in asymptomatic patients and if patients have symptoms such as seizures. Hypothyroidism is increased in this condition, and thyroid levels should be checked in symptomatic patients.

Cardiac disease: The treatment of congenital heart disease is the same as in other patients. All patients with a 22q11.2 deletion should have a cardiac evaluation including echocardiography regardless of symptoms. Patients have an increased incidence of carotid anomalies and vascular rings.

Immunologic disease: Although the classic descriptions of this syndrome include thymic aplasia and severe immunodeficiency, most patients with immune system involvement have mild deficiency resulting in frequent respiratory infections. Work up in symptomatic patients includes chest X-ray in infants, CBC, quantitative immunoglobulins with subtypes, and functional tests that are usually ordered in conjunction with an immunologist.

Otolaryngologic disease: Chronic otitis media with hearing loss is common and requires aggressive treatment. Patients may have standard cleft palate, submucous cleft palate, or occult submucous cleft palate. Submucous cleft palate may be suspected in a patient with bifid uvula, and is confirmed by palpation of the palate. Otolaryngologic examination for occult submucous cleft palate is indicated in patients with hypernasal speech. Endoscopic evaluation for nasopharyngeal hypotonia may be necessary for feeding or swallowing difficulty.

Consultations: The care of these patients often requires multiple subspecialty consults. A genetics consult may help with confirming the diagnosis, family testing, and prenatal counseling. Cardiology, ophthalmology, and otolaryngology consults are necessary for initial assessment. All other consults such as immunology, endocrinology, gastroenterology, neurology, and psychiatry depend on the patient's clinical presentation and needs at different stages of growth. Routine dental consults are essential to prevent periodontal disease in these patients and orthodontic issues are often seen in these children.

Therapy: Speech therapy is often necessary for patients, and occupational therapy may benefit infants with feeding problems.

Psychiatric: Attention deficit disorder is the most common behavioral abnormality in these children. Older patients may suffer from a wide range of psychiatric illness including obsessive compulsive disorder, bipolar disease, and schizophrenia. Treatment is similar to other patients with these conditions, although it is possible that more targeted therapies will emerge in the near future as the pathophysiologic basis of this condition is elucidated.

Social: Parents of these children may qualify for social security supplemental income benefit. Explore other medical and income benefits that may be available to these children and their families in your community and state.

> Parents can find internet support at:
> Velo-Cardio-Facial Syndrome Educational Foundation, Inc.
> P.O. Box 874
> Milltown, NJ 08850
> (214) 360-4740 (U.S./Canada) (732) 238-8803 (International)
> http://www.vcfsef.org

Monitoring: In addition to what is mentioned above, anticipate and monitor for the following: respiratory and/or feeding problems due to vascular rings; seizures due to hypocalcemia or strokes; renal anomalies, and ophthalmologic malformations. A renal ultrasound and ophthalmologic examination should be done after diagnosis.

There are a myriad of other malformations that may occur in this syndrome, including microcephaly, ear anomalies, brain malformations, malrotation, anal atresia, and vertebral anomalies.

Pearls and Precautions

Immunization: Patients with 22q11.2 syndrome and normal immunity or mild immunodeficiency should receive the full complement of vaccines to prevent illness, including an annual influenza vaccine. Patients with severe immunodeficiency should consult with an immunologist prior to receiving live virus vaccines.

Nutrition/Diet: Patients with 22q11.2 deletion syndrome usually do not need to follow any special diets.

School/Education: Patients often have problems with abstract reasoning, and require extra tutoring in addition to speech therapy.

References

Shprintzen RJ. Velo-cardio-facial syndrome: 30 Years of study. Dev Disabil Res Rev. 2008;14(1):3–10.
Kobrynski LJ, Sullivan KE. Velocardiofacial syndrome, DiGeorge syndrome: the chromosome 22q11.2 deletion syndromes. Lancet. 2007 Oct 20;370(9596):1443–52.

Turner Syndrome

Derek Wong

Etiology

Turner syndrome is a recognizable condition in females caused by the presence of one X chromosome with the absence of part or all of the second sex chromosome. This genetic imbalance causes a characteristic pattern of malformations, short stature, and behavior and learning difficulties.

Turner syndrome patients have one of several different karyotypes. The classic form is 45, XO, with a completely absent second chromosome. Although most of the second X is inactivated, several genes that are expressed on both X chromosomes in normal females are deficient in Turner patients. Patients with a second partial X chromosome may be indistinguishable from classic Turner patients. However, some patients have a partial X that cannot be inactivated, resulting in a much larger gene deficit and a more severe phenotype that may include mental retardation. Mosaic 45, XO/46, XX Turner syndrome patients may have a less severe phenotype than classic Turner patients. Finally, mosaic 45, XO/46, XY patients are important because they have a risk of gonadoblastoma.

Clinical Presentation and Prognosis

Demographics: Turner syndrome is the most common chromosomal abnormality in fetuses. However, many patients are lost in utero, and the incidence at birth is approximately 1 in 3,000. A mother with one Turner syndrome child is not at increased risk to have a second Turner child.

Presenting signs and symptoms: Turner syndrome causes edema of the neck, hands and feet, both in utero and after birth. Common features in the neonate include webbed neck, low posterior hairline, prominent ears, and broad chest with wide spaced nipples. Older patients present with the same findings, plus cubitus valgus (increased carrying angle). Turner syndrome should be considered in any female with unexplained short stature, especially with delayed or absent puberty.

Clinical course: Turner syndrome newborns often have congenital lymphedema, congenital heart disease, congenital hip dysplasia, renal malformations, and feeding difficulties. In addition to slow linear growth, Turner children have an increased incidence of strabismus, otitis media, hearing loss, and hypernasal speech. There is increased susceptibility to many autoimmune conditions, including hypothyroidism and celiac disease.

Older children and adolescents have an increased incidence of problems with visual spatial tasks, driving, and social interactions. Nearly all Turner patients have delayed or absent puberty and are at risk for early osteoporosis. Most, but not all patients are infertile. Patients have an increased risk of coronary artery disease, hyperlipidemia, stroke, diabetes, obesity, hypertension, and aortic root dilatation.

Prognosis: The average lifespan of a Turner female is approximately 10 years less than in the general population, presumably due to metabolic syndrome and congenital and acquired heart disease. Most have a normal IQ, and many attend college or professional school.

Diagnosis

Although Turner syndrome may be suspected on the basis of the clinical exam, a standard karyotype is the gold standard for the diagnosis.

Management

Growth: Growth hormone therapy is an option for Turner syndrome children. On average, Turner syndrome adults are 20 cm shorter than normal children, and growth hormone adds approximately 6 cm to final height. Estrogen therapy should be given to Turner syndrome patients with delayed or absent puberty to aid in development of secondary sex characteristics and prevent osteoporosis. Treatment should begin at approximately age 12 years in patients who are on growth hormone therapy, and at age 14 years in those who are not on therapy.

Cardiac disease: The incidence of congenital heart disease is markedly increased in Turner syndrome. Many of the common abnormalities, including bicuspid aortic valve, aortic coarctation, and aortic stenosis, increase the risk for aortic dilatation. An echocardiogram should be done on all patients with a new diagnosis, and at regular intervals (every 1–5 years). Blood pressure and lipid levels should be followed closely.

Endocrine disease: Thyroid function should be monitored annually after age 3 years, due to an increased incidence of autoimmune hypothyroidism. The incidence of type I and type II diabetes are increased, and should be screened in patients with additional risk factors such as obesity, family history, and acanthosis nigricans. Hormone replacement with estrogen followed by combination therapy is usually done through referral to a pediatric endocrinologist. The subject of infertility should be discussed during adolescence because of its importance to patients and the availability of options such as oocyte donation.

Renal disease: Turner patients have a high incidence of renal malformations, including horseshoe kidney, duplication of the collecting system, and hydronephrosis. A renal ultrasound should be done on all newly diagnosed patients.

Gastrointestinal disease: Feeding problems are common in Turner infants. There is an increased risk of celiac disease, and asymptomatic children should be screened with tissue transglutaminase (TTG) antibodies after the age of 3 years. Antibody positive patients should be referred to a gastroenterologist for endoscopic confirmation of the diagnosis. In addition, adolescents are at increased risk of inflammatory bowel disease.

Ophthalmologic disease: Strabismus is common and warrants ophthalmologic referral.

Otolaryngologic disease: Turner patients often have sensorineuronal hearing loss, which may be exacerbated by frequent episodes of otitis media. Early prophylaxis and referral to an otolaryngologist are indicated for recurrent otitis media.

Orthopedic disease: Spinal problems such as scoliosis, kyphosis, and lordosis are common. Patients have multiple risk factors for osteoporosis, and may require a bone densitometry study during adolescence or young adulthood.

Consultations: The care of these patients may require multiple subspecialty consults. A cardiology consult is usually necessary to look for congenital heart disease, and follow up is essential in case of complications such as hypertension and hyperlipidemia. An endocrinologist is essential to follow growth, hormonal replacement, osteoporosis, and thyroid disease. A genetics consult may help with confirmation of the diagnosis, especially in atypical cases. All other consults such as gastroenterology, nephrology, dental, otolaryngology, ophthalmology, and orthopedics should depend on the patient's clinical presentation and needs at different stages of growth.

Social: Parents of these children may qualify for social security supplemental income benefit. Explore other medical and income benefits that may be available to these children and their families in your community and state.

> Parents can find internet support at:
> Turner Syndrome Society of the United States
> 10960 Millridge North Drive
> Houston TX 77070
> Home page: www.turnersyndrome.org

Monitoring: In addition to what is mentioned above, anticipate and monitor for the following: Submucous cleft palate, gastroesophageal reflux, and GI bleeding (indicating a possible vascular malformation of the GI tract). As these patients enter puberty, as with all teenagers, sexual health, and fertility need to be discussed with the patients and their families to prevent sexual abuse, disease, or unwanted pregnancies.

Pearls and Precautions

Immunization: Turner syndrome patients should receive vaccines using the standard schedule. They should also receive an annual influenza vaccine, when available.

Nutrition/diet: Those who are not affected by celiac disease do not need to follow any special diets.

School/education: Many children have difficulty with non-verbal learning, and may require tutoring in subjects like mathematics. In addition, middle school and high school may be difficult due to social immaturity, lack of pubertal development, and somewhat impaired social functioning.

References

Gravholt CH. Clinical practice in Turner syndrome. Keil MF, Stratakis CA. Nat Clin Pract Endocrinol Metab. 2005 Nov;1(1):41–52.

Frías JL, Davenport ML; Committee on Genetics and Section on Endocrinology. Pediatrics. 2003 Mar;111(3):692–702

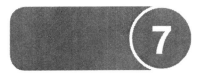

Hematologic Disorders

7

Table of Contents

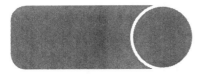

Neonatal and Infant Cytopenias

(Anemia, Neutropenia and Thrombocytopenia)

Stephen A. Feig, George B. Segel, Kenji Morimoto

Cytopenias of the infant and neonate may be due to decreased production (bone marrow failure or infiltration) or increased destruction. Likewise, they may be due to heritable or acquired disorders (also, see sections on *Hereditary Hemolytic Anemias*).

The bone marrow is the organ responsible for the production of the formed elements in the blood. Bone marrow failure conditions result in the inability to produce blood cells (erythrocytes, leukocytes, and platelets). These are a diverse group of conditions that may affect a single cell type (e.g., pure red cell aplasia) or multiple cell lines (e.g., aplastic pancytopenia). Decreased production of one or more blood elements results in deficiency of that type of cell in the circulation (anemia in the case of red cell aplasias, leukopenia in the case of white cell aplasias, and thrombocytopenia in the case of amegakaryocytosis, and aplastic pancytopenia in the case of trilineage hypoplasia) (see section on *Aplastic Pancytopenias*).

Anemias due to Lack of Red Cell Production

The red blood cell aplasias are a diverse group of congenital and acquired disorders that result in decreased red blood cell production and anemia.

Etiology

Approximately half of patients with Congenital Erythroid Hypoplasia (Diamond-Blackfan Syndrome, (DBS)) carry an identified mutation of the genes encoding for ribosomal proteins. DBS is presumed to result from malfunction of these proteins. DBS is a rare disorder that presents in the first year of life in 90% of patients. It may be variable in severity. Some consider this disorder to be a myelodysplastic disease that predisposes the patient to the development of acute myeloblastic leukemia.

The common forms of pure red cell aplasia are acquired; some are related to antecedent viral infection, particularly with parvovirus. In patients with an underlying hemolytic anemia, who are dependent upon a heightened reticulocyte count to maintain an adequate hemoglobin level, viral-induced red cell hypoplasia produces an acute anemia. In normal individuals, erythroid failure may occur without an apparent antecedent viral infection. In these patients, anemia develops slowly, and the patients may remain hemodynamically compensated at extremely low levels of hemoglobin (Transient Erythroblastopenia of Childhood (TEC)). The acquired forms of red cell aplasia are usually transient.

There are adult forms of red blood cell aplasia. These are more common in females, in whom the process is mediated by the presence of an auto-antibody to erythrocyte progenitor cells in the marrow. There is also a rare form of pure red cell aplasia that is associated with pregnancy.

Clinical Presentation and Prognosis

Presenting signs and symptoms: Pure red blood cell aplasias present with isolated severe anemia and an inadequate reticulocyte response. The white blood cell count, differential count, and platelet count are usually normal.

Clinical course: The congenital form, DBS, presents in infancy in the vast majority of patients, 90% in the first year of life. Physical abnormalities are observed in about 25% of patients with DBS, most commonly in the head and face. When red cell aplasia occurs in utero, it may lead to fetal hydrops. In utero red cell aplasia may result from either DBS or infection of the fetus with parvovirus. Most of the viral induced aplasias and TEC present later in childhood, with a peak incidence at 3–4 years of age. It is likely that many red cell aplasias of a transient nature are never diagnosed because they resolve before being brought to medical attention.

Prognosis: Patients with acquired red cell aplasia usually recover without sequelae. Patients with prolonged acquired red cell aplasia should be evaluated for immune dysfunction; some of these patients are unable to eliminate parvovirus, and respond to administration of monthly IVIg.

Patients with DBS require indefinite follow-up by a hematologist. About 1/3 of patients will recover with glucocorticoid therapy and require no further treatment, although the macrocytosis persists. Another 1/3 of patients will respond to glucocorticoid therapy, but remain dependent upon minimal doses (as little as 1–2 mg prednisone, twice per week). The remainder of DBS patients may or may not respond to prednisone, but if they do respond, will require continued high doses. This last group of patients is probably best managed with chronic transfusion therapy and chelation to prevent iron overload, and to avoid the toxicity of high dose, long-term glucocorticoid therapy. The use of other forms of immunosuppressive therapy, or hematopoietic stimulants, such as erythropoietin, IL-3, and Stem Cell Factor has not been beneficial. Hematopoietic stem cell transplants have been used successfully to treat DBS patients refractory to prednisone therapy. Unfortunately, many patients do not have a suitably matched donor. The risks of transplant may be increased because many of the DBS patients have been extensively transfused prior to making the decision to transplant; this may increase the risk of platelet refractoriness during the immediate post-transplant period, or even graft rejection.

Diagnosis

Differentiation between congenital and acquired red cell aplasia is usually simple. Most patients with DBS have significant macrocytosis that can be detected by the MCV and examination of a blood smear. By contrast, patients with acquired red cell aplasia have normocytic, normochromic RBC's. Examination of the bone marrow in either circumstance shows diminished or absent red cell precursors. In patients with parvovirus-induced disease, swollen, distorted erythroblasts may be seen, and parvoviral antigens may be demonstrated using special stains.

The presence of hypochromia and microcytosis should raise suspicion of concurrent iron deficiency or a thalassemia syndrome. Dietary history, history of blood loss, and testing for the presence of occult blood in the stool may be helpful in the presence of hypochromia and microcytosis.

The red blood cells in patients with DBS have fetal characteristics such as increased i antigen expression, decreased I antigen expression, fetal enzyme pattern and increased adenosine deaminase [ADA]. Mutated genes that encode for ribosomal proteins have been identified in some patients with DBS and provide a specific diagnosis, if they can be identified. Their specific relationship to the genesis of the anemia is not yet known.

The red cells of patients with TEC are normocytic and do not have the "fetal" characteristics described for DBS red cells. TEC patients tend to be older than DBS patients; the median age for TEC patients is 3–4 years, whereas 90% of DBS patients present before their first birthday.

Other causes of pure red blood cell aplasia are infrequent. An adult form, due to the presence of an auto-antibody, usually is seen in young adult females who often have other evidence of immune dysregulation. Pure red cell aplasia is also a rare complication of pregnancy.

Management

Transfusion: The management of patients with severe anemia due to pure red cell aplasia (hypoplasia) is transfusion. The details of transfusion management of severe anemia are described in the section of this chapter entitled Acute Management of Anemia. Patients with TEC rarely will require more than one, or at most two, transfusions. When additional transfusions are required for a patient with a diagnosis of TEC, an alternate diagnosis should be considered. Recurrent anemia should raise suspicion that the patient has DBS. Most patients with a chronic hemolytic anemia complicated by a viral-induced aplastic crisis will recover to their baseline state after transfusion.

Medications: DBS is treated initially with glucocorticoids. The usual starting dose is 2 mg/kg/day in divided dosage, and this dosage is slowly reduced to the minimum that will sustain the patient's hemoglobin. Patients who require continued immunosuppressive doses of prednisone are better managed with transfusion therapy. This may require placement of a venous access device (port-a-cath) and chelation of excess iron with deferasirox after the ferritin level exceeds 1000–1500 ng/mL.

Monitoring: The frequency with which DBS patients need to be followed depends upon the stability of their condition. Patients on high doses of corticosteroids or on a transfusion regimen must be seen frequently. Patients who are on minimal doses of steroids and have a stable hemoglobin may not require hematologic follow-up more often than once per year. TEC is a self-limited condition. It does not recur after marrow recovery and no special long-term follow-up is required.

Pearls and Precautions

1. Infants with DBS treated with <2 mg/kg/day of prednisone, or <20 mg/d for children weighing >10 kg, may be immunized with attenuated live virus vaccines, according to the recommendations of the American Academy of Pediatrics. Patients on higher doses of corticosteroids may develop hyperglycemia, hypertension, behavioral disorders, and all of the other complications of steroid therapy. Patients whose doses cannot be tapered to minimal doses without recurrence of anemia may be served best by discontinuation of the corticosteroids and institution of a transfusion program under the supervision of a Pediatric Hematologist.
2. Patients with DBS may have associated congenital anomalies that require special follow-up.
3. Support Groups and Registry:
   a. Diamond-Blackfan Anemia Registry, Director: Adriana Vlachos, M.D.: http://www.dbar.org
   b. Diamond-Blackfan Anemia Foundation (includes family resources): http://www.dbafoundation.org
   c. Daniella Maria Arturi Foundation (includes family resources): http://www.dmaf.org/html/home.html

References

Lipton JM, Ellis SR. Diamond-Blackfan anemia: diagnosis, treatment and molecular pathogenesis. Hematol Oncol Clin North Am 2009; 23: 261–282.

Lipton JM. Diamond-Blackfan anemia: New paradigms for a "not so pure" inherited red cell aplasia. Semin Hematol 2006; 43: 167–177.

Morimoto K, Lin S, and Sakamoto K. The functions of RPS 19 and their relationship to Diamond-Blackfan anemia: a review. Mol Genet Metab 2007; 90: 358–362.

Flygare JF, Karlsson S. Diamond-Blackfan anemia: erythropoiesis lost in translation. Blood 2007; 109: 3152–3160.

Vlachos A, Ball S, Dahl N, Alter BP, et al. Diagnosing and treating Blackfan-Diamond Anemia: Results of an international consensus conference. Br J Haematol 2008; 142: 859–876.

Anemias Due to Red Cell Loss or Destruction

Stephen A. Feig, George B. Segel, Kenji Morimoto

Neonatal anemia also may result from hemolysis or severe or prolonged blood loss. Hemolysis may be acquired (as in hemolytic disease of the newborn) or hereditary. Hemolytic conditions usually present in the neonatal period with significant and prolonged jaundice because of the inability of the neonatal liver to conjugate bilirubin. Hemolytic disease of the newborn is discussed in this section of the chapter. Hereditary hemolytic disorders are discussed in a separate section. Alternatively, neonatal anemia may be the result of intra-uterine hemorrhage, as seen with placental abruption, feto-maternal transfusion, or twin-twin transfusion.

Hemolytic Disease of the Newborn (HDN)

Stephen A. Feig, George B. Segel, Kenji Morimoto

HDN is an acquired immune hemolytic process in which a pregnant female is sensitized to an antigen on the surface of her fetus' red blood cells.

Etiology

In this condition, the mother's IgG antibody crosses the placenta, attaches to the fetal red cells, and causes their destruction. The fetus responds with increased erythropoiesis, but if the hemolysis is severe, anemia ensues. As a result of extreme erythroid hyperplasia, there may be extramedullary hematopoiesis (with hepatosplenomegaly), and circulating erythroblasts (nucleated RBC's). The common causes of HDN are materno-fetal incompatibility of the ABO or Rh (D) antigens, but incompatibility of minor blood group antigens also may cause HDN.

Clinical Presentation and Prognosis

Presenting signs and symptoms: The clinical presentation of HDN depends upon the severity of the hemolysis. The manifestations are anemia, hepatosplenomegaly, indirect hyperbilirubinemia, reticulocytosis, erythroblastosis, and, in the most severe cases, hydrops fetalis (congestive heart failure).

Clinical course: During pregnancy, the excess bilirubin produced by the fetus as a result of the hemolysis is transferred across the placenta to the mother, conjugated, and excreted. After delivery, the fetus accumulates unconjugated bilirubin because of the immaturity of the hepatic glucuronyl transferase mechanism; this causes a risk of kernicterus. Kernicterus develops after birth if the neonatal unconjugated bilirubin level reaches levels toxic to the brain.

Diagnosis

The manifestations of HDN may resemble those of any congenital hemolytic anemia. The severity of the hemolysis, not the cause, dictates the magnitude of the secondary manifestations (anemia, reticulocytosis, erythroblastosis, hepatosplenomegaly, and jaundice). The study that differentiates HDN from congenital hemolytic disorders (such as hereditary spherocytosis or pyruvate kinase deficiency), is the presence of a positive direct antiglobulin test (DAT, or Coombs' test). It is important to make the diagnosis of HDN because the risk of more severe hemolysis is increased in future pregnancies.

Obstetricians routinely test for the potential of Rh HDN early in pregnancy by blood typing the mother and, if she is Rh negative, assessing for the presence of anti-Rh (D) antibodies in her serum. In unsensitized females, sensitization to the D antigen can be prevented by the administration of anti-D serum (WinRho or RhoGam) during pregnancy and at delivery. In sensitized mothers, the fetus must be monitored closely; amniocentesis is used to assess the severity of hemolysis and ultrasound will detect organ enlargement and the edema of *hydrops fetalis*. Generally ABO hemolytic disease is less severe, but hemolysis due to minor group incompatibility may be severe.

Management

If severe, HDN is detected at an early stage of pregnancy (when delivery would create severe risk of the complications of prematurity). *Hydrops fetalis* can be prevented by intrauterine transfusion of packed red blood cells that do not carry the antigen to which the mother is sensitized. The baby should be delivered when the risks of prematurity are acceptable (i.e., less than the risk of intrauterine transfusion).

For the infant with HDN, the diagnosis must be made with the DAT. The bilirubin must be followed closely. Gradual increases in the bilirubin may be controlled by the use of phototherapy, "bili lights". The rate of hemolysis and the need for exchange transfusion may be diminished by the administration of IVIg. Severe elevation of the bilirubin causes an increased risk of kernicterus, which is exacerbated by prematurity and hypoalbuminemia. This should be prevented by exchange transfusion, the major benefit of which is the removal of sensitized red blood cells if the procedure is done early. In severe HDN, more than one exchange transfusion may be necessary.

Icteric babies managed with phototherapy will experience a normal nadir of erythropoiesis. The severity of resulting anemia may be exacerbated by the persistence of maternal antibody to the baby's red blood cells. Increased anemia is usually detected at 4–6 weeks of age, but the maternal antibody persisting in the baby may continue to diminish effective erythropoiesis until 10–12 weeks of age. This anemia develops slowly and may allow adequate hemodynamic compensation, even at remarkably low hemoglobins. Transfusion of compatible packed red blood cells will correct the anemia, but may also delay recovery of erythropoiesis.

Pearls and Precautions

1. HDN is distinguished from hereditary disorders of the red cell by the presence of a positive direct antiglobulin test (DAT, or Coombs' test).
2. Blood transfusions given to infants during the first three months of life must be compatible (cross-matched) with the mother's serum.
3. Blood transfusions to infants should be irradiated to prevent transfusion-induced graft-versus-host disease.

Reference

Roberts IA. The changing face of haemolytic disease of the newborn. Early Hum Dev 2008; 84: 515-523.

Neutropenias of the Infant or Neonate

Stephen A. Feig, George B. Segel, Kenji Morimoto

Neutropenias of childhood are a diverse group of disorders that may be hereditary or acquired; they may be the result of increased destruction in the periphery or diminished production by the marrow. Generally, when the absolute neutrophil count falls below 500/µL, a patient is considered at increased risk of infection. Patients with impaired granulocyte production have diminished "reserve" and are considered at greater risk of overwhelming infection than patients whose neutropenia is due to peripheral destruction.

Most infants are born with an elevated absolute neutrophil count (ANC) because the placenta is a source of granulocyte colony stimulating factor (G-CSF). After the umbilical cord is cut, the source of G-CSF is eliminated and the neonate's ANC decreases over the first few days of life. Infants usually have a normal white blood cell count (by adult standards), with relative lymphocytosis and neutropenia, but the latter is rarely severe (<500/µL). Serious neonatal infection may be associated with a diminished rather than a heightened ANC. Therefore, sepsis should be suspected when a sick infant is profoundly neutropenic.

When a low ANC is observed in an otherwise healthy infant, the most common cause is "benign neutropenia." This results from the destruction of circulating neutrophils, presumably by an antibody mediated autoimmune process. Sometimes these antibodies can be detected. Leukopoiesis, as seen on bone marrow aspirate, is normal, however, and these patients have sufficient myeloid reserve to combat infection. Alternatively, acquired neutropenia may result from viral infection or marrow suppression due to medications. Obviously, it is critical to differentiate between the benign and more severe forms of childhood neutropenia.

Neonates and infants with significant reduction in the ability to produce neutrophils do not have myeloid reserve and cannot combat infection. They suffer repeated bouts of severe infection. The ANC usually is fewer than 200/µL, and the marrow shows a promyelocyte arrest in the severe congenital neutropenias (SCN).

Etiology

The most severe forms of congenital neutropenia manifest themselves in early infancy. These patients have few, if any, circulating neutrophils and are susceptible to overwhelming sepsis. Examination of the bone marrow demonstrates a paucity of granulocyte progenitors at the myelocyte stage or beyond. The conditions may be inherited as autosomal dominant or recessive traits. About 60% of the patients have mutations that are presently identified. The original kindreds described by Kostmann have recessive mutations in a gene, HAX-1, which codes for the granulocyte colony stimulating factor receptor that is necessary for normal granulocyte maturation. Others with the dominant form of SCN have mutations in the neutrophil elastase gene, ELA2, or the GFI1 gene, which targets ELA2 and produces a similar picture.

Another condition that is associated with neutropenia early in life is the Schwachman-Diamond syndrome. In this illness, neutropenia is associated with exocrine pancreatic failure with secondary malabsorption and failure to thrive. The condition is autosomal recessive, and the gene has been identified and designated SBDS; clinical genetic testing is available. Other conditions leading to severe congenital neutropenia are known and associated with specific gene mutations, including the gene for glucose-6-phosphatase, glucose-6-phosphate transporter 1 (Glycogen Storage Disease, type 1b), and some variants of Wiskott-Aldrich Syndrome. Cyclic neutropenia is, as the name implies, associated with intermittent absence of circulating neutrophils that occurs in a regular pattern, usually in cycles of 15–28 days. It is due to a mutation in a region of the ELA2 gene different from the SCN mutations. At the nadir of the cyclic neutrophil count patients may be susceptible to pyogenic infection.

Acquired Neutropenia: The most common causes of acquired neutropenia are viral infection, marrow suppression from medications, and the development of neutrophil antibodies (autoimmune neutropenia). It is important to establish whether a neutropenic patient has ever had normal neutrophil counts in the past in an attempt to eliminate congenital conditions as the cause. The neutropenia related to viral infections will be transient and usually improves rapidly as the infection resolves. No specific treatment should be necessary for these patients, although antimicrobial agents often are administered. Similarly, those patients with antineutrophil antibodies and autoimmune neutropenia usually do not develop severe bacterial infections in spite of absolute neutrophil counts below 500/µL. Recurrent febrile illnesses in such patients may necessitate the use of granulocyte colony stimulating factor (G-CSF). The most effective management of patients with drug-induced neutropenia is cessation of the medication, if that is possible.

Clinical Presentation and Prognosis

Presenting signs and symptoms: Patients with severe neutropenia present with fever and are at high risk of bacterial sepsis. Although they may develop fever from routine viral infections, the blood count demonstrates severe neutropenia, and these patients must have multiple cultures and be treated promptly with antibiotics for presumed bacterial infection until the cultures are reported as negative.

Prognosis: The prognosis for patients with benign neutropenia is excellent. The neutrophil count usually returns to a normal level, but this may take years. Children with severe congenital neutropenic states are at risk of fatal infection when their counts are extremely low. If they respond to G-CSF, the risk of infection is averted. However, SCN patients remain at risk of future development of leukemia.

Diagnosis

These rare congenital neutropenic states must be differentiated from benign neutropenia, a condition in which the circulating neutrophil count may be very low, but the marrow shows full maturation of the myeloid cells. In this circumstance, there is adequate myeloid reserve and the ability to get neutrophils to a site of possible infection is preserved; this prevents the spread of bacterial infection. It is presumed that the circulating neutropenia is the result of an auto-immune process, although the presence of anti-neutrophil antibodies cannot be identified consistently. These patients present with neutropenia on a routine blood count done for other purposes. They have no history of severe infections, and fevers are not associated with bacterial infection although these children may have persistent, severe neutropenia. They may get some protection from the presence of monocytes.

By contrast, patients with cyclic neutropenia have fluctuating neutrophil counts, which can be documented by serial counts, performed twice per week for 3–4 weeks. The marrow of patients with severe congenital neutropenia is diagnostic; it shows severe paucity or absence of myeloid progenitors beyond the promyelocyte stage. This absence of "myeloid reserve" is what distinguishes the severe neutropenic states from benign neutropenia. For patients with the severe forms of neutropenia, analysis for mutations of the HAX-1, ELA2, and SBDS genes is available.

The history will reveal whether a patient is being treated with a medication that might suppress myelopoiesis. If exposure to such a medication or chemical is found, the first attempt at treatment should be to eliminate that exposure.

Common variable immunodeficiency, other immunodeficiency syndromes, and auto-immune diseases, like systemic lupus erythematosus, also may be associated with neutropenia.

Management

Medication: Patients with benign neutropenia require no special intervention, although it is frightening to just observe a febrile neutropenic patient. Patients with severe neutropenic states often respond to treatment with G-CSF; their absolute neutrophil counts can be brought into a safe range and their febrile episodes managed as normal children would be managed. When these children are neutropenic, febrile illnesses should be managed with caution; they should be carefully assessed, cultured and treated with empiric, parenteral, broad-spectrum antibiotics. These children may be at increased long-term risk of developing leukemia and require follow-up by a hematologist. If medication or chemical exposure is a potential cause of neutropenia, that exposure should be terminated.

Transplantation: The definitive treatment for patients with severe congenital neutropenia is hematopoietic stem cell transplantation, if a suitably matched donor can be identified.

Social support:
  a. Neutropenia Registry: http://depts.washington.edu/registry/
  b. Neutropenia Support Association: http://www.neutropenia.ca

Monitoring: Stable patients with severe neutropenia on G-CSF may be monitored at intervals of 3–6 months. The most important issue is that neutropenic patients must be evaluated promptly in the event they develop fever. Patients with benign neutropenia should be followed at 6–12 month intervals until the condition resolves.

Pearls and Precautions

1. The African-American population has lower WBC and neutrophil counts than the Caucasian population. The 95% reference ranges for WBC and absolute neutrophil count (ANC) for African-American males are 2800–9200/μL and 900–4200/μL, respectively. Afro-Caribbeans have an intermediate lowering of counts. It has been estimated that neutropenia (defined by an ANC<1500/μL) is five times more common in African-Americans than in Caucasians, but this is not accompanied by an increase in susceptibility to bacterial infections.
2. *Immunization:* Neutropenic patients without T- or B-cell impairment should receive immunization according to the schedule for normal children.
3. *Nutrition/Diet:* Patients with Schwachman-Diamond syndrome suffer from pancreatic insufficiency and therefore require close follow up of nutrition and growth. They require replacement of pancreatic enzymes.
4. *Dental care:* Neutropenia is often associated with chronic periodontal infection. Oral hygiene is critically important to diminish this potential portal for infectious entry and to prevent tooth loss.
5. *School:* Patients with SCN who have responded to G-CSF should attend school.

References

Welte K, Zeidler C. Severe congenital neutropenia. Hematol/Oncol Clin North Am 2009; 23: 307–320.

Boxer LA, Newburger P. A molecular classification of congenital neutropenia syndromes. Pediatr Blood Cancer 2007; 49: 609–614.

Segel GB and Halterman JS: Neutropenia in Pediatric Practice. Pediatrics in Review 2008, 29:12–24.

Thrombocytopenia

Stephen A. Feig, George B. Segel, Kenji Morimoto

The neonatal thrombocytopenias are a diverse group of conditions that may be of congenital or acquired origin. They may be due to failure of the marrow to produce platelets or to accelerated peripheral platelet consumption.

A. Thrombocytopenia Due to Decreased Platelet Production (Amegakaryocytic Thrombocytopenia)

Stephen A. Feig, George B. Segel, Kenji Morimoto

Amegakaryocytic thrombocytopenia is a very rare condition in which the marrow is severely depleted of megakaryocytes, resulting in severe thrombocytopenia. It must be distinguished from processes in which platelets are rapidly destroyed, such as immune thrombocytopenia.

Etiology

The etiology of this condition may be related to a mutation of the mpl gene or a part of syndromes such as Thrombocytopenia with Absent Radius (TAR) Syndrome or Radio-ulnar synostosis.

Clinical Presentation and Prognosis

Presenting signs and symptoms: Patients with pure amegakaryocytic thrombocytopenia present with bruising and petechiae early in life. They are at risk for life-threatening hemorrhage. The diagnosis is made by documenting the absence of megakaryocytes in the bone marrow. Other patients with amegakaryocytosis may have syndromes that can be recognized on physical examination. These include TAR Syndrome and Radio-ulnar synostosis.

Prognosis: Patients with TAR syndrome require supportive care early in life, but develop the ability to produce platelets during childhood, if they can be supported through the years of thrombocytopenia. Patients with Amegakaryocytic Thrombocytopenia have a guarded prognosis. They may require platelet transfusions to stop bleeding episodes and are at risk of becoming refractory to platelet transfusion.

Management

Transfusion: Acute bleeding is managed by the transfusion of platelets. Aminocaproic acid may be useful in the management of minor bleeding.

Transplant: Hematopoietic stem cell transplantation should be considered for patients with pure amegakaryocytic thrombocytopenia if a suitably matched donor can be identified.

Monitoring: Patients with Amegakaryocytic Thrombocytopenia may be followed at 3–6 month intervals, although they should be seen promptly for bleeding.

Pearls and Precautions

Immunization: Immunizations should be given at normal times, but it is recommended that they be given subcutaneously, rather than intramuscularly, to diminish the risk of bleeding.

Skin and dental care: Normal skin and dental care should be provided. Minor bleeding with dental prophylaxis should be managed, if possible, with aminocaproic acid or topical thrombin, to diminish the use of unnecessary platelet transfusion.

Education: School should be attended, but PE should be limited to activities that will avoid injury and the risk of bleeding (no contact sports or "off the floor" activities including e.g., rope climbing, pole vaulting, etc.).

Miscellaneous: Repeated platelet transfusions may induce subsequent refractoriness. Therefore, transfusions should be given only when necessary.

B. Thrombocytopenia due to Platelet Destruction

Stephen A. Feig, George B. Segel, Kenji Morimoto

Destructive thrombocytopenias are a varied group of acquired disorders that result from immunologic or mechanical causes.

Etiology

Neonatal thrombocytopenia is most commonly due to sepsis (DIC), Kasabach-Merritt syndrome (destruction of RBC and platelets associated with a hemangioma) or allo-immune disease. In the latter case, the surface antigens on the infant's platelets differ from those on the mother's platelets. If a sensitized mother carries a fetus with discordant paternal antigens, the resulting maternal IgG is passed across the placenta to the baby, destroying its platelets. The pathophysiology is analogous to allo-immune hemolytic anemia due to Rh incompatibility. Allo-immune thrombocytopenia occurs *in utero* and may be associated with prenatal intra-cranial hemorrhage. It is critically important to make this specific diagnosis by the detection of specific maternal antibodies to the disparate paternal platelet antigen because subsequent pregnancies may be more severely affected and require special obstetric care.

Neonatal thrombocytopenia also may result from the passive transfer of IgG antibody if the mother has or has had ITP or if she has systemic lupus erythematosus with immune thrombocytopenia. For unknown reasons, this type of immune thrombocytopenia causes less severe hemorrhage in the fetus and newborn. All neonatal allo-immune thrombocytopenias resolve within several months as the maternal IgG that had been transferred to the fetus is cleared.

Acute illnesses, such as Hemolytic Uremic Syndrome (HUS) and Thrombotic Thrombocytopenic Purpura (TTP) also may cause destructive thrombocytopenia. These, like Kasabach-Merritt Syndrome and "Waring Blender Syndrome" (turbulent blood flow due to cardiac malformations), are associated with microangiopathic changes of the red blood cells on the peripheral blood smear. TTP results from the lack of von Willebrand factor protease (ADAMTS13); this leads to an increase of the high molecular weight multimers of von Willebrand factor, which, in turn, activates platelets and induces consumption of coagulation factors, including platelets. This may result rarely from an inherited defect in ADAMTS13 or from an acquired antibody-mediated destruction of ADAMTS13.

There are mild forms of congenital thrombocytopenia, which may not require much intervention, such as the giant platelet syndromes (secondary to mutations of the MYH9 gene), Type 2b Von Willebrand disease, and Bernard-Soulier syndrome.

Management

The treatment of severe bleeding with allo-immune thrombocytopenia is the transfusion of compatible plate-lets. If the condition is anticipated and the maternal platelet type is known, some blood banks have walk in donors available for platelet pheresis. If the condition is not anticipated, or walk in donors are not available, transfusion of maternal platelets is appropriate (remembering that transfused blood products for infants must be irradiated to prevent transfusion-mediated graft-versus-host disease). If the patient has DIC, full supportive care with transfusion, and treatment of the underlying cause of DIC are indicated. Patients with Kasabach-Merritt syndrome may require support with transfusions and vascular imaging may provide information that allows intervention with ligation of feeder vessels or embolization.

HUS is often related to infection with E.coli (O157:H7) that produces a shiga toxin. This condition must be managed in close consultation with nephrologists. TTP is managed by plasmapheresis with administration of ADAMTS13-containing normal plasma. Care of these patients must be coordinated between various subspe-cialists, as needed according to the protean manifestations seen in the patient.

Reference

Bussell JB, Sola-Visner M. Current approaches to the evaluation and management of the fetus and neonate with immune thrombocytopenia. Semin Perinatol 2009; 33: 35–42.

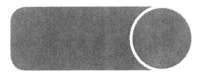

Childhood Anemias

Hereditary Hemolytic Anemias

Stephen A. Feig, George B. Segel, Kenji Morimoto

The mature red blood cell is a simple, effete cell. It has no nucleus, no mitochondria, and no protein synthesizing capability. Its only major function is to provide an envelope to carry enclosed hemoglobin for the exchange of oxygen and carbon dioxide in the lungs and body tissues. It has a complex membrane which is a lipid bilayer (with various inserted proteins), supported by an internal cytoskeleton. The major components of the red cell are the membrane, the enclosed hemoglobin, and the metabolic machinery required to maintain the integrity of the cell: Glycolytic enzymes for the production of ATP, hexose monophosphate shunt and glutathione pathway enzymes for resisting oxidant stress, and nucleotide retrieval pathway enzymes for the elimination of pyrimidine nucleotides that are toxic to the red cell.

Genetic alterations that affect the membrane, the hemoglobin, or the metabolic machinery of the red cell may result in alterations in the physiology of the red cell and its premature destruction (hemolysis). The effect of the hemolysis depends upon the degree of shortening of the red cell life span from the normal 100–120 days. As a result of reduced life span, there may be a decreased hemoglobin and decreased oxygen delivery to the tissues, increased production of erythropoietin, and increased eythropoiesis. Normal individuals can increase their erythropoiesis about six-fold above normal. This is reflected in the reticulocyte percentage. If the increased erythropoiesis can keep up with the increased destruction, there is compensated hemolysis, without anemia. If the hemolysis exceeds the capacity of the marrow to compensate, anemia ensues. If hemolysis occurs suddenly, as in the response to an oxidant stress, severe anemia may occur acutely, before the erythropoietic response can be mobilized.

The breakdown of red cells may occur in the cords of the spleen (extravascular), in the circulation (intravascular), or in the marrow (ineffective erythropoiesis). Most hereditary hemolytic processes involve a combination of these hemolytic sites, although one site or another may be prominent. Hereditary hemolytic anemias almost always manifest in the newborn by the presence of jaundice. The major exceptions to this rule are the β-globin chain hemoglobinopathies, which do not become symptomatic until the transition from γ chain (fetal hemoglobin) to β chain (adult hemoglobin) synthesis is well under way (at 6–12 months of age). Treatment of these hemolytic processes depends on the nature of the cause and the site of red cell destruction.

Red Cell Membrane Disorders

Stephen A. Feig, George B. Segel, Kenji Morimoto

These are a group of disorders that result from mutations of the genes that encode cytoskeletal or membrane proteins.

Etiology

The red cell membrane provides an envelope in which a high concentration of hemoglobin can be carried. It separates the intracellular environment (high hemoglobin, high potassium, low sodium) from the external plasma (no hemoglobin, high sodium, low potassium). The membrane contains ATPase's (Na+/K+ and Ca++) to maintain the internal cationic environment against the osmotic gradient. The various hereditary membrane disorders are the result of mutations in the genes involved in the plasticity of the membrane and/or the control of cation transport (Table 7.1).

The most common hereditary membrane disorder is Hereditary Spherocytosis (HS). It is caused by a variety of mutations in the membrane cytoskeleton, involving spectrin, ankyrin, and protein 4.1, among others. Most of the mutations are inherited as autosomal dominant traits, although some are recessive. As a result of the abnormal cytoskeleton, plasticity of the membrane is reduced and the red cells tend to take on sodium in excess of potassium lost. With each passage through the cords of the spleen, the relatively rigid cells lose small pieces of membrane until they become truly spherical. A sphere is the smallest envelope that can encompass a given volume; it is geometrically rigid. In contrast to the normal red cell that is about 7 microMeters (µ) in diameter, the diameter of the spherocyte may be about 5µ. Nevertheless, it must traverse the cords of the spleen, blind-ended pathways, at the end of which are basement membranes with apertures of about 3µ. Normal, plastic red cells are capable of twisting their way across the basement membrane, but rigid spheres cannot. Thus, as HS cells age, they become more spherical and are prematurely destroyed in the spleen.

Elliptocytosis is a similar disorder, but with less severe hemolysis. Pyropoikilocytosis is a rare disorder characterized by brisk hemolysis. Some neonates with elliptocytosis present with brisk hemolysis in the

Table 7.1: Red Cell Membrane Disorders

Disease	Localization	Cations Disrupted
Hereditary Spherocytosis	Cytoskeleton	Yes
Hereditary Elliptocytosis	Cytoskeleton	Yes
Hereditary Pyropoikilocytosis	Cytoskeleton	Yes
Hereditary Stomatocytosis	Membrane Protein	Yes

neonatal period and the blood smear demonstrates extreme poikilocytosis (fragmented forms, schistocytes, and helmet cells). During the first year of life, the morphologic appearance of their red cells gradually becomes classically elliptical and the severity of the hemolysis abates. Stomatocytosis is also rare; it is due to impaired ability to transport cations across the red cell membrane. Like HS, these disorders are inherited as autosomal dominant traits.

Clinical Presentation and Prognosis

Presenting signs and symptoms: Hereditary hemolytic anemias (except those due to β-globin abnormalities) may present in the newborn period with indirect hyperbilirubinemia. The neonatal liver usually is incapable of conjugating the excess bilirubin load. The anemia is variable because the rate of hemolysis may vary between individuals, as may the ability to compensate with increased erythropoiesis.

Clinical course: Anemia may be more pronounced during the physiologic erythropoietic nadir at 2–3 months of age. Some patients may pass through this period without diagnosis, although a family history of hemolysis may alert the physician to a possible hereditary anemia. Patients dependent upon a reticulocytosis to maintain hemoglobin are at risk of aplastic crises, especially those due to parvovirus infection. Splenomegaly may or may not be present. Severely affected patients may develop marrow hypertrophy with prominent maxilla, tower skull, thinning of cortical bone and splenomegaly. These children are at risk of splenic rupture and fractures of thin cortical bone after relatively minor trauma. Most patients do not have severe anemia, and only develop symptomatic anemia with aplastic crises. They are at risk of developing cholelithiasis and cholecystitis at a young age, secondary to the increased bilirubin production.

Prognosis: The long term outlook for the majority of patients with hereditary disorders of the red cell membrane is excellent. Patients should be observed for the late development of pulmonary hypertension, especially those who have undergone splenectomy.

Diagnosis

The diagnosis of red cell membrane disorders is suggested by careful examination of a good blood smear. Each of these disorders has a characteristic morphology that is usually apparent to the trained observer. In the case of HS, the osmotic fragility will demonstrate increased sensitivity to osmotic lysis, but it must be remembered that this is a characteristic of spherical cells and a spherical red cell may be due to conditions other than HS, especially autoimmune hemolytic anemia and hemolytic disease of the newborn secondary to ABO incompatibility. Certain research laboratories devoted to the study of membrane disorders are willing to perform physical studies of membrane plasticity (ektacytometry) or molecular studies of cytoskeletal proteins to make a specific diagnosis.

Management

Transfusion: Most patients do not require acute management. Neonatal hyperbilirubinemia is usually controlled well with phototherapy. Such patients may have more severe anemia during the physiologic nadir and may require transfusion. Occasionally, patients require chronic transfusion, but the need for transfusion may diminish or disappear as the patient gets older. Aplastic crises may require transfusion support. The approach to transfusion therapy is discussed in the section on Acute Management of Anemia.

Medications: As with all patients with chronic hemolysis, the administration of oral folic acid (1 mg per day) is recommended.

Surgery: Splenectomy is curative for HS and HE, and may be helpful for pyropoikilocytosis. The decision to perform splenectomy is an individual one and should be based upon relative risk and benefit analysis in the individual case. Generally, splenectomy should be reserved for the more severe cases, and should not be done before the patient is 5 years old. Before splenectomy, patients should be thoroughly immunized including pneumococcal and meningococcal vaccines. After splenectomy, patients should receive prophylactic antibiotics for at least one year to prevent overwhelming post-splenectomy infection.

Monitoring: Development of cholelithiasis and cholecystitis may result from any chronic hemolytic condition and should be managed according to standard practice. It is recommended that any patient undergoing cholecystectomy who has not had a prior splenectomy, undergo simultaneous splenectomy. This will reduce the hemolysis after surgery and diminish the risk of developing common duct stones in the future.

Pearls and Precautions

Immunization: Immunizations should be kept up to date.

Medications/situations/herbs that need to be avoided: Iron therapy should not be prescribed to patients with hemolytic anemia unless they are shown to be iron deficient. Hemolysis causes an increase in the absorption of iron from the gastrointestinal tract. Most patients with hemolytic anemia are replete with iron, even though they are anemic. Additional iron intake may increase the long term risk of hemosiderosis.

Counseling regarding protection of an enlarged spleen from rupture should be given.

References

An X, Mohandas N. Disorders of red cell membrane. Br J Haematol 2008; 141: 367–375.

Mohandas N, Gallagher PG. Red Cell Membrane: past, present and future. Blood 2008; 112: 3939–3947.

Bolton-Maggs PH, Stevens RF, Dodd NJ, et al. Guidelines for diagnosis and management of hereditary spherocytosis. Br J Haematol 2004; 126: 455–474.

Perrotta S, Gallagher PG, Mohandas N. Hereditary spherocytosis. Lancet 2008; 372: 1411–1426.

Red Cell Enzyme Deficiencies

Stephen A. Feig, George B. Segel, Kenji Morimoto

The mature RBC has limited metabolic capacity. It must produce ATP to meet its modest energy needs and metabolizes glucose via the Embden-Myerhof pathway to accomplish this. It must protect its proteins from oxidation and utilizes the hexose monophosphate shunt (HMPS) and glutathione pathways for this purpose. Virtually every enzyme in these pathways has been reported to be congenitally deficient in activity, leading to hemolytic disease.

Etiology

Deficiency of red cell pyruvate kinase (PK) activity is the most common defect in glycolysis. The clinical manifestations of hemolysis due to PK deficiency are similar to those of deficiency of the other glycolytic enzymes. Most of these conditions are inherited as autosomal recessive traits. The exception is deficiency of phosphoglycerate kinase (PGK) activity, which is X-linked. Most of the glycolytic enzyme deficiencies have their clinical manifestations limited to hemolysis, but PGK and Triose Phosphate Isomerase (TPI) deficiencies are associated with neurologic sequelae. The severity of hemolysis is variable.

Deficiency of Glucose-6-Phosphate Dehydrogenase (G6PD) is the most common abnormality in the HMPS, but deficiency of 6-Phosphogluconic Acid Dehydrogenase (6PGD) and the enzymes required for the synthesis and metabolism of glutathione have been reported. G6PD and 6PGD are inherited as X-linked recessive traits. Under conditions of oxidant stress, including by infection and various oxidant drugs and foods (see Table 7.2), sulfhydryl groups are oxidized, which results in inappropriate disulfide bonding. In particular, disulfide bonding between hemoglobin and the RBC membrane leads to the precipitation of hemoglobin (Heinz bodies). When this occurs, acute intra-vascular hemolysis may occur, with hemoglobinemia, hemoglobinuria, and acutely developing anemia. Numerous mutations in G6PD have been described; the common variant, A-, seen primarily in the African-American population, leads to hemolysis when patients are exposed to oxidant drugs. Chronic hemolysis and moderate anemia result commonly from chronic illness in patients with G6PD deficiency. Some rarer variants have sufficiently low enzyme levels that chronic hemolysis results. Some other variants are of little or no clinical significance.

A rare form of congenital hemolytic anemia is due to deficiency of Pyrimidine-5'-Nucleotidase. This results in increased content of pyrimidine nucleotides in the red blood cell. These nucleotides are toxic to the red cell and result in its early destruction.

Table 7.2: Agents Producing Hemolysis in G-6-PD Deficiency

Category	Agent
Antibacterials	Sulfonamides
	Trimethoprim-sulfamethoxazole
	Nalidixic Acid
	Cloramphenicol-Nitrofurantoin
Antimalarials	Primaquine
	Pamaquine
	Chloroquine
	Quinacrine
Others	Phenacetin-Vitamin K analogs
	Methylene Blue
	Probenecid
	Acetylsalicylic acid
	Phenazopyridine
Chemicals	Phenylhydrazine
	Benzene
	Naphthalene
Illnesses	Diabetic acidosis
	Hepatitis
	Sepsis
Foods	Fava beans

Clinical Presentation and Prognosis

Demographics: Hemolytic anemias secondary to deficiency of glycolytic enzymes have been reported in all populations. Presence of G6PD deficiency has been reported to be particularly common in individuals whose ancestors lived in Central Africa, the Mediterranean area, across the Middle East, and South East Asia. It is hypothesized that heterozygosity for G6PD deficiency may have provided a balanced polymorphism in which carriers had some protection against malaria. The A- variant is carried by almost 10% of African-Americans.

Presenting Symptoms: Deficiency of red cell enzymes may be associated with chronic hemolytic anemia. This is manifested in the neonatal period by hyperbilirubinemia which almost invariably requires treatment with phototherapy. For patients with chronic hemolysis, the symptoms and complications relate to the severity of hemolysis. In the more severely affected patients, especially those with PK deficiency, attempts to compensate for the anemia result in expansion of the marrow space and extra-medullary hematopoiesis. This, in turn, leads to maxillary hypertrophy, tower skull ("thalassemic facies"), hepatosplenomegaly, and increased risk of bone fractures. Long term sequelae include higher risk of cholelithiasis and cholecystitis as well as pulmonary hypertension.

Deficiency of G6PD and the other HMPS pathway enzymes usually is associated with neonatal hyperbilirubinemia. Undiagnosed patients, especially those with the A- variant, may present after exposure to an oxidant (infection, medication, or food) with hemoglobinemia, hemoglobinuria, and acute anemia. If the hemoglobinuria is severe, renal failure may ensue.

Clinical course: As with other hemolytic disorders, compensation is dependent upon accelerated erythropoiesis. Viral infections, especially parvovirus, may diminish red cell production and result in acutely developing anemia.

Prognosis: The prognosis for patients with mild hemolytic anemia is excellent. For patients with episodic hemolysis, such as with the A- variant of G6PD, the prognosis is also excellent. The avoidance of oxidant stress renders these individuals virtually asymptomatic. Patients with severe hemolysis are at risk of biliary disease and pulmonary hypertension and, if they require chronic transfusions, are at risk of all the complications of transfusion, especially blood-borne infections and iron overload. These patients will require iron chelation to prevent hemosiderosis.

Diagnosis

By contrast to membrane disorders and hemoglobinopathies, most red cell enzymopathies do not have distinctive morphology on the blood smear. Pyrimidine-5'-nucleotidase is an exception and is characterized by intense basophilic stippling. Acute hemolysis in G6PD deficiency may be characterized by "bite cells" that appear as if a small piece has been taken out of them.

Specific enzyme assays are available for the diagnoses of these deficiencies. Unless a specific deficiency is suspected, it is best to order a complete red cell enzyme panel. This will enable the assessment of red cell metabolism in its entirety, and is available from several research laboratories. G6PD and PK assays are available commercially.

Management

Acute management

The management of acute anemia is transfusion. See the Chapter entitled *Acute Management of Anemia* for specific details. Avoidance of oxidants (see Table 7.2) is essential for preventing ongoing hemolysis in patients with G6PD deficiency and the other disorders of the HMPS. Extreme intravascular hemolysis may result in renal failure.

Chronic management:

Medications: Folic acid (1 mg/day) is recommended for all patients with hemolytic anemia. Avoidance of oxidant medications and oxidant foods (e.g., fava beans) is recommended for patients with G6PD deficiency, and other enzyme deficiencies in the HMPS/glutathione pathways. Since infections may pose an oxidant risk, patients with HMPS/glutathione pathway disorders should be alert to the potential for increased hemolysis secondary to intercurrent infection.

Surgery: Patients with moderate to severe hemolysis secondary to deficiency of PK or other glycolytic pathway enzymes may benefit from splenectomy. Splenectomy of patients with severe PK deficiency often results in a dramatic increase in their reticulocyte count. This does not indicate an increase in hemolysis, but rather the improved survival of young cells that would have been destroyed by the spleen early after release into the peripheral circulation. Indeed, such patients often lose their dependence upon transfusion.

Monitoring: For patients who are transfusion dependent, careful matching of blood products will diminish the risk of sensitization and transfusion reactions. Iron chelation of transfusion-dependent patients is required to prevent iron overload. Such patients require careful monitoring of their iron status (ferritin, liver biopsy, and cardiac evaluation). They also should be observed for development of pulmonary hypertension and endocrinopathy secondary to iron deposition in the end organs.

References

Steiner, LA, Gallagher PG. Erythrocyte disorders in the perinatal period. Semin Perinatol. 2007; 31: 254–261.

Zanella A, Fermo E, Bianchi P, Valentini G. Red cell pyruvate kinase deficiency: molecular and clinical aspects. Br J Haematol 2005; 130: 11–25.

Cappellini MD, Fiorelli G. Glucose-6 phosphate dehydrogenase deficiency. Lancet 2008; 371: 64–74.

Beutler E. Glucose-6-phosphate dehydrogenase deficiency; a historical perspective. Blood 2008; 111: 16–24.

Segel GB, Hirsh MG and Feig SA. Managing Anemia in a Pediatric Office Practice: Part 2. Pediatrics in Review 2002 23(4):111–122.

Hemoglobinopathies

A. Thalassemias

Stephen A. Feig, George B. Segel, Kenji Morimoto

The thalassemias are anemias that result from unbalanced globin chain synthesis.

Etiology

When the balance between α and β globin synthesis is lost, it results in excess presence of the unaffected globin chain in erythroid progenitors. The excess chains form homotetramers that precipitate and cause ineffective erythropoiesis. The more severe the imbalance, the more severe the ineffective erythropoiesis and resulting anemia. Patients with severe thalassemia are transfusion dependent, develop expanded marrow space, extramedullary hematopoiesis, and are susceptible to bone fractures and iron overload.

The α globin genes are duplicated, so that normal individuals have two gene copies on each chromosome 16. Most patients with α-thalassemia have deletions of one or more of these genes. With each deletion, the patient loses approximately 25% of the capacity for α globin synthesis (see Table 7.3). The single deletions are indistinguishable from normal patients. Double deletions are clinically significant for their genetic implications and for their recognition in the differential diagnosis of a mild hypochromic, microcytic anemia. Patients with three deletions have sufficient imbalance in chain synthesis to develop significant anemia. In the newborn period, when babies are producing γ chains, the γ tetramers can be detected as Bart's hemoglobin on electrophoresis or HPLC. As the globin synthesis converts to β-chain during the first year of life, Bart's hemoglobin diminishes and β tetramers (hemoglobin H) can be seen on electrophoresis. The presence of four α gene deletions is incompatible with carrying a pregnancy to term. The fetus is dependent upon α chain synthesis for the production of fetal hemoglobin (Hgb F, $\alpha_2\gamma_2$). In the total absence of α chains, the erythroid progenitors produce only γ tetramers (Hgb Bart's). Bart's Hemoglobin is unstable and does not carry oxygen well. These mid-term fetuses become severely anemic and die of fetal hydrops *in utero*.

β-thalassemia is due to reduced synthesis of β chains. The β genes are not duplicated, so each individual carries one β gene on each 11th chromosome. In contrast to α-thalassemia, β-thalassemia is the result of various mutations rather than deletion. These mutations are numerous and varied; they result in variable degrees of diminished β-chain synthesis, from mild decrease to complete absence. Heterozygosity for β-thalassemia results in a mild hypochromic, microcytic anemia. Homozygosity results in a transfusion dependent anemia that becomes manifest during the latter half of the first year of life, due to the switch from γ (fetal) chain synthesis (Hgb F, $\alpha_2\gamma_2$) to β (Hgb A, $\alpha_2\beta_2$). β-thalassemia trait may interact with other β chain abnormalities, such as Hgb

Table 7.3: Alpha Thalassemia States

Gene Deletions	Condition
0	Normal
1	Silent carrier
2	α-thalassemia trait (cis or trans)
3	Hgb H disease
4	Fetal hydrops

S, to increase the severity of the other hemoglobinopathic trait. This is also true of the interaction between β-thalassemia and hemoglobin E; patients with homozygous hemoglobin E have a mild anemia, clinically similar to thalassemia trait, while patients doubly heterozygous for β-thalasssemia and Hgb E may have a severe, transfusion dependent anemia, more like thalassemia major.

Clinical Presentation and Prognosis

Demographics: Thalassemia is seen in patients of African, Mediterranean, and Southeast Asian descent. The heterozygous state offers protection against malaria which accounts for the high frequency with which it is seen in these populations. Among Southeast Asians with double deletion alpha thalassemia trait, the deletions are characteristically in the *cis* configuration (both deletions on the same chromosome). This results in a 25% risk that a mating between two such affected individuals will result in a hydropic baby. Among individuals of African descent, the deletions are typically in the *trans* configuration (the deletions on different chromosomes). A mating between two such affected individuals would have virtually no risk of producing a hydropic baby.

β-thalassemia mutations are passed in a simple Mendelian pattern. Matings between carriers of β-thalassemia carry a 25% risk that an offspring will be severely affected (thalassemia major).

Presenting signs and symptoms: Patients with β-thalassemia trait or α-thalassemia trait present with hypochromic, microcytic red cells. These conditions do not cause severe anemia or other symptoms. Patients with β-thalassemia trait who also carry a gene for another β-chain hemoglobinopathy, such as Sickle Cell Anemia, will develop symptoms more characteristic of the other hemoglobinopathy.

Patients with Hemoglobin H disease, three α gene deletions, present at birth with hypochromic, microcytic anemia, neonatal jaundice (secondary to ineffective erythropoiesis and hemolysis), and hepatosplenomegaly (secondary to extramedullary hematopoiesis). These patients may require chronic transfusion therapy, with the risk of iron overload. Splenectomy may be necessary to reduce hemolysis or improve the nutrition of some patients. Fetuses with deletion of four α genes develop heart failure and die in the second trimester, secondary to the inability to make fetal hemoglobin.

Patients with β-thalassemia major present in the second half of the first year of life. They are asymptomatic earlier because their ability to make hemoglobin F is unaffected. They present with anemia, the severity of which is dependent upon the residual ability to make β chains. The presence of concurrent α-thalassemia trait may improve the balance of chain synthesis and reduce the severity of the anemia.

Severe β-thalassemia major causes severe hypochromic, microcytic anemia, hepatosplenomegaly, and jaundice. Expansion of the marrow space causes thinning of the bones, susceptibility to fractures, and typical thalassemic facies (tower skull and prominent maxilla). Almost all of these patients require chronic hypertransfusion therapy for the anemia, and iron chelation, to prevent iron overload.

Prognosis: Patients with Hemoglobin H disease who do not require transfusion should do relatively well. They may require splenectomy with its attendant risk of overwhelming post-splenectomy infection. They tend to overabsorb dietary iron and if they require transfusions, may become iron overloaded. Therefore, iron therapy is contraindicated, unless iron deficiency is documented.

The only definitive treatment of β-thalassemia major is HSCT, if a matched donor is available. Patients with β-thalassemia major usually require chronic hypertransfusion. If they become sensitized to red cell antigens, splenectomy may improve the survival of transfused RBC's. Chelation, particularly with deferasirox, has been well-tolerated (with good compliance) and prevents or delays the secondary sequelae of iron overload (endocrine, liver, and cardiac failure).

Diagnosis

The thalassemias are characterized by hypochromia and microcytosis. The important differential is between thalassemia trait and iron deficiency. Patients with thalassemia trait have a low MCV, high red cell count, and mild or no anemia. Iron deficiency is characterized by a normal to low red cell count, low MCV, and anemia is a later manifestation. The distinction between mild-to-moderate iron deficiency anemia and thalassemia trait can be quantified by the Mentzer index:

$$\text{Mentzer Index} = \text{MCV/RBC.}$$

A value >13 suggests iron deficiency. A value <13 suggests thalassemia trait.

The diagnosis of thalassemia is made by hemoglobin analysis (electrophoresis or HPLC). Hemoglobin H and Bart's hemoglobin can be detected this way for the documentation of α-thalassemia. In patients with β-thalassemia trait, the A_2 hemoglobin is usually elevated, but this may be obscured in the presence of concurrent iron deficiency, which reduces the synthesis of δ chains to form Hgb A_2. Molecular testing is available to quantify the deletion of α genes, the position of the deletions (*cis* vs *trans*), and to test for many of the β-thalassemia mutations.

For pregnancies at risk, molecular diagnostic testing is available.

Management

Transfusion: The acute management of severe anemia is transfusion (see section on *Acute Management of Anemia*). The management of the more severe thalassemic conditions requires chronic hypertransfusion and chelation.

Consultations: These patients must be under the care of a hematologist for the management of the transfusions, the complications of transfusion (reactions, iron overload) and the management of chelation. For secondary complications and the sequelae of iron overload, consultation with endocrinologists, cardiologists, and possibly other specialists may be indicated. Patients with thalassemia trait should be counseled regarding whether there is a risk of a clinically significant thalassemia syndrome in their offspring.

Pearls and Precautions

Immunization: Vaccinations must be kept current, especially against hepatitis. Patients who are candidates for splenectomy should be immunized against polysaccharide bacterial antigens (Hemophilus influenza B, pneumococcus, and meningococcus) before splenectomy.

Medications: Iron therapy is contraindicated unless iron deficiency is documented.

References

Cunningham MJ. Update on thalassemia: clinical care and complications. Pediatr Clin North Am 2008; 55: 447–460.

Oliveiri NF, Muracca GM, O'Donnell A, et al. Studies in hemoglobin E-beta thalassemia. Br J Haematol 2008; 141: 388–397.

Schecter A. Hemoglobin research and the origins of molecular medicine. Blood 2008; 112: 3927–3938.

B. Sickle Cell Anemia

Stephen A. Feig, George B. Segel, Kenji Morimoto

Sickle cell anemia (SS disease) is a genetic hemoglobinopathy resulting in elongation of the shape of the erythrocytes (sickling), hemolysis, pain crises, and a variety of serious organ impairments that arise secondary to the vascular complications of sickling.

Etiology

Sickle cell anemia (SS disease) is a genetic hemoglobinopathy resulting from homozygosity for a mutation in the gene that changes the sixth amino acid in the beta chain of hemoglobin from valine to glutamic acid. This causes the mutated hemoglobin to gel in the deoxygenated state, resulting in elongation of the shape of the erythrocytes (sickling). Reduction in the partial pressure of oxygen in the blood causes sickling because this only occurs when hemoglobin S is in the deoxy configuration. This is a particular problem in patients with cyanotic congenital heart disease or pulmonary disease, and is further exacerbated by acidosis and dehydration.

The tendency of a cell to sickle is uniquely sensitive to dehydration, which increases the concentration of Hgb S in the red cell. The renal medulla, because of its acid, hypertonic milieu, is particularly prone to induce sickling of red cells as they pass through, and is damaged early in the childhood of patients with SS disease. As a result, these patients lose the ability to concentrate urine. This leads to enuresis and rapid development of dehydration in the event of fever, emesis, or extreme perspiration. Even patients with sickle trait develop isosthenuria and are at increased risk of dehydration.

The sickled RBCs are adherent and less deformable, leading to hemolysis, decreased regional blood flow and thrombosis. The vaso-occlusive events lead to vasculopathy and end-organ damage.

Clinical Presentation and Prognosis

Demographics: Sickle cell anemia is most prevalent among persons of Central African, Mediterranean, Saudi Arabian, and Indian origin, but Caucasians may be affected, particularly with Sickle-β-thalassemia. Sickle syndromes are being increasingly recognized in the Hispanic population. In most states, hemoglobinopathies are detected at birth by a newborn screening program. Over 90% of unscreened patients are diagnosed by 6 years of age while a small percentage of these patients present as early as 6 months of age. Prior to that time, infants are protected from vaso-occlusive symptoms because of the presence of Hgb F ($\alpha_2\gamma_2$).

Presenting symptoms/complications: Patients with sickle cell anemia are at increased risk of infections and end organ damage. They also experience a series of recurrent symptoms and complications. The following are the most commonly encountered complications and symptoms of sickle cell disease.

1. *Infection*: Patients with Sickle Cell Anemia develop functional asplenia in early childhood and subsequently infarct their spleens. There have also been reports of an associated opsonic defect. Thus, these patients are susceptible to overwhelming infections, especially with encapsulated bacteria. A high incidence of sepsis and early death in infants and toddlers with sickle cell anemia preceded the institution of neonatal screening programs which led to the administration of prophylactic antibiotics. Prophylactic antibiotics, and pneumococcal immunization (Prevnar and Pneumovax) have reduced the frequency of early death. Fever in these patients must be still viewed with caution as they continue to be at higher risk of overwhelming septicemia. A high frequency of salmonella osteomyelitis has also been reported.

2. *Vaso-occlusive crises*: Vascular occlusion is a common clinical problem in patients with severe sickle syndromes, and can occur in any organ.
   a. *Abdomen*: Abdominal pain crises are common. While most abdominal pain crises will resolve with hydration and pain management, an abdominal crisis may resemble an acute abdomen.
   b. *Bone*: Painful bone infarcts are frequent complications of sickle cell disease. In infants and toddlers, the metacarpals and metatarsals may be infarcted resulting in the Hand-Foot Syndrome (dactylitis), a common initial presentation of SS disease. In older patients, bony crises may occur in any bone or joint. These usually resolve with hydration and pain management, but because of the risk of infection, osteomyelitis must be considered. Staphylococcus and Salmonella are the most commonly involved organisms in sickle cell patients with osteomyelitis.
   c. *Central Nervous System (CNS)*: Strokes are another manifestation of sickle cell occlusive disease. The neurologic sequelae may be devastating. These events must be diagnosed and treated promptly to prevent further neurologic damage and recurrence. Mild, undiagnosed strokes may lead to more subtle CNS damage (e.g., learning handicaps).
   d. *Priapism*: Persistent and painful erections are a particularly troublesome complication. Conservative management and avoidance of surgical intervention are desirable to avoid permanent erectile dysfunction. Acute treatment may require urologic perfusion of the corpora with epinephrine.
   e. *Pulmonary*: The pulmonary complications of SS Disease include pneumonia and Acute Chest Syndrome (ACS). Patients present with fever, chest pain, and respiratory symptoms and may have either pneumonia or ACS. Pulmonary infiltrates on chest X-ray are present with either condition, and may be delayed in appearance if the patient is dehydrated on presentation. The infectious agents causing pneumonia include viruses, bacteria, and Mycoplasma, which causes a particularly severe pneumonia in patients with SS Disease. ACS frequently arises after several days of a pain crisis. It is thought to result from bone marrow infarction with embolization of fat to the lungs. The patient usually develops increasing respiratory distress with tachypnea, tachycardia, cough and the physical signs of pulmonary infiltration and oxygen desaturation. ACS carries a high risk of death in the year or two following the episode.

3. *Splenic sequestration*: The spleen is a major site of RBC destruction in infants and toddlers with SS disease, but by adolescence it has usually infarcted. While the spleen is still functional, it may become precipitously hyperactive and sequester circulating RBC. This results in a rapidly falling hemoglobin, rapidly enlarging spleen, and, potentially, hypovolemic shock. Sequestration must be recognized and treated quickly. While sequestration usually occurs in infants and toddlers with homozygous sickle cell disease or sickle-β-thalassemia, it may occur even in older patients with sickle-β-thalassemia, whose spleens may remain enlarged and active into adulthood.

4. *Anemia and aplastic crises*: The anemia in homozygous sickle cell disease may be severe, with a hemo-globin of 5–6g/dL and result in symptoms of chronic congestive heart failure, including dyspnea, fatigue, and limitation of activity. Such patients require treatment with a chronic transfusion pro-gram and iron chelation. Patients with severe hemolysis have increased reticulocyte counts reflecting increased hematopoiesis and RBC turnover in compensation for the shortened RBC life span. If erythropoietic activity becomes compromised, and the reticulocyte production falters, the hemoglo-bin and hematocrit will fall very quickly. This may occur after otherwise uneventful viral infections, such as parvovirus.

Prognosis is dependent on the prevention and control of infections and crises and the underlying severity of the disease. Severe sickle syndromes include SS, SC, SD, SOArab, and S-β-thalassemia. Patients heterozygous for both β-thalassemia and hemoglobin S have a clinical condition that closely resembles SS disease. The sever-ity of clinical manifestations in the double heterozygous condition is a function of how much normal β chain is produced by the thalassemia gene; the more hemoglobin A and F production, the milder the sickling. Hemoglobin C, D, and OArab interact with S to polymerize and hence produce a symptomatic phenotype. The more severe forms of this disease are life limiting but their life span and quality is improving. In addition, other factors, yet to be identified, impact upon the severity of the clinical outcome, since clinical severity varies among patients with SS disease.

Diagnosis

Although the clinical symptoms mentioned above may suggest sickle cell anemia, definitive diagnosis of this disease greatly relies on laboratory testing. The method of diagnosis is age dependent.

Prenatal testing: Chorionic villous sampling at 8–10 weeks of gestation; or, amniocentesis later in gestation, are the only reliable methods of prenatal diagnosis at this time.

Newborn screening: This is done with some variations in all 50 states. The possible reported results include: Hemoglobin F>S (homozygous sickle cell or sickle cell-β^0 thalassemia), F>A>S (sickle cell trait), F>S>A (sickle cell-β^+ thalassemia). If FAS and FSA are not distinguishable at birth, a repeat test at 3–6 months is rec-ommended. Often, the genotype of the child can be deduced from evaluating the parents' blood counts (MCV) and hemoglobin electrophoreses.

Undiagnosed children and adults: Diagnostic methods include complete blood counts, peripheral smear examination, cellulose acetate hemoglobin electrophoresis, citrate agar electrophoresis, thin layer isoelectric focusing, and solubility testing using dithionite. The "Sickledex," or dithionite solubility test, is positive if any sickle hemoglobin is present. Hence, it will not distinguish between sickle cell trait and more severe sickle syndromes.

Management

The management of these patients requires close observation, good access to care (primary, specialty, and acute care) and open communication between the patients and their physicians. The overall management of patients with clinically significant sickle syndromes should be under the supervision of a pediatric hematologist/oncol-ogist. The only "cure" for sickle cell anemia is hematopoietic stem cell transplantation. The following broad categories constitute most of the acute and chronic needs of these patients.

Acute management

1. *Fever*: Fever in patients with sickle cell anemia must be viewed with concern because of reduced or absent splenic function, potential opsonic defects, and the risk of septicemia. Knowledge of the immunization history, compliance with prophylactic antibiotic recommendations, recent exposures, specific foci of infection (e.g., otitis), and the general appearance of the child may allay some of the concern. Knowledge of the family, their proximity to the hospital, and the availability of transportation may influence the decision about hospital admission. If there is any possibility that the fever is due to septicemia, blood cultures are required. Antibiotics should be started empirically, and the child should be admitted for observation. Febrile patients should be adequately hydrated. Any patient with vomiting or compromised oral hydration requires parenteral hydration because of the inability to concentrate urine and conserve free water.

2. *Pain*: Pain crises must be managed with care. Hyper-hydration is essential with attention to avoid fluid overload and electrolyte imbalance. Young children are usually tolerant of increased fluid volume, especially since many of them start with some degree of dehydration secondary to isosthenuria, but as patients get older, the risk of fluid overload increases. Aggressive pain management is essential. While there is concern about the risk of addiction, most patients are well-educated with respect to pain management and by the time they come to the acute care clinic with a pain crisis, home analgesia has failed to alleviate their pain. Initial analgesic therapy should be provided and if rapid relief can be achieved, opiates can be tapered quickly and the patient released from the hospital. For patients with abdominal pain crises, there is the potential presence of other conditions that might be responsible for the symptoms (e.g., biliary disease or appendicitis). For patients with bone pain, the possibility of osteomyelitis must be considered.

3. *Stroke*: Patients with severe sickle cell syndromes should be enrolled in a program that monitors the blood velocity in their cerebral arteries by transcranial Doppler ultrasound (TCD). Accelerated flow indicates narrowing of vessels, recognition of which indicates the need for initiation of a hypertransfusion program to prevent the occurrence of an overt stroke. Stroke symptoms require rapid intervention to prevent further neurologic compromise. Exchange transfusion or erythrocytopheresis (erythrocyte exchange using the pheresis apparatus of the blood bank or pheresis service) are the methods of choice for reducing the percentage of hemoglobin S to 30% or less. If the patient has not been transfused recently and the blood bank does not know his/her complete red cell antigen phenotype, a blood specimen for this analysis should be sent with the type and cross match request. Most patients with sickle cell anemia are at increased risk of becoming sensitized to red cell antigens that are less frequent in patients of African extraction. Awareness of the complete red cell phenotype will make it simpler for the blood bank to obtain blood for future transfusions. These patients may require a program of hypertransfusion and iron chelation therapy indefinitely. Discontinuation of hypertransfusion may carry a high risk of recurrent stroke. For these patients hydroxyurea (to diminish the number of neutrophils, increase NO, and possibly increase the amount of hemoglobin F) may be beneficial.

4. *Priapism*: Priapism is a painful and embarrassing complication of sickle cell disease. It must be treated with hydration and analgesics. If it does not respond promptly, consider transfusion (not to exceed a hemoglobin >11g/dL). Epinephrine flushing of the corpora by a Pediatric Urologist may be useful in severe cases. Other surgical intervention may lead to permanent impotence.

5. *Pulmonary complications*: The initial management of pulmonary symptoms in the patient with SS Disease requires hydration and antibiotics, including azithromycin (for Mycoplasma). The development of progressive disease and respiratory compromise in the face of adequate hydration and antibiotic therapy

should increase the suspicion of ACS. Patients with ACS require full ICU support and reduction of the hemoglobin S in the blood to below 30%. This is accomplished most effectively with exchange transfusion or erythrocytopheresis (see above precaution regarding complete RBC antigen typing). Prolonged hypertransfusion therapy (with chelation) or hydroxyurea are indicated to prevent later complications. Once fluid homeostasis is established in the presence of ACS, over-hydration must be avoided to prevent worsening of the ACS. Ultimately, patients with a history of ACS may become candidates for hematopoietic stem cell transplantation, if a suitable donor is identified.

6. *Sequestration*: Splenic sequestration crisis is a true emergency. It is signaled by the presence of a rapidly enlarging spleen and a rapidly falling hemoglobin. Transfusion may be relatively ineffective as the spleen may not distinguish between sickle cells and normal cells in its destructive voracity. Caution is necessary as packed red cells are transfused since remobilization of the sequestered blood volume may precipitate congestive heart failure. Splenectomy is indicated as soon as the patient can be stabilized. Acute care physicians should be aware that patients with sickle-beta thalassemia may present with sequestration crises at a much older age than patients with homozygous sickle cell disease.

7. *Aplastic Crises*: Aplastic crises may occur in patients with sickle cell disease. These are no different from the aplastic crises that occur in other hemolytic anemias. The acute management of these crises with transfusion is discussed in the section with the other acute anemias.

Chronic management

1. *Vaccination*: All routine vaccines along with an annual flu vaccine are indicated. These patients should receive four conjugate pneumococcal vaccines (PCV-7) before 24 months of age and one Polysaccharide (PPV-23) vaccine every three to five years thereafter. The time interval between PCV-7 and PPV-23 should be a minimum of 8 weeks. Hyposplenic patients older than 2 years of age should be preferably vaccinated once with Meningococcal Conjugate vaccine (MCV-4). Those who have been previously vaccinated with the polysaccharide form (MPSV-4) should receive MCV-4 three years after their last dose of MPSV-4.

2. *Antibiotic prophylaxis*: Antibiotic prophylaxis against the encapsulated organisms is an essential part of these patients' management and should be started as soon as the sickle cell anemia is suspected. Oral Penicillin V is the recommended drug and should be prescribed at 125 mg twice daily until 3 years of age and then 250 mg twice daily indefinitely, if compliance is good. Prophylaxis for dental procedure is not indicated.

3. *Folic acid*: These children are at increased risk of folic acid deficiency due to enhanced utilization of folate for erythropoiesis. To prevent this problem, supplementation with 1 mg/day of oral Folic acid is recommended.

4. *Transcranial Doppler (TCD)*: All children with sickle cell anemia should receive an annual TCD to identify those at high risk for stroke. Those patients with confirmed excess velocity flow should subsequently receive preventive chronic transfusion. There are studies in progress to determine whether hydroxyurea therapy is equally effective.

5. *Ophthalmologic examination*: Children with severe sickle syndromes are at increased risk of proliferative sickle retinopathy and should have an annual eye examination starting at age 5.

6. *Cardiopulmonary*: Patients should be monitored for the development of pulmonary hypertension, as this may be a major cause of morbidity and mortality later in the course of the disease.

7. *Hydroxyurea*: There is growing evidence of beneficial effects of the use of hydroxyurea in patients with severe sickle syndromes. The benefits may result from suppression of the neutrophil count, increase in the hemoglobin F content of RBC, and increased availability of NO. There is a growing movement

toward a more widespread use of hydroxyurea to prevent or delay the onset and severity of complications in patients with milder or presymptomatic disease. Long-term therapy with hydroxyurea is usually well tolerated and is associated with few complications, but close monitoring for myelosuppression is required.

8. *Social*: NHLBI web site (includes family resources). http://www.sicklecell-info.org or Sickle Cell Disease Foundation www.scdfc.org.

Pearls and Precautions

School/education: Special services and educational resources are important for children with developmental impairments that are due to stroke or prolonged school absenteeism.

Sports: All sickle cell anemia patients should avoid strenuous exercise during hot days. The more severe patients should avoid trekking or climbing at high altitude. Patients with sickle trait should be encouraged to lead as normal lives as possible, but they develop isosthenuria, which creates a risk of dehydration, which, in turn, exacerbates sickling. Extreme exertion, especially in hot weather or at high altitudes may incur a risk of symptomatic sickling or rhabdomyolysis in patients with sickle trait. Coaches should be trained to watch for signs of dehydration and rhabdomyolysis. They should encourage athletes to maintain hydration during athletic training and competition.

Physical and occupational therapy (PT/OT): Like all stroke patients, these children may benefit from physical and occupational therapy.

References

Hagar W, Vichinsky E. Advances in clinical research in Sickle Cell Disease. Br J Haematol 2008; 141: 346–356.
Platt O. Hydroxyurea for the treatment of sickle cell anemia. N Engl J Med 2008; 358: 1362–1369.
Gladwin MT, Vichinsky E. Pulmonary complications of sickle cell disease. N Engl J Med 2008; 359: 2254–2265.

Acquired Hemolytic Anemias

A. Auto-Immune Hemolytic Anemias with Warm Antibodies (AIHA)

Stephen A. Feig, George B. Segel, Kenji Morimoto

Immune mediated hemolysis of the red cells may encompass allo- or auto-immune processes. Red cell destruction may occur in the spleen (extravascular) or the circulation (intravascular).

Etiology

There are several types of warm antibody auto-immune hemolytic anemias. The most common type occurs in younger children and is transient. The history may reveal an antecedent infection. Less frequently, chronic hemolysis is seen, as in older patients; these children are more likely to have an underlying immune dysregulation and destruction of other organs or blood cells may occur.

Various drugs may cause immune hemolytic anemia. Certain drugs bind to the red cell membrane and can be recognized by antibodies to the drug (hapten formation, as seen with penicillins and cephalosporins). Other drugs (e.g., quinidine) combine in a complex with a red cell antigen and an antibody that recognizes the drug and the red cell antigen. Other drugs (e.g., methyldopa) induce the production of true antibodies to red cell antigens.

Clinical Presentation and Prognosis

Demographics: AIHA is not specific to any race, but is more common in females than males.

Presenting signs and symptoms: The presentation of AIHA may be acute or subtle. The sudden, acute onset is manifested by weakness, fever, pallor, and jaundice, while the more subtle onset may only cause fatigue and pallor. The spleen may be enlarged with trapping of red cells coated with antibody.

Clinical course: The natural history of AIHA is variable. These children must be evaluated for the presence of an underlying disease process such as systemic lupus erythematosus, lymphoproliferative disease, or various acquired and congenital immunodeficiencies. The transient type usually responds to corticosteroid therapy during the early phase; treatment can be tapered as the patient responds, and eventually discontinued. The more chronic form may not respond well to corticosteroids and any underlying disease must be treated. This form of AIHA may have significant risk of mortality.

Prognosis: The transient forms of AIHA have a favorable prognosis, but the more chronic forms are associated with significant morbidity and mortality.

Diagnosis

The blood smear usually shows abundant spherocytic red blood cells and the direct antiglobulin test (DAT) usually is positive for IgG or complement coating of the red cells. When the amount of antibody present exceeds the target antigen on the surface of the red cells, excess antibody circulates in the plasma. This is detected by the indirect antibody test (IAT, or indirect Coombs' test). It is common for the antigen target of the antibody to be reactive against a "public" antigen, such as the Rh protein. This may make crossmatching of blood for transfusion difficult.

Management

A careful history of medications used is essential. Any potentially inciting medications should be discontinued immediately.

Mildly affected patients may require only observation, especially if their hemoglobin is maintained by increased erythropoiesis. More severe hemolysis, in which compensation cannot be maintained and anemia ensues, requires therapy with corticosteroids. Prednisone is usually begun at a dose of 2 mg/kg/day, although larger doses may be required in the face of extremely severe hemolysis. Treatment is continued at that dose until the rate of hemolysis subsides and the IAT is negative, at which time prednisone can be tapered, as tolerated.

The initial treatment of severe AIHA may require transfusion. Crossmatching of blood may be difficult if the antibody target is a "public" antigen. The blood bank may have to supply "the most compatible unit" and the physicians employ an "*in vivo* crossmatch." The efficacy of transfusion is transient, especially when the autoantibody recognizes the transfused cells. The treating physicians must work closely with the blood bank in the management of these patients. Plasmapheresis has been used to diminish the level of circulating antibody; it is of infrequent or transient benefit.

Treatment with prednisone can be discontinued when the DAT is negative. The DAT may remain positive after the hemoglobin has returned to normal levels. When prednisone fails to control the hemolysis or when high doses of prednisone are required for prolonged periods of time, alternative immunosuppression is preferable. Rituximab may be helpful in some of the patients with refractory disease. Therapy with intravenous immunoglobulin (IVIg) also may diminish hemolysis. Splenectomy may also be of benefit, but this approach must be used with caution because of the risk of overwhelming post-splenectomy infection. When splenectomy is considered, patients should be immunized with Hemophilus influenza type B vaccine, pneumococcal (pneumovax), and meningococcal vaccines before undergoing surgery. They should be treated with prophylactic antibiotics after surgery.

References

Packman CH. Hemolytic anemia due to warm antibodies. Blood Rev 2008; 22: 17-31.
Garvey B. Rituximab in the treatment of autoimmune haemolytic disorders. Br J Haematol 2008;141: 149–169.

B. Auto-Immune Hemolysis with "Cold" Antibodies

Stephen A. Feig, George B. Segel, Kenji Morimoto

This form of anemia is due to hemolysis following an infection that leads to the development of an IgM antibody to a public red cell antigen such as I or i. The antibody reacts with the red cell membrane and complement to induce intravascular hemolysis.

Etiology

"Cold" antibodies agglutinate red blood cells at temperatures below body temperatures. Maximum agglutination is at about 4°C, but the ability to lyse red cells *in vivo* depends upon the height of the antibody titer and the degree of residual activity at body temperature (thermal amplitude). These antibodies are of the IgM class, typically target the "public" I antigen system, and activate complement on the surface of the red blood cell. Neonatal red cells express the i antigen, which converts to I as the child matures. Typically, cold antibodies develop after infection with *Mycoplasma pneumoniae* or the Epstein-Barr virus (EBV), but may also be seen in association with lymphoproliferative disease. After Mycoplasma infection, the patient may develop high levels of anti-I antibody, sufficient to cause hemolysis. After EBV infection, patients may develop high titers of antibody to the i antigen. These rarely cause hemolysis because the red cell antigen has converted to I in most patients by the time they develop infectious mononucleosis.

Clinical Presentation and Prognosis

Demographics: Significant cold agglutinin hemolysis is more common in adults than in children.

Presenting signs and symptoms: In most adults this would be due to Mycoplasma infection or lymphoproliferative disease. If high titers of antibody are present and there is sufficient activity at body temperature, acute intravascular hemolysis may occur with hemoglobinemia and hemoglobinuria. Episodes of hemolysis may be triggered or exacerbated by exposure to cold (e.g., ingestion of cold liquids).

Diagnosis

The diagnosis is suggested by a falling hemoglobin, hemoglobinemia and hemoglobinuria. Red cell indices may be obscured by agglutination and rouleaux formation may be seen on the blood smear. The DAT will be positive for IgM and Complement. A "bed side cold agglutinin test" will often demonstrate reversible agglutination when a tube of anticoagulated blood is refrigerated.

Treatment

Glucocorticoid therapy is less effective in cold agglutinin disease than in warm antibody mediated hemolysis. Since the hemolysis is intravascular, splenectomy is rarely beneficial. Rituximab may be useful in reducing the production of the cold agglutinin and shortening the duration of hemolytic disease. Avoidance of exposure to cold diminishes hemolysis. Immunosuppression and plasmapheresis may be of benefit in severe cases. Any underlying illness should be treated.

Pearls and Precautions

Paroxysmal Cold Hemoglobinuria (PCH) is a unique immune hemolytic anemia in which an IgG cold-reactive auto-antibody (Donath Landsteiner Antibody) fixes complement at cold temperatures and lyses the red cells after the temperature is raised. This antibody has anti-P specificity. PCH is usually self-limited. It was associated with syphilis in the past, but now is seen mostly after viral infections. Treatment of severe cases requires transfusion and avoidance of cold temperatures.

Reference

Petz LD. Cold antibody autoimmune hemolytic anemias. Blood Rev 2008; 22: 1–15.

C. Paroxysmal Nocturnal Hemoglobinuria (PNH)

Stephen A. Feig, George B. Segel, Kenji Morimoto

PNH is an acquired disorder of hematopoiesis, in which a somatic mutation of the PIG-A gene reduces the membrane anchor protein that fastens the inhibitors of complement activation to the red cell surface. This renders the cells susceptible to complement lysis. The disease is in contrast to adults, rarely presents with night time intravascular hemolysis.

Clinical Presentation and Prognosis

Presenting signs and symptoms: Children with PNH usually present with thrombophilia or bone marrow failure. Thrombosis is believed to result from altered glycoproteins on the platelet surface which cause platelet activation. Thromboses may present with abdominal pain or headache. Bone marrow failure may be unilinear or trilinear. These patients are at risk of evolving into acute myelogenous leukemia.

Prognosis: This depends on the manifestations and the response to therapy.

Diagnosis

Previous clinical tests for PNH involved the activation of complement-mediated hemolysis in acid medium. These tests have been supplanted by reliable and sensitive detection of antigens (CD55 and CD59) on the surface of leukocytes by flow cytometry. PNH cells lack these complement-inhibitory surface proteins.

Management

The management of thrombophilia is covered in the section on *Thrombophilia*. Eculizumab, a monoclonal antibody against complement component C_5 has been reported to diminish hemolysis and thrombosis in adults. The management of bone marrow failure is covered in the section on *Bone Marrow Failure*. Hemolytic anemia may be controlled with glucocorticoids. Patients with significant chronic hemolysis may lose substantial iron as hemosiderin in the urine. Iron deficiency should be treated.

Nutritional Anemias

Stephen A. Feig, George B. Segel, Kenji Morimoto

These are a group of anemias that are due to nutritional deficiency in one or more of the components necessary for hematopoiesis.

Etiology

1. *Iron deficiency*: The most common nutritional anemia is due to iron deficiency. Anemia is a late manifestation of iron deficiency and iron stores must be depleted before a patient develops anemia. Iron deficiency may be aggravated by blood loss. Babies are born without iron stores. Since virtually all iron in the neonate is in the form of hemoglobin, premature infants are especially vulnerable to iron deficiency as they grow. This means that substantial iron intake is required to sustain growth of the red cell volume in parallel with body growth and that, in the absence of such intake, or the presence of iron loss, anemia will promptly occur. This occurs most often in toddlers whose main source of food is milk, which is poor in iron content, interferes with the absorption of iron, and may induce an enteropathy with malabsorption, protein loss, and bleeding. As children become anemic, they produce erythropoietin (EPO), which stimulates increased red cell production in the marrow. However, although more red cells are produced, increased hemoglobin production is not possible in the absence of iron. Thus, the characteristic hypochromic, microcytic, poikilocytic picture develops.

2. *Megaloblastic anemia (Vitamin B_{12} and Folic acid deficiency)*: Megaloblastic anemias are seen infrequently in children. Classical pernicious anemia is rarely seen in children. Deficiencies of vitamin B_{12} and folic acid may be the result of malabsorption, surgical loss of the stomach or terminal ileum, or extreme diets. Strict vegans will develop B_{12} deficiency and babies who drink only goat's milk will be at risk of folic acid deficiency. Vitamin B_{12} and folic acid are required for the conversion of homocysteine to methionine, and, ultimately, the production of the methyl donor, S-adenosyl methionine; B_{12} is required for the conversion of methylmalonyl-CoA to succinyl-CoA. Genetic disorders, such as methylmalonic aciduria, transcobalamin II deficiency, and orotic aciduria may also result in megaloblastic anemia. Megaloblastic anemia is a process of ineffective erythropoiesis in which erythroid progenitors in the marrow demonstrate dyskinetic maturation and nuclear maturation is slower than cytoplasmic maturation. Cells become larger as they fail to divide. White cell progenitors and megakaryocytes are affected; they become megaloblastic as well, and patients may develop leukopenia and thrombocytopenia. The blood smear shows macrocytosis, ovalocytosis, and hypersegmented neutrophils. Extreme ineffective erythropoiesis causes dramatic elevations of the serum AST and LDH.

3. *Vitamin E deficiency:* Another nutritional anemia is due to deficiency of Vitamin E. This is seen in patients with malabsorption including premature infants, children with celiac disease, cystic fibrosis, and abetalipoproteinemia. Vitamin E is a fat-soluble molecule that acts as an "oxidative sump" to protect red cell membrane unsaturated lipids from peroxidation. Red cells deficient in Vitamin E have more rigid membranes and are more susceptible to destruction. The peripheral blood smear is notable for extreme poikilocytosis.

Clinical Presentation and Prognosis

Presenting signs and symptoms: Patients present with the usual manifestations of anemia: pallor, lethargy, and reduced stamina. Children with severe iron deficiency may be extremely irritable. The classic presentation of Vitamin E deficiency in the premature infant is anemia, thrombocytosis and edema. Patients with Vitamin E deficiency may have sufficient hemolysis to become jaundiced. Patients with prolonged and severe Vitamin B_{12} deficiency may have neurologic symptoms.

Prognosis: The anemias of nutritional deficiency are correctable by replacement therapy. Underlying causes need to be treated. Sequelae of nutritional deficiencies such as neurologic impairment, may not be fully corrected by replacement therapy. Anemias due to genetic abnormalities of nutrient metabolism (very rare) may not be correctable.

Diagnosis

The differential diagnosis of a hypochromic, microcytic anemia is usually simple. The most common entity is iron deficiency. A history of excessive milk intake or bleeding may suggest this diagnosis. If the patient is severely anemic, the platelet count may be increased (suggesting the possibility of bleeding) or decreased. Other possible diagnoses of severe hypochromic microcytic anemia include β-thalassemia major, hemoglobin H disease (in which case hepatosplenomegaly is usually present), Hemoglobin E-thalassemia or one of the sideroblastic anemias (very rare). Studies of iron, iron binding capacity and ferritin should establish the diagnosis of iron deficiency. Basophilic stippling should raise the possibility of lead intoxication or β-thalassemia trait (see section on *Thalassemias*). The Mentzer index is often helpful in distinguishing between thalassemia trait and iron deficiency (See section on *Thalassemias*). If a diagnosis of iron deficiency anemia is made, the patient's stool should be tested for blood loss. While the anemia may be secondary to poor iron intake, it would be unfortunate to miss GI bleeding as an alternate cause. Other sources of blood loss (occult hemosiderinuria and pulmonary hemosiderosis) are rare and need be considered only in refractory or recurrent iron deficiency.

The presence of a megaloblastic anemia should not provide a major problem in diagnosis. It is important to establish the cause of the B_{12} or folic acid deficiency. If the B_{12} and folate levels are normal, testing for increased red cell adenosine deaminase (ADA) may suggest that the patient has Diamond-Blackfan Anemia. If the patient has diminished Vitamin E, the deficient vitamin can be replaced easily enough, but management of any underlying disease process will be critical to the outcome.

Management

Transfusion: As with other forms of severe anemia, the acute management of severe nutritional anemias requires transfusion (see section on Acute Management of Anemia).

Medications: Replacement of the deficient nutrient is necessary, but it is equally important to address the underlying cause, if possible. This would include institution of a gluten-free diet for patients with celiac disease, the administration of pancreatic enzyme replacement for patients with cystic fibrosis, resection of a bleeding Meckel's diverticulum, and the chelation of lead, to name a few instances of correctable underlying problems.

For iron deficient patients, the dose of supplemental elemental iron is 5–6 mg/kg/day. This usually is tolerated best in three equally divided doses of ferrous sulfate. Other preparations of polysaccharide iron may be given once per day. Milk intake should be restricted to a maximum of 16oz/day. Recovery from iron deficiency anemia occurs in the reverse steps in which it developed. Reticulocytosis is usually seen 4–7 days after the initiation of iron therapy. Thereafter, the hemoglobin usually increases by about 1g/week. The stores do not get replaced until after the hemoglobin has returned to normal. Iron therapy should be continued for 2–3 months after the hemoglobin has returned to normal.

Vitamin B_{12} deficiency is corrected with parenteral therapy. Various doses have been recommended. For children, a starting dose of 0.2µg/kg subcutaneously on two consecutive days has been recommended. Complete correction of the associated metabolic abnormalities must be monitored and doses adjusted accordingly. For patients with total inability to absorb B_{12}, monthly subcutaneous doses are recommended (100µg); an alternative regimen is 1000µg, every three months. For patients with inborn errors, such as deficiency of transcobalamin II, extraordinarily high doses of vitamin B_{12} are required, but may be administered orally.

Folic acid deficiency can be treated with oral folate (1 mg/day is more than sufficient). Dietary peculiarities should be corrected. Patients with underlying intestinal disease must have that treated. Vitamin E deficiency in premature infants should be avoided by the use of a Vitamin E containing formula. In older children, the underlying cause of fat malabsorption needs to be corrected.

References

Borgna-Pignotti C, Marsella M. Iron deficiency in infancy and childhood. Pediatr Ann 2008;37:329–337.

Whitehead VM. Acquired and inherited disorders of cobalamin and folate in children. Br J Haematol 2006; 134: 125–136.

Segel GB, Hirsh MG and Feig SA. Managing Anemia in a Pediatric Office Practice: Part 1. Pediatrics in Review 2002; 23(3):75–84.

Anemia of Chronic Disease

Stephen A. Feig, George B. Segel, Kenji Morimoto

This form of anemia is a secondary manifestation of many chronic disease states.

Etiology

The anemia of chronic disease is seen most frequently in association with end stage renal disease (ESRD) and chronic inflammatory states. In patients with chronic renal disease, the anemia is due, in part, to deficient production of erythropoietin (EPO), and this portion can be corrected by the administration of recombinant EPO.

There is another mechanism which has been elucidated recently, and is common to many chronic illnesses and inflammatory states. These patients produce excessive amounts of a small hepatic protein, hepcidin, which causes the internalization of an iron transporting protein, ferroportin, from the surface of cells. The internalized ferroportin is destroyed and this renders cells incapable of transporting iron. Thus, there is diminished iron absorption from the GI tract and reduced ability to effectively release iron recovered by the reticuloendothelial storage areas. Iron stores (ferritin) increase, serum iron is reduced, and iron-binding capacity (transferrin) is decreased.

Clinical Presentation and Prognosis

Presenting signs and symptoms: The clinical presentation of chronic anemia depends on the underlying problem. However, fatigue, pallor, lethargy, reduced stamina, and, if severe, irritability may occur.

Prognosis: The prognosis is that of the underlying condition.

Diagnosis

Anemia in the presence of an underlying chronic illness should suggest this diagnosis. Iron studies that document replete stores with low serum iron and normal or low transferrin in a patient with normal or hypochromic, microcytic red cell indices are consistent with the diagnosis. At present, measurement of hepcidin levels is not widely available, but increased hepcidin would be consistent with a diagnosis of anemia of chronic inflammatory disease.

Management

Transfusion: The treatment of the anemia of chronic disease is basically that of the underlying condition. In acutely symptomatic patients, the treatment of the anemia requires transfusion (see section on Acute Management of Anemias). Transfusion must be done with care to avoid problems of fluid overload, especially in patients with ESRD or borderline cardiac function.

Medications: Recombinant EPO is beneficial in patients with an inadequate natural EPO response to anemia (ESRD). Patients may require iron supplementation, in spite of the presence of normal iron stores, to provide an optimal response to erythropoietin.

References

Ganz T. Iron homeostasis: fitting the puzzle pieces together. Cell Metab 2008; 7: 288–290.

Nemeth E. Iron regulation and erythropoiesis. Curr Opin Hematol 2008; 15: 169–175.

Andrews NC. Forging a field. The golden age of iron biology. Blood 2008; 112: 219–230.

Methemoglobinemia

Stephen A. Feig, George B. Segel, Kenji Morimoto

Methemoglobinemia is a condition in which the heme iron of hemoglobin is in the ferric (Fe^{+3}) state, in which it is unable to bind oxygen. It is manifested by cyanosis in the presence of a normal arterial oxygen content (p_aO_2).

Etiology

In order to bind oxygen, the iron atoms in hemoglobin must be in the reduced, or ferrous (Fe^{+2}) state. In normal individuals, about 1% of the iron in hemoglobin is oxidized to the ferric (Fe^{+3}) state every day, producing methemoglobin, which is incapable of binding and carrying oxygen. Under conditions of oxidative stress, such as seen with the administration of oxidant medications, the production of methemoglobin increases. The process is reversed by a red cell enzyme, methemoglobin reductase (MHR, or NADH-Cytochrome b_5 Reductase), which reduces the ferric heme to the ferrous state.

In most cases, methemoglobinemia is due to a combination of increased oxidant stress and diminished red cell content of MHR. Newborns are normally deficient in MHR and are more susceptible to developing methemoglobinemia. Rarely, methemoglobinemia is the result of a hemoglobinopathy, the M hemoglobins. There are at least five mutant methemoglobins whose structure renders the heme iron more susceptible to oxidation. These proteins are unstable and cause some degree of concurrent hemolysis. At baseline, these patients have a higher methemoglobin level than those with methemoglobinemia due to MHR deficiency.

Clinical Presentation and Prognosis

Presenting signs and symptoms: Patients with methemoglobinemia are usually asymptomatic, in spite of cyanosis, and they may have no distress or signs of cardiac or pulmonary disease. This is the clue that should suggest the possibility of methemoglobinemia. The history may be helpful if there is a report of previous episodes of asymptomatic cyanosis on exposure to oxidant medications.

Methemoglobin has an absorption spectrum that differs from that of ferro-hemoglobin, and this produces the difference in color that results in clinical cyanosis. The intensity of cyanosis with methemoglobin is greater than with deoxy-hemoglobin. Cyanosis due to methemoglobin can be observed at concentrations of 2g/dL, while about 5g/dL of deoxyhemoglobin are required to produce clinically detectable cyanosis.

Prognosis: Methemoglobinemia is usually a benign condition. Patients are relatively asymptomatic and tolerate surprisingly high levels of methemoglobin well (see Table 7.4) The infant enzyme deficiency is transient, but the congenital forms of the disease persist throughout life.

Table 7.4: Symptoms of Methemoglobinemia

% Methemoglobin	Symptoms
15 – 40%	Cyanosis
40 – 60%	Headache, lethargy
60 – 75%	Stupor
>75%	Death

Diagnosis

The methemoglobin content of blood can be measured by a simple blood test. A presumptive test can be done at the bedside to differentiate the cyanosis of hypoxia from that of methemoglobinemia. Hypoxic blood exposed to air will reoxygenate quickly and become "pink," while methemoglobin will not oxygenate and remains a blue-brown color. This can be observed in a tube of anticoagulated blood or a drop of blood on a piece of filter paper. The important issue is to think of the possibility of methemoglobinemia in the cyanotic patient.

Treatment

Medication: Most patients with methemoglobinemia require no therapy other than diminution of any external oxidant stress. If therapy is required because of symptoms, administration of methylene blue is indicated. This increases the passage of glucose metabolism through the hexose monophosphate shunt and increases the availability of NADPH and reduced glutathione (GSH). There are alternate pathways of methemoglobin reduction using these substrates, although they are less efficient than the usual NADH-dependent enzyme. The dose of methylene blue is 1 mg/kg, administered slowly, intravenously. There are three issues to be considered when treating a patient with methylene blue:

1. Since methylene blue is an oxidant, excess administration may worsen the methemoglobinemia;
2. patients with concomitant G6PD deficiency may have a hemolytic reaction to the administration of methylene blue and fail to make the NADPH available for the alternate pathway of methemoglobin reduction; and,
3. Methylene blue may be excreted in the urine, resulting in the production of blue urine.

Transfusion: Those rare patients with methemoglobinemia who require therapy and in whom oxidant therapy is contraindicated, may be treated with exchange transfusion.

Pearls and Precautions

Methemoglobinemia is a remarkably well-tolerated condition. Oxidant medications and chemicals, such as those which cause hemolysis in patients with G6PD deficiency, may exacerbate the degree of cyanosis (see Table 7.2).

Reference

Percy MJ, Lappen TR. Recessive congenital methaemoglobinaemia: cytochrome b_5 reductase deficiency. Br J Haematol 2008; 141: 298–308.

Aplastic Pancytopenias

Stephen A. Feig, George B. Segel, Kenji Morimoto

Aplastic pancytopenias result when the marrow production of two or more of the formed elements in the blood are diminished.

Etiology

There are both acquired and congenital causes of general marrow failure in children. These result clinically in bicytopenia or pancytopenia. The acquired forms are most common and may be secondary to antecedent viral infection (most common), autoimmune (T-cell mediated) aplasia, or direct drug or chemical toxicity. Alternatively, aplastic pancytopenia may be the result of an inherited disorder (see Table 7.5). It is often impossible to identify a specific etiology for acquired aplasia.

Fanconi anemia is a rare disorder characterized by gradual onset of aplastic pancytopenia. The hematologic features may appear as early as the newborn period or as late as adulthood. It may be associated with a variety of dysmorphic anatomic features including short stature, radius and thumb anomalies, microcephaly, microphthalmia, renal anomalies, and others. As more patients have been entered into the International Fanconi Anemia Registry, it has been recognized that a third or more of patients with FA have no associated congenital anomalies. The disorder is due to mutation of one or more molecules which interact in the process of DNA repair. The hematologic manifestations may reflect a myelodysplastic disorder, and there is a strong predilection to the development of acute leukemia. There also is a risk of developing multiple other forms of cancer at a young age.

Table 7.5: Inherited Pancytopenias

Disease

- Fanconi Anemia (FA)
- Dyskeratosis Congenita
- Cartilage Hair Hypoplasia
- Reticular Dysgenesis
- Osteopetrosis
- Familial Marrow Dysfunction
- Dubowitz' Syndrome
- Seckel's Syndrome
- Pearson's Syndrome

Dyskeratosis congenita is an extraordinarily rare disorder characterized by reticulated hyperpigmentation of the skin, dystrophic nails, and leukoplakia, in addition to marrow aplasia. There are different genes involved since the inheritance pattern is varied; the disorder can be detected by the presence of telomere shortening.

Osteopetrosis is an inherited disorder in which osteoclasts fail to reabsorb bone. As a result, there is bone overgrowth which obliterates the marrow space and narrows bony neural foramina. Cranial nerves are damaged by the narrowing of the bony foramina. Hematopoiesis is shifted to extramedullary sites. This results in pancytopenia and often leukoerythroblastosis, i.e., the appearance of immature granulocytes, nucleated red cells, and tailed poikilocytes in the blood. A plain radiograph will document the density of the bones.

Clinical Presentation and Prognosis

Presenting signs and symptoms: The manifestations of aplastic pancytopenia are due to the presence of anemia, neutropenia, thrombocytopenia and (rarely) lymphopenia; the latter usually is only seen in Cartilage-Hair Hypoplasia and Reticular Dysgenesis. The cytopenias may arise suddenly or gradually, and they may manifest together or individually.

Anemia presents with pallor, lethargy, reduced stamina and, if severe, tachycardia and heart failure. Neutropenia results in increased risk of severe bacterial infection. Significant risk of infection increases with absolute neutrophil counts (total WBC x percent neutrophils and bands) below $500/\mu L$ and increases rapidly if neutropenia is more severe. Thrombocytopenia causes petechiae, purpura and bleeding from the nose, gums, gastrointestinal tract, genitourinary tract or wounds. These may occur at platelet counts below $20–30,000/\mu L$, but spontaneous, severe, life-threatening bleeding is not usually seen in children with platelet counts greater than $10,000/\mu L$. Lymphopenia results in defects of cell-mediated and humoral immunity, with increased susceptibility to viral and fungal infections, and poor antibody response to immunizations and infections.

Splenic enlargement may be seen in the presence of malignancy, or in case of extramedullary hematopoiesis. It is not seen in T-cell mediated immune aplasia.

Prognosis: The prognosis of aplastic pancytopenia is guarded. If the aplasia is severe, it is a life-threatening condition that requires both supportive and definitive therapy. It is essential to define a cause, if possible. In particular, the identification of exposure to a specific causative agent, such as a drug or toxin, may allow the condition to be reversed by eliminating exposure to that agent. The identification of specific genetic causes of aplasia, while rare, are indicative of the need for tailoring therapy to the specific disease. It is essential that patients with aplastic pancytopenia be under the care of a Pediatric Hematologist experienced in the supportive and definitive management of such patients.

Diagnosis

1. *History and physical examination:* A careful history is the first step in diagnosis of a specific cause of aplastic anemia. A history of drug exposure, chemical exposure, or hepatitis may suggest secondary disease. A detailed family history may reveal affected relatives, suggesting an inherited form of disease. A complete and careful physical examination is necessary and it is particularly important to look for those features which might characterize one of the congenital aplastic syndromes. However, even in patients with FA, 30–40% of patients may have none of the dysmorphic stigmata associated with the syndrome so that testing for chromosome fragility is indicated in all patients with bone marrow failure. If such patients are treated with hematopoietic stem cell transplantation (HSCT), the conditioning regimen must be

adapted to the presence of FA or DC because the defect in DNA repair puts them at risk of a deadly exfoliative response to alkylating agents.

2. *Laboratory examinations:* The CBC will determine the immediate severity of the cytopenias. A chemistry panel and serologies will assess the possibility of recent hepatitis. Selective cultures are required for the neutropenic patient who presents with fever. The bone marrow aspirate and biopsy are necessary to assess whether the cytopenias are due to aplasia, peripheral cell destruction, or marrow infiltration with malignancy, fibrosis, or a storage disease. Paroxysmal nocturnal hemoglobinuria (PNH) is a rare cause of aplastic pancytopenia in children; the diagnosis is made by the identification of deficient membrane CD55 and CD59 by flow cytometry (Table 7.6).

Management

Medication: The neutropenic, febrile patient should be evaluated with cultures and treated initially with parenteral broad-spectrum empiric antibiotics (e.g., ceftazidime) and ultimately with specific antibiotics. The use of hematopoietic growth factors such as erythropoietin or G-CSF, is not usually successful. Patients in whom exposure to a potentially causative agent has been identified should have that exposure terminated immediately.

Acquired aplastic pancytopenia usually is the result of a T-cell mediated auto-immune process, and immunotherapy is available for those patients who do not have a compatible donor for HSCT. Fifty to seventy percent of patients treated with anti-thymocyte globulin and cyclosporine show significant improvement in their blood counts and bone marrow cellularity within several months of starting treatment. In some cases the results are complete and lasting, but relapses occur in about thirty percent of responding patients.

Transfusion: The acute management of the patient with aplastic anemia is supportive. Anemia is treated with packed RBC transfusions. Thrombocytopenia is treated with platelet transfusions.

Transfusion products must be leukoreduced to diminish the risk of sensitization to major histocompatibility antigens. However, since even leukoreduced blood products may sensitize the patient to minor histocompatibility antigens, it is important to limit transfusions to the minimum necessary for safe supportive care, unless the possibility of HSCT has been ruled out. Transfusions from related donors should be avoided to diminish the risk of sensitization, in the event HSCT is required.

Transplant: The definitive treatment of aplastic pancytopenia is HSCT, if a matched donor is available. This is especially true for patients with congenital forms of aplasia, who are at increased risk of developing leukemia, but it is important to be certain that a sibling donor is unaffected, before proceeding with HSCT for congenital aplastic anemia. It is also true for patients with post-hepatitic aplasia and patients whose aplasia is due to PNH.

Table 7.6:   Work-up of Patient with Aplastic Pancytopenia

Laboratory Test

- Complete Blood Count, with differential, reticulocytes, indices and smear
- Chemistry Panel, including liver function tests
- Hepatitis serologies
- Bone marrow aspirate and biopsy
- Leukocyte CD 55 and CD 59
- Chromosome Fragility: If increased look for FANC mutations
- Telomere length assay: If short telomeres, assay for known Dyskeratosis mutations

Consultations: All patients with aplastic pancytopenia should be under the care of a pediatric hematologist, experienced in the care of these patients and with HSCT. For the patients with congenital syndromes of aplasia, or with other organ system involvement, appropriate additional subspecialty consultation may be indicated.

Social: Fanconi Anemia Research Fund (includes family resources) http://www.fanconi,org/index.htm
    International Fanconi Anemia Registry (Director: Arlene Auerbach, M.D.) http://www.rockefeller.edu/labheads/auerbach/description.php

Aplastic Anemia and MDS International Foundation (includes family resources) http://www.aamds.org/aplastic

Monitoring: Longitudinal follow-up for patients with marrow aplasia is necessary. This is particularly true for patients with congenital forms of aplasia, such as Fanconi Anemia, who are susceptible to other complications that are not corrected with resolution of the aplasia, such as secondary cancers.

References

Guinan EC. Acquired aplastic anemia in childhood. Hematol/Oncol Clin North Am. 2009; 23: 171–191.

Green AM, Kupfer GM. Fanconi anemia. Hematol Oncol Clin North Am 2009; 23: 193–214.

Tamary H, Alter BP. Current diagnosis of inherited bone marrow failure syndromes. Pediatr Hematol Oncol 2007; 24: 87–99.

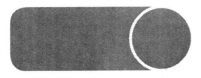 *Bleeding Disorders*

Congenital Factor Deficiencies (Hemophilioid States)

George B. Segel, Stephen A. Feig, Kenji Morimoto

Hemophilioid states include inherited deficiencies of one or more of the soluble clotting factors (proteins) that result in a propensity to bleed.

Etiology

Hemophilia A and B are the two most common inherited defects in the soluble clotting factors, factor VIII and factor IX, respectively. The functional deficiencies in these clotting factors result from abnormalities in their respective X-linked genes. Males are primarily affected, but carrier females may have excessive inactivation of the normal X-chromosome and hence low factor levels. Less commonly, a homozygous female or one with Turner syndrome may be symptomatic. The genes have been cloned and numerous gene alterations have been described. About half the patients with severe hemophilia A have a gene inversion that blocks the expression of factor VIII. Other gene mutations may result in dysfunctional Factor VIII and Factor IX proteins. Patients with severe hemophilia have less than 1% clotting factor activity; moderate hemophilics have 1 to 5% activity, and mild hemophilics have greater than 5% factor activity. Spontaneous bleeding usually occurs only in those patients with severe, or occasionally in moderate, hemophilia.

Other factor deficiencies are less common. Factor XI deficiency usually results in a much milder bleeding diathesis and is seen most often in patients of Ashkenazi Jewish extraction who are homozygotes or compound heterozygotes for this gene defect. It is inherited as an autosomal recessive trait. Deficiency of other factor activities are rare. Deficiencies in factors II, V, VII, X, and XIII also are inherited as autosomal recessive conditions and hetrozygotes rarely have any bleeding tendency.

The traditional view of the clotting cascade is shown in Figure 7.1. Activation of factor X can occur through the interaction of tissue factor and factor VII (extrinsic pathway) or through factors XII, XI, IX and VIII (intrinsic pathway). Activated factor X, in conjunction with factor V, then converts prothrombin to thrombin and, sequentially, fibrinogen to the fibrin clot. The question that arises is why the hemophiliacs bleed if the extrinsic pathway via tissue factor and factor VII is operative. This has been explained by demonstrating that hemostasis occurs on the surfaces of tissue factor bearing cells and on platelets. FVIIa/TF cannot make up for a lack of factor VIII or factor IX because it makes FXa on the wrong cell surface, i.e., the injured tissue, but not on the platelet surface. Activated factor VIII and factor IX are required to provide platelet surface factor X_a. Thus, the absence of either factor VIII or factor IX impairs the production of factor X_a on the platelet surface which is essential for adequate hemostasis.

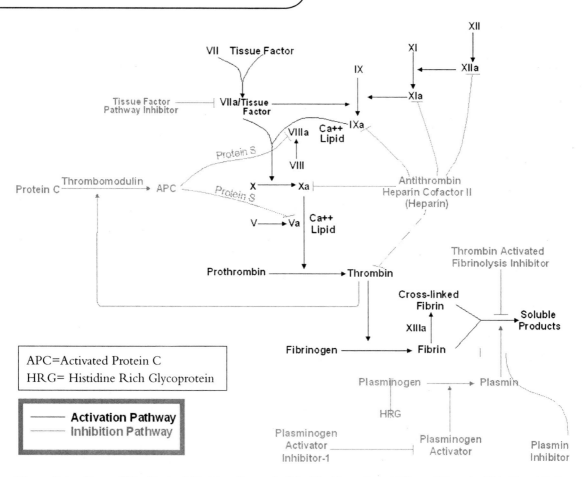

Figure 7.1: View of The Typical Clotting Cascade (Modified from Segel GB, and Francis CW. Blood Cells, Molecules and Diseases. 2000;26:542.)

Clinical Presentation and Prognosis

Demographics: The prevalence of hemophilia is 1/5000 males, and approximately 85% of these patients have factor VIII deficiency. It was classically described among the descendants of Queen Victoria, including the family of the last czar of Russia, Nicholas II.

Presenting signs and symptoms: Patients with hemophilia A or hemophilia B may have bleeding manifestations at birth. Vaginal delivery is recommended without vacuum extraction or the use of forceps. Intracranial hemorrhage occurs in 1–4% of babies regardless of the mode of delivery, and approximately one third of affected males bleed at circumcision. Excess bruising may occur with minor trauma, and the hallmark of severe hemophilia is the development of spontaneous hemarthroses. Less commonly, bleeding may occur into muscles, gastrointestinal tract, or central nervous system.

Clinical course: Bleeding manifestations usually are seen when the child becomes mobile as a toddler. Bleeding may be a particular problem if a mildly affected patient is undiagnosed and subjected to a surgical procedure. At the time of dental extraction, the bleeding may be well-controlled in the dental operatory because platelets and von Willebrand factor are normal, but the patient bleeds somewhat later because a definitive fibrin clot does not form.

Prognosis: The prognosis for hemophiliac patients has markedly improved with the development of recombinant factors, prophylactic treatment, comprehensive orthopedic care and new agents and techniques to deal with the development of inhibitors.

Diagnosis

The initial finding in a patient with a history of bleeding is a prolonged activated partial thromboplastin time (aPTT) with a normal prothrombin time (PT). The prolonged aPTT reflects a deficiency in factor VIII, IX, XI or XII. The definitive diagnosis of any of these factor deficiencies depends on the factor assays and molecular genetic diagnosis is not required. Factor XII deficiency does not cause a tendency to bleed, although it markedly prolongs the aPTT. Indeed, Factor XII deficiency may produce a thrombophilic state. Deficiency of factor XI results in a variable bleeding tendency.

If an inhibitor of factor VIII or IX is present, the prolonged aPTT will not be corrected if the patient's plasma is mixed with normal plasma. Factor deficiencies will be corrected with this mixing study.

Management

Routine Treatment: The treatment of hemophilia A and B requires administration of the appropriate recombinant factor preparation. For non-life threatening bleeding episodes such as tooth extraction, joint, muscle, or nose bleeding, correction to ~50% level is usually sufficient to control the bleeding. For life-threatening bleeding such as massive gastrointestinal or CNS (brain or spinal cord) bleeding, correction to 100% level is indicated. (Table 7.7)

Prophylactic treatment: With the availability of recombinant replacement products, prophylaxis has become the standard of care for most children with severe hemophilia to prevent spontaneous bleeding and early joint deformities. The results of prophylaxis have been impressive in the prevention of chronic joint disease. If target joints develop, "secondary" prophylaxis is often initiated.

Prophylactic administration of recombinant factor every 2–3 days may be appropriate for those patients with frequent and severe bleeding. The dose is adjusted to produce a factor level of 1–2% just before the administration of the next dose. Prophylactic factor administration is usually started after the first episode of bleeding into a joint and it is effective in preventing future joint damage. In young patients, this usually requires a venous access "port." Older children may be able to get prophylactic factor without placement of central venous access. While this approach is more expensive than episodic therapy, the improved quality of life and avoidance of future orthopedic surgery have made this the standard of care.

Patients with inhibitors: Patients with the most severe molecular defects such as inversions, nonsense mutations, or large deletions or insertions are most likely to develop inhibitors since they make no normal coagulation protein. The level of the inhibitor or antibody against a coagulation factor is measured in Bethesda units (BUs). One Bethesda unit is the amount of inhibitor that will neutralize 50% of factor activity. Patients with more that 5BUs are considered "high responders" of inhibitor activity, and tend to markedly increase this level if factor is given. Patients with less than 5BUs are "low responders" and can be treated with increased amounts of recombinant factor to overwhelm the inhibitor. For those patients who are high responders and are bleeding, preparations with bypassing activity are available to activate hemostasis.

These include recombinant factor VIIa, prothrombin complex concentrates and factor eight inhibitor bypassing activity (FEIBA). These preparations should only be used under the supervision of a pediatric

Table 7.7: Treatment of Hemophilia

Type of Hemorrhage	Hemophilia A	Hemophilia B
Hemarthrosis[*]	• 40 IU/kg factor VIII concentrateb[†] on day 1; then 20 IU/kg on days 2,3,5 until joint function is normal or back to baseline. Consider additional treatment every other day for 7–10 days. Consider prophylaxis.	• 60–80 IU/kg on day 1; then 40 IU/kg on days 2,4. Consider additional treatment every other day for 7–10 days. Consider prophylaxis.
Muscle or significant subcutaneous hematoma	• 50 IU/kg factor VIII concentrate; may need 20 IU/Kg factor VIII every-other-day treatment until resolved.	• 40-80 IU/kg factor IX concentratec[‡]; may need treatment every 2–3 days until resolved.
Mouth, deciduous tooth, or tooth extraction	• 20 IU/kg factor VIII concentrate; antifibrinolytic therapy; remove loose	• 40 IU/kg factor IX concentratec[‡]; antifibrinolytic therapyd[§]; remove loose deciduous tooth.
Epistaxis	• Apply pressure for 15–20 min; pack with petrolatum gauze; give antifibrinolytic therapy; 20 IU/kg factor VIII concentrate if this treatment fails.[**]	• Apply pressure for 15–20 min; pack with petrolatum gauze; antifibrinolytic therapy; 30 IU/kg factor IX concentratec[‡] if this treatment fails.
Major surgery, life-threatening hemorrhage	• 50–75 IU/kg factor VIII concentrate, then initiate continuous infusion of 2–4 IU/kg/hr to maintain factor VIII > 100 IU/dL for 24 hr, then give 2–3 IU/kg/hr continuously for 5–7 days to maintain the level at > 50 IU/dL and an additional 5–7 days at a level of > 30 IU/dL.	• 120 IU/kg factor IX concentratec, then 50–60 IU/kg every 12–24 hr to maintain factor IX at > 40 IU/dL for 5–7 days, and then > 30 IU/dL for 7 days.
Iliopsoas hemorrhage	• 50 IU/kg factor VIII concentrate, then 25 IU/kg every 12 hr until asymptomatic, then 20 IU/kg every other day for a total of 10–14 days.[||]	• 120 IU/kg factor IX concentratec; then 50–60 IU/kg every 12–24 hr to maintain factor IX at > 40 IU/dL until asymptomatic, then 40–50 IU every other day for a total of 10–14 days.[||]
Hematuria	• Bed rest; 1½ × maintenance fluids; if not controlled in 1–2 days, 20 IU/kg factor VIII concentrate; if not controlled, give prednisone (unless HIV-infected).	• Bed rest; 1½ × maintenance fluids; if not controlled in 1–2 days, 40 IU/kg factor IX concentratec[‡]; if not controlled, give prednisone (unless HIV-infected).
Prophylaxis	20–40 IU/kg factor VIII concentrate every other day to achieve a trough level of ≥ 1%.	30–50 IU/kg factor IX concentrate[‡] every 2–3 days to achieve a trough level of ≥ 1%.

NOTE: Adapted from Montgomery RR, Gill JC, Scott JP: Hemophilia and von Willebrand disease. In Nathan DG, Orkin SH (editors): Nathan and Oski's Hematology of Infancy and Childhood, 5th ed. Philadelphia, WB Saunders, 1998.

* For hip hemarthrosis, orthopedic evaluation for possible aspiration is advisable to prevent avascular necrosis of the femoral head.

† For mild or moderate hemophilia, desmopressin, 0.3 µg/kg, should be used instead of factor VIII concentrate, if the patient is known to respond with a hemostatic level of factor VIII; if repeated doses are given, monitor factor VIII levels for tachyphylaxis.

‡ Stated doses apply for recombinant factor IX concentrate; for plasma-derived factor IX concentrate, use 70% of the stated dose.

§ Do not give antifibrinolytic therapy until 4–6 hr after a dose of prothrombin complex concentrate.

** OTC coagulant-promoting products may be helpful.

|| Repeat radiologic assessment should be performed before discontinuation of therapy.

hematologist. Patients with inhibitors also can be treated by the regular administration of factor to induce immune tolerance and other immunosuppressive interventions.

Alternate therapy for mild hemophilia: With mild factor VIII hemophilia, the patient's endogenously produced factor VIII can be released by the administration of desmopressin acetate. In patients with moderate or severe factor VIII deficiency, the stored levels of factor VIII in the body are inadequate, and desmopressin treatment is ineffective. The risk of exposing the patient with mild hemophilia to transfusion-transmitted diseases and the cost of recombinant products warrant the use of desmopressin, if it is effective. A concentrated intranasal form of desmopressin acetate (Stimate) also can be used to treat patients with mild hemophilia A. The dose is 150 µg (1 puff) for children weighing <50 kg and 300 µg (2 puffs) for children and young adults weighing >50 kg. Most centers administer a trial of desmopressin to determine the level of factor VIII achieved after its infusion. Desmopressin is not effective in the treatment of factor IX–deficient hemophilia.

Social/support: NHLBI website, includes family resources:

> http://www.nhlbi.nih.gov/health/dci/Diseases/hemophilia/hemophilia_what.html
> National Hemophilia Foundation: http://www.hemophilia.org

Pearls and Precautions

Likely complications: Patients with hemophilia are susceptible to severe chronic arthropathy from repeated joint bleeding, the development of inhibitors to the infused corrective products, as well as to life-threatening hemorrhagic episodes. The issue of plasma-borne infections (i.e. hepatitis and HIV) has been markedly reduced by the availability of the recombinant factor products. Both their acute and chronic management still can be very complex and is best done in a comprehensive hemophilia or coagulation center. Patients who live at a distance from the Hemophilia Treatment Center may be cared for by a local physician with the assistance and consultation of a hematologist experienced in the care of hemophilia patients.

Skin and dental care: See Table 7.7.

School/education: Precautions appropriate to patients with a bleeding tendency are indicated, including avoidance of contact sports and "off the floor" activities (e.g., rope climbing, pole vaulting, etc.)

Medication avoidance: Medications that interfere with platelet function (e.g., NSAIDs and aspirin) should be avoided.

References

Hoffman M. A cell-based model of coagulation and the role of factor VIIa. Blood Reviews 2003; 17 Suppl 1: S1–5.

Hedner U, Ginsburg D, Lusher JM et al. Congenital Hemorrhagic Disorders: New Insights into the Pathophysiology and Treatment of Hemophilia. Hematology 2000; 241–265.

Hemorrhagic Disease of the Newborn

George B. Segel, Stephen A. Feig, Kenji Morimoto

Etiology

Hemorrhagic disease of the newborn results from a deficiency of vitamin K dependent coagulant factors in the newborn period. It may occur in the first few days of life or weeks later.

Clinical Presentation and Prognosis

Early hemorrhagic disease of the newborn: Factors II (prothrombin), VII, IX, and X require vitamin K for the final gamma glutamyl carboxylation step in their processing. These coagulation factors decrease during the first 3 to 4 days after birth and this results in bleeding. The administration of vitamin K tends to prevent this decrease, and effectively prevents classic, early occurring (first few days after birth) hemorrhagic disease of the newborn. Early occurring hemorrhagic disease is most often associated with maternal consumption of medications such as phenytoin (Dilantin) and warfarin, which reduce the vitamin K-dependent factors. Early hemorrhage can be prevented by administration of vitamin K to the mother in the 2–4 weeks prior to delivery. In rare cases, no contributing factor is found.

Late hemorrhagic disease of the newborn: Neonatal hemorrhage also may occur later at 2 to 12 weeks after birth, as a result of lack of vitamin K, and is called late hemorrhagic disease of the newborn or acquired pro-thrombin complex deficiency. The etiology of the deficiency of vitamin K is unclear but it may result from poor dietary intake particularly related to breast feeding, alterations in liver function with cholestasis and decreased vitamin K absorption, or a toxic or infectious impairment of hepatic utilization. Unfortunately, intracranial hemorrhage frequently is the presenting event in this condition. This problem can be prevented by parenteral or oral vitamin K, but the preferred route of administration remains controversial. The parenteral route rarely may result in neuromuscular complications. Oral administration, however, appears less reliable and may require repeated doses. The current recommendation of the American Academy of Pediatrics suggests that vitamin K_1, 0.5 to 1 mg, be administered intramuscularly at birth. Even the lower (0.5 mg) parenteral dose may be excessive for preterm (<32 week) infants, although no toxic effects have been reported as a result of high plasma values. Recent data suggest that 0.2 mg Vitamin K may be appropriate prophylaxis for infants delivered at fewer than 32 weeks gestation, but additional oral supplementation is needed when feeding is established.

Treatment: The treatment of bleeding infants requires the expertise of a pediatric hematologist. Vitamin K, 1–2 mg, should be administered intramuscularly or subcutaneously and supplemented with fresh frozen plasma, prothrombin concentrate or recombinant factor VIIa, depending on the severity of the hemorrhage.

Coagulopathy of Liver Disease

George B. Segel, Stephen A. Feig, Kenji Morimoto

Etiology

Liver failure from any cause may impair the synthesis of coagulation factors II, V, VII, IX and X.

The diminished factor V distinguishes this problem from vitamin K deficiency in which factors II, VII, IX and X are not carboxylated and hence are inactive, although the profactors are synthesized. Both the PT and PTT are prolonged in liver disease and in vitamin K deficiency.

Clinical Presentation and Prognosis

Presenting signs and symptoms: Bleeding from the upper GI tract is the most common type of bleeding seen in severe liver disease. This may be particularly severe if the liver disease is complicated by the presence of esophageal varicies. Other bleeding may occur from larger vessels and is characteristic of that seen in defects of the soluble coagulation factors. Capillary bleeding such as gum bleeding, superficial bruising and epistaxis is less of a problem, unless the liver disease is complicated by hypersplenism and thrombocytopenia.

Management

Medications: Vitamin K should be given, 1–2 mg SC or IM x 1, to correct any component of vitamin K deficiency. Alternatively, 2.5–5 mg, by mouth, per day, as needed, can be used for maximum PT and PTT correction. For the bleeding patient, slow infusion of IV vitamin K may be used. However, the patient must be observed for anaphylaxis.

Transfusion: For those patients who are actively bleeding or who require surgery, fresh frozen plasma may be used in an attempt to fully correct the PT and PTT. Adequate correction may not be possible because of the complicating volume overload induced by plasma infusion. Other factor preparations such as prothrombin concentrates or activated factor VII (Novoseven) are available, but should be administered under the supervision of a pediatric hematologist.

Pearls and Precautions

Consultations: Communication is required among the primary physician, the hematologist, gastroenterologist, and any other physicians caring for these complex patients.

Monitoring: Hemostasis should be monitored by measurement of the PT, aPTT, deficient factors (II, V, VII, IX, X, and Fibrinogen) and the platelet count, in conjunction with a hematologist.

Von Willebrand Disease

George B. Segel, Stephen A. Feig, Kenji Morimoto

Von Willebrand disease results from a hereditary or acquired deficiency of von Willebrand factor; this factor is required for initial hemostasis in the formation of a "platelet plug." The factor also adheres to Factor VIII and prevents its clearance from the plasma; therefore, patients deficient in von Willebrand factor also show diminished levels of circulating Factor VIII.

Etiology

The various types of von Willebrand disease usually result from inherited molecular changes in a large multimeric plasma protein that is synthesized in endothelial cells and megakaryocytes. It is stored in the Weibel-Palade bodies of endothelial cells and in the alpha granules of platelets. Von Willebrand factor adheres to platelets and binds to the damaged site in a blood vessel wall. Additional platelets are attracted to the site of injury, and blood coagulation proceeds in the tissue and on the platelet surface. Furthermore, von Willebrand factor serves as the carrier for Factor VIII, preventing its rapid clearance from the plasma. When there is diminished von Willebrand factor, there often is consequent diminution in the Factor VIII level. There are three major types and at least seven total subtypes of von Willebrand disease resulting from diminished quantity or poorly functional von Willebrand factor (Table 7.8).

Von Willebrand disease also may be acquired and result from antibodies directed against and inhibiting von Willebrand factor. Acquired von Willebrand disease has been associated with collagen vascular, myeloproliferative and B-cell disorders. There also may be loss of the large von Willebrand multimers in children with congenital heart defects. In these conditions, there is no family history of bleeding,

Clinical Presentation and Prognosis

Demographics: The prevalence of von Willebrand disease in the pediatric population may be as high as 1%, and it is likely the most common inherited bleeding disorder. Most of these patients have type 1 disease. All ethnic groups appear to be affected. An abnormal gene can be inherited from both parents, resulting in markedly diminished von Willebrand factor and factor VIII. In this, type 3 von Willebrand disease, the bleeding tendency is severe because it reflects the concurrence of defects in the formation of the primary platelet plug (due to deficiency of the von Willebrand factor) and the formation of the definitive fibrin clot (due to the secondary deficiency of factor VIII).

Presenting symptoms and complications: Patients with von Willebrand disease most often complain of excess bruising, epistaxis, menorrhagia and gum bleeding. Occasionally, petechiae are noted and excess bleeding may occur at the time of surgery, particularly at the time of tonsillectomy and adenoidectomy. The family history is important, as this is a dominant disorder, and multiple other family members may be affected.

Prognosis: The prognosis in the most common and mild form of von Willebrand disease is excellent, and a variety of therapeutic measures are available for treatment as well as prophylaxis when dental or surgical procedures are required.

Diagnosis

A personal and family history of mucocutaneous bleeding, postoperative bleeding or excessive bruising may suggest the diagnosis of von Willebrand disease. The key laboratory measurements are the immunological assay of the von Willebrand antigen and the ristocetin cofactor, which is the functional assay of von Willebrand factor activity (Table 7.8). Diminished levels of von Willebrand factor result in low levels of coagulation factor VIII, and the bleeding time or PFA100 closure time may be prolonged. The low factor VIII may prolong the aPTT, but the prothrombin time and INR are normal. High molecular weight multimers are decreased in type 2-A, 2-B, and platelet type disease. A ratio of ristocetin cofactor to von Willebrand antigen less than 0.6 suggests type 2 disease, and increased low dose ristocetin-induced aggregation is seen in type 2-B and platelet type disease. Persons who are blood type O often have levels of von Willebrand factor that are ~20–25% lower than persons with other blood types. The explanation for this is unclear and there are no data to suggest that they have a bleeding tendency. Patients often must be tested on multiple occasions before the diagnosis is clear. Von Willebrand factor, like Factor VIII, is an acute phase reactant. Therefore, external conditions such as inflammation and pregnancy, can heighten the levels of von Willebrand antigen and the functional activity. Many different mutations have been documented in the von Willebrand gene, and thus genetic testing is less useful at this time.

The details of the laboratory profiles of each of the von Willebrand subtypes are shown in Table 7.8.

In Brief

- *Type 1*: This is the most common variety of von Willebrand disease. There generally is a decreased level of von Willebrand protein, and all multimers are represented.
- *Type 2-A*: There are diminished high and medium molecular weight multimers. The response to DDAVP is variable.
- *Type 2-B*: There is a heightened affinity of the von Willebrand factor for platelets with resultant thrombocytopenia. The high molecular weight multimers are decreased. DDAVP may accentuate the thrombocytopenia and increase the tendency to bleed, and hence is not recommended.
- *Platelet-Type*: An abnormality in the platelet GPI-b protein causes heightened affinity for von Willebrand factor. There are decreased high molecular weight multimers as in type 2-B. Molecular studies of gene mutations in GPI-b distinguish this from type 2-B which is more common. Since the defect is not in the von Willebrand factor, transfusion of normal platelets is the treatment of choice.
- *Type 2-M*: There is decreased or absent binding of von Willebrand factor to GPI-b on platelets such that von Willebrand factor is functionally impaired.
- *Type 2-N*: There is decreased or absent binding of von Willebrand factor to factor VIII. Since von Willebrand factor is the carrier for factor VIII, the factor VIII longevity in the plasma is impaired and factor VIII levels are low.
- *Type 3*: Von Willebrand protein and functional activity are near zero, as is factor VIII activity.

Management

The management of bleeding in von Willebrand disease depends upon the site and severity of bleeding as well as on the type of von Willebrand disease present. Local measures including Gelfoam and topical thrombin with

Table 7.8: Von Willebrand Disease

	Factor VIII	Von Willebrand Antigen	Ristocetin Cofactor	RIPA Low Dose	Platelet Count	Bleeding or Closure Time	Treatments	Response to DDAVP	Frequency
Type 1: Decreased protein.	Normal or decreased	Decreased	Decreased	Absent	Normal	Normal or slightly long	DDAVP Amicar Humate-P Alphanate	Usually	70–80%
Type 2-A: Decreased HMW and MMW multimers	Decreased	Decreased	Moderate to severe decrease	Absent	Normal	Slightly long	Humate-P Alphanate Amicar Sometimes DDAVP	Sometimes	10–12%
Type 2-B: Increased interaction of VWF with platelets. Decreased HMW multimers.	Decreased	Decreased	Decreased	Increased	Decreased	Slightly long	Humate-P Alphanate Amicar	Contraindicated	3–5%
PT-VWD: Defect in platelet GPI-b. Increased interaction of platelets with VWF. Decreased HMW multimers.	Decreased	Decreased	Decreased	Increased	Decreased	Slightly long	Transfusion with normal platelets. May need Humate-P if VWF decreased	Contraindicated	0–1%
Type 2-M: Decreased interaction with platelets.	Normal	Decreased	Moderate to severe decrease	Absent	Normal	Slightly long	Humate-P Alphanate Amicar Sometimes DDAVP	Rarely	1–2%
Type 2-N*: Decreased interaction with Factor VIII.	Decreased	Normal or decreased	Normal or decreased	Absent	Normal	Normal (unless VWF decreased)	Humate-P Alphanate Amicar DDAVP	Sometimes	1–2%
Type 3**: No protein.	<10%	Absent	Absent	Absent	Normal	Very prolonged (BT> 15–20 minutes)	Humate-P Alphanate Amicar	Never	1–3%

High Molecular Weight (HMW)
Medium Molecular Weight (MMW)
* Most patients are compound heterozygotes with Type I.
** Patients are homozygous or compound heterozygotes with another VW defect.
Table was modified from RR Montgomery, JC Gill, and J Di Paola 2009. Hemophilia and von Willebrand Disease. In *Nathan and Oski's Hematology of Infancy and Childhood*. Orkin, Nathan, Ginsburg, Look, Fisher, and Lux, editors. Saunders Elsevier. Philadelphia. 1487–1524.

direct pressure may be useful for dental bleeding. Treatment of nasal allergy, local cautery and "Nosebleed QR" can help control epistaxis. Aminocaproic acid (Amicar), which is an inhibitor of fibrinolysis, can be used as [a] general inhibitor of bleeding, and it can be given orally or intravenously, usually at a dose of 50–100 mg/kg every 4–6 hours. A total dose of 30g/day is the upper limit for adults.

A DDAVP challenge test (Table 7.8) will establish whether correction of the closure time and normalization of the von Willebrand factor can be achieved in type 1 disease. DDAVP then can be used prophylactically for minor surgical procedures or dental extractions. It can be given 2-3 times (q 12 hours) before the stores in the endothelium are exhausted. A nasal preparation (Stimate) is useful on the first day of menses for those women with type 1 disease who have menorrhagia. It is important to remember that DDAVP is an antidiuretic hormone and can cause substantial hyponatremia if repeated doses are administered and fluid intake and output are not carefully monitored.

Treatment options for types of von Willebrand disease other than type 1 are outlined in Table 7.8. Humate-P is a pooled plasma product that contains factor VIII and von Willebrand factor, and it is the definitive product for severe bleeding in all types of von Willebrand disease except platelet type. In the latter, platelets are given and Humate-P also may be required if the von Willebrand factor is low.

Consultations: A hematology consultation is needed for establishing this diagnosis, particularly in mild Type I disease.

Monitoring: In order to adequately manage bleeding patients with von Willebrand disease, laboratory support for measurement of the ristocetin co-factor as the functional assessment of von Willebrand factor is essential. The factor VIII level also must be monitored, particularly if pooled plasma product such as Humate-P is used. Very high levels of factor VIII may predispose the patient to deep vein thrombosis.

Patients should be seen by the hematologist once per year. Additional input from the hematologist may be indicated in the event of trauma or surgery.

Pearls and Precautions

Skin and dental care: The patient's bleeding tendency should be communicated to dentists and surgeons so that appropriate prophylaxis can be given for procedures.

School/education: Precautions regarding physical activities and athletic participation are the same as for hemophilioid states (see section on Congenital Factor Deficiencies).

Medications: Treatment with DDAVP or Humate-P usually is required every 12 hours, but this regimen may be altered depending on the functional von Willebrand measurements. Medications that interfere with platelet function (e.g., NSAID's and aspirin) should be avoided.

Social: NHLBI website (information for health care professionals):
  http://.www.nhlbi.nih.gov/guidelines/vwd/index.htm/
  Project Red Flag for women with Von Willebrand Disease (VWD) is linked to the NHLBI web site.

References

Nichols WL, Hultin MB, James AH, Manco-Johnson MJ. Von Willebrand disease (VWD). evidenced-based diagnosis and management guidelines, the National Heart Lung and Blood Institute (NHLBI) Expert Panel Report (USA). Haemophilia 2008; 14: 171–232.

Montgomery RR. When it comes to von Willebrand disease, does 1+1=3? (comment). J Thromb Haemost 2006; 4: 2162–2163.

Sadler JE, Budde U, Eikenboom JC et al. Update on the pathophysiology and classification of von Willebrand disease: a report of the Subcommittee on von Willebrand Factor. J Thromb Haemost 2006; 4: 2103–2114.

Immune Thrombocytopenic Purpura (ITP)

George B. Segel, Stephen A. Feig, Kenji Morimoto

ITP is an immune mediated thrombocytopenia of variable etiology.

Etiology

The precise pathogenesis of childhood idiopathic immune thrombocytopenic purpura is not known, but the most appealing hypothesis invokes the concept of "molecular mimicry." This implies that there is a preceding illness one to three weeks before the onset of thrombocytopenia. Antigens on an infecting agent, usually a virus, initiate the production of an antibody response; these antibodies lack precise specificity and cross-react with antigens on the platelet surface that resemble the antigens on the virus. Antibodies with specificity to GPIIb/IIIa and GPIb/IX have been identified in plasma of patients with ITP, and they result in platelet destruction. Antibodies to GPIb/IX also can damage megakaryocytes and impair thrombopoiesis. Some time after the viral infection has cleared, the antibody titer falls, and the thrombocytopenia resolves.

Clinical Presentation and Prognosis

Demographics: ITP is among the most common causes of thrombocytopenia in children and affects 4–5 per 100,000 children per year. Most cases occur between two and four years of age in children, although it can occur at any age, and the male to female ratio is 1:1 in children compared to 1:3 in adults.

Presenting Symptoms and Complications: There usually is the rapid onset of thrombocytopenia with a petechial rash, increased bruising, and potentially epistaxis, oral mucosal bleeding and menometrorrhagia. Gastrointestinal hemorrhage, genitourinary hemorrhage and, rarely, intracranial hemorrhage can occur.

Prognosis: Resolution of the illness occurs in ~80% of children within six months of the onset. The likelihood of resolution is highest in those children with a clear history of a prior viral illness and an acute onset of the thrombocytopenic symptoms. Early remission is less common if there is a chronic history of easy bruising. Twenty percent of patients will remain thrombocytopenic beyond 8–12 months and [be] considered "chronic" after 12 months. These children need to be evaluated for an underlying autoimmune or immunodeficiency syndrome. Fewer than 5% of the original population of children will have platelet counts under 20,000/μl at 18 months from the onset of the illness. The best estimate of the incidence of intracranial hemorrhage is <0.2%, but the mortality with this complication is 50%.

Diagnosis

The presenting symptoms are noted above and include the rapid onset of a petechial rash and bruising. On physical examination, there may be large and palpable hematomas, general purpura, and petechiae if the platelet count is fewer than 20,000/ μL. Mucosal hemorrhage ("wet purpura") suggests an increased risk of more severe hemorrhage including intracranial hemorrhage.

The diagnosis of ITP requires consideration and exclusion of a number of other thrombocytopenic conditions. A detailed history will ascertain the use of drugs which may cause thrombocytopenia (heparin, quinidine). There usually is no lymphadenopathy or hepatosplenomegaly, and their presence may reflect malignancy, infectious mononucleosis, or Systemic Lupus Erythematosus (SLE) in the differential diagnosis. Hypertension suggests the possibility of renal involvement as seen in Hemolytic Uremic Syndrome (HUS), SLE, or Thrombotic Thrombocytopenic Purpura (TTP). Fever might reflect septicemia (with disseminated intravascular coagulation (DIC)), meningococcemia, or TTP.

Initial laboratory examination should include a CBC, reticulocyte percentage, blood smear and chemistry panel. The CBC will reflect the status of other cell lines and provide an assessment of platelet volume (usually increased in patients with destructive thrombocytopenias). Large platelets are newly-formed and usually have heightened function. The blood smear will corroborate the platelet count (platelet estimate), platelet size, and allow assessment of fragmentation (microangiopathic changes) of the red cells (seen in DIC, TTP, and HUS). The direct antiglobulin (DAT, or Coombs') test will detect whether the patient also has an auto-immune hemolytic anemia. This condition, Evans' Syndrome, implies the presence of multiple auto-antibodies and may suggest the presence of a more pervasive auto-immune disease. If a cause of secondary thrombocytopenia is identified, that cause should be promptly treated.

Generally, the risk of serious bleeding is very low in patients with platelet counts >20,000/μL. In the presence of platelet function abnormalities (as seen with several common medications or uremia) this risk may be increased.

Management

Acute

Generally, the risk of bleeding at any given platelet count is greater if the patient has a disorder of platelet production (an aplastic process, chemotherapy for cancer, etc.), as opposed to a disorder of platelet destruction (such as ITP). Trauma or exposure to drugs that impair platelet function (aspirin, non-steroidal anti-inflammatory agents, dipyridamole) may increase the risk of hemorrhage. This information may be obtained with a focused history.

The management of patients with acute ITP is controversial. There are no data to suggest that the institution of therapy has any effect on the risk of serious hemorrhage or the potential for the development of chronic ITP. Therefore, the decision to treat these patients is based on the immediate severity of bleeding, a need for surgery, the antecedent use of platelet inhibitors, concurrent trauma and a platelet count fewer than 10,000/μl. Other considerations such as the reliability of the caretakers and the distance of the family from the medical center also may influence the decision to treat.

The use of corticosteroids (prednisone, 2 mg/kg/day, in 2–3 divided doses) may increase the platelet count, but should not be used unless a marrow examination ensures the absence of leukemia, or a pediatric hematologist/oncologist has reviewed the entire clinical picture and decides that a marrow examination is not required. Alternate treatments include IVIg or AntiRhD which also increase the platelet count in patients with ITP. While these agents are substantially more expensive than corticosteroids and have significant side effects, they avoid the risk of the mistreatment of leukemia. The usual dose of IVIg is 1–2g/kg, given over 2–4 days. The dose of AntiRhD, which should not be used unless the patient's blood group is Rh positive, is

50–75 µg/kg as a single dose, intravenously. These agents require pretreatment with Tylenol and Benadryl or similar agents to minimize fever, chills, nausea and vomiting. AntiRhD will cause moderate hemolysis and a fall in hemoglobin of 1–2g/dL during the following few days, and this should be monitored. Rarely, antiRhD may cause massive hemolysis and renal damage. IVIg may cause an aseptic meningitis with severe headache, that often precipitates an evaluation with a head CT in a thrombocytopenic patient. Its use also has very rarely resulted in severe hemolysis (contains anti-A, anti-B and sometimes anti-D). Thus, in the minimally bleeding patient with ITP, and a platelet count >10,000/µL, we recommend watchful waiting. By contrast, those rare patients with severe, life threatening hemorrhage (e.g., G.I. or uterine) should receive platelet transfusions in addition to the treatments noted above. Platelet transfusion may provide hemostasis even if it does not increase the platelet count.

Chronic

Treatment of chronic ITP also is reserved for those patients who are symptomatic or at significant risk of bleeding. Treatment is necessary if bleeding symptoms are interfering with the patient's daily activities, but usually is not necessary if the platelet count remains above 20,000/µl. Some patients can be managed with intermittent courses of corticosteroids or periodic infusions of antiRhD or IVIg.

The treatment of a concomitant infection with H. Pylori has resulted in remission of chronic ITP in ~1/3 to ½ of patients so affected in Europe and Asia. However, its success rate in the U.S. appears lower. Alternative treatments include Rituximab (anti CD-20) which is an anti B-cell agent that markedly reduces the B-cell population for 12–18 months. This agent is given at 375 mg/m² weekly for four weeks and results in 25–30% sustained responses. Other immunosuppressive agents have been used but are not the standard of care.

The most recent additions to the armamentarium of treatment are the thrombopoietin receptor agonists. These include Romiplostim (AMG531, Nplate) which is administered starting at 1µg/kg subcutaneously once a week, and escalated at 1µg/kg until the platelet count reaches 200,000/µl (maximum dose 10µg/kg). Seventy-nine percent of treated patients achieved a platelet count of >150,000/µl. Alternatively, the oral thrombopoietin receptor agonist, Eltrombopag, is administered at 50–75 mg per day with similar results. These agents are approved by the FDA, but their long term safety is not yet established and they are very expensive. Patients should be monitored for myelofibrosis and myelodysplastic changes by a hematologist.

Pearls and Precautions

1. Acute ITP in children is a benign disease that usually resolves by itself.
2. Treatment should be reserved for those children with significant bleeding or the potential of significant bleeding.
3. There are no data to substantiate that any treatment prevents the major bleeding complications of ITP or prevents the disease from becoming chronic.
4. Treatment with antiRhD or IVIg is expensive and has major side effects.
5. The management of chronic ITP is more complicated and should be supervised by a Pediatric Hematologist.
6. New agents are available for treatment of symptomatic patients with chronic ITP.

References

Segel, GB and Feig SA: Controversies in the Diagnosis and Management of Childhood Acute Immune Thrombocytopenic Purpura. Pediatric Blood and Cancer. 2009; 53: 318–324.

Stasi R, Evangelista ML, Amadori S. Novel thrombopoietic agents: A review of their use in idiopathic thrombocytopenic purpura. Drugs 2008; 68: 901–912.

Platelet Function Disorders

George B. Segel, Stephen A. Feig, Kenji Morimoto

This designation is used for a heterogeneous group of bleeding disorders that are caused by defects of platelet function. This results in impairment of the primary platelet plug in establishing hemostasis. The severity of the bleeding tendency depends upon the extent to which platelet function is impaired.

Etiology

The disorders of platelet function are classified as those that are inherited, and those that are acquired (Table 7.9).

Congenital Disorders of Platelet Function: The inherited abnormalities include platelet membrane disorders such as Glanzmann's thrombasthenia and Bernard-Soulier syndrome; and, those with impaired platelet secretion; such as storage pool disease, including those with decreased alpha granule contents (grey platelet syndrome); decreased dense granule contents (delta storage pool deficiency); those with other defective secretion mechanisms; or cytoskeletal disorders (Table 7.9). Glanzmann's disease is a disorder of membrane glycoprotein IIb-IIIa that results in impaired fibrinogen-dependent platelet aggregation during formation of the primary platelet plug. In Bernard-Soulier Syndrome, there is diminished membrane glycoproteins Ib, V and IX. This results in impaired adhesion of platelets to the endothelium in conjunction with the von Willebrand antigen.

Glanzmann's disease and Bernard-Soulier Syndrome are transmitted by autosomal inheritance and affected patients are either homozygous or double heterozygotes for the respective gene defects. Of the alpha granule disorders, the grey platelet syndrome is inherited in an autosomal recessive manner, but the Quebec platelet disorder with abnormal proteolysis of alpha granule proteins is inherited as an autosomal dominant condition. Platelet abnormalities with impaired secretion and delta storage pool disease also may be autosomal recessive conditions. Delta storage pool deficiency may be associated with other granule-related inherited disorders such as Hermansky-Pudlak syndrome, Chediak-Higashi syndrome, and with the Wiskott-Aldrich syndrome.

The inherited platelet disorders are rare, but in ethnic groups where consanguinity is common, they may occur more frequently.

Acquired Disorders of Platelet Function: Acquired thrombasthenia results from a variety of underlying medical conditions (Table 7.9). Medications such as aspirin, non-steroidal anti-inflammatory medications, dipyridamole, or clopidogrel affect platelet function directly. Aspirin inhibits cyclooxygenase-1, the enzyme required to produce thromboxane A-2 which is required for normal platelet function. Dipyridamole blocks the platelet uptake of adenosine and increases its local concentration, inhibiting platelet aggregation.

Table 7.9: Disorders of Platelet Function

Platelet Membrane Disorders
- Glanzmann Thrombasthenia: Impaired platelet aggregation.
- Bernard Soulier Syndrome: Impaired adhesion of platelets to endothelium.

Platelet Secretion Disorders
- Storage Pool Disease
  - Alpha Storage Pool Deficiency
  - Grey Platelet Syndrome: Markedly decreased alpha granules.
  - Quebec Syndrome: Increased u-PA (urokinase-type plasminogen activator).
  - Delta Storage Pool Deficiency: Decreased dense granules.
    - Primary Delta Storage Pool Deficiency
    - Chediak Higashi Syndrome; Hermansky-Pudlak Syndrome
    - Other Defects in the Secretion Mechanism
  - Receptor Defects in G-protein signaling

Platelet Cytoskeletal Disorders (Congenital)
- MYH9 disorders
  - May-Hegglin anomaly
  - Fechtner syndrome
  - Epstein syndrome
  - Sebastiani syndrome
- Duchenne muscular dystrophy

Platelet Cytoskeletal Disorders (Acquired)
- Medications
- Uremia
- Liver disease
- Anti-[p]latelet antibodies
- Dysproteinemia
- Myeloproliferative Disorders
- Acute Myeloid Leukemia
- Acquired Storage Pool Disease
- Acquired von Willebrand Disease

Clopidogrel blocks the ADP receptor and prevents amplification of platelet aggregation. Metabolic disease such as hepatic or renal failure results in impaired platelet function through retention of metabolites or intermediate metabolic products that inhibit platelet function. Acquired von Willebrand disease may result from antibodies directed against von Willebrand factor; anti-platelet antibodies also may alter platelet function as well as cause thrombocytopenia. Myeloproliferative disorders and acute myeloid leukemia may have associated abnormalities of platelet function secondary to the underlying molecular defects in each disorder.

Clinical Presentation and Prognosis

Presenting signs and symptoms: The clinical features of platelet dysfunction in order of frequency in Glanzmann's thrombasthenia, for example, are menorrhagia, bleeding after circumcision, bruising and bleeding from minor lacerations, spontaneous gingival bleeding, epistaxis and gastrointestinal bleeding. Most patients with disordered platelet function have similar presenting symptoms (Table 7.10).

Prognosis: The prognosis depends upon the severity of the platelet function defect and the degree of impairment of the formation of the primary hemostatic plug. Bleeding may be episodic or related to trauma or surgery.

Diagnosis

Platelet membrane disorders

Glanzmann's Thrombasthenia: The platelet count is normal, but bleeding and closure times are long. The platelets do not aggregate in response to any of the usual agents including ADP, epinephrine, collagen or thrombin. Ristocetin (and von Willebrand factor) induced platelet aggregation is normal. Clot retraction usually is markedly reduced.

Bernard–Soulier: Most patients have thrombocytopenia. The syndrome is also characterized by the presence of giant platelets, and a long bleeding or closure time. In contrast to Glanzmann's thrombasthenia, clot retraction is normal and aggregation to ADP, epinephrine, and collagen are normal, but ristocetin aggregation is diminished.

Platelet secretion disorders

Alpha Storage Pool Deficiency: The grey platelet syndrome is characterized by mild thrombocytopenia, a long bleeding or closure time and usually normal platelet aggregation to ADP and epinephrine. Some patients have poor aggregation to thrombin, collagen and ADP. The most notable abnormality is a markedly decreased or absent number of alpha granules when the platelets are examined by electron microscopy.

Quebec Platelet Syndrome: The platelets in the Quebec platelet syndrome have markedly impaired aggregation responses to epinephrine and reduced response to ADP and collagen. The bleeding and closure times are prolonged, and the platelet count usually is normal with normal platelet morphology. There is an excess of urokinase-type plasminogen activator (u-PA), with degradation of proteins in the alpha granules.

Delta Storage Pool Deficiency: The platelet count is normal, but bleeding and closure times are long. The second wave of platelet aggregation induced by ADP, epinephrine and collagen usually is markedly diminished or absent. However, some patients may have minimal or no alterations in platelet aggregation. Electron microscopic examination of the platelets reveals decreased dense granules, and the dense granule contents such as ADP are consequently diminished.

Platelet Receptor Defects: Platelet functional defects also may occur when there are diminished receptors for various platelet agonists such as epinephrine, collagen, ADP or thromboxane A2.

Defects in Signal Transduction: Several patients have been reported who had abnormal aggregation to ADP, epinephrine and collagen, but normal aggregation to arachidonic acid and normal phospholipase A2 activity, suggesting a defect in arachidonic acid release from phospholipids. Other defects in the signal transduction pathway include cyclooxygenase deficiency and thromboxane synthase deficiency.

Platelet cytoskeletal defects

May-Heggelin anomaly, Fechtner syndrome, Epstein syndrome and *Sebastiani syndrome* are associated with the presence of large platelets on the blood smear. They have a characteristic appearance on electron microscopic examination. There may be leukocyte inclusions (Dohle bodies) seen in the May-Heggelin anomaly, while Fechtner and Epstein syndromes are associated with hearing loss, renal disease, and cataracts. These syndromes are associated with the presence of mutations in the MYH9 (myosin heavy chain) gene. MYH9 gene defects are associated with cytoskeletal abnormalities, defective platelet production, and megathrombocytes, but clinical bleeding, when present, is usually mild.

Table 7.10: Laboratory Diagnosis of Platelet Function Disorders

	Platelet count	BT (Closure time)	Platelet Aggregation					Clot Retraction	Morphology	Other
			ADP	Epinephrine	Collagen	Thrombin	Ristocetin			
Glanzmann	N	↑	0	0	0	0	N	↓	N	Deficiency of GPIIb +/or GPIIIa
Bernard Soulier	↓	↑	N	N	N	—	↓	N	Mega-thrombocytes	Deficiency of GPIb/IX/V
αSPD Grey Platelet	↓	↑	N or ↓	N	N or ↓	N or ↓	N	N	Pale platelets by LM	↓α granules by EM
αSPD Quebec	N	↑	↓	0	↓	—	N	N	N	↓ Excess u-PA
δSPD	N	↑	↓ 2°	↓ or 0	↓ or 0	—	N	N	N	↓δ granules by EM
Platelet receptor defects	N	↑	N	↓	↓	—	N	N	N	—
Signal transduction	N	↑	↓ 2°	N or ↓	N or ↓	—	N	N	N	—
MYH9 Disorders	↓	N or ↑	NCD	NCD	In Epstein syndrome	NCD	N	N	Mega-thrombocytes	Cytoskeletal Defect Clinical bleeding mild Dohle bodies in wbc.
Aspirin	N	↑	↓ 2°	↓	↓ or 0	—	N	N	N	Inhibits cyclo-oxygenase

NOTE:
No Consistent Defect (NCD)
Storage Pool Defect (SPD)
Light Microscopy (LM)
Electron Microscopy (EM)
White Blood Count (wbc)
The data were compiled from multiple sources including http://referencelab.clevelandclinic.org/images/PlateletAggregationTable.PDF and Sharathkumar AA, Shapiro A. Platelet Function Disorders (Second Edition) World. Federation of Hemophilia (2008).

Management

Transfusion: The principal mode of treatment for disorders of platelet function is platelet transfusion, when required. Platelet transfusion should be reserved for treatment of bleeding and for pre-operative prophylaxis. Platelets are available as random units prepared from individual units of blood or single donor units prepared by plateletpheresis. The complications of platelet transfusion include the risk of infectious diseases transmitted in blood and the sensitization of patients so that they become refractory to future platelet transfusions. In this regard, patients with Glanzmann's thrombasthenia are particularly susceptible to developing antibodies to platelet membrane proteins IIb-IIIa.

Medications: A DDAVP challenge test may be warranted as some patients with intrinsic platelet abnormalities achieve correction of their bleeding or closure times with infusion of DDAVP. DDAVP increases the levels of factor VIII and von Willebrand factor in the plasma, but its salutary effect on platelet function is not fully explained. DDAVP may be useful in selected patients for elective surgical procedures such as tonsillectomy and adenoidectomy or dental extractions. The intranasal preparation (Stimate) may be useful on the first and second days of menses in those patients with menorrhagia. For minor mucosal bleeding or dental procedures, topical thrombin and/or amino-caproic acid may be useful.

Consultations: Consultation with otolaryngology, gynecology, and nephrology may be helpful in the management of selected patients.

Monitoring: Monitoring should be tailored to the needs of the specific patient and the severity of the platelet function defect.

Pearls and Precautions

School/education: Physical activities should be limited the same as for hemophilioid states (see section on congenital factor deficiencies).

Likely complications: For Glanzmann's thrombasthenia, the long term risks are quite severe, especially after the patient has become sensitized to IIb-IIIa antigens, which markedly impairs the efficacy of platelet transfusion, and bleeding may require control with clotting factors (such as recombinant factor VII$_a$ or prothrombin complex concentrate). Some hematologists advocate hematopoietic stem cell transplantation before this occurs.

Reference

Freson K, Labarque V, Thys C, et al. What's new in using platelet research? To unravel thrombopathies and other human disorders. Eur J Pediatr. 2007; 166: 1203–1210.

Harrison P, Robinson M, Liesner R et al. The PFA-100: a potential rapid screening tool for the assessment of platelet dysfunction. Clin Lab Haematol. 2002; 24: 2005

Poon MC, d'Oiron R, von Depka M, et al. Prophylactic and therapeutic recombinant factor VIIa administration to patients with Glanzmann's thrombasthenia: Results of an international survey. J Thromb Haemost 2004; 2: 1096.

Thrombophilia and Childhood Thrombosis

George B. Segel, Stephen A. Feig, Kenji Morimoto

Thromboembolic disease is less frequent in children than it is in adults, but may cause profound morbidity and mortality when it occurs. The risk factors that are seen in adults such as atherosclerosis, congestive heart failure, and paralysis usually are not problems in children. Rather, childhood thrombophilia is related to either acquired or inherited conditions that impair the anticoagulant mechanisms that balance the normal clotting processes or that more directly promote abnormal coagulation (see Table 7.11). Acquired conditions include: (1) Antiphospholipid antibodies, (2) vascular damage or injury, particularly from the presence of intravenous central catheters, (3) taking estrogen-containing oral contraceptives, (4) immobilization, (5) acute phase responses, and (6) severe dehydration. Inherited conditions include factor V_{Leiden}, which is a mutated clotting factor that is not cleaved (inactivated) by the anticoagulant proteins C and S, protein C or protein S deficiency, antithrombin deficiency, increased plasma levels of procoagulants, and elevated lipoprotein a or homocysteine. When two or more of these predisposing conditions occur in the same individual at the same time, the risk of thrombosis is increased beyond the additive risk of each individual factor.

Etiology

Acquired conditions

Endothelial cell damage usually occurs in children as a result of an indwelling central venous catheter. These catheters are the single most common cause of venous thrombosis. They often are used in prothrombotic, inflammatory conditions such as inflammatory bowel disease (IBD) or cystic fibrosis, in which multiple procoagulant factors are increased, including fibrinogen, factor VIII and von Willebrand factor. This combination of prothrombotic factors, in combination with reduced free protein S, heightens the risk of thrombosis in the catheterized vessel.

The lupus anticoagulant and antiphospholipid antibodies bind phospholipids, and prolong the PTT. They actually are not an "anticoagulant," but rather activate platelets by binding to lipids on the platelet membrane, activating the coagulation cascade, and thus predisposing to thrombus formation. They are seen in some patients with systemic lupus erythematosus, but may also be present in other conditions such as inflammatory bowel disease, pregnancy, and in association with some medications such as phenothiazines, phenytoin, hydralazine, quinine, amoxicillin, and birth control pills.

Immobilization in children from paralysis or plaster casts also predisposes to thrombosis, similar to adults. Adolescent women taking estrogen-containing oral contraceptives are at risk for thrombosis as are certain patients receiving chemotherapeutic agents such as asparaginase. A number of specific underlying conditions such as sickle cell disease and hyperleukocytic leukemias also predispose patients to thrombosis.

Table 7.11 Causes of Thrombophilia

Slow Blood Flow	• Obstructed vein:
	  – Prolonged sitting
	  – Immobilization
	  – Obstructing mass
	  – Venous access device
	• Dehydration
	• Hyperleukocytic leukemia

Vascular Endothelial Damage	• Vasculitis • Trauma • Venous access device • Sickle cell anemia

Biochemical	• Increased levels of procoagulants
	  – Fibrinogen (acute phase reactant)
	  – Factor VIII (acute phase reactant)
	  – Von Willebrand factor (acute phase reactant)
	  – Prothrombin (G20210A mutation)
	  – Factor XI
	  – Lipoprotein a
	  – Homocysteine (MTHFR mutations)
	• Reduced circulating anticoagulant
	  – Factor V Leiden (resistant to activated Protein C)
	  – Protein S deficiency
	  – Protein C deficiency
	  – Antithrombin (AT) deficiency
	  – Decreased thrombomodulin
	  – Inflammation (decreased free Protein S)
	• Other
	  – Pregnancy
	  – Estrogen-containing oral contraceptives
	  – Anti-cardiolipin and Lupus anticoagulant
	  – Fibrinolytic defects
	  – Decreased plasminogen activator
	  – Increased plasminogen activator inhibitor

Inherited conditions

The inherited conditions that impair endogenous anticoagulation may involve four major anticoagulant pathways. These include the mechanism of fibrinolysis, the protein C pathway, the antithrombin pathway and the tissue factor inhibitor pathway. Other inherited problems are related to increased levels of coagulation factors and increased homocysteine.

- *Fibrinolysis:* Defects in the fibrinolytic pathway are very rare and include decreased plasminogen activator or increased plasminogen activator inhibitor. Both conditions result in diminished generation of plasmin and predispose to venous thrombosis. The reported cases have been autosomal dominant in inheritance. An impairment in plasminogen synthesis also would generate a similar risk.

- *Protein C pathway:* Thrombomodulin acts with thrombin to activate protein C. Decreased thrombomodulin very rarely has been associated with pulmonary embolism and myocardial infarction in adults. A mutant form of Factor V, Factor V$_{Leiden}$, is resistant to proteolysis and inhibition by activated protein C. Patients who are heterozygous for this factor have a 4-fold increase in thrombotic risk, while those rare patients with homozygous factor V_{Leiden} have an even higher risk. The heterozygous condition affects about 5% of the Caucasian population, and hence is a common risk factor for thrombosis, particularly if it is coupled with other acquired or inherited conditions. Alternatively, and less frequently, a deficiency in protein C or protein S may be inherited, compromising the effectiveness of the protein C anticoagulant pathway. Protein S is partially bound to complement component 5 in the plasma. When complement is increased in inflammatory states, the free protein S is diminished, and this may increase the risk of thrombosis.

- *Anti-thrombin pathway:* Antithrombin inhibits activated factors XI, IX, and X as well as thrombin. Its inhibitory activity is greatly enhanced by heparin. Persons who are heterozygous for antithrombin deficiency usually have few symptoms until adulthood. However, the rare patient with two abnormal genes usually develops severe venous and arterial thrombi in the first decade of life. Acquired antithrombin deficiency has been reported in patients with nephrotic syndrome, secondary to urinary protein loss.

- *Tissue factor pathway inhibitor:* This factor is involved in inhibition of activated factor VII and X. However, defects in this factor are not clearly related to thrombotic risk.

- *Increased prothrombin and other coagulation factors:* Although the prothrombin gene mutation, G20210A affects 1–1.5% of the population and may produce hyperprothrombinemia in adults, it rarely causes hyperprothrombinemia in children. Elevations of factor XI also may predispose the patient to thromboembolism and factors VIII, von Willebrand factor and fibrinogen often are elevated in patients with chronic inflammatory disease as noted above.

- *Hyperhomocysteinemia:* Patients with cystathionine beta synthase deficiency have hyperhomocysteinemia and homocysteinuria. They have a Marfan-like phenotype with bony abnormalities and ectopic displacement of the optic lens as well as developmental delay. They are predisposed to thromboembolism, including deep venous thrombosis, pulmonary embolism, myocardial infarction, stroke and peripheral vascular disease. Methylene tetrahydrofolate reductase (MTHFR) deficiency affects as many as 5% of the population who are homozygous for this gene abnormality. It results in hyperhomocysteinemia in adults and is associated with venous thrombosis and arteriosclerosis.

Clinical Presentation and Prognosis

Presenting Signs and Symptoms: Venous and arterial thromboses have distinctly different signs and symptoms. Thrombosis of veins draining the extremities may cause swelling from increased venous pressure, subsequent pain and change in skin color, and more chronically, trophic changes of the skin. A thrombosed vein may be palpated as a cord, and a positive Homan's sign (calf pain when the ankle is passively dorsiflexed) may be present. When the superior vena cava is involved, the patient develops suffusion of the head and neck and swelling of the face. Thrombosis in the inferior vena cava may result in lower extremity edema and threaten intra-abdominal organs, such as the kidneys. Intracranial venous sinus thrombosis may cause seizures or various neurologic deficits depending on the location of the thrombus. By contrast, the signs and symptoms of arterial thrombosis reflect acute tissue ischemia of the affected organ or area.

Clinical course

Purpura fulminans occurs primarily in newborn infants who have inherited homozygous protein C, protein S or antithrombin deficiency. It results in extensive venous and arterial thrombosis resulting in widespread purpura, skin necrosis, renovascular damage and renal failure. Death may result from extensive thrombosis in other vital organs. This condition also may occur in gram-negative septicemia, and classically meningococcemia, with disseminated intravascular coagulation. The rapid progression of this condition and high risk of death make early recognition and prompt therapeutic intervention critical.

Catheter related thrombosis is a common complication among hospitalized patients and those with chronic illness requiring frequent venous access for blood studies or for medication, blood product or nutritional infusion. Catheter types include Hickman, Broviac, percutaneous intravenous central catheter (PICC) and Porta-Cath access devices. All of these are inserted to reach the deep venous system, and they are prone to initiate thrombus formation, particularly where they may be traumatizing the vessel wall. If, in addition, the patient has any of the inherited or acquired prothrombotic conditions, such as factor V_{Leiden} or a chronic inflammatory condition, there is heightened likelihood that the thrombus will extend from the catheter into the vessel. The signs and symptoms of the deep vein thrombosis depend on the location of the catheter. For example, the superior vena cava syndrome, with suffusion of the head and neck, may result from thrombus on a catheter in the subclavian vein that extends into the larger vessels. Ileofemoral thrombosis from femoral lines may extend into the inferior vena cava and threaten the renal veins. Deep venous thrombosis in any area predisposes the patient to clot embolization to the lungs with potentially dire consequences. Lesser degrees of vascular occlusion may result in the development of venous collaterals seen as a *caput medusa* in the region drained by the catheterized vein.

Thrombosis related to combined factors may occur in patients without obvious predisposing conditions (chronic inflammatory disease, catheters, casts and immobilization). For example, approximately 5% of the population is heterozygous for factor V_{Leiden} and would be asymptomatic without confounding factors. When such a patient takes estrogen-containing oral contraceptives and then is immobilized in an airplane or automobile for a prolonged time, the combination of factors markedly heightens the risk of a thrombus forming in her legs, with the additional risk of pulmonary embolization. Although the increased risk of either heterozygosity for Factor V_{Leiden} or the use of estrogen-containing oral contraceptives is 4-fold, the combination increases the thrombotic risk to 30-fold. Unfortunately, this is not a hypothetical risk, as patients with this combination of factors are frequently seen. Combined factors also may include the occurrence of multiple gene defects in the anticoagulant proteins in the same patient. More than 10% of the children with deep vein thromboses in a large series had combinations of factor V_{Leiden} and protein S deficiency, antithrombin deficiency or elevated lipoprotein a.

Other clinical settings for spontaneous thrombosis include conditions that result in severe dehydration such as severe gastroenteritis, diabetes mellitus and diabetes insipidus. Spontaneous thrombus formation in the ileofemoral veins, renal veins or intracranial veins may occur in this setting. As noted above, chronic inflammation results in increases in a number of coagulation factors, and it may be associated with diminished free protein S, heightening the risk of thrombosis. In patients with nephrotic syndrome, loss of anticoagulant proteins occurs in the urine, and these patients also are prone to thrombus formation, particularly if vascular access catheters are placed.

Diagnosis

The initial step in diagnosis is the confirmation of the venous or arterial thrombosis. The presenting signs and symptoms mentioned above may locate the site of thrombus formation.

Delineation of the thrombus nearly always requires imaging studies such as Doppler ultrasound, CT or spiral CT, lung ventilation-perfusion scanning, MRI, or angiography. Clinical assessment alone has a low predictive value in establishing the diagnosis of a deep venous thrombosis or pulmonary embolism.

A negative D-dimer test may indicate a lower likelihood of a deep venous thrombosis, but a positive test has little predictive value. If a pulmonary embolism has occurred, the patient may be in severe respiratory distress, have considerable chest pain, diaphoresis, and the condition may progress to cardiovascular collapse. The electrocardiogram may show a right axis shift, and the oxygen saturation may be reduced. The most definitive study for diagnosis of a pulmonary embolus is a pulmonary arteriogram, but this has been superseded by spiral CT. Although a ventilation-perfusion scan has been used in the past to evaluate a potential embolism, many scans are not diagnostic, and a low-probability scan does not rule out a pulmonary embolus.

The acquired and inherited conditions that are described above should be considered in patients who develop thrombi. Usually, an anti-nuclear antibody, anti-cardiolipin antibody and a lupus anticoagulant are ordered to assess acquired procoagulant conditions. Factor V_{Leiden} is quite common in the general population, as is hyperprothrombinemia (in adults) due to the prothrombin mutation, G20210A. In addition, it is helpful to obtain measurements of protein C, protein S, and anti-thrombin—which may be diminished—and, of lipo-protein a and homocysteine, which may be increased.

Treatment

General treatment

The treatment goals for patients with deep venous thrombosis include eliminating extension of the thrombus and preventing thrombus fragmentation and pulmonary embolization. Predisposing conditions should be eliminated. Central venous catheters should be removed and oral contraceptive medication discontinued. The mainstay of treatment is prompt anticoagulation. The usefulness of the following recommendations is valid for most thrombotic conditions. However, although the value of anticoagulation for sinovenous thrombosis has been established in adults, it is less certain in children. Treatment should be considered in children who do not have any evidence for intracranial hemorrhage.

Unfractionated heparin may be administered as soon as the diagnosis is established if there is no compelling contraindication to this therapy, such as an actively bleeding gastric ulcer. Unfractionated heparin is given intravenously at a total dose of 75 units/kg for the initial 10 minutes, and then at a dose of 20 units/kg/hour to maintain the activated partial thromboplastin time at twice normal or an anti-factor Xa level between 0.35 and 0.7. These levels should be initially monitored ate least every six hours. Younger children may require increased doses to achieve therapeutic levels. Low molecular weight heparin at 1 mg/kg administered every 12 hours subcutaneously is as effective as the unfractionated heparin continuous infusion. The anti-Xa level should be determined 4 hours after the second or third dose to ensure that it is between 0.4 and 0.8, indicating adequate anticoagulation. Further testing is necessary if the patient is growing rapidly. Failure to achieve adequate anticoagulation with heparin should raise the suspicion of antithrombin deficiency.

Warfarin should be prescribed for children older than one year after the initiation of heparin or low-molecular weight heparin anticoagulation at a starting warfarin dose of 0.2 mg/kg/day. The dose then is adjusted by 20% after three day intervals to produce a prolonged prothrombin time with an international normalized ratio (INR) of 2–3. Heparin must be continued until the INR is in the therapeutic range. Children younger than one year of age may be difficult to manage on warfarin. For these patients, low-molecular weight heparin may be used safely for the continued treatment at 1 mg/kg given subcutaneously every 12 hours. Deep vein thromboses and pulmonary emboli should be treated for at least 3 and preferably 6 months. At this time, re-imaging should be performed to ensure that the thrombus has resolved before discontinuing therapy. If there is residual thrombus or evidence of severe endothelial damage, anticoagulation should be continued for an additional 6 months before re-imaging and re-evaluation.

Thrombolytic therapy with agents such as tissue plasminogen activator (TPA) is used most frequently in femoral artery thrombosis, usually secondary to catheter placement. Rarely, TPA is used in venous thromboses such as bilateral renal vein thrombosis with renal failure, acute superior vena cava syndrome, or to save vessels that are needed for future organ transplantation. It also has been used to clear arterio-venous fistulae or in low dosage to clear central venous lines. For major clot lysis, TPA is administered at 0.1 to 0.6 mg/kg/hour systemically for 6 to 12 hours. Longer infusions may deplete plasminogen and fibrinogen. This therapy should be monitored with measurements of fibrinogen, a thrombin clotting time, prothrombin time and activated partial thromboplastin time. Heparin should be given during or immediately after completion of the TPA treatment. There is a risk of significant hemorrhage with the use of TPA.

Specific treatment

Protein C concentrate is available as recombinant protein C (Xigris) or as a fractionated preparation from human plasma (Ceprotin). It also is present in prothrombin complex concentrates used for factor IX replacement and in plasma. It is indicated primarily in patients with homozygous protein C deficiency who develop neonatal purpura fulminans, and these patients may require long-term treatment. Anticoagulant treatment as described previously is the appropriate treatment for thrombosis in patients heterozygous for protein C deficiency.

Antithrombin concentrates and recombinant antithrombin (ATryn) are available for treatment of patients with homozygous antithrombin deficiency and for those with insufficient antithrombin to allow effective heparinization. They may be used prophylactically in patients with inherited heterozygous deficiency in high risk circumstances such as pregnancy, or in patients with homozygous deficiency.

There is as yet no available concentrate or recombinant preparation of protein S. Replacement requires the use of fresh frozen plasma or prothrombin complex concentrate.

Monitoring:

The PT and INR should be monitored weekly in stable patients on warfarin therapy.

Pearls and Precautions

Diet/nutrition: A stable diet is helpful in regulating the dose of warfarin. Foods rich in Vitamin K (e.g., green vegetables) may counteract the anticoagulant effect of warfarin and should be eaten in a consistent pattern.

Complications: The most important complication of anticoagulation therapy is, of course, bleeding. This is a particular problem with the use of TPA. Bleeding complications can be minimized by careful laboratory monitoring of the anticoagulation as described above. Each of the anticoagulants has additional potential complications. The administration of unfractionated heparin may initiate the formation of antibodies to the combination of heparin and platelet factor 4 and produce heparin-induced thrombocytopenia (HIT). These antibodies are prothrombotic and can precipitate worsening of the thrombotic problem for which the heparin was initially given. This should be suspected if the platelet count falls precipitously (a fall to one half the baseline value is considered suspicious of reflecting HIT), particularly if there is evidence of heightened thrombosis. In HIT, heparin should be discontinued, and an alternative anticoagulant administered. Drugs such as Argatroban and Bivalirudin (antithrombins) are short acting anticoagulants and fondaparinux (anti-factor Xa) is a longer acting anticoagulant (like low molecular heparin) that can be used in this setting under the supervision of a Pediatric Hematologist. Unfractionated heparin given for prolonged periods of time inhibits the function of osteoblasts and results in osteoporosis. Low molecular weight heparin less frequently is complicated by HIT and appears to produce less osteoporosis.

In addition to bleeding, there are two additional potential complications with the use of warfarin. Warfarin therapy should not be initiated in patients with thrombi who are not first anticoagulated with heparin.

Warfarin causes a fall in anticoagulant proteins, such as protein C, prior to adequately reducing the clotting factors, II, VII, IX and X, and can produce extensive tissue necrosis. Patients with inherited defects in protein C, protein S and anti-thrombin are most susceptible to this complication, although others have been affected. Warfarin also must never be given to pregnant patients as it is teratogenic, and can cause loss of the pregnancy or severe fetal anomalies. A number of new oral anticoagulants are in clinical trials, and these drugs such as Rivaroxiban or Dabigatran may prove to be as effective as warfarin, have as good or better therapeutic/toxicity ratio and require little or no monitoring.

References

Segel GB and Francis CW. Anticoagulant proteins in childhood venous and arterial thrombosis: A Review. BCMD 2000; 26:540–560.

Ehrenforth S, Junker R, Koch HG et al. Multicentre evaluation of combined prothrombotic defectes associated with thrombophilia in childhood. Eur J Pediatr 1999; 158 (suppl. 3) S97–S104.

Seligsohn U, Lubetsky A. Genetic susceptibility to venous thrombosis. N Engl J Med 2001; 344: 1222

Acute Management of Severe Anemia

Stephen A. Feig, George B. Segel, Kenji Morimoto

General Issues: The treatment of severe anemia in the acute care setting must be tailored to the patient's diagnosis, the degree of physiologic impairment, and the presence of other conditions such as cardiac or pulmonary disease that might impact upon the need for urgent therapy. The acuity of the situation depends upon the rapidity with which the anemia has developed. Gradually developing iron deficiency anemia may be tolerated well by infants and children whose hemoglobin has fallen to 4–5 g/dL, while a patient who has bled acutely to a level of 7–8 g/dL may be quite unstable because of hypovolemia. However, when the hemoglobin is <4 g/dL, there is little or no reserve, and the development of an arrhythmia or congestive heart failure may be fatal.

Assessment of the patient and the cause of the anemia

History and physical: The first issue to address is the cause of the anemia (Figure 1). Past medical history and family history may reveal clues to the etiology. A history of neonatal jaundice or the presence of anemia, jaundice or cholelithiasis in relatives may suggest a congenital hemolytic process. Dietary history may suggest iron deficiency secondary to excessive milk intake or milk-induced enteropathy. A history of dark, loose or overtly bloody stools suggests gastrointestinal bleeding. The physical exam will reveal the degree of physiologic impairment. Tachycardia, respiratory distress and hepatomegaly may suggest congestive heart failure. The presence of splenomegaly may suggest red cell sequestration, extramedullary hematopoiesis, or the presence of a malignancy such as leukemia. The diagram in Figure 7.2 provides an approach to the differential diagnosis of anemia in children.

Laboratory

The complete blood count (CBC) will provide data on the severity of the anemia and the nature of the anemia through the hemoglobin, hematocrit, RBC indices and the reticulocyte percentage.

1. *Mean Corpuscular Volume (MCV):* A low MCV suggests severe iron deficiency or a thalassemic state. Lead intoxication alone is an unlikely cause of a severe hypochromic, microcytic anemia, but may be associated with severe iron deficiency. A high MCV indicates the possibility of marrow failure or ineffective erythropoiesis (e.g., myelodysplasia or a megaloblastic anemia).
2. *Reticulocytes:* The reticulocyte percentage reflects how the patient's bone marrow responds to the presence of severe anemia. It is best to calculate the absolute reticulocyte count which normally is ~50,000/μL (1% of $5x10^6$ RBC). Normal marrow potentially can reach absolute reticulocyte counts of 400,000/μL or more. An elevated absolute reticulocyte count reflects an attempt to compensate for either a hemolytic process or chronic blood loss.

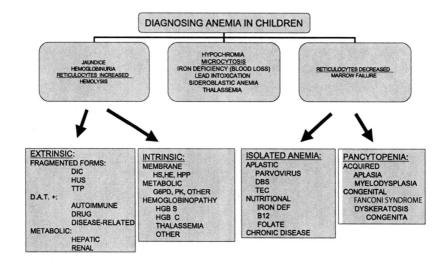

Figure 7.2: Diagnosing Anemia in Children

3. Both acquired and congenital hemolytic anemias may be complicated by the presence of an aplastic crisis, such as seen after parvovirus infection, and the clue to this possibility is an absolute reticulocyte count less than the patient's baseline (see Figure 7.2). If the reticuloctye count is depressed, the hemoglobin will fall precipitously when the RBC lifespan is short (i.e., in hemolytic diseases).

4. *Blood smear:* It is essential to have a reliable interpretation of a good blood smear. The smear can reveal the presence of sickle cells, hemoglobin C inclusions, target cells (suggestive of liver disease, hemoglobin C or thalassemia), fragmented schistocytes and helmet cells (suggestive of hemolytic uremic syndrome (HUS), disseminated intravascular coagulation (DIC), Thrombotic Thrombocytopenic Purpura (TTP) and pyropoikilocytosis), spherocytes (seen in auto-immune hemolysis and hereditary spherocytosis), basophilic stippling (lead intoxication, pyrimidine-5'-nucleotidase deficiency, thalassemia and unstable hemoglobins), elliptocytes, or stomatocytes.

5. *Platelets:* The platelet count may be depressed in marrow failure syndromes, such as aplastic anemia or leukemia, or in destructive processes, such as immune cytopenias (Evan's Syndrome [immune hemolytic anemia and thrombocytopenia]), or mechanical destruction such as Disseminated Intravascular Coagulopathy, Hemolytic Uremic Syndrome, Kasabach-Merritt Syndrome or Thrombotic Thrombocytopenic Purpura.

6. *Leukocytes:* The leukocytes may be elevated or diminished in leukemia, and there may be abnormal white cells on the peripheral smear.

7. *Leukoerythroblastosis:* The presence of immature myeloid cells, nucleated red blood cells, and teared poikilocytes on the peripheral blood smear suggests the presence of something in the marrow which should not be there (leukemia, metastatic tumor, or fibrosis). It indicates the need to perform a marrow aspirate and biopsy.

Treatment

Transfusion

The acute treatment of severe anemia is transfusion of packed red blood cells. The decision to transfuse should be individualized, based upon the patient's ability to compensate for the severity of the anemia hemodynamically, and the likelihood of spontaneous recovery (based upon the reticulocyte count). A patient's other medical conditions must be taken into consideration in this decision. For instance, a patient with cyanosis secondary to heart disease or pulmonary disease may be more severely compromised and require transfusion at a higher level of hemoglobin.

Consider the following steps before transfusing these patients.

1. *RBC antigen testing:* If the clinical picture suggests a chronic anemia in which the patient may require ongoing transfusion therapy, it is important that the blood bank perform complete RBC antigen typing before initiating transfusion therapy. Chronic transfusion may induce antibodies to minor blood group antigens, which could create future difficulty in obtaining suitably matched blood.

2. *Save extra blood samples:* If the diagnosis is not known and the status of complete blood typing is unknown, specimens for these studies should be drawn before transfusions are given to avoid contamination of test specimens with transfused blood.

3. *Avoid fluid overload:* Transfusions have increased risk in the severely anemic patient. Attempts to correct chronic anemia with simple transfusion may induce congestive heart failure as a result of fluid overload. The more severe the anemia, the more slowly blood products should be administered to avoid this complication. As a simple rule of thumb, for patients with hemoglobins below 5 g/dL, the volume of the first transfusion, in mL of packed RBC (PRBC) should be:

$$mL\ PRBC = hemoglobin\ (in\ g/dL) \times body\ weight\ (in\ kg)$$

administered over 30–60 minutes. After equilibration, transfusion may be repeated as needed. Once the patient is stabilized, and not in heart failure, with a hemoglobin greater than 5 g/dL, larger volumes of PRBC may be administered.

4. *Assure same donor unit:* For the transfusion of small children, the blood bank should provide progressive aliquots of blood from the same donor unit, to minimize the risks of infection and antigen sensitization.

5. *Irradiated blood:* Infants receiving large volume transfusions and all patients receiving transfusions from first-degree relatives should receive irradiated blood.

6. *Fresh blood:* It is advantageous to use the freshest blood available for patients who are to be chronically transfused. This will diminish the iron burden.

There are unusual circumstances in which a rapid increase in hemoglobin is required. This might occur in the severely anemic patient, in whom emergent surgery is indicated, such as for appendicitis or after trauma. In this situation, emergency exchange transfusion with packed RBC's can rapidly correct the anemia, without the risk of heart failure. This can be done manually or by erythrocytopheresis, if this is available.

References

Fasano R, Luban NLC. Blood component therapy. Pediatr Clin North Am 2008; 55: 421-445.

Segel G, Hirsch M, Feig SA. Managing anemia in pediatric office practice. Pediatrics in Review 2002; 23: 75-84 and 111–122.

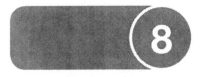

Immunologic Disorders

Table of Contents

Ataxia-Telangiectasia (AT)

Sean A. McGhee

Ataxia-telangiectasia is a degenerative neurologic disorder that presents with ataxia and is associated with immune deficiency.

Etiology

This disorder is caused by mutations in the ATM gene. The ATM protein senses double stranded breaks in DNA and signals for their repair.

Clinical Presentation and Prognosis:

Demographics: The disorder is autosomal recessive and affects males and females equally. Most patients are diagnosed in the early school years, when the neurologic disease becomes evident. About 1:40,000 births have AT.

Presenting signs and symptoms: The ataxia may be misdiagnosed as cerebral palsy, since it is so slowly progressive that it may seem static over short term follow-up. Telangiectasias, particularly on the sclera, are characteristic of the disorder, though not diagnostic. Although there is an immune disorder and patients may have recurrent infections, the neurologic disease is far more prominent, and infection is usually not the primary concern in therapy. Most infections are respiratory; fungal and opportunistic infections are uncommon. Some patients have lower T-cell counts, suggesting T-cell immunodeficiency, although antibody deficiencies are the primary manifestation of immune deficiency. Radiation sensitivity is also characteristic of the disorder, and radiologic procedures should be minimized.

Clinical course: The disorder is slowly progressive without remission with respect to the neurologic manifestations. Children with AT learn to walk at a normal age, but have ataxia beyond the usual toddler period. Eye movements provide an excellent screen for the disorder, as AT children have difficulty with smooth pursuit of an object fixed in gaze. Telangiectasias appear between ages 3–6 and occur on the bulbar conjunctiva and sun-exposed skin.

AT patients are highly susceptible to malignancy, possibly due to the defect in DNA repair. These malignancies are mostly non-Hodgkin's lymphoma, leukemias, and Hodgkin's lymphoma, but other solid tumors occur as well.

Prognosis: Many textbooks suggest a life-expectancy less than 25 years, but this is not true in all cases, and some patients have lived into their 50s with medical care. Eventually, almost all become wheelchair dependent for mobility.

Diagnosis

Screening for the disorder can be done by measuring serum alpha-fetoprotein levels, which are elevated greater than 10 ng/ml in 95% of AT patients. This must be measured after 8 months of age, as infant levels are normally elevated, and can sometimes remain elevated in normal infants to age 2. Diagnosis can be confirmed by sequencing of the gene, or by immunoblotting for the ATM protein.

Management

Medications: IVIG should be given (400 mg/kg q 3–4 wks titrated to maintain trough levels greater than 600 mg/dL) if patients have hypogammaglobulinemia or difficulty with recurrent infection. Daily vitamin E is suggested for patients. Though there is little objective evidence of effect for vitamin E therapy, there is little harm.

Therapy: Physical and occupational therapy is critical to both maximize available function and to provide adaptive resources for the patient. Swallowing disorders are common and occupational therapy and nutritional consultation may help in managing this complication. Speech therapy is also useful for many individuals. Respiratory therapy for pulmonary hygiene is helpful for those with bronchiectasis.

Social: Despite significant physical disabilities as patients age, AT patients have normal intelligence throughout their lives, and many finish college or university. The neurologic defect is purely extrapyramidal. Genetic counseling is indicated for parents, as there is typically a recurrence risk of 25% for a given couple.

Pearls and Precautions

Immunization: Live virus vaccines should be avoided, although the immunodeficiency is usually mild.

Miscellaneous: Growth and sexual maturation may be delayed, with ovarian dysgenesis and testicular atrophy. AT patients may also have premature aging and graying of the hair. Periodic clinical assessment for bronchiectasis and malignancy is important, but ionizing radiation (i.e., radiographs) should be minimized. If malignancy develops, patients must be evaluated for radiation sensitivity prior to any radiation therapy.

References

Swift M, Morrell D, Massey RB, Chase CL. Incidence of cancer in 161 families affected by ataxia-telangiectasia. N Engl J Med 1991;325:1831–1836.

Lavin MF. Ataxia-telangiectasia: from a rare disorder to a paradigm for cell signaling and cancer. Nat Rev Mol Cell Biol 2008;9:759–769.

Congenital Agammaglobulinemia

Sean A. McGhee

This condition is defined as failure to produce IgG and other immunoglobulins due to a developmental abnormality in B cells.

Etiology

The vast majority of cases are due to mutations in the Bruton's tyrosine kinase (BTK), which prevents B cells from developing. Other genes also exist that cause a lack of B-cell development; these cause autosomal recessive forms of the disorder.

Clinical Presentation and Prognosis

Demographics: Almost all patients are male because BTK is found on the X chromosome. A few girls may be affected due to the rare autosomal recessive forms of the disorder.

Presenting signs and symptoms: Most patients present with recurring sinopulmonary infections, but patients may also present with arthritis and autoimmune disease. The first signs of disease do not occur in the first 6 months of life because maternally transferred IgG is present. Common infections include S. pneumoniae, H. influenzae, S. aureus, Pseudomonas spp., Salmonella and Campylobacter.

Clinical course and prognosis: Once receiving IVIG therapy, the overall prognosis is good, though it is still possible for patients to develop bronchiectasis. Patients who are not on IVIG may develop severe complications including chronic enteroviral disease and encephalitis. This was previously among the leading cause of fatalities in this disorder. Chronic gastroenteritis is common and may be due to Giardia lamblia, rotavirus or Campylobacter, but frequently no specific infectious cause is found.

Diagnosis

The diagnosis is made by demonstrating low levels of all classes of immunoglobulin and an absence of B cells (CD19+ or CD20+ cells). The absence of B cells with normal numbers of other lymphocytes is pathognomonic. Patients usually make some IgG (up to 200 mg/dL), although the level is markedly reduced from normal. On physical examination, there are hypoplastic tonsils and lymph nodes, despite the recurrent infections.

Management

Medications: IVIG should be given (400 mg/kg q 3–4 wks titrated to maintain trough levels greater than 600 mg/dL). Subcutaneous infusion of IVIG is also an option and allows greater independence for the patient. IVIG extends survival and virtually eliminates complications such as encephalitis. There is some concern that IVIG may not always prevent the ultimate onset of bronchiectasis, so yearly monitoring of pulmonary function is necessary to identify changes in lung function early. Antibiotic prophylaxis against organisms causing pulmonary disease is used by some centers. Opportunistic infections, such as Pneumocystis jiroveci, are not a feature of the disorder.

Therapy: Attention to the musculoskeletal system is important because inflammatory arthritis is common. Arthritis is managed as for juvenile rheumatoid arthritis. If bronchiectasis is present, appropriate pulmonary hygiene with respiratory therapy is important.

Surgery: Surgery for central line placement is possible, if necessary, but should be discouraged because the need for therapy will be life-long and indwelling catheters present significant infection risks.

Social: There should be no restriction on activities and X-linked Agammaglobulinemia (XLA) patients should be encouraged to participate in all aspects of life. Quality of life is slightly lower than healthy controls, but much higher than for those with rheumatic diseases.

Pearls and Precautions

Education on the importance of IVIG therapy and the need for life-long treatment is key to the success of therapy. Efforts should be made to minimize the effect of infusions on the patient's life. The decision to use subcutaneous infusion or intravenous infusion should be based primarily on the patient's preference.

Genetic counseling is indicated for parents to determine recurrence risk, which for families with the X-linked disorder is generally 0% for girls and 50% for boys. If the patient has an autosomal recessive form, the recurrence risk is 25%.

Immunization: Vaccination of these patients is not worthwhile, as no immunoglobulin can be produced. Live attenuated poliovirus has caused fatal vaccine-associated polio.

Miscellaneous: Prior to the use of IVIG, chronic enteroviral infections with echovirus and coxsackievirus, as well as chronic encephalopathy due to enterovirus were common. The onset may be acute or subacute, and can still occur despite IVIG therapy, although it is much less common. XLA has occasionally been diagnosed in adulthood when childhood infections were mild.

Neutropenia may also be a feature of the disease. This may resolve with IVIG therapy.

It is critical to realize that in agammaglobulinemic patients, antibody titers are of no value in investigating the cause of infection. Patients do not produce antibody in response to infection and when on IVIG, titers only reflect the immunologic experience of the donor pool.

References

Soresina A, Renata N, Bomba M, Cassani M, Molinaro A, Sciotto A, et al. The quality of life of children and adolescents with X-linked agammaglobulinemia. J Clin Immunol 2008;29:501–507.

Ochs HD, Smith CE. X-linked agammaglobulinemia: A clinical and molecular analysis. Med 1996;75:287–299.

Chediak-Higashi Syndrome

Sean A. McGhee

This syndrome is caused by a defect in granule function and release that results in a syndrome of immune deficiency, albinism, and tumor susceptibility.

Etiology

Defective granule production results in inability to effectively kill phagocytosed pathogens. The defect is caused by mutations in the gene LYST.

Clinical Presentation and Prognosis

Demographics: Most are diagnosed at age three or four, as albinism becomes more apparent.

Presenting signs and symptoms: Many patients are diagnosed incidentally when a routine blood smear shows the highly characteristic giant granules found in the disorder. This finding is effectively pathognomonic. Frequent abscesses and periodontal disease are found in the disorder. In addition, the hair and skin pigmentation is light and silvery. This partial albinism becomes more pronounced as the patient ages. Patients may also be found with peripheral and cranial nerve neuropathies. Patients are frequently neutropenic.

Clinical course and prognosis: Patients early on have a susceptibility to infection. At some point, however, most patients undergo an accelerated phase, in which there is a transformation into a hemophagocytic syndrome with fever, hepatosplenomegaly, elevated ferritin and triglycerides as well as other inflammatory markers, anemia, and cytopenias.

Diagnosis

The blood smear is usually sufficient, but sequencing of LYST may also be performed to document the disorder.

Management

Medications: Antibiotic prophylaxis and IVIG may be used.

Surgery: Surgical intervention may be needed for deep or persistent infections.

Stem cell transplant: Stem cell transplant is indicated because it prevents the accelerated phase, which can arise at any time. It does not correct the albinism, but does prevent the recurring infections.

Therapy: Since neuropathies are common, signs of neuropathy should be sought on follow-up visits and occupational and physical therapy may be of benefit for those affected.

Social: Patients should not engage in yard work, mulching, raking leaves, etc., as this is a high-risk activity for acquiring Aspergillus infections.

Pearls and Precautions

Immunization: Live vaccines, such as attenuated influenza vaccine, measles, mumps, rubella, oral polio, varicella, or BCG, should not be given.

Nutrition: Chediak-Higashi syndrome does not have any specific nutritional issues.

Miscellaneous: Infections may appear less severe than they are and be associated with fewer systemic symptoms.

References

Kaplan J, De Demonico I, Ward DM. Chediak-Higashi syndrome. Curr Opin Hematology 2008;15:22–29.

Nagle DL, Karim MA, Woolf EA, Holmgren L, Bork P, Misumi DJ, et al. Identification and mutation analysis of the complete gene for Chediak Higashi syndrome. Nature Genet 1996;14:307–311

Chronic Granulomatous Disease (CGD)

Sean A. McGhee

Immune deficiency due to defective neutrophil function leads to chronic granulomatous disease.

Etiology

Inability by neutrophils to create superoxide anion leads to ineffective killing of some intracellular organisms, particularly bacteria and fungi. The exact mechanism by which lack of superoxide prevents killing is not fully understood. The defect is in components of the NADPH oxidase that generates superoxide anion. Deficiency of gp91phox is X-linked, p22phox, p47phox, and p67phox are autosomal recessive.

Clinical Presentation and Prognosis

Demographics: Majority of the patients are diagnosed in childhood, but many may not be recognized until adulthood. Most, but not all, are male.

Presenting signs and symptoms: Patients have recurrent and severe abscesses and infections, particularly involving the lung, skin lymph nodes and liver. Osteomyelitis is also common. Common organisms in CGD include Aspergillus, Serratia marcescens, Staphylococcus aureus, Burkholderia cepacia, and Nocardia species. Note that many of these are unusual organisms in healthy patients and their occurrence in a previously healthy individual should prompt evaluation for the disease.

Clinical course and prognosis: Patients have recurrent infections as described above. In addition, granulomas can develop that lead to gastric outlet obstruction or urinary tract obstruction. Delayed wound healing following trauma or surgery is common. Severe acne may also be a problem. Growth is delayed in children with CGD, but most usually achieve predicted adult height. Carriers of CGD mutations are not affected unless the number of granulocytes expressing functional oxidase activity is less than 10%. This can occasionally happen in females with gp91phox due to abnormal X chromosome inactivation. There is increased risk for autoimmune disease, particularly lupus, in people with CGD.

Mortality is usually due to Aspergillus or B. cepacia. With current prophylaxis, many patients live into the third and fourth decade or beyond, but they continue to have a high risk of potentially lethal infections.

Diagnosis

Dihydrorhodamine flow cytometry has generally replaced the nitroblue tetrazolium test, but both are acceptable ways of screening for the diagnosis. Molecular methods can be used to confirm the diagnosis. Any healthy patient with an invasive aspergillus infection should be presumed to have CGD until proven otherwise. CGD patients can have significant infections despite a minimum of symptoms and lab findings. G6PD deficiency can occasionally mimic CGD. If necessary, sequencing of all four genes responsible for CGD is available.

Management

Medications: For preventing staphylococcal infections, trimethoprim/sulfamethoxazole prophylaxis, 5 mg trimethoprim/kg daily, may be used. Prophylaxis of fungal infections should be used, usually with itraconazole (200 mg PO daily for those over age 13, 100 mg PO daily for those under 13). IFN-γ (for body surface area (BSA)) ≤ 0.5 use 0.05 mg/m^2 SQ thrice weekly, and for BSA >0.5 use 0.0015 mg/m2 SQ thrice weekly) improves superoxide production and decreases the incidence of infection. Obstructing granulomatous lesions can be treated with prednisone 1 mg/kg/day for several days followed by a taper, but prolonged low dose steroids are often needed for maintenance. For acute infections, granulocyte transfusions may be used, though their efficacy is unclear.

Surgery: Hepatic abscesses may be particularly problematic and almost always require aggressive surgical management. Postoperatively, wound healing may be delayed.

Stem cell transplant: Bone marrow transplantation can be successful and may help in the setting of refractory infections. It remains a high-risk procedure for CGD patients though, so decisions about the need for and timing of transplantation are difficult. Gene therapy is under active investigation with promising early results.

Therapy: There is no specific occupational or physical therapy indicated for patients with CGD.

Social: Patients should not engage in yard work, mulching, raking leaves, etc, as this is a high-risk activity for acquiring Aspergillus infections. Genetic counseling is advised, because of the variety of inheritance patterns and differing recurrence risks.

Pearls and Precautions:

Immunization: BCG vaccination should not be given, though other routine vaccines may be used.

Nutrition: There are generally few nutritional issues for patients with CGD.

Miscellaneous: All infections must be aggressively treated. The erythrocyte sedimentation rate is a useful sign of developing infections. Lung function should be followed yearly and as needed. Regular ophthalmology visits should be scheduled to screen for chorioretinitis.

References:

Seger RA. Modern management of chronic granulomatous disease. British J Haematology 2008:140;255–266.

Martire B, Rondelli R, Soresina A, Pignata C, Broccoletti T, Finocchi A, et al. Clinical features, long-term follow-up and outcome of a large cohort of patients with chronic granulomatous disease: An Italian multicenter study. Clin Immunol 2008;126:155–164.

Heyworth PG, Cross AR, Curnutte JT. Chronic granulomatous disease. Curr Opin Immunol 2003;15:578–584.

Common Variable Immunodeficiency (CVID)

Sean A. McGhee

Failure to produce IgG and possibly other immunoglobulins despite normal total numbers of B cells is called Common Variable Immunodeficiency (CVID).

Etiology

CVID is found sporadically and in families, and is thought to be due to a genetic defect. However, only 10% of CVID patients have any of the few known mutations described to cause CVID. Even when cases are clustered familially, the mutation usually cannot be identified.

Clinical Presentation and Prognosis

Demographics: Men and women are equally affected. The onset is typically in young adulthood, but the disorder can be found in younger children as well. There is commonly a significant delay (years) between the onset of symptoms and diagnosis.

Presenting signs and symptoms: Most patients present with recurrent sinusitis and pulmonary infections. However, there is a broad spectrum of disorders that may develop during the course of CVID, and sometimes these may be the presenting sign. Granulomatous disease may be found in CVID patients. Others may present with lymphoma. Gastric cancer may also be seen. Autoimmunity, usually in the form of hemolytic anemia, also occurs at a higher frequency in patients with CVID. Enteropathy presenting with malabsorption and diarrhea is also common.

Clinical course and prognosis: The clinical course varies markedly. Some patients never have disease more significant than recurrent sinusitis, which usually resolves with IVIG therapy. Those with granulomas, enteropathy, lymphoma or autoimmunity have a more morbid clinical course as these entities do not usually improve on IVIG therapy.

Diagnosis

The diagnosis may be made by demonstrating low IgG levels in the presence of normal numbers of total B cells. Some patients may have low levels of switched memory B cells, which may herald a worse prognosis. If vaccination is performed, patients will respond poorly.

Management

Medications: The mainstay of therapy is IVIG (400 mg/kg q 3–4 wks titrated to keep trough levels at least 600 mg/dL), which improves the infectious complications. However, other manifestations of the disease do not respond to IVIG. Subcutaneous infusion of immune globulin is also an option. Currently, granulomas are usually treated with high dose steroid, with variable success. Autoimmunity is managed similarly to the non-syndromic counterpart.

Therapy: There is no specific occupational or physical therapy required.

Social: Genetic counseling is optional, as the inheritance mechanism is unknown except for those rare cases where the specific genetic defect is identified. The recurrence risk for other children is quite small, but not predictable.

Pearls and Precautions

Immunization: Vaccination is usually not helpful in these patients as response to vaccination is poor. Some patients do respond to vaccines though, and, if known to respond, this may allow patients to receive vaccines such as seasonal influenza, which are not well represented in IVIG.

Miscellaneous: Careful monitoring for the non-infectious complications is important. Patients may develop bronchiectasis, and the usual monitoring for this is yearly pulmonary function tests with high resolution CT scanning if these are abnormal. Because many patients have lymphadenopathy at presentation, it should be carefully documented and followed, since a change in the size or distribution of these lymph nodes may suggest lymphoma and a need for biopsy.

References

Cunningham-Rundles C, Bodian C. Common variable immunodeficiency: clinical and immunologic features of 248 patients. Clin Immunol 1999;92:34–48.

Mechanic LJ, Dikman S, Cunningham-Rundles C. Granulomatous disease in common variable immunodeficiency. Ann Int Med 1997;127:613–617.

Grimbacher B, Hutloff A, Schlesler M, Glocker E, Warnatz K, Dräger R, et al. Homozygous loss of ICOS is associated with adult-onset common variable immunodeficiency. Nature Immunol 2003;4:261–268.

Complement Deficiencies

Sean A. McGhee

Failure to produce one or more components of complement, resulting in susceptibility to infection and auto-immunity.

Etiology

Almost all are due to mutations within the individual complement genes.

Clinical Presentation and Prognosis

Demographics: Most of the complement genes are autosomal recessive so males and females are equally affected. The one exception is deficiency of properdin, which is located on the X chromosome and occurs primarily in males.

Presenting signs and symptoms: Serious infections are common in complement deficiencies. Pneumococcal and H. influenzae infections are the most common infections in those with complement deficiencies that result in an inability to activate C3 (C3 deficiency). C1, C2, and C4 deficiencies also result in infection with encapsulated organisms, but less frequently. These deficiencies are more associated with rheumatic disease including lupus, dermatomyositis, scleroderma and vasculitis. Those with deficiencies of C5, C6, C7, C8, or C9 (terminal complement deficiencies) are susceptible to Neisseria infections (though not other gram negative organisms). Those with terminal complement deficiencies have less rheumatic disease than those with early complement deficiencies. The most common infections in all complement deficiencies are blood borne: Sepsis, meningitis, or osteomyelitis. Complement deficient patients may have increased sinopulmonary infections as well, but these are less common.

Clinical course and prognosis: Many patients have infrequent infection but have severe presentations of streptococcal or neisserial infections when these do occur.

Diagnosis

Because there are many possible components of complement that result in the same general phenotype, the CH50 should be used as a screening test. If any component is defective, the CH50 will be reduced. If the CH50 is reduced, functional and quantitative measurements of the individual complement components will need to be performed.

Management

Medications: Generally, no ongoing antibiotic prophylaxis is provided.

Therapy: There is no specific occupational or physical therapy required.

Social: Genetic counseling may be offered. Most disorders are autosomal recessive, suggesting a recurrence rate of 25%.

Pearls and Precautions

Immunization: Vaccination against N. meningitidis and S. pneumoniae should be given. These patients may receive live virus vaccines.

References

Unsworth DJ. Complement deficiency and disease. J Clin Path 2008;61:1013–1017.

Mathew S, Overturf GD. Complement and properdin deficiencies in meningococcal disease. Ped Infect Dis J 2006;25:255–256.

Hyper-IgM Syndrome (HIGM)

Sean A. McGhee

This syndrome is caused by a defect in the ability of B cells to switch from making IgM to making other classes of immunoglobulin (IgG, IgM or IgA). As a result, there may be increased levels of IgM in association with low levels of other immunoglobulins, and a susceptibility to infection.

Etiology

Although the defect may appear to be a B-cell disorder, the mutated gene is most commonly CD154 (CD40 ligand). This is a T-cell receptor that is involved in the communication with B cells to trigger class switching. However, the gene has other roles in T-cell activation so patients are at risk for opportunistic infections and other infections that are more characteristic of T-cell disorders. The disorder is genetically heterogeneous, and there are other genes within the class switching pathway that cause hyper-IgM syndrome.

Clinical Presentation and Prognosis

Demographics: Because CD154 is an X chromosome gene, most patients are male. However, other genes, such as AID, CD40 or UNG, may also cause the syndrome so girls can be affected. Patients are usually detected early in life because of the characteristic set of infections they are likely to suffer.

Presenting signs and symptoms: Patients usually present as infants with recurring respiratory infections. Almost all will be symptomatic by age 4. However, a common presenting infection is Pneumocystis jiroveci infection, suggesting the T-cell deficiency that also exists in this disease. Patients may develop diarrhea, both from Giardia lamblia or Cryptosporidium parvum infection. In addition, sclerosing cholangitis is common in those with HIGM. A neutrophil production defect resulting in intermittent neutropenia also occurs. Thrombocytopenia and anemia have been observed. With parvovirus B19 infection, a pure red cell aplasia may develop. This can be managed with IVIG therapy. On physical examination, lymphadenopathy is often present, in contrast to those with X-linked agammaglobulinemia.

Clinical course and prognosis: The severity of infections, as well as liver disease from sclerosing cholangitis or chronic parenteral nutrition results in reduced survival, but can be improved by stem cell transplantation. Gastrointestinal tumors may develop by adolescence.

Diagnosis

Increased levels of IgM in the presence of low levels of other classes is characteristic of the disorder, but may not be present in patients less than 2 years old. The disorder may be specifically diagnosed by sequencing CD154 gene or measuring the level of the CD154 expression on T cells by flow cytometry. This test should be performed in the setting of a young boy with characteristic infections, neutropenia, or elevated IgM levels with reduced IgG.

Management

Medications: Patients should be given IVIG (400 mg/kg q 3–4 wks adjusted to keep levels greater than 600 mg/dL). Subcutaneous IVIG may be used as well. Trimethoprim-sulfamethoxasole prophylaxis (5 mg/kg trimethoprim PO BID) is essential. Granulocyte colony stimulating factor (Filgrastim 5 mcg/kg/day given daily, with adjustment of the dose to keep the absolute neutrophil count greater than 1000 cells/mm^3) may be given to those with neutropenia.

Surgery: Liver transplantation for sclerosing cholangitis may be associated with relapse.

Stem Cell Transplantation: Hyper-IgM syndrome patients are candidates for stem cell transplant which improves survival. They remain at risk for malignancy.

Therapy: There is no specific occupational or physical therapy required.

Social: Education about IVIG therapy is an important part of the success of the therapy, including the need for ongoing treatment prior to transplantation. Genetic counseling is indicated for parents.

Pearls and Precautions

Immunization: HIGM patients may safely receive live virus vaccines, but the response may be minimal.

Nutrition: Enteropathy with malabsorption, whether due to infection or other causes can necessitate parenteral nutrition.

Miscellaneous: Precautions to avoid Cryptosporidium infection (primarily assuring an uncompromised water supply with bottled water) are warranted. Patients should be regularly monitored for the noninfectious complications of disease such as GI malignancy, neutropenia, or lymphoma.

References

Levy J, Espanol-Boren T, Thomas C, Fischer A, Tovo P, Bordigoni P, et al. Clinical spectrum of X-linked hyper IgM syndrome. J Pediatr 1997;131:47–54.

Durandy A, Peron S, Fischer A. Hyper-IgM syndromes. Curr Opin Rheumatol 2006;18:369–376.

Selective IgA Deficiency

Sean A. McGhee

This condition is a deficiency of IgA production, which may result in recurrent sinopulmonary infections.

Etiology

The disorder can result from both genetic and environmental causes. For example, phenytoin is a known cause of IgA deficiency, but the disorder may also result from a genetic inability to produce IgA. Most cases do not have a clear etiology, though the disorder does run in families.

Clinical Presentation and Prognosis

Demographics: IgA deficiency is most prevalent in Caucasians, and is the most common primary immune deficiency. Males and females are equally affected.

Presenting signs and symptoms: IgA deficiency is often detected only on laboratory testing, since the majority of those with the disorder do not appear to have clinical symptoms. When it is associated with symptoms, the primary infections are sinopulmonary infections, particularly recurrent sinusitis.

Clinical course and prognosis: The disorder is usually not progressive, though in some cases patients may go on to develop common variable immunodeficiency, especially if IgG subclasses are also abnormal. Families with CVID also have a higher incidence of selective IgA deficiency.

Diagnosis

Measurement of IgA levels establishes the diagnosis. Though many people may have levels > 2 standard deviations from the mean, there is rarely any association with infections unless the IgA level is fully absent. Since other immunoglobulin levels are normal, there is little need to enumerate B cells.

Management

Medications: Most patients do not have recurrent infections and require no therapy. Follow-up to monitor for changes in infection frequency or severity is useful because a small number may develop CVID. IgA deficient patients should not receive IVIG, since some preparations contain IgA and can trigger anaphylaxis.

Surgery: Surgical interventions are not required unless needed for the management of infection (i.e., tympanostomy tubes).

Therapy: There is no specific occupational or physical therapy required.

Social: Since the disorder is rarely clinically significant, it is important to assess patients for unrealistic ideas about their medical fragility. Parents may hinder the child's development by unnecessarily restricting activities. There should be no restrictions on activity. Genetic counseling is generally not needed as recurrence is of low clinical significance.

Pearls and Precautions

Immunization: IgA deficient patients may receive any and all vaccines.

Nutrition: Nutritional concerns are minimal.

Miscellaneous: A wide range of other disorders have been associated with IgA deficiency. However, it is unclear if this is simply the co-occurrence of two common diseases or ascertainment bias. Such associations include allergy, autoimmune disease, malignancy and epilepsy.

References

De Laat PCJ, Weemaes CMR, Gonera R, Van Munster PJJ, Bakkeren JAJM, Stoelinga GBA, et al. Clinical manifestations in selective IgA deficiency in childhood. Acta Pediatr 2008;80;798–804.
Cunningham-Rundles C. Physiology of IgA and IgA deficiency. J Clin Immunol 2001;21:303–309.

Severe Combined Immunodeficiency (SCID)

Sean A. McGhee

A disorder of adaptive immunity that results in a near complete absence of T- and B-cell function. As a result, both cellular and humoral immunity are compromised.

Etiology

SCID is a genetically heterogeneous condition, with at least 10 different genes known to cause the syndrome, including lack of the common gamma chain (the cause of X-linked SCID), adenosine deaminase deficiency, and recombinase activating gene (RAG) deficiency. Most of the genes causing SCID prevent the development of functional T-cells. The lack of adequate T-cell function inhibits B-cell function as well, resulting in a lack of humoral immunity.

Clinical Presentation and Prognosis

Demographics: SCID is diagnosed before the age of two, as untreated cases almost always die before this age. The preponderance of cases are male because the most common form is X-linked. However, there are many autosomal recessive forms as well.

Presenting signs and symptoms: Patients may present in several ways. Most commonly, patients will present with severe infections, especially viral or fungal infections. Frequently, the presenting infections will be an opportunistic pathogen, such as Pneumocystis jiroveci. However, recurrent or opportunistic infection is only one manner of presentation. Patients may also present with failure to thrive and chronic diarrhea. The initial presentation may also be one of severe erythroderma from graft vs. host disease caused either by a blood transfusion or maternal lymphocytes that are found in the infant. Another presentation may be through dissemination of a live virus vaccine. This happens most frequently in countries in which Bacille Calmette-Guerin vaccination is given for tuberculosis. Finally, patients may be detected as part of a newborn screening program, as some U.S. states currently screen for SCID as part of the newborn screening process.

Clinical course and prognosis: Patients with SCID will eventually develop severe opportunistic, viral and fungal infections, which will be difficult to clear with standard antibiotic therapy. Though their life may be extended with antibiotic prophylaxis and IVIG therapy, they will require stem cell transplantation for long-term survival. Following successful transplant, though, long-term survival is expected.

Long-term survival data has demonstrated that most SCID patients do well following transplant. The immune system is generally not completely reconstituted though, and they retain some susceptibility to infection. About 60% of patients will require IVIG therapy because B-cell function is not completely restored. This is particularly true of those with common gamma chain deficiency, because the common gamma chain also plays a role in B-cell function, but is not required for B-cell development. As a result, most transplanted patients with this disorder engraft T-cells from their donor, but not B-cells. In addition, cutaneous viral infections such as resistant verrucae can be found in post-transplant patients. Finally, there appears to be some advanced senescence of the immune system, with fewer naïve T-cells and recent thymic emigrants. The clinical consequence of this senescence is not yet clear, but does not appear to compromise long-term survival.

Diagnosis

The best screening test for SCID is an absolute lymphocyte count. In infants, a normal ALC will be greater than 4000 cells/mm^3. In SCID infants, this will be usually < 2000 cells/mm^3. Enumeration of T- and B-cells by flow cytometry will identify a marked reduction in T-cell numbers and possibly B-cell numbers. If necessary, the lack of T-cell function can be demonstrated by lymphocyte proliferation studies. An absence of T-cell function is definitive. These studies should be followed by sequencing of candidate genes based on the presence or absence of B- and NK-cells to provide a molecular diagnosis.

Management

Medications: Once a low lymphocyte count is detected, the infant should be given trimethoprim/sulfamethoxasole prophylaxis (5 mg trimethoprim/kg BID) and IVIG (400 mg/kg q 3–4 wks adjusted to keep IgG trough level greater than 600 mg/dL). If the diagnosis has been made because of a presenting infection, the presenting infection must be aggressively treated to prepare the infant for stem cell transplantation. Only irradiated and filtered blood products should be used to prevent graft-vs-host disease.

Surgery: There are no surgical interventions specifically for SCID. Prior to transplant, infants will require excellent venous access, and a long-term tunneled catheter is indicated. Following transplant and engraftment, long-term catheters should be avoided if possible to eliminate the risk of catheter-associated infection.

Stem cell transplant: Immune reconstitution through stem cell transplant is required for all SCID. The protocol used depends on the institution performing the transplant. For most protocols, engraftment is slow and prolonged, with T-cell function not becoming evident until 6–9 months following transplant. Prophylaxis with trimethoprim/sulfamethoxasole and IVIG should be continued during this time. Patients should be kept outpatient as much as possible to avoid iatrogenic infection.

Therapy: There is no specific physical or occupational therapy indicated, though prolonged hospitalization is common around the time of transplant so attention to developmental concerns must be paid during this time.

Social: Genetic counseling is warranted for parents as there is a recurrence risk for most forms of SCID. Following engraftment, children should be encouraged to attend school and undertake normal activities.

Pearls and Precautions

Immunization: BCG vaccination should not be given nor should other live vaccines be used. Once T-cell function has been demonstrated post-transplant, the patient should be vaccinated according to a standard catch-up schedule.

Nutrition: For infants prior to transplant there may be malabsorption and chronic diarrhea complicating nutrition. Parenteral nutrition is indicated if adequate caloric intake cannot be maintained by mouth. Following transplant, this is typically not required.

References

Fischer A, Le Deist F, Hacein-Bey-Abina S, André-Schmütz I, de Saint Basile G, de Villartay JP, et al. Severe combined immunodeficiency. A model for molecular immunology and therapy. Immunol Rev 2009;203:98–109.

Buckley RH. Molecular defects in severe combined immunodeficiency and approaches to immune reconstitution. Ann Rev Immunol 2004;22:625–655.

Transient Hypogammaglobulinemia of Infancy (THI)

Sean A. McGhee

An exaggerated physiologic drop in IgG levels in early infancy that resolves with further development. It is distinguished from CVID by resolution of the problem with age.

Etiology

THI may develop as a result of incomplete transfer of IgG from the mother to the infant during the last trimester of pregnancy, such as may occur with premature birth. With a lower starting level of IgG, the physiologic drop is exaggerated, and may reach a point at which infections start to occur. In other infants, the etiology is not clear.

Clinical Presentation and Prognosis

Demographics: By definition, the disorder presents in infancy and affects both males and females. There is an increased risk in premature infants.

Presenting signs and symptoms: These infants are distinct from those with other immune deficiencies in that they appear relatively healthy. Some, but not all, infants will manifest recurrent infections, generally sinopulmonary or gastrointestinal infection. They do not have opportunistic infections.

Clinical course and prognosis: This disorder is defined by its clinical course and the ultimate resolution of the laboratory abnormality. The time to resolution may extend even into early school age, but most will resolve by 2–3 years of age. It should be distinguished from the normal physiologic nadir in immunoglobulin levels, which occurs from 3–6 months of age and resolves by a year. This occurs as immunoglobulin from the mother is metabolized while the infant's immunoglobulin is just beginning to be produced. In contrast to physiologic hypogammaglobulinemia, THI is more pronounced and longer lasting.

Diagnosis

Infants have a level of IgG less than 2 standard deviations below the mean for age. They should have B-cell numbers checked to exclude X-linked and autosomal recessive agammaglobulinemia due to deficiency of B cells. Infants can be further classified by their response to vaccination. Those who make good responses to their vaccines, as measured by an increase in titer to a protective level, are not candidates for IVIG therapy.

Management

Medications: Most infants with THI will not require IVIG therapy. If recurring sinusitis or otitis media is a problem, short-term antibiotic prophylaxis may resolve the issue long enough to allow recovery of the IgG level. A variety of antibiotics have been used for this purpose including azithromycin, bactrim, and sulfamethoxasole. If there is poor response to vaccination and a history of infection, IVIG therapy may be useful. These patients may be more likely to be cases of common variable immunodeficiency and may be less likely to resolve their hypogammaglobulinemia.

Surgery: Surgical interventions are not required, unless needed for the management of infection (i.e., tympanostomy tubes).

Therapy: There is no specific occupational or physical therapy required.

Social: For infants who are healthy and have good responses to vaccines, the good prognosis should be stressed to parents. They should not be restricted from participating in public activities such as schooling or day care.

Pearls and Precautions

Immunization: Infants may receive routine childhood vaccinations including measles, but response to vaccination should be determined. As mentioned, if there is poor response to vaccination and recurrent infection, IVIG may be warranted temporarily until the problem resolves. Children should be revaccinated after resolution if there has been no response to initial vaccination.

Nutrition: Nutrition may be managed as for any other healthy infant.

Miscellaneous: Careful follow-up is important to distinguish this disorder from common variable immunodeficiency, which also manifests as low immunoglobulin levels with normal B cell numbers. For this reason, the documentation of resolution of the hypogammaglobulinemia is required. If there is no resolution by early school age, the diagnosis must be reconsidered, with CVID as the most likely alternative.

References

Dressler F, Peter HH, Müller W, Rieger CHL. Transient hypogammaglobulinemia of infancy. Five new cases, review of the literature and redefinition. 2008;78:767–774.

Dalal I, Reid B, Nisbet-Brown E, Roifman C. The outcome of patients with hypogammaglobulinemia in infancy and early childhood. J Pediatr 1998;133:144–146.

Wiskott-Aldrich Syndrome (WAS)

Sean A. McGhee

Wiskott-Aldrich Syndrome (WAS) is a genetic disorder that results in thrombocytopenia, eczema, autoimmunity and immune deficiency.

Etiology

WAS results from mutations in a single gene, the Wiskott-Aldrich Syndrome Protein (WASP). Reduction in WASP function results in abnormal signaling and cytoskeletal function, leading to the observed defects.

Clinical Presentation and Prognosis

Demographics: WAS is generally detected early because of the bleeding disorder and severe eczematous rash, often before a year. The disorder is X-linked and so occurs almost exclusively in males.

Presenting signs and symptoms: Although caused by a single gene, there is a wide range of severity in WAS, with some patients having only thrombocytopenia, while others have the full spectrum of thrombocytopenia, eczema, recurrent infection and autoimmunity. Most patients present with bleeding, and abnormal bleeding following circumcision is a common presentation or historical point. A key diagnostic point is that the platelets will be small in this disorder, while they are large in destructive platelet disorders such as ITP.

Clinical course and prognosis: Because of the heterogeneity in the severity of the disorder, it is difficult to predict the clinical course for an individual patient. However, because there is a limited time window for successful stem cell transplantation, close follow-up and monitoring of clinical progress is critical. A decision on transplant must be reached before age 5, and preferably earlier. Those with mild disease may have only manageable thrombocytopenia, while those with severe disease may have uncontrollable autoimmunity and frequent infections.

Pneumocystis jiroveci has been reported in WAS patients, as have candidal infections, in addition to otitis media and frequent viral infections. Autoimmune diseases that have occurred in patients with WAS include Coombs positive hemolytic anemia, vasculitis, Henoch-Schönlein purpura and IgA nephropathy.

Diagnosis

The platelet count and size are key screening parameters for identifying this disorder early. If the clinical scenario is suggestive, WAS protein may be directly measured by flow cytometry, and sequencing of the WASP gene may be performed. A reduction in WASP protein is diagnostic.

Management

Medications: For those with recurrent infection, prophylaxis with IVIG may be useful. Autoimmunity is managed according to the specific type of autoimmunity, and the management strategy generally does not differ from the idiopathic form of the autoimmunity. For example, autoimmune hemolytic anemia is managed with steroid and high-dose IVIG. Eczema is treated with topical steroid, topical tacrolimus and skin hydration, but may be resistant to therapy. Blood products should be CMV negative, filtered and irradiated. Platelet transfusions should be reserved for life-threatening bleeding.

Surgery: Splenectomy is commonly considered in WAS. The thrombocytopenia will improve following splenectomy, but the risk for blood-borne infection will increase. Life-long penicillin prophylaxis is indicated following splenectomy.

Stem Cell Transplant: SCT is curative, but peri-transplant survival is limited. The outcome is much better for those transplanted prior to age 5. Hence, a decision on this point is required by this time. SCT relieves the autoimmunity as well as the infections and thrombocytopenia. Transplantation requires a matched donor. Haploidentical transplants are not used.

Therapy: There is no specific occupational or physical therapy required.

Social: Genetic counseling is indicated for this disorder.

Pearls and Precautions

Immunization: Killed vaccines are acceptable, but live vaccines, such as attenuated influenza vaccine, measles, mumps, rubella, oral polio, varicella, or BCG, should be avoided.

Nutrition: Nutrition is generally maintained PO and is usually not a concern.

Miscellaneous: Wiskott-Aldrich syndrome patients are frequently misdiagnosed as having idiopathic thrombocytopenic purpura. The platelet volume is small in WAS and large in ITP, and the thrombocytopenia in WAS does not respond to IVIG or steroids.

WAS patients may require higher doses or more frequent doses of IVIG to maintain adequate levels. Avoid aspirin, NSAIDs, or other platelet inhibitors.

References

Ochs HD, Thrasher AJ. The Wiskott-Aldrich syndrome. J Allergy Clin Immunol 2006;117:725–738.

Symons M, Derry JM, Karlak B, Jiang S, Lemahieu V, McCormick F, Franck U, Abo A. Wiskott-Aldrich syndrome protein, a novel effector for the GTPase CDC42Hs, is implicated in actin polymerization. 1996;84:723–734.

Notarangelo LD, Miao CH, Ochs HD. Wiskott-Aldrich syndrome. Curr Opin Hematology. 2008;15:30–36.

Meer S, Liu A. Isolation of a novel gene mutated in Wiskott-Aldrich syndrome. 1995;96:411

Kim AS, Kakalis LT, Abdul-Manan N, Liu GA, et al. Autoinhibition and activation mechanisms of the Wiskott-Aldrich syndrome protein. Nature 2000;404:151–58.

Snapper SB, Rosen FS, Mizoguchi E, Cohen P, et al. Wiskott-Aldrich syndrome protein-deficient mice reveal a role for WASP in T-cell but not B-cell activation. Immunity 1998;9:81–91.

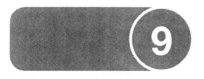

9 Infectious Diseases

Table of Contents

Congenital Cytomegalovirus (CMV) Infection

Natascha Ching

Etiology

CMV is a double stranded DNA and is a member of the *Herpesviridae* DNA virus group.

Clinical Presentation and Prognosis:

Demographics: The incidence of congenital CMV disease is estimated at 1% which accounts for about 30,000 to 40,000 cases per year in the United States. Approximately 10–15% of patients with congenital CMV are symptomatic at birth while 80–90% of patients are asymptomatic at birth. Of those with symptomatic congenital CMV infection, about half will go on to have sensorineural hearing loss (SNHL), mental retardation and microcephaly.

Presenting signs and symptoms: Symptomatic congenital CMV infection may present with signs of sepsis, pneumonia, colitis, hepatitis, chorioretinitis, intrauterine growth retardation (IUGR), central nervous system (CNS) disease with intracerebral and periventricular cerebral calcifications and/or involvement of reticuloendothelial system. Patients may have hepatomegaly, splenomegaly, microcephaly, jaundice, neutropenia, anemia, thrombocytopenia, purpura or petechial rash. Asymptomatic congenital CMV infants may have a silent disease with no signs or symptoms at initial presentation, but develop neurological impairment later in life.

Transmission: Women of childbearing age may acquire CMV from their young children who were infected from an outside source. CMV is transmitted in utero transplacentally, at birth via passage through infected maternal genital tract (cervical infection), or postnatally via breast milk. In utero infections can be from primary or recurrent maternal infections. There is a greater risk to the fetus in the first half of gestation.

Clinical course: Symptomatic congenital CMV infection with multisystem organ disease may have significant morbidity and mortality along with long term SNHL and neurodevelopmental sequelae. Asymptomatic neonates may have more subtle sequelae that manifest later in life as significant mental retardation, cerebral palsy or SNHL or progression of developmental disabilities.

Prognosis: The mortality rate is approximately 5% for symptomatic congenital CMV. About 10% of symptomatic neonates may have poor outcomes with hearing loss and mental retardation. For asymptomatic infants, about 10% may develop SNHL, 5% may have microcephaly and neuromuscular defects and 2% may have chorioretinitis later in childhood. Abnormal neuroradiographic findings such as intracranial calcifications and ventriculomegaly along with increased cerebral spinal fluid protein in symptomatic congenital CMV disease are prognostic indicators of adverse neurodevelopmental outcomes.

Diagnosis

The diagnosis of congenital CMV infection requires isolation of CMV from urine, stool, respiratory tract secretion or cerebral spinal fluid within the first 2–3 weeks of life. This timeframe is utilized to determine in utero versus perinatal infection, unless there is significant CNS disease with intracerebral calcifications or chorioretinitis. The first priority in the diagnosis of congenital CMV infection is to determine the severity of clinical disease. Detailed clinical examination at initial diagnosis should be performed along with laboratory evaluation of complete blood counts, liver enzymes, neuroradiologic imaging, and audiological evaluation. Laboratory diagnostic monitoring should be performed with molecular tests to check CMV viral load. Molecular testing with CMV DNA hybridization or PCR has become the more standard method of quantifying viral load and is also used for monitoring disease. Serological diagnosis of strongly positive CMV IgM in cord or peripheral blood in the first 2–3 weeks can be indicative of congenital CMV infection but not definitive and further workup as described previously should be initiated.

Management

There is no current literature to suggest that treatment with antiviral therapy for asymptomatic congenital CMV will prevent or possibly alter SNHL or neurodevelopmental outcomes.

In regards to treatment of symptomatic congenital CMV disease in infants involving the CNS, there has been a phase III, randomized, controlled trial that treated infants with 6 weeks of intravenous ganciclovir. The investigators found improved hearing function (or maintenance of normal hearing function) and prevention of hearing deterioration at 6 months. There was also the possibility of prevention of hearing deterioration at or beyond 1 year. Although this study has provided encouraging information about the use of antiviral therapy in congenital CMV disease to limit neurodevelopmental injury, the antiviral medication is not without side effects. There is also potential for long-term gonadal toxicity or carcinogenicity, effects that are being studied by the NIH-NIAID Collaborative Anti-viral Study Group (CASG).

Ganciclovir intravenous therapy for 6 weeks may be considered for patients with severe symptomatic congenital CMV but consultation with a Pediatric Infectious Disease specialist should be obtained to determine treatment course, monitor toxicities and long-term follow-up. If patients are placed on this therapy, complete blood counts, liver enzymes and renal function should be followed along with close monitoring for central venous catheter infections. Molecular testing should also be followed to monitor CMV DNA viral load. Some Pediatric Infectious Disease experts may consider long-term suppressive antiviral therapy for neonates with symptomatic CMV disease with CNS involvement but this is still being investigated. Therapeutic options should be discussed with parents to evaluate the risks and benefits of antiviral therapy.

Medications

Ganciclovir (Cytovene®): Ganciclovir is a synthetic acyclic nucleoside analog similar to guanine that is given intravenously. This drug has been used for the treatment of severe CMV disease in those with CMV retinitis and end-organ disease in immunosuppressed patients. Symptomatic patients with congenital and perinatal CMV infection have been treated with a total daily dose of 12 mg/kg/day divided twice a day given intravenously through a central venous catheter. The duration of treatment in clinical trial was for a treatment course of 6 weeks. The oral formulation of ganciclovir has poor oral bioavailability and has not been studied for long term use in pediatric patients to prevent neurodevelopmental adverse outcomes.

The toxicities associated with ganciclovir are myelosuppression with reversible neutropenia, anemia and thrombocytopenia, but can recover with discontinuation of the drug. Granulocyte colony stimulating factor or granulocyte-monocyte colony stimulating factor is often considered to help with neutropenia. The dose should be adjusted with renal insufficiency due to renal clearance. Catheter related infections should be closely monitored during intravenous administration of medication.

Valganciclovir (Valcyte®): Valganciclovir is a prodrug of ganciclovir that is available in an oral formulation and is licensed for the treatment of CMV retinitis in HIV-infected adults and the prevention for CMV disease in high risk transplant recipients. Studies are currently in progress to evaluate the short- vs. long-term therapy with valganciclovir for symptomatic congenital CMV infections.

Long-term follow up care: Growth parameters, neurological examination, auditory evaluations, and ophthalmologic evaluation should be performed to monitor for neurodevelopmental outcome. Developmental and intellectual assessments should also be performed with standard psychometric tests based on the age of the patient as time progresses to determine extent of learning disabilities.

Surgery: Neurosurgical intervention may be necessary for ventricular peritoneal shunts for those with severe hydrocephalus.

Therapy: Physical, occupational and speech therapy should be offered with enrollment in early intervention programs.

Pearls and Precautions

Likely complications: Neurodevelopmental disabilities may be SNHL, vision difficulties, cerebral palsy, or mental retardation. Congenital CMV is progressive so close follow-up should be provided for SNHL and these neurodevelopmental outcomes. In asymptomatic congenital CMV, the hearing loss may also be progressive or be delayed in onset. SNHL may result in a bilateral deficit and can vary from mild to high frequency loss to profound impairment. Ongoing audiological evaluation is critical to determine if hearing aids and speech therapy should be provided. Ophthalmologic evaluation should monitor for CMV chorioretinitis and assess optic neuritis, cataract formation or colobomas.

School/Education: Special educational services and early intervention resources are critical for children who are at risk for neurodevelopmental disabilities. Developmental delay, SNHL, learning disabilities and motor deficits should be evaluated. Students should have speech and language therapy and special seating in the classroom.

Infection control: Children with CMV should not be kept out of day care. Although patients with congenital CMV infection may have asymptomatic shedding, individuals should not be treated differently. However, when caring for children with CMV infection, attention should be paid to proper hand hygiene, especially after diaper changes. Pregnant women with children younger than 2 years of age should assume that children may shed the virus and therefore, should perform careful hand hygiene when in contact with secretions and excretions.

Early Diagnosis: Infants who fail their newborn hearing screen should be evaluated for congenital CMV infection as a possible cause.

References

American Academy of Pediatrics. Cytomegalovirus Infection. In: Pickering LK, Baker, CJ, Long SS, McMillan JA, editors. Red Book: 2006. Report of the Committee on Infectious Diseases. Elk Grove Village, IL: American Academy of Pediatrics; 2006. p. 273–277.

Kimberlin DW, Lin CY, Sanchez PJ, Demmler GJ, Dankner W, Shelton M, et al. Effect of ganciclovir therapy on hearing in symptomatic congenital cytomegalovirus disease involving the central nervous system: a randomized, controlled tril. J. Pediatr 2003; 143(1):16–25.

Ross SA, Boppana SB. Congenital cytomegalovirus infection: outcome and diagnosis. Semin Pediatr Infect Dis 2005;16(1):44–9.

Schleiss MR. Antiviral therapy of congenital cytomegalovirus infection. Semin Pediatr Infect Dis 2005;16(1):50–9.

Hepatitis B infection (HBV)

Natascha Ching

Etiology

Hepatitis B virus (HBV) is a DNA virus from the hepadnavirus family.

Clinical Presentation and Prognosis

Demographics: Due to the high prevalence of this disease in Asia (which includes Southeast Asia, East Asia and Northern Asia), the Pacific Islands, South America, Eastern Europe, the Middle East and Africa, children born to immigrants or adopted from these countries are at risk for perinatal transmission of HBV. Adolescents and adults in the U.S. are at risk of acute HBV if they are or have ever been an injection-drug user, are men who have sex with men or have multiple heterosexual partners. Adolescents and adults with HBV may also have associated other sexually transmitted infections. Institutionalized individuals such as those with severe developmental disabilities and patients who undergo hemodialysis may also be at risk of HBV.

Transmission: Perinatal infection is acquired when virus is transmitted from a mother with chronic Hepatitis B surface antigen (HBSAg) or acute HBV infection. Risks of transmission are greater with a mother who is Hepatitis Be Antigen (HBeAg) positive or has high HBV DNA viral load. HBV is transmitted through blood or direct contact with other infected body fluids such as wound exudates, saliva, semen, or cervical secretions. Modes of transmission may include percutaneous or mucosal contact with these fluids through open cuts or sores, non-sterile needles, syringes or medical equipment or sexual exposure. Patients with chronic HBV may be a source of infection, and universal precautions should be followed for household contacts.

Presenting signs and symptoms: Infants and children less than 5 years of age may present with asymptomatic infection. Older children may have mild constitutional symptoms or fulminant hepatic failure with jaundice, encephalopathy or coagulopathy. Adults may present with symptoms of icterus after an incubation period of 6 weeks to 6 months. Acute hepatitis in adulthood may present as an acute exacerbation of chronic HBV infection that occurred in childhood. The incubation period for acute HBV infection is 45 to 160 days.

Perinatal Hepatitis B: Perinatal transmission to the newborn may be asymptomatic, but signs may present at 2–6 months of age. Infants may have non-specific signs of low-grade fever, lethargy, poor feeding, or they may present with mild jaundice with a varying degree of mild to fulminant hepatitis. Infants with perinatal infection have been described to be "immune tolerant" with high HBV DNA viral loads and normal alanine-amino-transferase (ALT). These individuals may develop HBeAg positive chronic HBV with increased ALT later in life.

Acute Hepatitis B Symptoms: Fatigue, poor appetite, nausea, vomiting, abdominal pain, low-grade fever, jaundice, dark urine and light colored stool.

Signs: jaundice, liver tenderness, hepatomegaly, or splenomegaly

Extrahepatic clinical manifestations such as arthritis, arthralgias, macular rashes, thrombocytopenia, or papular acrodermatitis (Gianotti-Crosti syndrome) and membranous glomerulonephritis can occur.

Chronic Hepatitis B: Chronic HBV infection occurs when patients continue to have detectable hepatitis B surface antigen (HBsAg) and do not develop HBsAb. These individuals may be asymptomatic for years.

Clinical course

Acute HBV: Patients may have acute hepatitis with asymptomatic seroconversion with signs and symptoms dependent on age. Duration may be up to 6 months.

Chronic Hepatitis B: Patients with chronic HBV may be asymptomatic for years and present with serious liver disease with chronic hepatitis, cirrhosis or hepatocellular carcinoma later in life.

Prognosis: The age of the patient is an important predictor for development of chronic HBV infection. Untreated infants with perinatally transmitted HBV from a mother who is HBeAg positive have about a 90% risk of chronic HBV. For children 1–5 years of age, there is a 25–50% chance, while children greater than 5 years of age and adults have a 5–10% chance of chronic HBV. Up to 25% of infants and older children with chronic HBV are at risk of developing HBV related hepatocellular carcinoma and cirrhosis. Patients who remain HBeAg positive are at risk for progressive liver disease. Patients with immunosuppression or other chronic illnesses may have an increased risk of developing chronic infection with HBV. In addition, if patients become immunosuppressed, patients with resolved chronic HBV may have reactivation of HBV.

Diagnosis: Serological testing for hepatitis B surface antigen (HBsAg), hepatitis B surface antibody (HBsAb), IgM-antibody to Hepatitis B core antigen (IgM anti-HBcAg), total antibody to Hepatitis B core antigen, hepatitis Be antigen and hepatitis B antibody provide information about the different phases of acute and chronic HBV infection. (See Tables 9.1 and 9.2)

Diagnosis

Molecular tests: Polymerase chain reaction (PCR) assays for HBV DNA can detect and quantify viral load in serum and tissue, and be used to monitor response to treatment.

- The diagnosis of chronic HBV is confirmed with positive HBsAg on 2 episodes separated by a 6 month period.
- High levels of HBV DNA and HBeAg indicate active viral replication and increased infectivity in either acute or chronic HBV infection.

Management

Immunoprophylaxis of perinatally exposed infant: For infants born to a mother with a positive HBsAg, HBV vaccine and Hepatitis B Immune Globulin (HBIG) should be given within 12 hours of birth simultaneously, but at 2 separate sites. The infant should receive the 2nd dose at 1 month and 3rd dose at 6 months of age. The

Table 9.1:   Different Phases of Hepatitis B

HBV surface antigen (HBsAg)	Protein on surface of HBV. Can be positive in acute or chronic HBV infection
HBV surface antibody (HBsAb)	Denotes resolved HBV infection or protective immunity after immunization
IgM-antibody to Hepatitis B core antigen (IgM anti-HBCAg)	Indicates acute infection in window period ≤6 months (except in perinatally infected infants)
Total antibody to Hepatitis B core antigen (Total anti-HBcAg)	May appear at onset of acute infection and persist for life; may indicate previous or ongoing infection
Hepatitis Be Antigen (HBeAg)	Product of nucleocapside gene of HBV found in acute and chronic HBV Means virus is replicating and person is infectious
Hepatitis Be Antibody (HBeAb)	May be produced during or after viral replication

Table 9.2:   Types and Phases of Hepatitis B

HBV Disease	HBS Ag	HBs Ab	IgM-anti –HBcAg	Total anti- HBcAg	HBe Ag	HBe Ab	HBV DNA	Notes
Susceptible	–	–	–					
Immune-natural infection	–	+		+				
Immune-HBV vaccine	–	+		–				
Acute HBV	+	–	+	+				
Chronic HBV	+	–	–	+				
Chronic HBV – HbeAg positive	+	–	–	+	+	–	+++	High HBV DNA likely transmit
							±	Low HBV DNA inactive-chronically infected
Chronic HBV – HbeAg negative	+	–	–	+	–	+	+++	
Resolved infection **	–	+	+					Clearance HBsAg; usually normal LFTs and develop HBsAb

**Can also be false positive anti-HBc total (susceptible), low level chronic infection or resolving acute infection.

infants should have testing of HBsAb and HBsAg after completion of the immunization series, at 9–18 months of age. If there is no detectable HBsAb and the HBSAg is negative, a repeat hepatitis B series of 3 doses (0, 1 and 6 month schedule) may be repeated. HBsAb and HBSAg should be rechecked one month after the 3rd dose. In order to further evaluate for perinatal HBV infection (despite immunoprophylaxis due to intrauterine infection or vaccine failure), referral to a pediatric infectious disease specialist should be made if (a) there is no detectable HBsAb; and (b) HBSAg is positive.

Acute HBV: Supportive care, no medication available.

Chronic HBV: Medical evaluation necessary to monitor and determine whether disease is progressing and determine if therapy is indicated.

Clinical monitoring

Children and adolescents with chronic HBV should be followed closely to evaluate for complications of serious liver disease, cirrhosis and hepatocellular carcinoma as they mature. There are no established pediatric guidelines for monitoring pediatric patients, but some specialists extrapolate from the Adult guidelines. Complications in patients with chronic HBV should be monitored with serum liver transaminase tests (specifically ALT or Serum glutamic pyruvic transaminase (SGPT)), HBV DNA viral load, alpha-fetoprotein concentration (AFP) (as a marker to detect hepatocellular carcinoma) and abdominal ultrasonography to evaluate the liver for any signs of tumors. The testing interval for patients with chronic HBV varies with each individual patient and specialist, but would be more frequently checked in patients with abnormal results or reactivation of HBV. Liver biopsy is used to evaluate the extent of liver damage and rule out other etiologies of liver disease.

Medications

Adults with chronic HBV have FDA approved medications such as interferon-alfa, lamivudine, adefovir and entecavir. Currently, the pediatric treatment options in the United States consist of 2 FDA approved drugs for children with chronic hepatitis B: interferon alpha-2b and lamivudine. Adefovir has only been approved for children 12–17 years of age. The goal of treatment in chronic HBV is to induce seroconversion (loss of HBeAg and HBSAg and the development of HBeAb and HBsAb), achieve viral suppression of HBV DNA replication, normalization of transaminase enzymes and eventually decrease inflammation as determined by liver histology. Studies of children with chronic HBV found that between about 20–58% of patients responded to treatment with interferon alfa2b compared to 8–17% of controls. Treatment with lamivudine for children with chronic HBV has been shown to be associated with higher rates of seroconversion from HBeAg to HBeAb, normalization of ALT and viral suppression of HBV DNA in 23% of patients as compared to 13% of controls.

Patients diagnosed with acute or chronic HBV should be evaluated by a physician who specializes in chronic HBV infection to determine whether treatment for chronic HBV should be initiated. If serum ALT is persistently greater than 2 times the upper limit of normal, AFP is elevated or abdominal ultrasound is abnormal, initiation of therapy may be considered. However, the advantages and disadvantages of therapy must be carefully considered for each case, as therapy produces significant side effects.

Interferon alpha-2b (Intron®A) has anti-viral, anti-proliferative and immunomodulatory effects. It is an intramuscular injection usually given three times a week for 4–6 months at a dose of $6x10^6$ Units/m^2 or max $10x10^6$ Units/m^2. Adverse effects include fever, headache, myalgia, neutropenia, worsening hepatitis, depression, or irritability.

Lamivudine (Epivir-HBV®) is a nucleoside analog that inhibits HBV polymerase and prevents viral replication which in turn reduces viral load, liver damage and inflammation. However, there is a risk of selecting lamivudine resistant mutations with longer duration of treatment. While on lamivudine, liver enzymes are monitored every 3 months and HBV DNA is monitored every 3–6 months. HBeAg and HBeAb are tested at the end of 1 year of treatment and every 3–6 months thereafter. Total duration of therapy for pediatric patients should be until 6 months after HBeAg positive patients seroconvert and for 6 months or until HBSAg clearance for HBeAg negative patients.

Adefovir dipivoxil (Hepsera®) is a nucleotide analog reverse transcriptase inhibitor. This drug has been used in adults with chronic HBV as first line therapy as well as for those with lamivudine-resistance. This drug was found to be safe and efficacious in children between 12–17 years of age for treatment of chronic HBV.

Surgery: Liver biopsy may be performed in chronic hepatitis to determine the extent of inflammation by histology and to monitor therapy.

Pearls and Precautions

Nutrition: No specific dietary measures have been shown to affect progression of chronic HBV, but alcohol use should be avoided as a risk factor for development of cirrhosis.

Likely complications: Chronic HBV may lead to cirrhosis, hepatocellular carcinoma, liver failure or death.

Medications/situations that need to be avoided/infection control etc.: Universal precautions should be initiated to prevent person to person spread of HBV in the setting of a patient with acute or chronic HBV in households. Young children are at risk, and spread from child to child can occur. Exact mechanisms for transmission are unknown, but contact with skin or mucous membranes with blood-containing secretions or saliva may be a source. Personal care items such as washcloths, towels, razors or toothbrushes should not be shared. Household bleach diluted 1:10 with water can be used to clean the environment to inactivate the HBV. Guidance should be offered on prevention through close contact or sexual behavior. All patients with chronic HBV should receive 2 doses of Hepatitis A vaccine separated by 6 months apart if not already immune to Hepatitis A. Hepatotoxic drugs such as acetaminophen should be avoided, and non-steroidal anti-inflammatory drugs should be used instead for analgesic or antipyretic needs.

References

American Academy of Pediatrics. Hepatitis B. In: Pickering LK, Baker CJ, Long SS, McMillan JA, editors. Red Book: 2006 Report of the Committee on Infectious Diseases. Elk Grove Village, IL: American Academy of Pediatrics; 2006. p. 335–355.

Lok AS, McMahon BJ. Chronic hepatitis B. Hepatology 2007;45(2):507–39.

Kurbegov AC, Sokol RJ. Hepatitis B therapy in children. Expert Rev Gastroenterol Hepatol 2009;3(1):39–49.

Slowik MK, Jhaveri R. Hepatitis B and C viruses in infants and young children. Semin Pediatr Infect Dis 2005;16(4):296–305.

Weinbaum CM, Williams I, Mast EE, Wang SA, Finelli L, Wasley A, et al. Recommendations for identification and public health management of persons with chronic hepatitis B virus infection. MMWR Recomm Rep 2008;57(RR-8):1–20.

Neonatal Herpes Simplex Virus (HSV) Infections

Natascha Ching

Etiology

Herpes simplex virus (HSV) types 1 and 2 are double-stranded DNA viruses from the Herpesviridae family which can cause neonatal or congenital infection.

Clinical Presentation and Prognosis

Demographics: In the United States, neonatal HSV disease occurs in about 1 in 3200 deliveries with an estimated 1500 cases annually. The majority of newborn HSV infections (85%) are from transmission of HSV from maternal genital tract secretions during delivery. Infants may also acquire this infection by the intra-uterine route in 5% of cases or post-partum via maternal or other close contacts in 10% of cases. Infants born to mothers with primary genital herpes late in pregnancy or at delivery may be at high risk of transmission.

Clinical Course:

1. Disseminated disease involving multiple organs such as the brain, lung, liver, adrenal glands, skin, and/or eye.
2. Central Nervous System disease can present with encephalitis with or without skin involvement. Patients with CNS disease may have significant brain destruction with acute neurological and autonomic abnormalities. Neonatal HSV can involve any or multiple areas of the brain as compared to the temporal lobe CNS disease that occurs in children outside the neonatal period.
3. Localized disease limited to skin, eye, and/or mouth disease (SEM disease). Approximately 80–85% of patients with SEM disease may present with vesicular lesions.

Presenting signs and symptoms: Symptoms may include fever, temperature instability, lethargy, cutaneous lesions, seizures, disseminated intravascular coagulopathy (DIC), hepatitis, and pneumonitis. Seizures and skin vesicles are clinical features suggestive of neonatal HSV disease. Vesicular lesions may develop in 39% of neonates with disseminated disease, 32% in CNS disease, and 17% in SEM disease.

The clinical presentation of neonatal HSV may vary depending on type of disease:

- Patients with disseminated disease may present with signs of sepsis, respiratory failure, liver failure, DIC, hepatitis, or pneumonitis.

- Infants with CNS disease may present with focal or generalized seizures, lethargy, poor feeding, temperature instability or bulging fontanelle. About 60–70% of these patients with CNS disease may have skin vesicles during the course of their disease.

Patients with disseminated disease or SEM may present at 10–12 days of life as compared to those patients with CNS disease who may present at 16–19 days of life.

Prognosis: Patient mortality is usually related to disseminated disease with severe DIC, liver failure or pulmonary involvement. Prior to the antiviral era, 85% of patients with disseminated disease died by 1 year of age while 50% died with CNS disease. However, with the high dose acyclovir treatment regimen, mortality has decreased to 29% for disseminated disease and 4% for CNS disease. Factors associated with mortality are lethargy and severe hepatitis for those with disseminated disease, and prematurity and seizures for those with CNS disease. There is a slightly improved neurological outcome—from 50%, to 83%—in patients having disseminated disease in the post antiviral era. Those patients with SEM disease during the antiviral era have had fewer developmental delays than those with SEM disease prior to antiviral use.

Diagnosis

Infants with suspected HSV infection should be evaluated for disseminated disease, CNS disease and SEM disease. Viral cultures should be performed of skin lesions, and of the CSF, urine, blood, and stool. In addition, viral cultures of skin lesions or vesicles, mucous membranes and surface cultures of oropharynx, nasopharynx, conjunctivae and rectum prior to antiviral therapy should also be performed to determine extent of neonatal HSV disease. It is best to obtain CSF studies with cell indices and chemistry along with CSF viral cultures and CSF HSV PCR. There may be a pleocytosis in the CSF with 20–100 WBC/ml and elevated protein. However, this may not be seen in early neonatal HSV disease. CSF viral cultures may be positive in less than 50% of viral cultures so molecular testing of CSF is essential.

Molecular testing by HSV polymerase chain reaction (PCR) should be sent from CSF and blood. HSV PCR from the CSF is critical to diagnose extent of disease. However, the PCR result should be correlated with the clinical presentation of the infant so in some cases a negative test does not always eliminate possibility of neonatal HSV disease.

HSV Direct Fluorescent Antibody (DFA) tests can be performed on cutaneous lesions or vesicles in some microbiology laboratories. This test is performed by unroofing the vesicle or lesion, scraping the lesion base with a sterile dacron swab, smearing a glass slide with specimen and sending it to a lab for further staining so as to look for the HSV virus. Serologic testing is useful in some cases. While a positive HSV IgM or four fold change in HSV IgM may help in diagnosis, HSV IgG is usually not helpful because of transplacental transfer of maternal IgG.

Management

Medications

Parenteral acyclovir dosed at 60 mg/kg/day divided every 8 hours (20 mg/kg/dose) should be given intravenously for neonatal HSV disease. Premature infants need adjustment of dosing interval. Treatment duration for disseminated or CNS disease is 21 days. Localized SEM disease can be treated for 14 days. CSF fluid studies should be repeated at the end of therapy to document negative HSV PCR and evaluate CSF cells indices and other studies. It has been recommended that if HSV PCR is positive after 21 days of therapy, intravenous acyclovir should be continued until it is negative. While on acyclovir, complete blood counts should be monitored for absolute neutrophil counts. If absolute neutrophil count is below 500, Granulocyte colony-stimulating factor (GCSF) use is considered in some instances.

There is concern of HSV reactivation leading to relapse of HSV disease involving skin, eyes, mouth and CNS with recurrent damage. Currently, the use of suppressive oral acyclovir therapy is under evaluation in an NIH-NIAID Collaborative Anti-viral Study Group (CASG) phase III placebo-controlled trial of suppressive oral acyclovir for 6 months in neonates with CNS disease after initial treatment for neonatal HSV. The study is evaluating the neurological impairment and cutaneous recurrence of HSV. Some experts may consider long-term suppressive antiviral therapy for neonates with SEM, but this is still being investigated. One should consult with a pediatric infectious diseases specialist for individualized long term management of these patients.

Therapy: Physical and occupational therapy may be indicated, particularly for those with CNS disease.

Pearls and Precautions

- Septic neonates with a negative bacterial work-up should be evaluated and empirically treated for neonatal HSV disease while viral work-up is pending.
- Relapse of CNS and SEM disease can occur after completion of treatment.
- Acyclovir dose for HSV disease in neonates and infants from birth to 3 months should be 20 mg/kg/dose every 8 hours.
- Acyclovir dose for HSV encephalitis for children 3 months to 12 years of age should be 20 mg/kg/dose every 8 hours.
- Acyclovir dose for HSV encephalitis for adults and adolescents ≥12 years is 10 mg/kg/dose every 8 hours.

Likely complications: Complications include ocular sequelae, motor delay, speech delay, microcephaly, hemiparesis, spastic quadriplegia, persistent seizures, chorioretinitis, blindness, and developmental delay. For this reason, neurologic and developmental assessment should be followed closely. Ophthalmologic evaluation should also be obtained to monitor for eye involvement and recurrence of HSV keratitis. Close monitoring should also evaluate for any recurrent skin lesions or vesicles.

School/education: Early intervention programs should be comprehensive and include physical therapy, occupational therapy, and speech therapy.

Infection control: Neonates with mucocutaneous lesions should have contact precautions initiated; otherwise, standard precautions should be followed for those with CNS disease.

References

American Academy of Pediatrics. Herpes Simplex. In: Pickering LK, Baker CJ, Long SS, McMillan JA, editors. Red Book: 2006 Report of the Committee on Infectious Diseases. Elk Grove Village, IL: American Academy of Pediatrics; 2006. p. 361–371.

Enright AM, Prober CG. Neonatal herpes infection: diagnosis, treatment and prevention. Semin Neonatol 2002;7(4):283–91.

Kimberlin DW. Herpes simplex virus infections of the newborn. Semin Perinatol 2007;31(1):19–25.

Kimberlin DW, Lin CY, Jacobs RF, Powell DA, Corey L, Gruber WC, et al. Safety and efficacy of high-dose intravenous acyclovir in the management of neonatal herpes simplex virus infections. Pediatrics 2001;108(2):230–8.

Pediatric Human Immunodeficiency Virus (HIV) Disease/ AIDS

Karin Nielsen-Saines

Etiology

HIV-infection is the cause of a chronic, eventually fatal illness (in the absence of treatment), caused by a human retrovirus, Human Immunodeficiency Virus type 1 (HIV-1). Human retroviruses include human T-cell lymphotropic viruses (HTLV-I, HTLV-II, HTLV-III and HTLV-VI), also known as oncoviruses, and lentiviruses (HIV-1 and HIV-2). Retroviruses are RNA viruses capable of transforming themselves into DNA viruses and integrating into the host cell genome. Prior to 1980, retroviruses were only known to cause disease in animals. However, shortly thereafter HTLV-I and II were shown to be associated with human disease. The virus responsible for the newly identified human acquired immunodeficiency syndrome (AIDS) was described by a number of investigators worldwide in 1983. It was initially termed human lymphotropic virus III or lymphadenopathy associated virus, but further identification revealed the syndrome was caused by a single novel virus renamed HIV. Two species of HIV were later identified, HIV-1 and HIV-2. Both are lentiviruses responsible for the development of AIDS. However, transmission patterns, demographics and disease progression differ. HIV-2 is closely related to Simian Immunodeficiency Virus (SIV), and is not generally responsible for pediatric HIV disease, as it has lower rates of mother to child transmission and a very protracted disease course. In children, HIV-1 is responsible for pediatric disease.

Pathogenesis: HIV-1 is a viral quasispecies, with multiple viral strains circulating in an infected individual at a given moment. The virus requires the expression of CD4+ receptors and specific cell surface co-receptors such as CCR5 and CXCR4 for viral entry and cell infection. HIV-1 infects CD4+ cells, monocytes, macrophages and glial cells. Immune activation, particularly in the gut, is a required phenomenon in viral pathogenesis. The destruction of CD4+ cells is a hallmark of HIV disease. Declining CD4+ cells and development of opportunistic infections characterize the tail end of HIV disease, also known as Acquired Immunodeficiency Syndrome (AIDS).

Origin and transmission: HIV originated in Central Africa where it infected non human primate species for centuries. It is thought that the virus spread to humans in the first half of the twentieth century through blood exposure from the hunting and processing of bush meat. The virus is transmitted in humans through sexual contact, exposure to blood or blood products, and from mother to child during pregnancy, labor and delivery or postpartum through breastfeeding. In the absence of treatment, approximately 8–10% of infants are infected during pregnancy; an additional 10–15% at birth; and, an estimated 16% during breastfeeding. Thus, the overall risk of HIV transmission from an untreated mother to her child in the first year of life is approximately 40%.

Epidemiology: It is estimated that approximately 36 million individuals worldwide are infected with HIV-1. Over the course of the last 28 years, since the epidemic was first described, approximately 24 million individuals succumbed to the disease. HIV/ AIDS is the second leading cause of global disease burden and the leading cause of death in sub-Saharan Africa. The HIV pandemic has reversed all health care benefits brought to the developing world in the last 30 years. Life expectancy in countries where HIV is endemic has decreased by 30–40% within the last two decades. Approximately 5 million children are infected with HIV worldwide and 50% of these will die due to the illness before age 5 years.

Clinical presentation: Children who are born with HIV or acquire it shortly after birth have a faster pace of disease progression than adults. Infants infected in utero are particularly susceptible to rapid disease progression. In developed countries, prior to availability of effective treatment, approximately 20% of infected children developed AIDS or died by 2 years of age (rapid progressors); 60–70% developed AIDS symptoms by age 7–8 years (intermediate progressors); and, a remaining 10–20% showed minimal symptoms of HIV disease until adolescence (slow progressors). A subpopulation of adolescent slow progressors is equivalent to the so-called adult elite controllers, patients capable of controlling their HIV illness and maintaining an undetectable virus load without the use of antiretrovirals. It is estimated, however, that these are less than 5% of the total number of infected pediatric patients. Rapid progression of HIV disease is generally the rule in children and one of the reasons for rapid disease progression is the coexistence of an immature immune system and an extraordinarily high peak viremia during primary infection. HIV viral dynamics in infants are such that peak viremia is reached between 5–10 weeks of life and persists for approximately 6 months, which is different from the viral dynamics in adults. The presence and quantity of HIV RNA at birth and the magnitude and duration of viremia are predictors of disease outcome. In developing countries, where the environmental burden of disease is significantly higher, and malnutrition and anemia coexist, chances of survival with untreated HIV disease are exceedingly lower. In such a scenario, with a compromised immune system, children do not develop the necessary immunity to surrounding illnesses and vaccines most frequently do not generate protective titers. Regular childhood illnesses soon become unmanageable with chronic diarrhea and growth delay highly prevalent. Natural history studies conducted in sub-Saharan Africa indicate that 40% of HIV-infected infants die within the first year of life and that by approximately age 3–5 yrs., this figure escalates to 60%. According to the World Health Organization's (WHO) moderate to severe disease (MSD) classification, if infants are symptomatic in the first year of life, their chance of dying is 90%.

Presenting signs and symptoms: Disease manifestations in HIV infected children vary according to the stage of disease progression and environmental conditions (resourceful versus resource-limited settings). Generalized lymphadenopathy, parotid enlargement and hepatosplenomegaly are frequent features in symptomatic children. Recurrent bacterial infections in childhood and rapid onset of Pneumocystis carinii pneumonia (P. jiroveci) in the first six months of life are very common in untreated children. In very advanced progressors, however, lymphadenopathy may no longer be present. Chronic diarrhea, recurrent thrush, and particularly failure to thrive are extremely common features in rapid disease progressors. As such, growth parameters have been shown to be very useful clinical surrogates in assessing disease progression, especially in the developing world. The presence of coinfections such as tuberculosis and disseminated atypical mycobacterial infections are also frequent, especially in older children. Recurrent infections with herpes family viruses is a frequent finding in children with advanced HIV; and with patients suffering from recurrent HSV-1 lesions, recurrent varicella, or shingles. In sub-Saharan Africa, HHV-8 infections with Kaposi sarcoma in children are not as rare as in the developed world. Epstein-Barr virus (EBV) disease with Burkitt lymphomas in young HIV-infected African children is also not uncommon. EBV associated illness in HIV infected children also manifests itself as lymphoid interstitial pneumonitis (LIP), a chronic lung disease with characteristic radiological findings. With the advent of effective antiretroviral therapy, however, LIP—a late complication of HIV disease in children—has virtually disappeared in pediatric HIV-infected patients. Concurrent CMV infection has been shown to accelerate the HIV disease course in infants. However, CMV retinitis occurs only in approximately 5% of children and is generally a more frequent complication of late stage disease in adults. Other manifestations of HIV disease include HIV encephalopathy, which tends to develop in approximately 10% of perinatally infected children, particularly rapidly progressing children. HIV encephalopathy is characterized by a predominant motor illness with hyperspasticity, hyperreflexia, rigidity, and increased muscle tone. Loss of developmental milestones is a hallmark. By contrast, HIV dementia which is very frequently found in adults, is not as prevalent in children. Nephrotic syndrome is a late complication of advanced HIV disease, generally seen in untreated adolescents or patients who fail therapy. Congestive heart failure in patients with advanced HIV disease has been described. However, the role of HIV in the pathogenesis of heart disease is not well understood. Other findings in HIV-infected children, particularly those who survive many years without treatment are AIDS-related lymphomas. In the western world, non-Hodgkin lymphomas are rarely seen in untreated HIV-infected children.

Laboratory abnormalities: The most frequent laboratory abnormalities in untreated HIV infected children include anemia, neutropenia, and thrombocytopenia. Increase in liver transaminases due to HIV hepatitis is also frequent. Hypergammaglobulinemia is a common finding in HIV+ children as opposed to hypo-gammaglobulinemia, more frequently seen in adults. Anergy on skin testing and failure to develop anti-bodies post vaccination are common features in patients with advanced HIV disease. Decreased absolute CD4 cell counts and percentages for age as well as inverted CD4/ CD8 ratios are surrogate markers for HIV disease.

Diagnosis

Early diagnosis of HIV-infection is critical for prompt initiation of treatment. Recent studies of early versus deferred antiretroviral treatment initiation have shown it is impossible to predict which infants, even if asymptomatic, are at risk of rapid disease progression and death in the first year of life. As a consequence, antiretroviral treatment guidelines recommend treatment of all HIV-infected infants identified under one year of age. Since all HIV-exposed infants carry maternal antibodies until 12–18 months of age, serology is not a reliable diagnostic parameter for younger infants. The identification of HIV-1 through molecular tests is the preferred diagnostic method. HIV-1 DNA Polymerase Chain Reaction (PCR) in peripheral blood mononuclear cells (PBMC) is the preferred diagnostic test. Quantitative HIV-1 RNA PCR in plasma, although mainly used for treatment monitoring, is an acceptable alternative. Branched DNA assays (bDNA) are suitable tests for monitoring of virus load; however, because of a high false positive rate, they should be avoided for diagnostic purposes. HIV-1 can also be isolated through PBMC co-culture; however, at high cost. The extended length of time for retrieval of results and increased laboratory requirements for this assay preclude its use beyond that of research purposes. The timing of performance of diagnostic assays in infancy is also critical. For diagnosis of *in utero* infection, it is standardized that a positive PCR result should be available in specimens collected in the first 48 hours of life. In the absence of breastfeeding, a negative PCR result in the first 48 hours of life followed by a positive PCR result between 7 days of age until 3 months of life is suggestive of *intrapartum* acquisition of infection. In breastfed infants, earlier negative PCR assays followed by a positive result in the first year of life are indicative of late postnatal transmission. For practical purposes, it is difficult to differentiate *intrapartum* infections from early postnatal infections through breastfeeding. One important caveat is that a negative PCR result in the first two weeks of life does not rule out HIV-infection. In order for *intrapartum* acquisition of HIV disease to be completely ruled out, non breastfed infants should have a negative PCR result between 3–4 months of age. All positive PCR results should be immediately repeated on a separate specimen drawn on a separate date for confirmatory purposes. Beyond 18 months of age, the testing algorithm is the same as in adults. Serologic testing is the norm, either via traditional EIA assays on serum or rapid test blood assays, with confirmatory testing performed via western blot assays or immuno fluorescence.

Prevention: Most pregnant women with HIV infection are asymptomatic during pregnancy, particularly in the developed world. Universal screening for HIV infection during pregnancy, regardless of risk perception, is the norm. Most states in the U.S. have currently an opt-out approach to HIV testing during pregnancy which has significantly facilitated screening and uptake of testing. Since 1994, the first intervention clinical trial of the antiretroviral agent zidovudine taken during pregnancy demonstrated effective reduction—from 25% to 8%—using that agent. One of the ultimate challenges in the area of HIV prevention of mother-to-child transmission (MTCT) is prevention of postnatal transmission via breastfeeding. In certain areas of the world, replacement for-mula feeding is not an option. Observational studies have demonstrated significant success in MTCT reduction to less than 2% with the use of HAART in mothers while breastfeeding until the weaning period is completed. Other studies have evaluated the use of antiretroviral prophylaxis in exposed infants during breastfeeding in untreated mothers, with encouraging results thus far. One additional consideration is that HIV-exposed infants borne to mothers with advanced disease are at higher risk of other congenital infections such as CMV, toxo-plasmosis, or HSV as mothers with advanced HIV disease may reactivate the disease during pregnancy. It is also not uncommon in areas of high prevalence for syphilis, HTLV-1 or hepatitis C, for mixed infections to occur.

Treatment: Used in combination, a number of agents of different classes were developed for treatment of HIV-infection in the last two decades and have definitively improved disease prognosis and the outlook on HIV disease from a fatal illness to a chronic infection. These include agents that work on viral enzymes such as reverse transcriptase inhibitors, protease inhibitors and integrase inhibitors. Other therapeutic targets include fusion inhibitors and co-receptor inhibitors. Extensive and detailed treatment guidelines are available for antiretroviral management of infants, children and adolescents with HIV-1 infection [3]. There are significant differences in treatment guidelines between the U.S. Department of Health and Human Services and WHO guidelines, as well as differences in individual country guidelines across the western world. Nevertheless, most strongly recommend treatment of infants below one year of age and treatment of older children based on CD4 cell count and percent-age, symptoms, and if possible, HIV-1 virus load. Early versus deferred treatment is a continuous debate in the HIV arena, but it is well accepted that particularly in children, effective treatment early on likely reduces viral replication before genetic mutations develop; potentially reduces viral set point with less circulating viral strains; prevents immunologic demise; and, decreases seeding of CD4 cell latent reservoirs. Because of resource con-straints on laboratory monitoring, international guidelines generally do not base changes in therapy on virus load monitoring. However, it is well established that monitoring of HIV-1 virus load has revolutionized the care of HIV disease in both children and adults. Because of virus load monitoring, it is possible to change antiretroviral therapy in patients prior to a significant decline in CD4 cells and well before symptomatic disease is established. The continuation of antiretrovirals in patients with detectable viremia fosters development of antiretroviral resis-tance. Thus, if at all possible, it is critical that virus load monitoring be available for prevention of development of resistance and for evaluation of adherence issues, a common problem in adolescents with HIV disease.

Monitoring: Treatment of HIV disease requires continuous laboratory monitoring including toxicity monitor-ing of antiretrovirals (anemia, neutropenia, increase in transaminases, jaundice, increases in amylase or lipase, lipid levels, glucose levels) and also monitoring of effectiveness of treatment through surrogate markers includ-ing HIV-1 virus load (measured through quantitative RNA PCR or bDNA) and CD4 cell subsets. In the presence of elevated virus load levels, further testing with genotypic or phenotypic evaluations for antiretroviral resistance mutations may be required. The best way to prevent development of antiretroviral resistance is the maintenance of an undetectable virus load: i.e., no replication, no mutation. During the first weeks of treat-ment, a characteristic immune reconstitution syndrome may develop, particularly in patients with advanced

HIV disease. This syndrome is characterized by appearance of latent, previously undiagnosed opportunistic infections, such as tuberculosis. Temporary interruption of highly active antiretroviral therapy may be warranted in conjunction with treatment of the underlying illness.

In summary, prevention and treatment of pediatric HIV infection entails interruption of infection to mothers and their partners; diagnosis and treatment of women during pregnancy; early diagnosis and treatment of their infants; clinical and laboratory monitoring of this treatment; and, the provision of a continuous supply of drugs and second or third line treatments, a major challenge in resource limited settings. Laboratory infrastructure for diagnosis and management of treatment is of the essence, as well as motivation of patients to adhere to their treatment. Continuous research and knowledge of antiretroviral side effects is critical as we guide a new generation of perinatally HIV-infected children into adulthood, an unthinkable phenomenon little more than a decade ago.

References:

Newell ML, Coovadia H, Cortina-Boria M, et al. Mortality of infected and uninfected infants born to HIV-infected mothers in Africa: a pooled analysis. Lancet. 364:1236–1243, 2004.

Nielsen K, McSherry G, Petru A, Frederick T, Wara D, Bryson Y, Martin N, Hutto C, Ammann AJ, Grubman S, Oleske J, Scott G. A descriptive survey of pediatric human immunodeficiency virus-infected long term survivors. Pediatrics. 99(4): pe4, 1997.

Working Group on Antiretroviral Therapy and Medical Management of HIV-Infected Children. Guidelines for the Use of Antiretroviral Agents in Pediatric HIV Infection. pp 1-139,2009; http://aidsinfo.nih.gov/ContentFiles/PediatricGuidelines.pdf.

Kawasaki Disease

David Bronstein

Kawasaki disease is an acute systemic vasculitis which has surpassed acute rheumatic fever as the most common cause of acquired heart disease in children in the United States. While Kawasaki disease is self-limited even without treatment, sequelae such as coronary artery abnormalities with long-term implications may occur among untreated and a smaller percentage of treated patients. The cause of Kawasaki disease is unknown. However, clinical and epidemiological features suggest an infectious etiology.

Clinical Presentation and Prognosis

Demographics: While Kawasaki disease is most common in Japanese children and in children of Japanese ancestry, it has been reported in all racial and ethnic groups. Approximately 85% of patients are younger than 5 years and there is a male-to-female ratio of 1.5:1.

Presenting signs and symptoms: Children with Kawasaki disease typically present with a high-spiking and remittent fever, usually greater than 39°C in addition to some or all of the following principal clinical features: (1) Bilateral conjunctival injection; (2) changes in the lips and oral cavity (erythema, cracking of lips; oropharyngeal erythema; strawberry tongue); (3) polymorphous exanthem; (4) peripheral extremity changes (erythema and swelling of hands and feet; later periungual desquamation, Beau lines (transverse depressions on the fingernails)); and (5) cervical lymphadenopathy (at least 1.5cm in diameter). These features are often not all present at the same time, and in cases of incomplete Kawasaki disease, certain characteristic signs or symptoms may be absent completely.

Clinical course: In general, the signs and symptoms of Kawasaki disease are self-limited, evolving over the first 10 days of illness with gradual spontaneous resolution in most children even without specific therapy. Approximately 15–25% of untreated children with Kawasaki disease develop coronary artery aneurysms or ectasia, which may lead to myocardial infarction, sudden death, or ischemic heart disease. Timely treatment reduces the risk of coronary artery abnormalities to approximately 5%, usually transient coronary artery dilatation.

Prognosis: Children without known coronary artery abnormalities during the first month of Kawasaki disease typically return to their previous state of health without clinical evidence of cardiac impairment. The prognosis for children with aneurysms depends primarily on the initial size of the lesion. Overall, approximately 50% of coronary aneurysms have been shown to resolve 1–2 years after disease onset, with smaller aneurysms regressing more commonly. Children with giant aneurysms more frequently experience thrombotic complications. The peak mortality occurs between 15 and 45 days after the onset of fever. However, sudden death from myocardial infarction may occur many years later, sometimes into adulthood.

Diagnosis

The diagnosis of Kawasaki disease is based on clinical criteria, as there is no specific diagnostic test. The diagnosis is confirmed by the presence of fever for at least 5 days and four of the five principal clinical features described previously, assuming no other known disease process explains the illness. To identify coronary artery abnormalities, echocardiography is performed at the time of diagnosis and at 2 and 6 weeks after disease onset. Incomplete Kawasaki disease may be diagnosed in patients with fever, but fewer than 4 of the principal clinical features. More common in young infants, a diagnosis of incomplete Kawasaki disease is supported by the presence of coronary artery abnormalities on echocardiogram or by supplemental laboratory criteria, such as elevation of acute phase reactants (erythrocyte sedimentation rate and C-reactive protein), thrombocytosis after 7 days, hypoalbuminemia, anemia, elevation of alanine aminotransferase, leukocytosis, or sterile pyuria.

Management

Medications: Standard treatment for Kawasaki disease is the combination of aspirin and intravenous immunoglobulin (IVIG), which appear to have an additive anti-inflammatory effect. High-dose aspirin (80–100 mg/kg per day in 4 doses) is given during the acute phase of Kawasaki disease, usually until day 14 of illness, provided that there are no abnormalities on initial echocardiogram. By contrast, some clinicians stop the high dose aspirin after the child has been afebrile for 48–72 hours. Low-dose aspirin (3–5 mg/kg per day) is subsequently given until no evidence of coronary artery abnormalities are seen on follow-up echocardiogram by 6–8 weeks after the onset of illness. IVIG (2g/kg in a single infusion) is given during the acute phase concomitantly with aspirin. While studies have demonstrated greatest efficacy when given within the first 10 days of illness, IVIG should also be administered to children diagnosed after the 10th day of illness if they have persistent fever, laboratory evidence of ongoing systemic inflammation, or aneurysms. In children who develop coronary artery abnormalities, therapy depends on the severity of the lesions and may include long-term antiplatelet therapy with aspirin, with or without clopidogrel, anticoagulant therapy with warfarin or low-molecular-weight heparin, or a combination of antiplatelet and anticoagulant therapy.

Surgery: Coronary artery bypass grafts have been the mainstay of surgical therapy for coronary artery aneurysms, as attempts at aneurysm excision or placation have been less successful. Catheter interventions such as balloon angioplasty, rotational ablation, and stent placement, are being used more frequently, and a relatively small number of patients with severe myocardial dysfunction have undergone cardiac transplantation.

Follow-up: Follow-up is determined by the level of cardiac involvement. Assessment and counseling about cardiovascular risk factors is recommended at 5 year intervals for patients with no coronary artery changes, and at 3–5 year intervals for patients with transient coronary artery ectasia or dilatation which resolves in the initial 6–8 weeks after onset of illness. Patients with isolated small to medium coronary artery aneurysms should undergo annual follow-up by a pediatric cardiologist with an echocardiogram and an electrocardiogram, in addition to stress tests with myocardial perfusion imaging every 2 years after 10 years of age. Echocardiograms and electrocardiograms are performed at 6 month intervals for patients with large, multiple or complex coronary artery aneurysms and in patients with coronary artery obstruction, as well as cardiac catheterization with selective coronary angiography when clinically indicated. Reproductive counseling is recommended for women of childbearing age.

Pearls and Precautions

School/education: As with follow-up, limitations on physical activity are determined by the extent of cardiac involvement. Patients with no or transient coronary artery ectasia or dilatation have no restrictions on physical activity after 6–8 weeks. Patients with small or medium coronary artery aneurysms also have no restrictions on physical activity after 6–8 weeks during the first decade of life; however, recommendations for restrictions in the second decade are often based on stress tests with myocardial perfusion evaluation. Recommendations for patients with large or complex aneurysms or with coronary artery obstruction are based primarily on annual stress tests; collision or high impact sports are discouraged due to the potential for bleeding.

Prevention: Due to the potential for severe complications in untreated patients, physicians should have a low threshold to consider the diagnosis of Kawasaki disease and begin the workup in patients with unexplained fever. While Kawasaki disease itself is not preventable, associated complications may be avoided or mitigated by the timely initiation of therapy.

References

Burns JC, Glode MP. Kawasaki Syndrome. Lancet 364:533–44, 2004.

Newburger JW, Takahashi M, Gerber MA, et al. Diagnosis, treatment, and long-term management of Kawasaki disease: a statement for health professionals from the Committee on Rheumatic Fever, Endocarditis and Kawasaki Disease, Council on Cardiovascular Disease in the Young, American Heart Association. Pediatrics 114:1708–33, 2004.

Congenital Rubella Syndrome (CRS)

Karin Nielsen-Saines

Etiology

Congenital rubella syndrome is caused by maternal infection with rubella virus during the first trimester of pregnancy. Rubella virus is the only viral species in the genus Rubivirus, of the Togaviridae virus family (which also includes the genus Alphavirus). The rubella virion is a spherical RNA virus measuring approximately 60 nm. It contains a capsid protein (C) and two glycoproteins (E1 and E2). Rubella virus has only a human reservoir. For many centuries, rubella was confused with measles or scarlet fever, and so it was described in the medical literature as rubeola, rubeola scarlatinosa, bastard measles or bastard scarlatina, among other eponyms. The first clinical description of rubella as a specific exanthematous illness was in the mid-1700s by two German physicians. As such, it was originally coined German measles. It was not until the early 1940s that congenital defects were linked to prenatal infection with rubella virus [1].

Postnatal Rubella: Outside of the prenatal period, rubella is responsible for a very mild, self-limited characteristic exanthematous illness which can be subclinical in one fourth to nearly half of the cases. When clinical disease is apparent, typical findings include a generalized erythematous maculopapular rash which starts on the face and then disseminates over 24 hours. The rash tends to coalesce and form pinpoint papules (a reason why rubella has been confused with scarlet fever in the past). In a few days, the rash disappears first from the face and then from the remainder of the body. Lymphadenopathy (particularly suboccipital and post auricular) is characteristic and can precede the rash and usually a low grade fever is present. Disease generally lasts for about a week (5–8 days) and is preceded by an incubation period of approximately 16–18 days. Approximately 7 days following exposure, the virus can usually be isolated from nasopharyngeal secretions and is usually present until 14 days after the rash onset. Most children do not have prodromal symptoms, although mild coryza and diarrhea have been reported in young infants. Adults and adolescents not infrequently report a prodrome which can include eye pain, headaches, sore throat, cough, coryza, fever, muscular pain and nausea. Conjunctivitis and palatal enanthems are occasionally present in the early stages of rubella. The vast majority of children have no additional symptoms. However, adolescents and adults, particularly females, not infrequently develop polyarthralgias or polyarthritis one week after the onset of rash with pain and morning stiffness persisting for one to four weeks. Chronic arthritis is not caused by rubella [2]. Rare complications include encephalitis (1:5000) and thrombocytopenia (1:3000 cases). There are reports of myocarditis, pericarditis, hepatitis, hemolytic anemia and hemolytic uremic syndrome in association with rubella.

Transmission and Pathogenesis: Rubella infection is transmitted by the respiratory route via direct droplet contact. Infected individuals shed virus from nasopharyngeal secretions for an extended period of time, even prior to the development of rash. Once the host is infected, viral replication occurs in the lymphoid tissue of the respiratory tract with subsequent hematogenous spread. Maternal viremia in the absence of neutralizing antibody leads to transplacental hematogenous passage of the virus to the fetus. The virus induces cytopathic damage to fetal blood vessels leading to ischemia and tissue/organ damage. The risk of congenital defects following maternal infection with rubella correlates with the period of fetal organogenesis. It is highest in the first eight weeks of gestation (85%), followed by a 52% risk between 9 to 12 weeks and a 16% risk up to 20 weeks of gestational age. No congenital defects have been reported in mothers infected after 20 weeks of gestation although intra-uterine growth retardation can still occur. Fetal infection with rubella virus can happen until the time of delivery but in the third trimester of pregnancy clinical repercussions are generally not significant. Maternal rubella infection immediately prior to conception does not increase the risk of congenital rubella syndrome.

Clinical Presentation and Prognosis

Epidemiology: Before the availability of rubella vaccine in 1969, rubella occurred in epidemic cycles, approximately every 6–9 years, with children being most frequently affected. The United States suffered a rubella pandemic in 1964 which resulted in approximately 12.5 million cases, resulting in 11,000 fetal deaths and 20,000 cases of congenital rubella syndrome. With the widespread use of rubella vaccine, the incidence of rubella declined 99% from the pre-vaccine era. There are less than 25 cases reported annually in the U.S. and most cases are in foreign born or unimmunized individuals. Studies demonstrate, however, that approximately 10% of the U.S. born population over 5 years is susceptible to the virus with higher susceptibility rates among foreign born individuals. Internationally, rubella is still endemic in a number of countries particularly in Asia and sub-Saharan Africa. In Nigeria, for example, a study reported that one quarter of women of childbearing age were susceptible to rubella. In countries where immunization policies were originally selective to girls and young women, a large pool of susceptible individuals has remained. Subsequent outbreaks demonstrated this strategy is ineffective for prevention of CRS, as was the case of a large outbreak in Greece in 1993. Efforts are under way for elimination of rubella from the Caribbean, Central and South America.

Clinical course and prognosis: Fetal infection with rubella virus can result in devastating disease leading to fetal death with ensuing spontaneous abortion or stillbirth, a number of characteristic fetal defects and/or intra-uterine fetal growth retardation. One third of CRS patients present with the most common findings in congenital rubella syndrome including ophthalmologic abnormalities such as cataracts, microphthalmia, congenital glaucoma or pigmentary retinopathy. Ten to twenty percent will have cardiac malformations: Patent ductus arteriosus or peripheral pulmonary stenosis while myocarditis can be seen in neonates with multisystem involvement and is frequently the cause of death. Another 10–20% have neurological disorders including mental retardation, behavioral disorders or meningoencephalitis. Almost all patients have some form of sensorineural hearing deficits with most suffering some degree of deafness. Other neonatal findings in CRS include intrauterine growth retardation (most common manifestation), microcephaly, radiolucent bone disease, interstitial pneumonitis, hepatosplenomegaly as well as thrombocytopenia with purpura and dermal erythropoiesis (which underlie the characteristic blueberry muffin skin lesions). There are gradients in symptomatology and as such, neonates with mild forms of disease may have very limited to no clinical findings at birth.

Late manifestations of disease include neuromotor deficits, pneumonitis, diabetes mellitus, thyroid abnormalities, and progressive panencephalitis. Cell mediated immunodeficiencies are not uncommon in children with CRS, and specific cell mediated immune responses against rubella are generally decreased in this population. There is no link between CRS and autism, and no association between MMR immunization and autism. Viral shedding in infants with CRS occurs for several months to years, and virus can be isolated from the throat, urine and also from lens aspirates in children with congenital cataracts. These children can transmit infection to susceptible contacts.

All birth defects suggestive of congenital rubella syndrome should be investigated appropriately and reported to the Centers for Disease Control (CDC) through county or state health departments. A case of

CRS is defined as the presence of any of the characteristic clinical findings confirmed by laboratory results such as isolation of rubella virus, demonstration of IgM antibody or persistently elevated IgG titers which fail to decline by a two-fold dilution each month.

Diagnosis

Identification of the virus through isolation or PCR is the best diagnostic method. Appropriate specimens for viral identification include nasopharyngeal secretions (nose or throat swabs), urine, buffy coat of blood, and CSF. Since virus is shed for prolonged periods of time, viral isolation should not be difficult. Rubella virus culture entails an indirect procedure where growth of the virus in specific cell lines (African green monkey kidney) is followed by an echo-11 virus challenge. If the cell line does not demonstrate the characteristic cytopathic effect (CPE) following challenge, then rubella virus is present [3]. Serologic diagnosis is complicated by maternal passage of IgG antibodies. Nevertheless an IgM antibody response is usually present in the infant, although it can be delayed. False positive and false negative IgM results also can occur. If infant IgG antibodies to rubella result from maternal passage of virus, those should drop four to eightfold over the first 3 months of life and become undetectable in the second semester of life. In some cases, however, the immune derangements caused by congenital infection can affect antibody profiles, and as such, negative antibody levels are not completely reliable in excluding rubella infection. IgG antibody avidity studies can be helpful in some circumstances. Rubella antibodies can be measured by enzyme linked immunoassays (EIA), immunofluorescent antibody assays, complement fixation, passive hemagglutination, latex agglutination and hemagglutination inhibition. Viral isolates can be typed during epidemic times.

A greater challenge is the diagnosis of CRS in older children, particularly in late infancy and second year of life. By that time, a large proportion of children may no longer be shedding virus, and antibody levels may be difficult to interpret. Antibody avidity assays may be helpful in this scenario as children with CRS have been shown to have low avidity of rubella-specific IgG levels. For prenatal diagnosis, rubella virus can be identified through PCR of amniotic fluid specimens or chorionic villous samples. Evaluation for congenital infections should be strongly considered in fetuses shown to have intrauterine growth retardation by ultrasound. Maternal serologic screening for rubella is standard obstetric practice. In patients who are recent immigrants from developing countries, a positive rubella IgG result in the first prenatal visit may reflect recent infection as opposed to prior immunization. This possibility should be considered in further evaluations of such patients.

Prevention: Immunity from vaccine or wild type infection is generally longstanding. Reinfection is very rare and generally asymptomatic, but has been associated (also very rarely) with cases of CRS. The vaccine available in the U.S. is the live virus RA 27/3 strain grown in human diploid cells. One dose of live virus rubella vaccine confers longstanding, likely lifelong immunity to 90% of vaccine recipients. Ninety-five percent of 12 month olds receiving combination MMR vaccine seroconvert to rubella on the first immunization. Since current guidelines recommend two doses of MMR during childhood, protective levels of antibody are present in an even larger number of vaccine recipients. Rubella vaccine should not be administered to pregnant women as there is a theoretical risk to the fetus. It is recommended that patients receiving rubella vaccine abstain from becoming pregnant within 28 days of receipt of the vaccine. In cases where vaccine was inadvertently provided to pregnant women, no congenital defects were ever reported; although in a very small number of cases infection of the offspring did occur. Therefore, inadvertent rubella immunization is not an indication for pregnancy termination. Breastfeeding is not a contraindication to rubella immunization nor is immunization of children of pregnant women. Although the virus can be isolated from the nasopharynx of children between 7–28 days following immunization, there is no evidence of transmission of vaccine virus from a child to an adult. Administration of live virus vaccine can prevent disease if provided within 3 days of exposure. However, it is only recommended for nonpregnant susceptible individuals.

If a pregnant woman is exposed to rubella, serologic testing for rubella-specific IgG and IgM should be performed with sera stored for later batched testing. If IgG antibodies are present, it is likely that there is prior immunity. If no antibodies are detectable, repeat serologic testing should be performed 2–3 weeks later and tested concurrently with the earlier specimen. If tests are negative, repeat testing six weeks after initial exposure is again recommended. In exposed susceptible individuals, there is data demonstrating that intramuscular immunoglobulin can decrease rates of viremia, viral shedding and clinical disease. Thus, immunoglobulin can be considered in the management of postexposure prophylaxis of pregnant susceptible individuals exposed to confirmed cases early in pregnancy. Absence of clinical disease in a pregnant woman receiving immunoglobulin, however, does not reassure that infection did not occur, as asymptomatic infection leading to CRS can still ensue. Further monitoring of maternal infection is warranted in these cases and evaluation of IgG antibodies will not be helpful because of prior immunoglobulin use.

Management

There is no specific antiviral treatment for rubella. Infants with congenital rubella are actively infected and should be isolated, being cared for only by individuals immune to rubella. In the home setting, since virus shedding is prolonged, precautions against exposure to susceptible pregnant women should be taken and contact isolation is recommended until at least one year of age. For neonates with significant manifestations of CRS indicating severe viral infection, intravenous immunoglobulin should be considered. Ophthalmologic evaluation is imperative to rule out glaucoma, cataracts or retinopathy. The management of respiratory distress due to pneumonitis is not different from that of other respiratory viruses and assisted ventilation, monitoring of blood gases and adequate critical care support is warranted. Structural cardiac anomalies should be treated surgically and in the same manner as other congenital heart diseases. Hepatosplenomegaly is a clinical finding usually with no major repercussions in CRS.

Pearls and Precautions

Long-term disabilities: Sensorineural deafness is the most frequent long-term disability from CRS, occurring in at least 80% of infected infants. Deafness should be promptly diagnosed in infants with CRS to ensure appropriate referral to an educational program before the second year of life. Use of auditory amplification devices are recommended and evaluation for conduction defects by ENT specialists should also be performed as a high number of older children also have concurrent conduction defects. Appropriate follow-up by ophthalmology and cardiology is warranted. Mental impairment should not be diagnosed before extensive evaluation for vision and hearing deficits have been performed and addressed. A subgroup of children with CRS is at risk for hypogammaglobulinemia, particularly low IgG levels. Provisions for intravenous immunoglobulin therapy may be warranted in this setting.

References

Gregg NM. Congenital cataracts following German measles in the mother. Trans Ophtalmol Soc Aust, 3:35–46, 1941.

Frenkel L, Nielsen K, Garakian A, Cherry JD. A search for persistent measles, mumps, and rubella vaccine virus in children with Human Immunodeficiency Virus type 1 infection. Archives of Pediatric and Adolescent Medicine, 148:57–60, 1994.

Nielsen K, Garakian A, Frenkel L, Cherry JD. The in vitro growth and serial passage of RA27/3 in cord blood mononuclear leukocytes from normal babies. Pediatric Research, 37(5): 623–5, 1995.

Congenital Toxoplasmosis

David Bronstein

Etiology

Toxoplasmosis is caused by the obligate intracellular protozoan *Toxoplasma gondii*, transmitted to humans through consumption of raw or inadequately cooked infected meat or inadvertent ingestion of oocysts passed in cat feces. Congenital toxoplasmosis occurs when a newly infected pregnant woman transmits the infection transplacentally to her fetus.

Clinical Presentation and Prognosis

Demographics: *Toxoplasma gondii* occurs worldwide with an increased incidence in tropical areas. Approximately 85% of child-bearing age women in the United States have no laboratory evidence of previous infection with *T. gondii* and are therefore susceptible to infection when pregnant. An estimated 400–4000 cases of congenital toxoplasmosis occur annually in the United States. The risk of congenital disease is lowest (10–25%) when acute maternal infection occurs during the first trimester and highest (60–90%) when maternal infection occurs during the third trimester.

Presenting signs and symptoms: Maternal infection is usually asymptomatic or with nonspecific signs or symptoms. The severity of fetal infection is inversely related to the gestational age during which maternal infection occurs. Infection acquired in the first trimester is usually most severe and can mimic disease caused by other congenitally acquired organisms such as herpes simplex virus, cytomegalovirus, and rubella. Infants diagnosed with congenital *T. gondii* at birth may present with the classic triad of chorioretinitis, hydrocephalus, and intracranial calcifications. However, other less specific clinical signs include microcephaly, seizures, a maculopapular rash, generalized lymphadenopathy, hepatosplenomegaly, jaundice, and thrombocytopenia. By contrast, infection acquired in the third trimester is often asymptomatic in the newborn period, with a substantial number of undiagnosed infants developing signs or symptoms weeks, months, or years later.

Clinical course: If untreated, as many as 85% of children born with the subclinical form of infection will develop signs and symptoms of the disease, mostly chorioretinitis or delays in development. While the initial signs and symptoms of active infection may be relieved within weeks of initiating appropriate therapy, treated individuals remain at risk of recurrent chorioretinitis, often at primary school entry age (5–7 years) and adolescence.

Prognosis: When untreated, infants with generalized or neurologic manifestations of infection in the neonatal period have a poor prognosis, with substantial cognitive and motor dysfunction, seizures, visual impairment, and profound hearing loss. Outcomes are generally better for infants treated in utero and for 1 year with pyrimethamine-sulfadiazine and leucovorin. Cerebral calcifications diminish in size or resolve for most of these children, and over time, normal cognitive function may be achieved. Infants with high CSF protein levels or hydrocephalus with delayed or unsuccessful shunt placement may experience irreversible neurologic damage despite therapy.

Diagnosis

In a pregnant woman, Toxoplasmosis is diagnosed by antibody detection, with IgG and IgM antibody levels rising within one to two weeks of infection. Since IgM antibodies may persist up to 18 months after infection and false-positive reactions are possible, IgM-positive test results should be confirmed by a Toxoplasma reference laboratory which uses additional testing to narrow the time of infection. To determine if the fetus is infected, parasite DNA may be detected in amniotic fluid. If congenital toxoplasmosis is suspected postnatally, ophthalmologic, auditory, and neurologic examinations, including a lumbar puncture for *T. gondii* polymerase chain reaction and a head computed tomography scan, in addition to serologic testing of the newborn and the mother are performed. Congenital infection is confirmed serologically by persistently positive IgG titers beyond the first 12 months of life. While routine screening of pregnant women is not recommended in the United States, human immunodeficiency virus-infected pregnant women should be screened for toxoplasmosis, along with women with suspicious ultrasonographic findings, including hydrocephalus, intracranial calcifications, microcephaly, fetal growth restriction, ascites, or hepatosplenomegaly.

Management

Medications: A pregnant woman with a confirmed acute *T. gondii* infection is treated with spiramycin to prevent transmission to the fetus. If toxoplasmosis is diagnosed in the fetus via amniocentesis, maternal treatment with pyrimethamine-sulfadiazine and leucovorin is recommended after the 18th week of gestation. After birth, the infant is continued on these same medications for at least 1 year. Corticosteroids are recommended as adjunctive therapy for infants with elevated CSF protein or with active chorioretinitis that threatens vision. Maintenance antiparasitic therapy is recommended for children with HIV and congenital Toxoplasma coinfection.

Surgery: In patients with hydrocephalus, ventriculoperitoneal shunt placement, in conjunction with the above antiparasitic therapy, is often necessary and may result in dramatic brain cortical expansion and growth.

Follow-up: Regular ophthalmological examinations, hearing tests, neuroradiology studies, and, if indicated, CSF analyses are used to monitor response to therapy. Following completion of 1 year of initial therapy, 3 monthly retinal examinations are suggested, followed by quarterly examinations until the child is able to describe visual symptoms accurately. The examinations may then be performed twice yearly, or sooner if any acute visual symptoms develop.

Pearls and Precautions

Likely complications: The recommended antiparasitic agents are generally well tolerated, as the supplemental leucovorin minimizes the potential pyrimethamine-associated hematologic toxicity. As in all patients with ventriculoperitoneal shunts, children with congenital toxoplasmosis who undergo shunting are at risk of obstruction and infection, usually due to coagulase negative Staphylococci. Such signs and symptoms as headaches, papilledema, emesis, mental status changes, fever, and meningismus must be evaluated immediately.

School/education: Special services and educational resources are important for children with such potential sequelae as learning disabilities, developmental delay, visual impairment, deafness, and epilepsy.

Prevention: Pregnant women with unknown or seronegative status for *T. gondii* should avoid contact with cat feces, either through changing litter boxes or gardening, and avoid consumption of undercooked meat or unwashed fruits and vegetables.

References

Jones J, Lopez, A, Wilson M. Congenital toxoplasmosis. Am Fam Physician 67:2131–8, 2003.

McLeod R, Boyer K, Karrison T, et al. Outcome of treatment for congenital toxoplasmosis, 1981–2004: the National Collaborative Chicago-Based, Congenital Toxoplasmosis Study. Clin Infect Dis 42:1383–94, 2006.

Preventing congenital toxoplasmosis. Centers for Disease Control and Prevention. MMWR Morb Mortal Wkly Rep 49 (RR02):57–75, 2000.

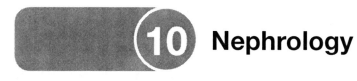

10 Nephrology

Table of Contents

Bartter's Syndrome

Katherine Wesseling Perry

Bartter's syndrome is an inherited defect of the thick ascending loop of Henle causing a phenotype of polyuria, failure to thrive, and normotensive, chloride resistant metabolic alkalosis.

Etiology

Genetic defects in ion transporter or channels in the thick ascending limb of the loop of Henle are responsible for the signs and symptoms associated with Bartter's syndrome. These defects are detailed in Table 10.1.

Clinical Presentation and Prognosis:

Presenting signs and symptoms: Polyhydraminos may be present in utero and polyuria, polydypsia, metabolic alkalosis, and failure to thrive are evident from birth. Hypokalemia is typical of Bartter's syndrome. However, some forms of Neonatal Bartter's may present with hyperkalemia.

Clinical course: Untreated, these children fail to thrive and may have debilitating weakness secondary to chronic hypokalemia. Nephrocalcinosis may result from chronic hypercalciuria and renal cysts occur from chronic hypokalemia. Over time, nephrocalcinosis and renal cysts may lead to progressive renal failure (chronic kidney disease (CKD)).

Prognosis: Treatment improves quality of life in a number of ways: Urine output can be decreased with indomethacin (1–2 mg/kg/day divided bid), allowing children to escape from diaper usage; final adult height may

Table 10.1: Signs and Symptoms of Bartter's Syndrome

Name	Bartter Type	Defect
Neonatal Bartter's	1	Na-K-2Cl symporter
Neonatal Bartter's	2	Thick ascending limb potassium channel
Classic Bartter's	3	Chloride channel
Bartter's with sensorineural deafness	4	Barttin (cofactor for chloride channel)
Bartter's with autosomal dominant hypocalcemia	5	Calcium-sensing receptor

be improved, although many children continue to be short in comparison with their peers; muscle strength improves with the administration of supplemental potassium; and cognitive development improves.

Early treatment of Bartter syndrome may improve growth and cognitive development, but children typically remain small. Chronic hypokalemia may result in renal cysts while long-standing hypercalciuria may result in nephrocalcinosis and chronic kidney disease.

Diagnosis

The overall diagnosis for Bartter's syndrome is made clinically: A dehydrated, normotensive, alkalotic, and hypokalemic child with an elevated urinary chloride concentration (greater than 15 mEq/L) and hypercalciuria (urine calcium/creatinine ratio greater than 0.6 in an infant) is suspicious for Bartter's syndrome. Loop diuretic use (identical serum and urinary findings), cystic fibrosis (differentiated by low urinary chloride and urinary calcium excretion), and hyperaldosterone states (differentiated by the presence of hypertension) should be considered in the differential for Bartter's syndrome. Genetic testing to define the specific type of Bartter's is available at select labs throughout the world: www.genetests.org.

Management

Sodium chloride and potassium chloride supplementation improve electrolyte abnormalities (dosage is generally based on weight; the typical starting dose is 1 mEq/kg/d and the dose is titrated up based on serum electrolyte concentrations. Daily dose may be divided into bid to tid). Indomethacin therapy may decrease polyuria.

Pearls and Precautions

Disease complications: Polyuria is significant and may require the use of diapers in school aged and older children, interfering with social functioning.

Consultations: Nephrology should be consulted at diagnosis for management of electrolytes, polyuria, and renal function.

Monitoring: Serum electrolytes, urinary calcium excretion, and growth should be monitored routinely (every 3–6 months) in all patients with Barrter's syndrome.

References

Naesens, M., P. Steels, R. Verberckmoes, Y. Vanrenterghem, and D. Kuypers. 2004. "Bartter's and Gitelman's syndromes: from gene to clinic." *Nephron Physiol* 9665–78.

Chronic Kidney Disease (CKD)

Katherine Wesseling Perry

Chronic kidney disease is a term applied to an irreversible loss of renal function. It is staged according to glomerular filtration rate (GFR).

- Stage 1: GFR >90 ml/min/1.73 m² with signs of renal damage (i.e., proteinuria).
- Stage 2: GFR 60–90 ml/min/1.73 m².
- Stage 3: GFR 30–60 ml/min/1.73 m².
- Stage 4: GFR 15–30 ml/min/1.73 m².
- Stage 5: GFR <15 ml/min/1.73 m² or treatment with maintenance dialysis (End-stage renal disease).

In children, GFR is calculated from the Schwartz formula. The calculation is based on serum creatinine and patient height, gender, and pubertal development. The formula used to calculate Schwartz formula varies on whether serum creatinine concentration is determined by the Jaffe method or by an enzymatic method.

GFR (Jaffe)

- Infants: 0.45*ht (cm)/serum creatinine (mg/dl).
- Pre-pubertal children and adolescent girls: 0.55* ht (cm)/serum creatinine (mg/dl).
- Adolescent boys: 0.7* ht (cm)/serum creatinine (mg/dl).

GFR (enzymatic creatinine)

- 0.41*ht(cm)/serum creatinine (mg/dl).

Etiology

Loss of renal function in childhood may be due to congenital structural abnormalities of the kidney (obstruction, reflux, and/or dysplasia). Progressive conditions such as glomerulonephritis (immune mediated), progressive nephrotic syndrome (focal segmental glomerulosclerosis), or hereditary disease (Alport's syndrome, cystinosis) may also lead to chronic deterioration of kidney function.

Clinical Presentation and Prognosis

Demographics: Obstructive/dysplastic uropathy disproportionately affects boys. Autoimmune disease (such as lupus nephritis) is more common in girls. Overall, a predominance of males are affected by pediatric CKD.

Presenting signs and symptoms: As renal function declines, many children experience such constitutional symptoms as nausea and anorexia. Damage to the renal medulla often results in a urinary concentrating defect with subsequent polyuria and nocturia.

Hypertension: Hypertension may occur, and is either renin-mediated (from renal scarring) or due to volume overload.

Electrolyte abnormalities: Develop in the late stages of CKD. Acidosis, hyperkalemia, hyperphosphatemia, and hypocalcemia all develop as patients near dialysis.

Proteinuria: Occurs with progressive renal scarring.

Anemia: Anemia, due to declining erythropoietin production, develops as kidney function declines to about $1/3^{rd}$ of normal.

Renal osteodystrophy: Bony deformities, resulting from renal osteodystrophy, occur early in the course of CKD and progress as renal function declines. Short stature occurs due to a combination of factors including acidosis, renal osteodystrophy, and resistance of the growth plate to growth hormone.

Cardiovascular disease: The major cause of death of both adults and children with CKD is cardiovascular disease, due to a combination of factors including poorly controlled hypertension and the development of vascular calcifications.

Cognitive impairment: School performance also declines as uremic toxins accumulate.

Clinical course: The rate of decline in renal function varies between diseases and between patients. Typically, renal function declines more quickly during adolescence as decreased renal mass is unable to keep up with the demands of increased body mass. Although there is variability in the rate of progression, many pediatric patients with chronic kidney disease will progress to end-stage renal disease. Untreated CKD results in severe anemia, growth failure, and boney deformities.

Prognosis: With optimal treatment, initiated early in the course of the disease, progression to end-stage renal disease can be delayed. Many of the comorbidities that result in decreased life span and poor quality of life can also be mitigated.

Anemia: Anemia can be prevented with iron and erythropoietin therapy.

Renal osteodystrophy: Boney deformities and fractures can be prevented by optimal control of serum calcium, phosphorus, PTH, and vitamin D levels.

Growth: Growth hormone therapy increases final adult height in patients with chronic kidney disease.

Cardiovascular disease: Control of hypertension and prevention of excessive calcium intake can limit cardiovascular disease.

Management

Medications

Hypertension: Virtually all classes of antihypertensives are used to control blood pressure in CKD patients. Each have their benefits and down-sides (see "Pearls and Precautions").

Proteinuria: Angiotensin Converting Enzyme Inhibitor (ACEI) therapy reduces proteinuria and delays deterioration in kidney function while controlling blood pressure. ACEI may prolong the time until dialysis and should be administered in anyone with proteinuria and/or hypertension.

Anemia: Erythropoietin and Iron therapy are initiated when hemoglobin levels decline below the normal range.

Renal osteodystrophy: Dietary phosphate restriction, phosphate binder medications, and vitamin D sterols are the mainstays of therapy of renal osteodystrophy. Phosphate binder therapy should be initiated when serum phosphorus levels rise above the normal range despite dietary phosphate restriction. Several phosphate binders are available including calcium containing salts, sevelamer hydrochloride, aluminum hydroxide, and lanthanum carbonate. Vitamin D sterols are used to suppress serum parathyroid hormone levels and control complications of renal osteodystrophy. Several active vitamin D sterols are available for use including calcitriol, doxercalciferol, and paricalcitol.

Growth: Recombinant Growth hormone (GH) is FDA approved for use in children with growth failure due to CKD. Although GH improves linear height, it should only be used in well nourished children in whom acidosis and renal osteodystrophy have been well controlled.

Consultations: To improve outcomes such as nutrition, growth, and delay of renal function deterioration, a Nephrologist should be included in the care of all children early in the course of CKD.

Surgical consultation is required when renal function deteriorates to the point that dialysis catheter access is required. Particularly in young children and infants, G-tube placement may also be necessary to ensure proper nutrition and facilitate medication administration. Orthopedic surgical expertise may be required if boney deformities are present at diagnosis.

Therapy: Renal osteodystrophy, chronic illness, and often multiple hospitalizations make all children with chronic kidney disease physically and emotionally at high risk for disability. Physical therapy is warranted in all children in whom gross or fine motor delay or muscle weakness is noted either on history or physical exam. Occupational therapy should be considered, particularly in infants and younger children, when an abnormal feeding and/or swallowing history are obtained.

Psychiatry: All children with chronic kidney disease are at high risk for emotional problems. Short stature, chronic illness, and repeated hospitalizations tend to isolate these children from their peers. Many uremic children have trouble learning and; when combined with multiple school absences related to their illness, school success is often limited. Thus, a psychosocial assessment is warranted in EVERY child with chronic kidney disease.

Social: Support for chronic kidney disease: www.nephcare.com

Regional kidney camps are available for children with all forms and stages of kidney disease throughout the United States. Contact the local National Kidney Foundation for information in your area.

Monitoring: Serum electrolytes, BUN, creatinine, hematocrit, and iron studies, along with urine protein excretion should be monitored routinely (q3 to 6 months, more often in late stages of CKD) in all patients with CKD. Blood pressure and growth parameters (height and weight) should also be followed closely.

Pearls and Precautions

Blood pressure medications: ACE inhibitors are particularly useful in patients with renin-mediated hypertension (i.e., renal scarring) and are useful in decreasing proteinuria. Side effects include hyperkalemia, and increase in serum creatinine levels (typically less that 15–20%) that is reversible by stopping the medication, and a dry cough.

Calcium channel blockers may cause peripheral edema.

Beta blockers may cause exercise intolerance, asthma exacerbation, and decreased sensing of hypoglycemia in diabetics.

Alpha 1 agonists (central alpha agonists) may result in drowsiness.

Peripheral vasodilators may result in peripheral edema and may have side effects including hirsutism and lupus-like syndromes.

- *Hypertensive emergencies:* Intravenous drips of nitroprusside, labetalol, and nicardipine are typically used in hypertensive emergencies. Oral clonidine is also effective. Cyanide levels should be monitored during the use of nitroprusside.
- *Neonates:* Beta blockers should not be used in infants who depend on heart rate for cardiac output.

Phosphate binders: Aluminum hydroxide, although an effective phosphate binder, should be used with caution as it may induce encephalopathy and bone disease. Calcium containing salts may worsen cardiovascular disease—the leading cause of death in both pediatric and adult patients with CKD. Sevelamer, as a metal and calcium free agent is safer, but twice as much medication is required to bind as much dietary phosphate as calcium salts.

Contraindications to growth hormone therapy: Growth hormone therapy should not be initiated until children are adequately nourished and acidosis, anemia, and renal osteodystrophy are controlled. Prior to starting growth hormone, an ophthalmologic exam (for increased ICP) and cardiac echo should be performed. Growth hormone should not be administered if the epiphyses are closed or if bony deformities are present. Growth hormone therapy should be stopped when the child reaches the 50% for height and/or the mid-parental height.

References

KDOQI practice guidelines: http://www.kidney.org/professionals/KDOQI/.
KDIGO practice guidelines: http://www.kdigo.org/.

Cystic Kidney Disease

(Polycystic Kidney Disease and Multicystic Dysplastic Kidneys)

Katherine Wesseling Perry

As opposed to solitary cysts (simple cysts) which may occur in asymptomatic individuals, Cystic Kidney Disease refers to several conditions, all of which can lead to renal failure or bilateral renal cysts.

Etiology

Cystic kidney disease may either occur from a genetic cause, from dysplastic renal development, or may be acquired. Genetic forms of Cystic Kidney Disease include:

1. *Autosomal dominant polycystic kidney disease (ADPKD)*: A defect in the gene encoding polycystin 1 or polycystin 2 is associated with the disease in the vast majority of patients. Both polycystin 1 and polycystin 2 localize to renal primary cilia, implicating altered urinary flow sensing as contributing to cyst development.
2. *Autosomal recessive polycystic kidney disease (ARPKD):* ARPKD is due to a mutation in the gene *nephrocystin* (also knows as *polyductin*). Three types of ARPKD have been described, depending on the age at presentation. Perinatal/neonatal ARPKD affects between 60–90% of renal tubules. Infantile ARPKD presents at 3–6 months of age with 25% of renal tubules affected by cysts. Juvenile ARPKD, in which 10% of renal tubules are involved, presents between ages 6 months and 5 years.
3. *Familial juvenile nephronopthesis* may have either a childhood or adult presentation (from 1st to 4th decades of life). Renal cysts occur in the cortex and corticomedullary junction.
4. *Multicystic dysplastic kidney (MCDK)* is a developmental abnormality. Typically, one kidney is affected with large, dysplastic cysts. This kidney is completely non-functional and involutes over time while the other kidney is normal.
5. *Acquired cysts* may also develop in the kidneys of long-term dialysis patients and have a risk of malignant transformation.

Clinical Presentation and Prognosis

Demographics: The demographics of cystic kidney disease depend on the specific type. ADPKD has an autosomal dominant inheritance pattern and occurs in 1 in 500 individuals of both genders and all ethnicities. ARPKD has an autosomal recessive inheritance pattern and occurs in 1:6000 to 1:40,000, depending on the ethnic group sampled. An increased prevalence is found amongst the Finish and Afrikaaners. Sixty-seven percent of Nephronopthesis cases have an autosomal recessive inheritance pattern. The disease occurs in 1 in 500 individuals of both genders and all ethnicities.

Presenting signs and symptoms and natural history

ADPKD: Patients are born with normal appearing and functioning kidneys; cysts develop, one at a time, throughout childhood and adulthood. Cysts also may develop in the liver, pancreas, CNS, spleen and ovaries. Eventually, cyst-laden abdominal organs become massively enlarged, leading to discomfort. Cyst rupture is typically painful and causes episodes of gross hematuria. Hypertension, proteinuria, and renal failure are common as more and more cysts develop with time. Ultimately, many patients progress to end-stage renal disease and require renal replacement therapy (dialysis and/or transplantation). End-stage renal disease typically occurs in adulthood (50% of patients by age 60). Although cysts may be present in childhood, end-stage renal disease is uncommon in pediatric patients. Intracranial aneurysms occur in 10–15% of patients, typically in the anterior circulation. Rupture may occur, even at small sizes (50% rupture at less than 10 mm in size).

ARPKD presents in infancy or childhood as large, hyperechoic ("bright") kidneys, renal failure, hepatic fibrosis, and hypertension. Unlike ADPKD, individual cysts may not be appreciated on renal ultrasound. Up to 50% of children with perinatal/neonatal ARPKD die in infancy from pulmonary failure. Infantile ARPKD presents at 3–6 months of age and, while hypertension is common early, renal failure develops later in childhood. Renal function is typically preserved in patients with juvenile ARPKD, but many of these children develop portal hypertension and bleeding varices in adolescence.

Familial juvenile nephronopthesis (medullary cystic disease) is associated with hyposthenuria, growth failure and anemia. Renal cysts occur in the cortex and corticomedullary junction. Nephronopthesis is associated with congenital hepatic fibrosis, neurological ("Joubert" syndrome) and ophthalmologic ("Senior-Loken" syndrome) abnormalities, and skeletal dysplasia ("Bardet-Biedl").

Multicystic dysplastic kidney (MCDK) presents either as an incidental finding on prenatal or post-natal ultrasound or as a neonatal abdominal mass. An increased incidence of reflux is observed in the contralateral kidney, but the majority of patients have normal blood pressure and kidney function.

Prognosis: Although deterioration of renal function may be slowed with strict blood pressure control and the use of ACE inhibitors, dialysis therapy and renal transplantation are ultimately necessary in the majority of patients with ADPKD, ARPKD, and nephronopthesis.

Patients with a solitary MCDK do well, typically maintaining normal kidney function throughout life.

Diagnosis

Renal imaging, including ultrasound is critical in evaluating cystic kidney disease. ADPKD presents as multiple large cysts in both kidneys; ARPKD presents as enlarged, hyperechoic kidney, while nephronopthesis presents as small, fibrotic kidneys with cortical cysts. Multicystic dysplastic kidney can be visualized on ultrasound; assessment of kidney function is then typically performed by MAG-3 scan.

Genetic diagnosis can be performed in some centers (www.genetests.org) for genetic forms of PKD. Genetic diagnosis, while useful for counseling, rarely affects medical management.

A voiding cystourethrogram should be performed in patients with MCDK to assess for reflux into the normal kidney.

Management

In patients with ADPKD, strict control of blood pressure and proteinuria (preferable with ACE inhibitors) may slow progression to end-stage renal disease. Patients with a family history of stroke and any patients with a severe headache should have periodic MRI evaluations for intracranial aneurysms. Although pain is a significant problem (due to cyst rupture and recurrent cyst infections), care should be taken in the management of pain. NSAIDS should be avoided as they may have a deleterious effect on kidney function. Opioids and acetaminophen are preferable alternatives.

Patients with ARPKD have significant hypertension, often necessitating the use of multiple antihypertensive medications or bilateral nephrectomies. Nephronopthesis is often complicated by severe anemia, requiring the early use of iron and erythropoietin, and a urinary concentrating defect, requiring free access to water and electrolytes.

Dialysis patients with acquired cysts should undergo surgical resection of the cysts, due to the potential for malignant transformation.

Consultations: All patients with cystic kidneys should be referred to a Nephrologist at diagnosis. Surgical consultation should be obtained for unilateral or bilateral nephrectomy in infants with ARPKD who have uncontrollable hypertension or respiratory distress or feeding intolerance due to compression by enlarged kidneys. Surgical consultation is also required for vascular access or peritoneal dialysis placement when renal failure is severe (uremia, electrolyte abnormalities, and volume overload).

Social: PKD foundation: http://www.pkdcure.org/

Monitoring: Renal ultrasound should be performed periodically (often annually) in most patients with PKD. Cyst size is monitored in ADPKD. Involution of the dysplastic kidney (which has a small, but increased risk of malignant transformation) and growth of the normal kidney are assessed in MCDK. Renal ultrasounds are performed yearly in dialysis patients to assess for the development of acquired cysts which have the potential for malignant transformation.

Pearls and Precautions

Disease complications: Kidney biopsies should be avoided in patients with renal cysts as the biopsy needle may cause cyst rupture and massive bleeding.

References

Grantham, J. J. 2008. "Clinical practice. Autosomal dominant polycystic kidney disease." *N.Engl.J.Med.* 3591477–85.

Hildebrandt, F. and W. Zhou. 2007. "Nephronophthesis-associated ciliopathies." *J.Am.Soc.Nephrol.* 181855–71.

Rossetti, S. and P. C. Harris. 2007. "Genotype-phenotype correlations in autosomal dominant and autosomal recessive polycystic kidney disease." *J.Am.Soc.Nephrol.* 181374–80.

Bisceglia, M., C. A. Galliani, C. Senger, C. Stallone, and A. Sessa. 2006. "Renal cystic diseases: a review." *Adv. Anat.Pathol.* 1326-56.

Cystinosis

Katherine Wesseling Perry

Cystinosis is an autosomal recessive lysosomal storage disorder resulting in cystine crystal deposition in multiple tissues including kidneys, cornea, thyroid, and heart. It typically presents in infancy and childhood (infantile form). Very rarely, a mild form, sparing the kidney and affecting only the cornea, may present in adulthood. This is termed "benign" cystinosis (adolescent or adult forms).

Etiology

Cystinosis is an autosomal recessive lysosomal storage disease due to a defect in cystonin—the lysosomal transporter for cystine. Intralysosomal cystine levels accumulate and crystals develop in a variety of tissues.

Clinical Presentation and Prognosis

Demographics: This autosomal recessive disorder affects between 1–2 in 100,000 newborns. Cystinosis is often seen in fair-skinned Caucasians. However, it may be seen in people of non-European origin as well. The male to female ratio in this disease is 1.4:1.

Presenting signs and symptoms: Cystinosis often presents with polyuria and short stature. Fanconi syndrome (renal wasting of phosphate, bicarbonate, uric acid, glucose, and amino acids) is highly suggestive of cystinosis. Photophobia is also common, due to intracorneal accumulation of cystine crystals.

Clinical course: Without treatment, patients with infantile cystinosis have a decline in renal function during childhood, resulting in end-stage renal disease by age 10. Progressive accumulation of cystine crystals in the cardiac conduction system and endocrine organs may result in arrhythmias, hypothyroidism, hypogonadism, diabetes, and neurological disease, typically in adulthood. Blindness may result from untreated eye disease.

Patients with "benign" cystinosis do not develop renal disease; these patients have corneal cystine deposits only.

Prognosis: Regular, consistent, treatment with oral cysteamine can halt the accumulation of cystine crystals within body tissues. If started in infancy (before 4 months of age) and used routinely, this medication may potentially prevent Fanconi syndrome, prevent deterioration of renal function, endocrine, and cardiac complications, and improve growth. However, treatment does not necessarily reverse existing systemic—including renal—disease.

Cystinotic patients do well after kidney transplantation. The transplanted kidney, with functioning cystonin, transports cystine well and Fanconi syndrome does not recur. However, transplantation does not ameliorate the symptoms in other organs so cysteamine therapy must be continued to halt progression of cardiac, eye, and endocrine disease.

Diagnosis

Accumulation of cystine in white blood cells is diagnostic of this disease. This test is performed in only a few specialized centers world-wide.

Management

Fluids: Children with cystinosis are polyuric, and daily urine output can exceed 10 liters per day. Cystinotic patients who must be made "NPO" MUST receive sufficient maintenance fluids to accommodate this obligate polyuria. The best assessment of maintenance fluids needs are typically ascertained from asking the parents the typical quantity of the child's daily fluid intake.

Electrolytes: Potassium and bicarbonate (typically in the form of potassium citrate: see below) and phosphate supplementation (potassium phosphate or sodium phosphate) are essential in these patients to maintain normal serum electrolytes.

Treatment: Cysteamine (cystagon) reduces cystine accumulation by undergoing disulphide exchange with cystine to form the cysteine-cysteamine mixed disulphide, which can be transported out of the lysosome. Long term cysteamine treatment in patients with cystinosis reduces the rate of progression of renal damage and improves growth. Treatment is foul tasting and must be given every six hours for life to prevent further crystal accumulation. Dosage is based on weight as listed in Table 10.2.

Cysteamine eye drops, (0.55% solution, administered every 2 hours), reduce photophobia.

Consultations: Nephrology and ophthalmology should be consulted at diagnosis. Endocrinology and cardiology should become involved when thyroid and cardiac abnormalities (i.e., conduction defects) develop.

Social: Numerous patient and family support groups are available.

Cystinosis research network:

http://www.cystinosis.org/support.html

Table 10.2: Cysteamine (Cystagon) Dosage

Weight (kg)	Dose
> 50	500 mg/dose cysteamine free base/dose
41.4–50	450 mg/dose
32.3–40.9	400 mg/dose
23.2–31.8	350 mg/dose
18.6–22.7	300 mg/dose
14–18	250 mg/dose
9.5–13.6	200 mg/dose
5–9	150 mg/dose
< 4.5	100 mg/dose

302 Whytegate Court
Lake Forest, IL 60045 USA
Toll Free: 1-866-276-3669 Tel: (847) 735-0471
Fax: (847) 235-2773 e-mail: CRN@cystinosis.org

Monitoring: Thyroid function tests and echocardiograms should be monitored on a regular (yearly basis) in all patients with cystinosis. Routine biochemical parameters including electrolytes, BUN and creatinine should be performed frequently (every 3 months). Yearly thyroid function tests, echocardiograms, and eye exams should also be performed. Height and weight should be monitored at every visit.

References

Gahl, W. A., G. F. Reed, J. G. Thoene, J. D. Schulman, W. B. Rizzo, A. J. Jonas, D. W. Denman, J. J. Schlesselman, B. J. Corden, and J. A. Schneider. 1987. "Cysteamine therapy for children with nephropathic cystinosis." N.Engl.J.Med. 316971–7.

Gahl, W. A., J. G. Thoene, and J. A. Schneider. 2002. "Cystinosis." N.Engl.J.Med. 347111–21.

Kleta, R., I. Bernardini, M. Ueda, W. S. Varade, C. Phornphutkul, D. Krasnewich, and W. A. Gahl. 2004. "Long-term follow-up of well-treated nephropathic cystinosis patients." J.Pediatr. 145555–60.

Diabetes Insipidus (DI)

Katherine Wesseling Perry

Diabetes Insipidus (DI) is characterized by polyuria (large amounts of dilute urine) and polydypsia. Polyuria and dilute urine persist when fluid intake is restricted. Hypernatremia is common in infants, the elderly and others without unrestricted access to water.

Etiology

DI may be either central or nephrogenic. Central DI consists of a deficiency in antidiuretic hormone (ADH) production by the posterior pituitary gland—frequently due to trauma or tumors. Nephrogenic DI (NDI) is an inability of the kidney to appropriately respond to ADH, either through an X-linked recessive defect in the vasopressin (V2) receptor (most commonly) or due to an autosomal recessive deficiency in the gene for aquaporin (AQP2) (rare).

Clinical Presentation and Prognosis

Presenting signs and symptoms: Infants with diabetes insipidus present with dehydration, hypernatremia, irritability and failure to thrive. Hypernatremia is common. Older patients may present with polyuria, nocturia, or bed-wetting.

Demographics: Nephrogenic DI is more common in boys than in girls and typically is detected in infancy.

Prognosis: Infants with NDI are at risk for growth failure and neuro-developmental delay.

Diagnosis

The diagnosis of DI is made in polyuric, polydypsic patients by the water deprivation test. Patients are continuously observed for 6–8 hours of water deprivation. Patient weight, serum sodium, serum osmolality, and urine osmolality are measured at hourly intervals. DI is diagnosed in patients who have a decrease in body weight and increase in serum osmolality and sodium despite a persistently dilute urine. A dose of ddAVP is then administered to assess whether the problem is central (urine concentrates in response to ddAVP) or nephrogenic (no response to ddAVP).

Management

Medications: Desmopressin acetate (ddAVP) is effective in treating central DI. Free access to water is essential for patients with NDI. Infants with NDI should ingest a low-solute formula, preferably breast milk.

Consultations: Nephrology should be consulted at first diagnosis of Nephrogenic DI to ensure electrolyte management and proper growth. Surgery may be required for G-tube placement in infants with Nephrogenic DI who are not able to consume sufficient oral free-water intake.

Monitoring: Serum electrolytes and growth parameters should be monitored routinely (at least every 3–6 months) in all children with DI.

Pearls and Precautions

Disease complications: Poor growth, particularly in infancy, is a significant problem for patients with DI. Achieving adequate nutrition in combination with adequate volume intake is challenging.

References

Knoers, N. and L. A. Monnens. 1992. "Nephrogenic diabetes insipidus: clinical symptoms, pathogenesis, genetics and treatment." *Pediatr. Nephrol.* 6476–82.

Knoers, N. V. and P. M. Deen. 2001. "Molecular and cellular defects in nephrogenic diabetes insipidus." *Pediatr. Nephrol.* 161146–52.

Hypophosphatemic Rickets

Katherine Wesseling Perry

Hypophosphatemic rickets is characterized by chronically low serum phosphorus levels, normal 25(OH)vitamin D levels, normal kidney function, and inappropriately normal or low 1,25(OH)$_2$vitamin D levels.

Etiology

Hypophosphatemic rickets may occur from any one of a number of genetic conditions, the majority of which are associated with increased circulating levels of the phosphaturic hormone, fibroblast growth factor (FGF) 23. These conditions include X-linked hypophosphatemic rickets (XLH), caused by a mutation in phosphate regulating endopeptidase homologue (PHEX); autosomal dominant hypophosphatemic rickets (ADHR) due to stabilizing mutation of FGF-23; or autosomal recessive hypophosphatemic rickets (ARHR) due to a mutation in dentin matrix protein 1 (DMP1). Mutations in the renal transporter, sodium-phosphate contransporter 2c (NaPi2c) will also result in hypophosphatemic rickets. This condition is termed "hereditary hypophosphatemic rickets with hypercalciuria" (HHRH).

Diagnosis

The diagnosis of hypophosphatemic rickets is made by characteristic clinical (short stature, bony deformities) and biochemical (hypophosphatemia, low 1,25(OH)$_2$vitamin D levels with normal 25(OH)vitamin D stores). Genetic testing can also be performed by a few research laboratories throughout the world.

Clinical Presentation and Prognosis

Demographics: Due to the X-linked pattern of inheritance, only boys are affected by XLH. Other forms of hypophosphatemic rickets affect males and females similarly.

Presenting signs and symptoms: Children with hypophosphatemic rickets present with short stature and deformities—typically bowing—of the long bones. Skeletal X-rays reveal diffuse osteopenia, often with horizontal hyperdense Looser's lines and fraying of the epiphyses. Serum biochemical evaluation reveals low serum phosphate levels, normal serum calcium, normal 25(OH)vitamin D stores, and inappropriately normal or low

1,25(OH)$_2$vitamin D. Urinary phosphate excretion is high, despite hypophosphatemia. Serum FGF-23 levels are elevated in most individuals. However, this test is only performed in research laboratories.

Clinical course and prognosis: Hypophosphatemia and rickets are difficult to control, even with massive doses of inorganic phosphate and 1,25(OH)$_2$vitamin D. Indeed, in patients with HHRH, nephrocalcinosis is common and its progression may be hastened by the administration of active vitamin D analogues, resulting in end-stage renal disease in some of these patients.

Management

Medications: Medical therapy relies on the administration of inorganic phosphate (orally in the form of neutraphos) and active vitamin D sterols. Dosages are titrated to maintain normal or near-normal serum phosphorus and alkaline phosphatase (a marker of skeletal mineralization) levels.

Consultations: Nephrology should be consulted in all patients who develop nephrocalcinosis and renal failure. Orthopedic Surgery should be consulted if/when bony deformities are noted.

Monitoring: Serum phosphorus, alkaline phosphatase and creatinine levels, along with urinary calcium excretion should be routinely checked (every 3–6 months) in all patients with hypophosphatemic rickets. Renal ultrasounds (to evaluate for nephrocalcinosis) should be performed yearly.

Pearls and Precautions

Nutrition/diet: A high phosphate diet should be encouraged (dairy products, particularly)

Likely complications: Chronic bone deformities may accompany hypophosphatemic rickets, even with high amounts of phosphate and vitamin D supplementation. Secondary hyperparathyroidism may also develop over time.

References

Bastepe, M. and H. Juppner. 2008. "Inherited hypophosphatemic disorders in children and the evolving mechanisms of phosphate regulation." *Rev.Endocr.Metab Disord.* 9171–80.

Juppner, H. 2007. "Novel regulators of phosphate homeostasis and bone metabolism." *Ther.Apher.Dial.* 11 Suppl 1S3–22.

Nephrosis

(Nephrotic Syndrome (NS))

Katherine Wesseling Perry

Nephrotic syndrome (NS) is a constellation of symptoms including proteinuria at a rate greater than or equal to 40 mg/m^2/day, edema, hypoalbuminemia, and hypertriglyceridemia.

Etiology

This syndrome has a myriad of causes. The most common etiology in children is Minimal change disease (MCNS), but a variety of pathologies may result in NS; treatment and prognosis depend on underlying etiology.

Minimal Change Nephrotic Syndrome (MCNS) is so named due to a normal appearing glomerulus under light microscopy. This is the most common cause of NS in pre-pubescent children.

Focal segmental glomerulonephritis (FSGS) becomes more common in older children (adolescents). This diagnosis is made by findings of focal scarring in the glomeruli. Underlying etiologies vary from idiopathic to genetic defects of the glomerulus or basement membrane. Genetic defects resulting in FSGS may result in isolated renal disease or may be part of a syndrome. These defects are listed below:

Podocyte

a. *Podocin (NPHS2):* Autosomal recessive mutations in this protein may either cause congenital nephrotic syndrome or childhood FSGS.
b. *Alpha actinin 4:* Autosomal dominant mutations result in FSGS in late childhood and/or adulthood.
c. *Phospholipase PLCE1 (NPHS3):* Autosomal recessive mutations result in childhood NS, some of which may respond to steroid therapy.
d. *Basement membrane LAMB2:* Autosomal recessive defects in this protein result in FSGS as part of the Pierson Syndrome.

Transcription factors

a. Wilm's tumor suppressor gene (WT1): Mutations in WT1 may result in FSGS alone or as part of the WAGR (Wilm's tumor, aniridia, and growth retardation), Denys-Drash, or Frasier Syndromes
b. LMX1B: Autosomal dominant defects result in FSGS as part of the Nail-Patella syndrome

Congenital nephrotic syndrome: Presents in the first year of life, and is due to inherited mutations of the podocyte or TORCHS infections. Genetic mutations associated with congenital nephrotic syndrome are located in NPHS1 (nephrin gene) or in NPHS2 (podocin).

Membranous nephropathy: Defined by thickened basement membranes with sub-epithelial immune deposits that often occurs as a consequence of autoimmune diseases (systemic lupus erythematosis), but may be idiopathic or secondary to chronic Hepatitis B or C infection.

Clinical Presentation and Prognosis

NS presents with massive proteinuria (>40 mg/m^2/hr), hypoalbuminemia, edema, and hyperlipidemia.

Demographics: This depends on the type of NS as described below.

Minimal change: MCNS affects both genders. This disease tends to affect younger children (age 2–10 years). No specific gene has been implicated, although there is a propensity to run in families. This condition is more common in patients with allergies and asthma and may occur secondary to T-cell lymphomas.

FSGS: FSGS occurs in older children and teenagers and may be either a primary (idiopathic) disease or secondary to obesity, infection (HIV or parvovirus), or familial causes.

Congenital Nephrotic Syndrome (CNS): CNS presents in the first year of life. CNS may be genetic or due to a congenital infection (classically, syphilis).

Membranous Nephropathy: Membranous nephropathy is rarely idiopathic in childhood. It is more frequently associated with systemic lupus erythematosis (in teenage girls) or chronic infection (hepatitis B).

Presenting signs and symptoms: The definition of nephrotic syndrome includes the presence of heavy proteinuria (over 40 mg/m^2/hr), edema/anasarca, hypoalbuminemia, and hypercholesterolemia/lipidemia. Hypertension is not common in patients with MCNS, but often occurs with other forms of NS. Microscopic hematuria is not typical of minimal change NS, though it may be present in 25% of cases. Hematuria more frequently accompanies FSGS and lupus nephritis. Pleural effusions are present on chest X-ray, but pulmonary edema is NOT a typical feature of pure nephrotic syndrome. Systemic signs such as rash, oral lesions, iritis, and arthritis are associated with autoimmune disease.

Patients with syndromic forms of FSGS also present with characteristics individual to their syndrome:

- *WAGR*: NS due to congenital nephrotic syndrome (diffuse mesangial sclerosis), Wilm's tumor, aniridia, and growth retardation
- *Frasier Syndrome*: NS due to FSGS, delayed kidney failure and complete gonadal dysgenesis
- *Denys Drash*: NS due to congenital nephrotic syndrome (diffuse mesangial sclerosis), pseudohermaphroditism, and Wilms tumor
- *Nail-Patella syndrome*: NS due to FSGS, renal failure, finger and toe-nail dysplasia, dislocation of the radial head and iliac horns, hypoplastic or absent patella, and glaucoma
- *Pierson syndrome*: NS, severe ocular maldevelopment, and neurological defects

Clinical course and prognosis

Minimal Change Nephrotic Syndrome: 70–80% of children with nephrotic syndrome respond to steroid therapy with complete remission of their symptoms within 4 weeks of initiating therapy. Those that respond do not undergo a kidney biopsy and are considered to have MCNS. Of those that respond, the majority will experience at least one recurrence of the disease. Children whose disease remits with steroids have an excellent prognosis; relapses become less frequent with time, disappearing by puberty. Children who do not respond to steroids, those who have a relapse of symptoms while on steroids, and those who have frequent relapses (>3/yr) should undergo a kidney biopsy to establish diagnosis.

Focal Segmental Glomerular Sclerosis (FSGS): FSGS and on renal biopsy confers a worse prognosis, irrespective of treatment, with many patients progressing to end-stage renal disease in childhood. Nephrotic syndrome may recur after renal transplantation, although not in genetic forms of FSGS (vide infra).

Nephrotic Syndrome due to Systemic Lupus Erythematosis: The majority of lesions associated with lupus nephritis can be treated and kidney function saved if aggressive therapy (typically consisting of cyclophosphamide and steroids) is promptly initiated.

Hereditary forms of NS, including Congenital NS: Genetic forms of nephrotic syndrome do not respond to therapy and progress to end-stage renal disease over months to years. NS does not typically recur after renal transplantation in these patients (a small minority of patients (<5%) with complete lack of NPHS1 mutation may develop NS or Anti-GBM disease post-renal transplantation.)

Viral associated NS: NS responds to antiviral therapy in many patients with Hepatitis B and C.

Diagnosis

Minimal Change Nephrotic Syndrome (MCNS): MCNS is a clinical diagnosis. Children ages 2–10 yrs. with the typical presenting symptoms (edema, hypoalbuminuria, and proteinuria with no hypertension or hematuria) who remit with prednisone therapy are considered to have MCNS. Those who do not remit or have atypical features should undergo kidney biopsy to establish a diagnosis.

Focal Segmental Glomerular Sclerosis (FSGS): FSGS is diagnosed by the presence of segmental glomerular scarring on renal biopsy. Patients presenting with atypical symptoms of nephrotic syndrome (age greater than 10 years, renal failure, hematuria, or hypertension), and patients who do not respond to steroid therapy in 4 weeks should undergo a kidney biopsy. Hereditary forms are diagnosed by genetic testing (www.genetests.org).

Systemic Lupus Erythematosis: Lupus Nephritis is also diagnosed by renal biopsy, where light microscopy reveals proliferative lesions and immunofluorescence highlights immune complex deposits. Low serum complement levels (C3 and C4) may also suggest the diagnosis, along with elevated ANA and dsDNA. Any patient with systemic lupus and the presence of renal failure and/or an active urinary sediment (i.e., proteinuria and/or hematuria) should undergo a kidney biopsy.

Viral Associated Nephrotic Syndrome: Serological evidence of TORCH infection or Hepatitis B or C along with typical features on renal biopsy, confirm the diagnosis of viral-associated NS.

Management

Minimal Change Nephrotic Syndrome (MCNS): Untreated MCNS self-remits in months to years. However, edematous patients are at increased risk for spontaneous bacterial peritonitis (SBP) (most commonly due to Streptococcus Pneumoniae infection) and thrombosis. Standard prednisone therapy (2 mg/kg/day for one month, followed by 2 mg/kg/every other day for another month) will typically induce remission within weeks of the treatment. However, up to 70% of MCNS patients may experience relapse. Treatment of a relapse also relies on prednisone therapy (2 mg/kg/day until proteinuria resolves, followed by 2 mg/kg/every other day for 2 weeks, followed by a slow taper, decreasing the dose every two weeks until off). Salt restriction is also of the utmost importance in these patients, since excess salt intake will exacerbate edema. To prevent GI irritation, antacids are an important adjunct to prednisone therapy. Treatment with albumin and diuretics (typically furosemide) in the acute phases of nephrotic syndrome is warranted for severe edema, particularly in the case of significant pleural effusions and scrotal edema.

Of note, diuretics should not be administered without albumin if the serum albumin level is less than 2g/dl as this may exacerbate vascular contraction and induce thromboembolic events. Albumin should not be administered in a nephrotic child without chest X-ray for confirmation of hypovolemia (small cardiac silhouette and the absence of pulmonary edema). Some forms of nephritis (see post infectious acute glomerulonephritis) may present with nephrotic range proteinuria and low serum albumin levels in the face of volume overload. A chest X-ray in these patients will show a full cardiac shadow and pulmonary edema. The administration of albumin in these patients may worsen pulmonary edema and cause respiratory compromise.

Focal Segmental Glomerular Sclerosis: Since some FSGS patients remit with steroid therapy, initial treatment for FSGS is identical to that for MCNS (i.e., prednisone as above, along with salt restriction). For patients who do not remit with steroids, cyclophosphamide (2 mg/kg/d for 12 weeks) may induce remission. Children who fail cyclophosphamide therapy may have a response to a calcineurin inhibitor (cyclosporine or tacrolimus) or to mycophenolate mofetil.

Systemic Lupus Erythematosis: Treatment of Lupus nephritis depends on pathological diagnosis. Focal segmental (FSGN) and diffuse proliferative (DPGN) lesions may be rapidly progressive unless treated promptly with steroids (initially 2 mg/kg/day weaning as tolerated) and cyclophosphamide (Induction: Monthly IV pulse dose of $1g/m^2$ for 6 months. Followed by Maintenance: $1g/m^2$ once every 3 months for a total of 2 years). In some patients, mycophenolate mofetil (up to 2 g/day in divided doses in adult-sized individuals) may be substituted for cyclophosphamide in the maintenance phase of treatment. Membranous lupus nephropathy tends to be resistant to treatment. However, it tends to progress to renal failure slowly. Therapy for membranous nephropathy typically relies on prednisone. Cyclophosphamide and/or mycophenolate mofetil may also be used.

Hereditary Forms of Nephrotic Syndrome: Genetic forms of Nephrotic Syndrome progress to end-stage renal disease over time, regardless of therapy. Thus, supportive therapy centers on controlling edema with salt restriction, periodic albumin infusions, and ACE inhibitor therapy. Unilateral or bilateral nephrectomy may be needed to control the edema associated with severe nephrotic syndrome. After nephrectomy, these patients do well on dialysis.

Infectious Forms of Nephrotic Syndrome: Antiviral medications for Hepatitis B and C are effective in controlling NS in affected patients.

Pearls and Precautions

Disease complications: The two most dreaded complications of nephrotic syndrome are: (1) Spontaneous bacterial peritonitis (most commonly due to streptococcus pneumonia); and (2) thrombosis secondary to urinary losses of antithrombin III and volume contraction. Abdominal pain in any patient with NS should be evaluated immediately. Moreover, diuretics should not be administered without concomitant albumin infusion in patients with serum albumin levels less than 2 mg/dl.

Medications: Immunosuppressant medications are the mainstay of therapy for non-genetic, non-infectious forms of NS. **Steroids** are the mainstay of therapy. Those who do not exhibit a response to steroids may be treated with cyclophosphamide, calcineurin inhibitors (cyclophosphamide or tacrolimus), or mycophenolate mofetil. Side effects of these medications include:

- *Steroids:* Weight gain (abdominal, facial, and at the base of the neck—so called "buffalo hump"), bone disease (decreased growth and osteopenia), skin changes (striae), and mood changes (irritability and sometimes significant changes in personality).
- *Cyclophosphamide:* Infertility, hemorrhagic cystitis, SIADH, heart failure, and neutropenia.
- *Calcineurin inhibitors (cyclosporin A and tacrolimus):* Chronic renal scarring, progressive renal failure, electrolyte abnormalities (type IV RTA: hyperkalemia and acidosis).
- *Mycophenolate mofetil:* Diarrhea, GI upset, and neutropenia.

Immunizations: While the administration of killed vaccines is safe, they may not induce immunity. Live attenuated vaccines are contraindicated in patients treated with immunosuppressive agents. In addition to the Prevnar vaccination that is recommended for all children, administration of Pneumovax, the 23-valent vaccine, is recommended in all children with NS over 2 years of age.

Consultations:

Nephrology: While consultation with a Nephrologist is recommended at the first diagnosis of any child with Nephrotic Syndrome, it is imperative that children with an atypical presentation (age greater than 10 or less than 1 year, hypertension, renal failure, or hematuria) be referred.

Surgery may be required for the following:

1. *Nephrectomy* may be required to limit proteinuria and edema and improve nutrition in forms of NS that do not respond to therapy. Unilateral nephrectomy is commonly performed in infants with congenital forms of NS to allow for improvement in symptoms and growth until the child is ready for kidney transplantation, at which time the second native kidney is removed.
2. *G-tube* placement is commonly required in small infants to ensure adequate nutrition and for the administration of medications.
3. *Central line* (Broviac or PICC) placement is useful in small infants and in some older children with NS that is refractory therapy and who require frequent albumin infusions and blood draws.
4. *PD or HD catheter* (see sections on PD or HD) placement is required when renal function deteriorates.

Rheumatology: Combined care by a Nephrologist and Rheumatologist is warranted in patients with Systemic Lupus Erythematosis with renal involvement.

Hepatology: Consultation and co-follow with a Hepatologist should be initiated as soon as Hepatitis B or C is diagnosed.

Social: The Nephcure Foundation: www.nephcure.org

Monitoring: Lab tests: 25(OH)vitamin D levels (urinary loss of vitamin D binding protein), thyroid function tests (urinary loss of thyroid binding protein), lipids and cholesterol panels.

Imaging: Gonads and kidneys should be monitored routinely (yearly) with ultrasound and/or CT scan in all patients with WAGR, Denys-Drash, and Frasier syndromes (i.e., all patients with defects in WT1) for the development of Wilm's tumor and/or gonadoblastoma.

References

Niaudet, P. 2004. "Genetic forms of nephrotic syndrome." *Pediatr. Nephrol.* 191313-8.
Chesney, R. W. 1999. "The idiopathic nephrotic syndrome." *Curr. Opin. Pediatr.* 11158-61.

Nephritis

A. Post Infectious Acute Glomerulonephritis (PIAGN)

Katherine Wesseling Perry

PIAGN is an immune complex nephritis which occurs after an infection.

Etiology

Infection with group A beta-hemolytic streptococcus (either as a throat or skin infection) is the most common etiology, but essentially any other infection can produce a similar syndrome. The pathology is believed to be Type III hypersensitivity reaction. Immune complexes (antigen-antibody complexes formed during an infection) become lodged in the glomerular basement membrane. Subsequent complement activation leads to destruction of the basement membrane.

Clinical Presentation and Prognosis

This condition may occur at any age, but is prevalent in childhood (age 2–12) and affects males and females equally.

Gross (visible to the naked eye) hematuria, occurring 7–10 days after a strep throat (or 4–6 weeks after strep cellulitis), is often the presenting sign. The urine is typically described as "coca-cola" or "tea-colored." Proteinuria is common and may be nephrotic range. Hypertension occurs due to volume overload. Increased creatinine indicating acute renal failure, also occurs.

Clinical course: PIAGN is a self-limited disease. Hypertension is common and must be aggressively managed as it can result in seizures, even at only mildly elevated pressures.

Prognosis: The prognosis for PIAGN is excellent. Renal function returns to normal and hematuria and proteinuria resolve in the vast majority of patients.

Diagnosis

PIAGN is a clinical diagnosis. Hematuria, proteinuria with a suppressed C3 level, but normal C4 value and a positive ASO or Anti-DNase B after a group A strep infection are highly suggestive for the condition. Patients in whom a depressed C4 level does not return to normal within 6 weeks of presentation should undergo a renal biopsy to evaluate for other conditions (membranoproliferative glomerulonephritis (MPGN), or lupus nephritis) associated with hypocomplementemia.

Management

Since hypertension is due to salt and water overload, diuretics are the treatment of choice. Patients should be evaluated with a chest X-ray to determine volume status. A large heart size and pulmonary congestion are characteristic of PIAGN. Albumin should not be administered to patients with such characteristic X-ray findings as it may result in pulmonary edema and respiratory failure. Group A streptococcal throat infection should be treated with antibiotics to prevent the development of rheumatic heart disease. Treatment of the pharyngitis does not prevent the development of nephritis.

Pearls and Precautions

A chest X-ray must be performed prior to albumin infusion, regardless of degree of hypoalbuminemia. An enlarged heart and pulmonary edema on chest X-ray is a contraindication for IV albumin as it may result in respiratory failure.

Consultations:

Nephrology: Consultation with/referral to a Nephrologist is imperative if both C3 and C4 are depressed at diagnosis or if C3 does not return to normal within 6 weeks of diagnosis.

Surgery: PD or HD catheter (see sections on PD or HD) placement is rarely required if PIAGN presents with severe renal dysfunction and uremia, volume overload, and/or electrolyte abnormalities.

Monitoring: Lab tests: Serum complement (C3 and C4) levels should be obtained 6–8 weeks after presentation. At this point, both should be within the normal range. Abnormal complement levels at this stage are not consistent with PIAGN; immediate referral to a Nephrologist for kidney biopsy (rule out MPGN and Lupus Nephritis) is warranted.

References

Carapetis, J. R., A. C. Steer, E. K. Mulholland, and M. Weber. 2005. "The global burden of group A streptococcal diseases." *Lancet Infect. Dis.* 5685–94.

Vijayakumar, M. 2002. "Acute and crescentic glomerulonephritis." *Indian J. Pediatr.* 691071–5.

B. Hemolytic Uremic Syndrome (HUS)

Katherine Wesseling Perry

HUS is characterized by a triad of renal failure, hemolysis, and thrombocytopenia.

Etiology

HUS is most commonly associated with gastroenteritis due to E. coli O157:H7 (called Diarrhea + (or D+) HUS), which produces a verotoxin leading to the production of microthrombi throughout the body, particularly in the kidney and brain. HUS may also be secondary to other infections (most notably, streptococcus pneumonia). In 5–10% of cases, recurrent HUS occurs from a congenital (genetic) deficiency of Factor H, Factor I, or membrane complex protein 1.

Clinical Presentation and Prognosis

Typical (D+) HUS presents with bloody diarrhea, pallor (from hemolysis) and irritability. Biochemical abnormalities include hemolytic anemia, renal failure (increased serum creatinine), thrombocytopenia, leukocytosis, increased levels of LDH (due to hemolysis) and a positive stool culture E. coli O157:H7.

Atypical (D-) HUS presents with similar symptoms, excluding the bloody diarrhea. In Streptococcal HUS, a Coombs test is typically positive. Genetic forms of HUS are associated with low serum levels of complement (C3, C4, CH50).

Demographics: D+ HUS occurs most commonly in young children, typically between the ages of 2 and 5 years.

Clinical course and prognosis: The clinical course of HUS depends on the etiology. D+ HUS is often self-limited, although many children need extensive supportive care, including dialysis, for a period of time. The length of required dialysis therapy is an indicator of long-term prognosis; prolonged anuria and dialysis therapy (greater than 5–10 days) portend a worse outcome. Despite normalization of serum creatinine, children who have HUS often have some residual damage and may develop chronic kidney disease or hypertension later in life.

Streptococcal HUS also tends to resolve, albeit with a higher rate of subsequent chronic kidney disease.

Genetic forms of HUS have the worst prognosis. These forms respond to therapies such as apheresis and plasma infusions, but recur and often lead to end-stage kidney disease.

Diagnosis

The triad of hemolytic anemia, renal failure, and thrombocytopenia are diagnostic for HUS. A stool culture positive for E. coli O157:H7 confirms D+ HUS. A positive Coombs test with a source of streptococcal infection signify streptococcal HUS. Low complement levels suggest genetic forms of HUS. Definitive diagnosis can be made by Factor H and I activity or genetic mutation analysis for Factors H, I or MCP. These tests have a long turn-around time and are performed in only a few research laboratories.

Management

Loop diuretics (e.g., furosemide) may be beneficial in the acute phase to maintain urine output. Dialysis is required for anuric renal failure. Blood transfusions are often required until the rate of hemolysis slows and washed RBCs should be considered for pneumococcal HUS.

Pearls and Precautions

Medications: Antibiotic therapy is typically NOT recommended for bloody diarrhea as it has been associated with an increased risk for the development of HUS.

Plasma therapy (cryoprecipitate or FFP) is indicated in genetic forms of HUS, as it will replace factor deficiencies. However, FFP is CONTRAINDICATED in streptococcal HUS as it may worsen the hemolysis and overall prognosis.

Consultations:

Nephrology: Consultation with a Nephrologist is suggested for all children with HUS. Even children with apparent "complete" recovery should have long-term renal follow-up as residual scarring may lead to chronic renal failure later in life.

Surgery: Surgical consultation may be required for PD or HD catheter in the event of anuria, volume overload, or electrolyte imbalances.

Social: see section in "chronic kidney disease."

Monitoring: All patients with a history of HUS should have routine (yearly) blood pressure, serum creatinine, and urinalysis (for proteinuria) performed. Serum LDH levels and complement levels should be monitored in patients with HUS as decreasing C3 and C4 levels and/or rising LDH levels portend a relapse.

References

Ruggenenti, P., M. Noris, and G. Remuzzi. 2001. "Thrombotic microangiopathy, hemolytic uremic syndrome, and thrombotic thrombocytopenic purpura." *Kidney Int.* 60831–46.

Trachtman, H. and E. Christen. 1999. "Pathogenesis, treatment, and therapeutic trials in hemolytic uremic syndrome." *Curr. Opin. Pediatr.* 11162–8.

C. Henoch-Schonlein Purpura (HSP)

Katherine Wesseling Perry

HSP is a vasculitic condition characterized by palpable purpura, arthritis, and abdominal pain. Renal involvement is also common.

Etiology

Deposition of IgA is found in numerous tissues. The renal findings in HSP are similar to those seen in IgA nephropathy.

Clinical Presentation and Prognosis

HSP tends to afflict children ages 2–5 and presents with palpable purpura of the lower extremities, arthritis of the ankles and feet. Abdominal pain may be severe and may progress to intussusception. Renal manifestations of HSP include proteinuria and hematuria.

Clinical course and prognosis: HSP is typically self-limited and therapy is aimed at reducing discomfort (i.e., with pain medications). However, serious complications may ensue and should be dealt with promptly. Intussusception is a worrisome consequence of HSP; thus, steroid therapy is indicated in the face of abdominal pain. Renal manifestations of HSP are typically confined to microscopic hematuria which self resolves over 1–2 years. However, severe crescentic glomerulonephritis occurs occasionally. Nephrotic range proteinuria, hypertension, and renal failure confer a poor prognosis for long-term renal function.

Diagnosis

The triad of palpable purpura, arthritis, and abdominal pain are diagnostic for HSP.

Management

Medication: Pain control with non-steroidals is typically sufficient to control arthritis although steroids (1 mg/kg/d for 2 weeks, followed by a 2 week taper) are indicated for abdominal pain. A kidney biopsy is warranted in the face of significant proteinuria; findings on biopsy dictate treatment. Patients with active glomerular disease often require immunosuppressive therapy including steroids and/or cyclophosphamide, in addition to ACE inhibition.

Consultations:

Nephrology: A nephrologist should be consulted if any hematuria, proteinuria or renal failure are present either at initial presentation or if they develop later.

Surgery: Surgical consultation is indicated if intussusception is suspected and barium enemas are <u>contraindicated</u> as they may result in bowel perforation.

Social: See section in "chronic kidney disease."

Monitoring: Urinary findings may develop after the rash and arthritis have resolved. Thus, urinalysis should be followed after HSP, even in patients with no initial urinary findings.

Pearls and Precautions

Medications: As above.

Immunizations: While the administration of killed vaccines is safe, they may not induce immunity in patients treated with immunosuppressive agents. Live attenuated vaccines are contraindicated in this patient population.

References

Sanders, J. T. and R. J. Wyatt. 2008. "IgA nephropathy and Henoch-Schonlein purpura nephritis." *Curr. Opin. Pediatr.* 20163–70.

Davin, J. C., Berge Ten, I, and J. J. Weening. 2001. "What is the difference between IgA nephropathy and Henoch-Schonlein purpura nephritis?" *Kidney Int.* 59823–34.

D. IgA Nephropathy

Katherine Wesseling Perry

IgA nephropathy is an immune complex glomerular disease characterized by the deposition of IgA in glomerular mesangium.

Etiology

The underlying etiology of IgA Nephropathy is incompletely understood, but has strong familial associations. Although it may occur in any ethnic group, it is most common in Asians. Acute exacerbations often accompany infections.

Clinical Presentation and Prognosis

The classic presentation of IgA nephropathy is an episode of "syn-pharyngitic" (i.e., at the same time as an infection) gross hematuria.

Demographics: IgA Nephropathy is the most common cause of glomerulonephritis worldwide. Its prevalence varies by ethnicity and is much higher in Asia (32–42% of all primary nephritis) than in Northern Europe (2–10%).

Clinical course and prognosis: IgA Nephropathy has a variable clinical course as some patients have microscopic hematuria alone and maintain normal renal function long-term. Others develop proteinuria and renal failure in childhood, progressing to end-stage renal disease requiring dialysis and renal transplantation. Although IgA Nephropathy may recur after transplantation, the clinical course is often milder than the original disease.

Diagnosis

IgA nephropathy is diagnosed on renal biopsy by identification of IgA deposits in the glomerular mesangium.

Management

Management varies based on the severity of the disease. Hematuria, in the absence of proteinuria, hypertension, or renal failure, is conservatively managed with observation alone.

Medication: Patients who develop proteinuria or an increase in serum creatinine are typically treated with ACE inhibitors and steroids. Rapidly progressive renal failure due to IgA Nephropathy is treated with high dose steroids and cytoxan (see RPGN).

Consultations: A Nephrologist should be consulted in all patients with IgA Nephropathy who have proteinuria and/or increased serum creatinine levels.

No specific surgical intervention is needed until end-stage renal disease (see sections on peritoneal and hemodialysis).

Social: IgA Nephropathy Support Group: http://www.igan.ca/

Monitoring: All patients with IgA nephropathy should have routine monitoring (frequency varying between yearly and q3 months depending on degree of renal impairment) of blood pressure, urinalysis (for proteinuria: trace and 1+ are often negative; 2+ and 3+ are usually real, but it depends on the concentration of the urine), and serum creatinine. Those with microscopic hematuria alone may be monitored yearly; those who develop proteinuria should be treated as above and followed more frequently.

Pearls and Precautions

Immunizations: While the administration of killed vaccines is safe, they may not induce immunity. Live attenuated vaccines are contraindicated in patients treated with immunosuppressive agents.

References

Davin, J. C., Berge Ten, I, and J. J. Weening. 2001. "What is the difference between IgA nephropathy and Henoch-Schonlein purpura nephritis?" *Kidney Int.* 59823–34.

Andreoli, S. P. 1995. "Chronic glomerulonephritis in childhood. Membranoproliferative glomerulonephritis, Henoch-Schonlein purpura nephritis, and IgA nephropathy." *Pediatr. Clin. North Am.* 421487–503.

Churg, J. 1993. "Large vessel vasculitis." *Clin. Exp. Immunol.* 93 Suppl 111–2.

E. Membranoproliferative Glomerulonephritis (MPGN)/Mesangiocapillary Glomerulonephritis (MCGN)

Katherine Wesseling Perry

MPGN (MCGN in older literature) is an immune complex glomerulonephritis characterized by varying degrees of hematuria and proteinuria. There are three types, termed types I, II (a.k.a. Dense Deposit Disease) and III.

Etiology

MPGN type I may be primary (idiopathic) or secondary to chronic infection. MPGN type II may either be idiopathic or associated with partial lipodystrophy. MPGN type III is always idiopathic.

Clinical Presentation and Prognosis

Demographics: The reported incidence of MPGN is difficult to establish, but is estimated to be between 1 to 2 per 1,000,000 pediatric patients. Type I is the most common form (55%), followed by types III (25%) and II (20%). MPGN affects older children and adolescents (average age: 9 years). Males and females are equally affected.

Presenting signs and symptoms: Patients with MPGN typically present with one of three scenarios: Nephrotic syndrome (33%); nephritic syndrome (gross hematuria) (25%); or asymptomatic hematuria and proteinuria (40-50%). Complement levels (C3 and C4) are typically very low. Approximately 25% of patients with type I MPGN present with antecedent constitutional complaints (fatigue, weakness, or weight loss).

Clinical course and prognosis: Prognosis varies according to the type of MPGN. 70–80% of patients with type I and type III MPGN respond to steroid therapy with preserved renal function 10 years after diagnosis. In those who progress to end-stage renal disease, these forms of MPGN recur in approximately 20–30% after renal transplantation. By contrast, the majority of patients with type II (dense deposit disease) progress to renal failure with the disease recurring in nearly 100% of patients who undergo renal transplantation.

Diagnosis

Hematuria, proteinuria, and low serum complement (C3 and C4) levels are suspicious for MPGN. Subtypes of MPGN cannot be distinguished by clinical features; a renal biopsy is required for diagnosis. Sub-endothelial immune deposits, cellular proliferation, and basement membrane "tram-tracking" are consistent with MPGN. Types I and III MPGN are distinguished from type II by immunofluorescence.

Management

Steroids (as for treatment of minimal change nephrotic syndrome) are the first line of treatment for MPGN. ACE inhibitors should also be used in patients with proteinuria. Other immunosuppressants, including cyclophosphamide, calcineurin inhibitors, and antimetabolites (mycophenolate mofetil) have all been used as adjuvant therapy.

Pearls and Precautions

Immunizations: While the administration of killed vaccines is safe, they may not induce immunity. Live attenuated vaccines are contraindicated in patients treated with immunosuppressive agents.

Consultations: All patients with MPGN should be closely followed by a Nephrologist and referral should be made at first diagnosis.

Surgical consultation may be required for PD or HD catheter if the disease progresses to end-stage renal disease and anuria, volume overload, or electrolyte imbalances ensue.

Social: See section in "chronic kidney disease."

Monitoring: All patients with MPGN should be followed carefully with serum creatinine levels, blood pressure, and urinalyses for blood and protein.

References

Andreoli, S. P. 1995. "Chronic glomerulonephritis in childhood. Membranoproliferative glomerulonephritis, Henoch-Schonlein purpura nephritis, and IgA nephropathy." *Pediatr. Clin. North Am.* 421487–503.
Licht, C. and V. Fremeaux-Bacchi. 2009. "Hereditary and acquired complement dysregulation in membranoproliferative glomerulonephritis." *Thromb. Haemost.* 101271–8.

F. Alport Syndrome (Hereditary Nephritis)

Katherine Wesseling Perry

Alport Syndrome is a genetic disorder characterized by Nephritis, end-stage renal disease, and hearing loss.

Etiology

Mutations in type IV collagen lead to alterations in the basement membrane of the kidney, inner ear, and eye in Alport Syndrome. The most common inheritance pattern is X-linked (80% of all cases) and is due to a mutation in the alpha 5 chain (COL4A5) of type IV collagen. Autosomal recessive Alport Syndrome occurs in 10–15% and is due to mutations in the alpha 3 or alpha 4 (COL4A3 or COL4A4). The remaining 5% of cases are due to autosomal dominant mutations in COL4A3 or COL4A4.

Clinical Presentation and Prognosis:

Demographics: Due to the predominance of an X-linked inheritance pattern, boys are more commonly affected than girls.

Presenting signs and symptoms: Hematuria may be present as early as infancy. Microscopic hematuria is common, although episodes of gross hematuria (red, pink, or brown) may also occur at the time of infection and last for days. Proteinuria and progressive renal failure typically develop in childhood. Although hearing is normal at birth, many experience high frequency hearing loss which coincides with the onset of declining renal function during childhood. Anterior lenticonus, an abnormal shape of the eye lens, affects 15–20% of patients with X-linked and AR Alport Syndrome. A minority of patients (with deletion of COL4A6 in conjunction with COL4A5) may experience Leiomyomas (benign smooth muscle neoplasms) that present as dysphagia.

Clinical course: Proteinuria and progressive renal failure accompany hearing loss in childhood. Renal function declines with time and most patients progress to end stage renal disease.

Prognosis: There is variability in the rate of progression as the majority of patients develop end-stage renal disease by the teenage to young adult years. However, some do not require dialysis until middle age. Patients with autosomal dominant disease have a slower progression with end-stage renal disease developing in middle-age.

Diagnosis

Alport's syndrome should be on the differential diagnosis of a child or adult with hematuria, proteinuria and/ or renal dysfunction. A family history of hearing loss and renal failure is typical. Definitive diagnosis requires a tissue biopsy. A skin biopsy may be sufficient in patients with X-linked (COL4A5 mutation) Alport syndrome. Since the alpha 5 chain of collagen 4 is found in dermal tissue, the absence of staining is diagnostic for Alport syndrome. However, normal skin biopsy findings do not rule out Alport syndrome and require a renal biopsy. Upon renal biopsy, areas of thinned basement membrane, alternating with thickened, disorganized ("basket weaving") basement membrane is consistent with Alport syndrome. Immunofluorescence for collagens 4A3, 4A4, and 4A5 can be performed on renal tissue and is diagnostic for the condition.

Management

Angiotensin Coverting Enzyme Inhibitor (ACEI) therapy controls hypertension, reduces proteinuria and protects kidney function. ACEI may prolong the time until dialysis in Alport patients and should be administered in anyone with proteinuria and/or hypertension. Some centers have also advocated the use of calcineurin inhibitors to decrease proteinuria (Charbit et al. 2007). Little else is effective in treating this syndrome; management of the complications of chronic kidney disease (anemia, renal osteodystrophy, and acidosis) becomes important as renal function declines.

As renal function declines, management of electrolytes, anemia, and osteodystrophy should be performed as routine for chronic kidney disease (see Chronic Kidney Disease).

Medications: ACE inhibitors are routinely used to control hypertension and proteinuria. Calcineurin inhibitors (cyclosporin) have also been used by some physicians to decrease proteinuria and control progression (Charbit et al. 2007); its mechanism of action is incompletely understood.

Consultations: All patients with Alport's syndrome—and all siblings of Alport's patients who have hematuria— should be referred to a Nephrologist as soon as they are identified.

Yearly follow-up by an ophthalmologist for lens abnormalities and corrective lenses are indicated. Otolaryngology should be involved to provide annual ear exams and prescribe hearing aids when hearing loss becomes significant.

Patients with dysphagia should be evaluated by gastroenterology and pediatric surgery for achalasia and esophageal lyomyomas.

Social: Alport Syndrome Foundation: https://www.alportsyndrome.org/links-sub/links_support.html

Monitoring: Vision and hearing should be monitored yearly. Blood pressure, serum creatinine, and urinalysis (for protein and creatinine) should also be followed routinely in all patients with Alport's.

Pearls and Precautions

Medications to be avoided: NSAIDS and nephrotoxic medications should be avoided in all patients with renal impairment. This is not specific to Alport's. NSAIDS should REALLY be avoided in all children with dehydration.

Likely complications: Same as for progressive renal failure. In addition, progressive hearing loss.

References

Charbit, M., M. C. Gubler, M. Dechaux, M. F. Gagnadoux, J. P. Grunfeld, and P. Niaudet. 2007. "Cyclosporin therapy in patients with Alport syndrome." *Pediatr. Nephrol.* 2257–63.

Turner, A. N. and A. J. Rees. 1996. "Goodpasture's disease and Alport's syndromes." *Annu. Rev. Med.* 47377–86.

Flinter, F. 1997. "Alport's syndrome." *J. Med. Genet.* 34326–30.

Obstructive Uropathy

(UPJ Obstruction, UVJ Obstruction, Ureteroceles, and Urethral Obstruction, and Neurogenic Bladder)

Katherine Wesseling Perry

Obstruction of the urinary tract leads to high pressures in the urinary system, urinary stasis, infections, and renal scarring. Structural obstruction may occur at the following locations: Urethra, bladder/ureteric junction, or ureteric/kidney junction. Functional obstruction occurs due to a failure of the bladder to empty appropriately and is termed "neurogenic bladder."

Etiology

Posterior urethral valve (PUV) is caused by an obstructive flap of tissue at the junction of the prostatic and penile urethra and is believed to be a developmental failure to completely recanulate the urethra. Uretero-pelvic junction (UPJ) obstruction occurs as a stricture just distal to the renal pelvis and is believed to be due to an in-utero vascular accident. Ureterovesicular junction (UVJ) obstruction is secondary to a stricture at the junction of the ureter and bladder. Neurogenic bladder is a condition in which the bladder does not properly empty either due to lack of neural stimulation (as in tethered cord and spina bifida) or due to behavioral issues (non-neurogenic neurogenic bladder or Hinman syndrome). Ureteroceles are developmental outpouchings of the distal end of the ureter, which, inside the bladder, obstruct urinary flow from the ureter to the bladder.

Clinical Presentation and Prognosis

Demographics: Urethral obstruction, most commonly in the form of posterior urethral valves (PUV), affects boys exclusively. Uretero-pelvic junction (UPJ) and ureterovesicular junction (UVJ) obstructions as well as neurogenic bladder affect males and females equally. Ureteroceles more commonly affect girls.

Presenting signs and symptoms: Urinary tract obstruction may present as hydronephrosis or as urinary tract infection (pyelonephritis). Hydronephrosis is often detected on prenatal ultrasound. It may also be detected in early infancy as an abdominal mass.

Clinical course/natural history: Obstruction results in chronic pooling of urine, which, in turn, is a set up for recurrent infections. Chronic, unrelieved obstruction may also lead to progressive, irreversible kidney damage. If drained early, renal function may be preserved to varying degrees.

Prognosis: Prognosis depends on the severity of obstruction and length of time the obstruction is present before being surgically corrected. Patients with unilateral obstruction or those with minor degrees of bilateral obstruction and who have preserved renal function do well, with near-normal long-term kidney function. Patients with severe bilateral obstruction and renal failure may not recover kidney function, despite surgical correction.

Diagnosis

A renal ultrasound is warranted in any pediatric patient with a 1st episode of pyelonephritis or any infant with an abdominal mass. Hydronephrosis found on ultrasound suggests obstruction, but may also be due to reflux. Thus, further imaging is warranted including a voiding cystourethragram (VCUG), which identifies reflux as well as obstruction from posterior urethral values and a Tecnetium 99 labeled mercapto acetyl tri glycine (MAG-3), intravenous pyleogram (IVP), or computed tomographic urogram (CT Urogram) which identify the level of a UPJ or UVJ obstruction. Urodynamic studies, performed by a Urologist, are useful in assessing neurogenic bladders, and a spinal MRI should be performed in this group of patients to evaluate for tethered spinal cord even if an obvious neural defect is not present.

Management

Some obstructions, particularly neurogenic bladders and urethral obstructions, may be temporarily relieved with foley-catheter drainage.

Surgery: Surgery (fulguration of the valve) is required to permanently relieve PUV obstruction. UPJ and UVJ obstructions are also relieved by surgery. The degree of obstruction and the size of the patient often determine the urgency of surgical repair (i.e., small infants with mild obstructions are often allowed to grow before repair is attempted. Larger children or those at risk for sustaining long-term kidney damage typically undergo surgery more promptly). Nephrostomies (drainage tubes directly from the renal pelvis to the exterior) and vesicostomies (bladder drainage) and/or foley catheters (bladder drainage) may provide temporary decompression before definitive repair.

Consultations: Urology consultation is necessary when obstruction is identified.

Nephrology referral is warranted at the time of diagnosis if renal failure, hypertension, or proteinuria is noted.

Monitoring: Blood pressure, serum creatinine levels, and urine protein excretion should be monitored routinely every 3–6 months depending on the degree of renal failure in all patients with a history of obstructive uropathy.

Pearls and Precautions

Disease Complications: After severe obstruction is relieved, some patients waste fluids and electrolytes (so-called post-obstructive diuresis). Electrolytes in these patients should be monitored regularly and fluids and electrolytes replaced as they are lost in the urine.

References

Becker, A. and M. Baum. 2006. "Obstructive uropathy." *Early Hum. Dev.* 8215–22.
Quintero, R. A. 2005. "Fetal obstructive uropathy." *Clin. Obstet. Gynecol.* 48923–41.

Oxalosis

Katherine Wesseling Perry

Oxalosis ("primary hyperoxaluria") is a disease of excess calcium oxalate crystal accumulation throughout the body, particularly in kidneys, bone, and cardiac tissue, leading to nephrocalcinosis and end-stage renal disease.

Etiology

Primary hyperoxaluria results from a defect in one of the hepatic enzymes that converts poorly soluble oxalate to more soluble biproducts, glycolate and glycerate. Type I primary hyperoxaluria is caused by a deficiency in alanine-glyoxylate aminotransferase (AGXT). Type II is due to a deficiency in glyoxylate reductase/hydroxypyruvate reductase (GR/HPR). Both types of oxalosis are autosomal recessive.

Diagnosis

The evaluation of primary hyperoxaluria includes the evaluation of blood and urine samples for oxalate (increased in oxalosis), glycolate (decreased), and glycerate (decreased). Renal ultrasound reveals bilateral nephrocalcinosis and/or urinary tract stones. Definitive diagnosis and differentiation between types I and II hyperoxaluria is accomplished by measurement of enzyme activity in liver biopsy specimen.

Clinical Presentation and Prognosis

Demographics: Autosomal recessive inheritance pattern is the most common inheritance pattern, thus, primary oxaluria affects boys and girls equally.

Clinical course: Patients with partial deficiencies in AGXT or GR/HPR (those who present in late childhood or adolescence) may have increased enzyme activity with pyridoxine therapy. In these individuals, oxalate deposition may decline and nephrocalcinosis and renal function stabilize with pyridoxine treatment combined with high fluid intake. The majority of patients who present in infancy have complete absence of enzyme, do not respond to therapy, and go on to require combined liver and kidney transplantation.

Prognosis: Untreated primary oxaluria leads to end-stage renal disease anywhere from infancy to adulthood. The severity of the phenotype is related to the amount of functioning AGXT or GR/HPR; patients with some functioning enzyme fair better than those with absolutely none.

Management

Urinary oxalate is best solubilized by *increased water intake* (3-4 liters/1.73 m^2/day).

Medications: Thiazide diuretics may be used to decrease urinary calcium excretion. Magnesium, neutral phosphate, and sodium citrate may all be helpful in solubilizing calcium oxalate stones.

Pyridoxine (0.5 grams/1.73 m^2/day) may stimulate hepatic enzyme activity in those with only partial decrease in enzyme activity.

Dialysis: In patients with renal failure due to primary oxaluria, dialysis and transplant become essential for the management of end-stage renal disease. Daily hemodialysis is the dialysis modality of choice in children with oxalosis as this method removes considerably more systemic oxalate than does peritoneal dialysis.

Transplant: Combined hepatic and renal transplantation is necessary to completely "cure" oxalosis. Without a liver transplant, oxalate reaccumulates in the transplanted kidney.

Social: Patients and their families may find support at the Oxalosis and Hyperoxaluria Foundation: http://www.ohf.org/.

Monitoring: Routine echocardiogram and ophthalmologic exam may show abnormal oxalate deposits in the heart and eyes, respectively, and should be performed yearly in patients with primary hyperoxaluria. Urinary oxalate concentration should be monitored frequently and fluid intake adjusted to maintain urinary concentrations less than 22 mg/dl (250 mole/L).

Family screening: If primary hyperoxaluria is suspected, siblings should also be tested.

Pearls and Precautions:

Nutrition and diet: These patients should be advised to avoid oxalate containing foods such as vitamin C, chocolate, and rhubarb.

Consultations: Nephrology should be consulted immediately. A renal dietician should also be consulted. A surgeon will be needed for G-tube placement and HD catheter placement. Ultimately, a transplant surgeon may be needed to perform a combined liver and kidney transplant.

References

Milliner, D. S. 2005. "The primary hyperoxalurias: an algorithm for diagnosis." *Am.J.Nephrol.* 25154–60.

Cochat, P., A. Liutkus, S. Fargue, O. Basmaison, B. Ranchin, and M. O. Rolland. 2006. "Primary hyperoxaluria type 1: still challenging!" *Pediatr.Nephrol.* 211075–81.

Bobrowski, A. E. and C. B. Langman. 2008. "The primary hyperoxalurias." *Semin.Nephrol.* 28152–62.

Potter's Syndrome

Katherine Wesseling Perry

Potter's Syndrome, more accurately termed Potter's Sequence or Oligohydramnios Sequence, refers to a physical appearance including a beaked nose, redundant skin, and low-set ears that are pressed against the skull. Lung development, which relies heavily on adequate amounts of amniotic fluid, is also abnormal, resulting in reduced numbers of alveolar sacs and small lung volumes. Typically, the bladder is small and non-distensible and abnormalities of the genital tract may also be present. Infants with Potter's syndrome are often born prematurely and are small for gestational age.

Etiology

Typical features result from in-utero compression.

Clinical Presentation and Prognosis

Demographics: Classically, this sequence is found in children with bilateral renal agenesis, but may also occur in any condition with decreased urine output since fetal urine is the primary constituent of amniotic fluid.

Clinical course: Lung hypoplasia is the major obstacle to viability in infants with Potter's sequence. Difficulties in maintaining long-term dialysis axis may also occur in very small, anuric babies as vascular access is limited in infants weighing less than 3 kg. Peritoneal dialysis is often possible, but problems that arise (including infections, leaks, and hernias) are difficult to manage with limited access for hemodialysis.

Prognosis: Children whose lung function is sufficient to survive the neonatal period can often be successfully dialyzed until they reach a large enough size to undergo renal transplantation (see section on transplantation).

Diagnosis

Potter's sequence is a clinical diagnosis. Renal failure, a history of low amniotic fluid, and the typical appearance (see above) define the condition.

Management

Difficulties in ventilation immediately after birth result in death in the majority of these infants, despite treatment with dialysis. The extent of pulmonary disease may not, however, be apparent for some time as pulmonary vascular resistance decreases in the first few weeks of life, facilitating ventilation.

Dialysis: Anuric infants require renal replacement therapy (i.e., dialysis). Complications associated with access, including difficulties in placing hemodialysis access, and infections and hernias associated with peritoneal dialysis, may limit its effectiveness. However, infants who survive the neonatal period have a good chance of surviving and, once they have grown to a sufficient size (7–10 kg, typically 1 year of age or older) are candidates for renal transplantation (see section on dialysis).

Consultations: Nephrology should be consulted at the identification of any child with renal failure (i.e. immediately in all children with Potter syndrome).

Pulmonology should be consulted for the long-term management of hypoplastic lungs.

General Surgery should be consulted for the placement of dialysis access if renal function is insufficient to maintain normal serum electrolytes or provide adequate clearance.

Urology should be consulted immediately for any child with obstructive uropathy.

Orthopedic Surgery should be consulted in any child born with arthrogryposis.

Monitoring: See monitoring in "Chronic Kidney Disease" and "Obstructive Uropathy".

Pearls and Precautions

Disease Complications: Respiratory distress and failure and pneumothoraces may accompany hypoplastic lungs.

References

Kurjak, A., V. Latin, G. Mandruzzato, V. D'Addario, and B. Rajhvajn. 1984. "Ultrasound diagnosis and perinatal management of fetal genito-urinary abnormalities." *J. Perinat. Med.* 12291–312.

Rapidly Progressive Glomerulonephritis (RPGN), Pulmonary-Renal Syndrome

(Goodpasture's, Wegener's Granulomatosis, Microscopic Polyangiitis, and Systemic Lupus Erythematosis)

Katherine Wesseling Perry

Pulmonary-renal syndrome is characterized by the simultaneous occurrence of diffuse alveolar hemorrhage and rapidly progressive glomerulonephritis (RPGN).

Etiology

Pulmonary-renal syndrome can occur as a result of one of three underlying diagnoses: (1) Immune complex disease (systemic lupus erythematosis); (2) anti-glomerular basement disease (Goodpasture's disease); and (3) pauci-immune disease (Wegener's, and Microscopic Polyangiitis).

Clinical Presentation and Prognosis

Demographics: The Pulmonary-renal syndrome occurs predominantly in older adolescents and adults. Lupus has a 3:1 female to male ratio.

Presenting signs and symptoms: Classically, the pulmonary-renal syndrome presents with hemoptysis and renal failure (increased creatinine). Early stages of Wegener's may be characterized by apparent recurrent upper respiratory infections (recurrent sinusitis), hematuria, and proteinuria, with or without hypertension. Initial constitutional symptoms include fever and weight loss. 33% of patients have arthralgia/arthritis at presentation, and 9% have a rash. 10–35% ultimately have some neurologic involvement.

Clinical course: Untreated, RPGN goes to complete renal failure in days to weeks and pulmonary hemorrhage may be massive and rapidly fatal. Thus, untreated patients have an average survival of 5 months, with 82% succumbing to the disease in 1 year.

Prognosis: With aggressive therapy (high dose of steroids, cytoxan, with or without plasmapheresis) 80–90% of patients are alive at 4 years.

Diagnosis

An active urine sediment (proteinuria and hematuria) in combination with renal failure and respiratory symptoms is suggestive of the pulmonary-renal syndrome. Sinus films and/or CT scans may confirm the presence of sinusitis, while a chest X-ray or chest CT may confirm a pulmonary process. Circulating anti-glomerular basement antibodies may be detectable in patients with Goodpasture's. Definitive diagnosis depends on renal biopsy to characterize the subtype of disease; crescentic glomerulonephritis is consistent with the diagnosis of RPGN. The presence of linear anti-glomerular basement (anti GBM) IgG staining on immunofluorescence is consistent with the diagnosis of Goodpasture's disease. Full-house (IgA, IgG, IgM, C3, and C1q) staining on immunofluorescence is consistent with immune complex-mediated (systemic lupus erythematosis) RPGN. A lack of immunostaining is consistent with pauci-immune GN (Wegener's granulomatosis, Polyarteritis).

Management

Medications: Early and aggressive immunosuppressant therapy is crucial to salvaging lung and kidney function in all types of pulmonary-renal syndrome. The mainstay of therapy relies on steroid therapy (typically initially given in pulse doses of 1 g/day for 3 days followed by daily oral prednisone at 60 mg/day) and cyclophosphamide (cytoxan) (given either as pulse, intravenous induction therapy given in doses of $1g/m^2$/dose monthly for six months or as oral therapy, given in a dose of 2 mg/kg/day). Oral cyclophosphamide therapy is generally considered to be more effective than IV therapy; however, side effects (including reproductive sterility) are more prevalent during oral therapy.

Plasmapheresis may also be warranted, particularly in patients with Goodpasture's disease.

After 6 months of intensive induction therapy as above, patients with pulmonary-renal syndrome receive an additional 2 years (at the least) of maintenance therapy consisting of steroids in combination with cytoxan, immuran, or mycophenolate mofetil. This maintenance therapy is imperative—even in patients who progress to end-stage renal disease—in order to reduce the risk of severe (often deadly) pulmonary hemorrhage.

Consultations: A Nephrologist should be consulted immediately if RPGN is suspected.

A Rheumatologist and/or Pulmonologist should be immediately consulted in all patients with pulmonary symptoms—particularly in patients with hematuria. Surgery should be consulted if complications of acute renal failure (fluid overload, uremia, and/or electrolyte abnormalities) necessitate HD or PD catheter placement.

Social: See section in "chronic kidney disease."

Monitoring: ANCA levels, serum creatinine, urinary protein excretion, and pulmonary function tests should be followed regularly (every 1–3 months) in all patients treated for RPGN.

Pearls and Precautions

Immunizations: While the administration of killed vaccines is safe, they may not induce immunity. Live attenuated vaccines are contraindicated in patients treated with immunosuppressive agents.

Disease complications: Fatal pulmonary hemorrhage may accompany any of the pulmonary-renal syndromes. Prompt evaluation and treatment of hemoptysis is warranted in all patients with these conditions.

Patients who are receiving either induction or maintenance therapy for the pulmonary-renal syndrome are significantly immunosuppressed. Infection should be high on the differential diagnosis for all complaints in this population, even in the absence of classical signs of infection (including fever). Antibiotic therapy should be initiated promptly if the diagnosis of infection is entertained.

References

Ozen, S. 2002. "The spectrum of vasculitis in children." *Best. Pract. Res. Clin. Rheumatol.* 16411–25.

von Vigier, R. O., S. A. Trummler, R. Laux-End, M. J. Sauvain, A. C. Truttmann, and M. G. Bianchetti. 2000. "Pulmonary renal syndrome in childhood: a report of twenty-one cases and a review of the literature." *Pediatr. Pulmonol.* 29382–8.

Roberti, I., L. Reisman, and J. Churg. 1993. "Vasculitis in childhood." *Pediatr. Nephrol.* 7479–89.

Renal Tubular Acidosis (RTA)

Katherine Wesseling Perry

Renal Tubular Acidosis (RTA) is defined as a metabolic acidosis that is due to the kidneys' failure to appropriately acidify the urine.

Etiology

RTA may occur from either a failure of the kidneys to reclaim bicarbonate in the proximal tubule (type II RTA) or a failure to excrete hydrogen ion in the distal tubule (types I and IV RTA). Type I RTA may be autosomal recessive or dominant. Type II RTA in childhood is typically associated with phosphaturia, glucosuria, aminoaciduria, and uric aciduria (together, termed "Fanconi syndrome"). Causes of Fanconi syndrome include: Cystinosis, galactosemia, tyrosinemia, hereditary fructose intolerance, Lowe's syndrome, Wilson's disease, and ifosphamide chemotherapy. Type IV RTA is typically caused by an autoimmune disease (lupus nephritis) or urinary tract obstruction.

Clinical Presentation and Prognosis

Demographics: Genetic forms of RTA present in infancy or early childhood and affects boys and girls equally. The condition may be autosomal dominant, recessive, and sporadic.

Presenting signs and symptoms: Short stature with or without concomitant rickets may call the clinician's attention to the potential for RTA. The diagnosis is made by the following biochemical abnormalities: (1) A normal anion-gap metabolic acidosis; (2) hyperchloremia, and (3) hypokalemia (in types I and II). Sensorineural deafness and nephrocalcinosis may also accompany type I RTA. Hyperkalemia, rather than hypokalemia, is present in type IV RTA.

Clinical course: Untreated, chronic metabolic acidosis from RTA may lead to rickets (growth failure and bone deformities), chronic hypercalciuria, nephrocalcinosis, and, ultimately, renal failure.

Prognosis: With citrate or bicarbonate therapy, growth and bone disease improves. Timely therapy will offer these children improved growth and minimal sequelle.

Diagnosis

The presence of a hyperchloremic, non-gap metabolic acidosis, in the absence of diarrhea or gastrointestinal fistula, is diagnostic of RTA. Urinary pH may help to distinguish distal (type I or IV) RTA from proximal (type II) RTA. An acidotic urinary pH (pH < 5.5) suggests an intact distal tubule able to acidify the urine (hence, the presence of a proximal RTA); while an alkalotic urine suggests a distal RTA. A urinary anion gap ($U_{Na} + U_K - U_{Cl}$) of greater than 0, or a urinary osmolar gap ($U_{osmoles(measured)} - (2U_{Na} + 2U_K)$) less than 100 suggests a distal tubular defect (i.e., Type I or Type IV RTA). Hyperkalemia accompanies Type IV RTA; hypokalemia suggests Types I or II RTA.

Management

Correction of acidosis (with bicarbonate or citrate) and correction of hypokalemia (with potassium) are the mainstays of therapy. The amount of base required to correct the acidosis is much less for types I and IV RTA (typically 1–2 mEq/k/d) than for type II RTA (5–10 mEq/kg/d).

Medications: Polycitra (a combination of sodium citrate and potassium citrate) or Polycitra K (potassium citrate alone) at a dose of 1–2 mEq/kg/d is effective in treating type I RTA; higher doses (5–10 mEq/kg/d) are required for type II. Bicitra (sodium citrate) or sodium bicarbonate (baking soda) at a dose of 1–2 mEq/kg/d is useful for treating type IV RTA. Patients with type IV RTA due to aldosterone deficiency (Addison's disease) will benefit from aldosterone replacement therapy.

Resistant hyperkalemia can be ameliorated with daily doses of lasix.

Consultations: Nephrology consultation at the time of the diagnosis is highly recommended. Audiology screening should be performed shortly after diagnosis.

Monitoring: A renal ultrasound is necessary in patients with types I and IV RTA. In type I RTA, increased urinary calcium excretion may lead to nephrocalcinosis and, if untreated, progressive renal disease. Type IV RTA may be secondary to urinary tract obstruction, which may be visualized as hydronephrosis on renal ultrasound.

Response to treatment (i.e. serum electrolytes and urine calcium/creatinine levels) should be followed routinely (every 3–6 months) in all children on a stable therapeutic regimen for RTA.

Pearls and Precautions

Disease Complications: Growth failure is due to rickets rather than due to growth hormone deficiency or resistance to growth hormone. Thus, the majority of children display catch-up growth after correction of acidosis and growth hormone therapy is not warranted in the majority of patients. Children who do not have catch-up growth despite 1–2 years of normal serum bicarbonate concentrations should be referred to an endocrinologist for evaluation.

Medication interactions: Drugs that exacerbate acidosis, including sodium chloride, ammonium chloride, and Arginine chloride should be avoided.

References

Laing, C. M. and R. J. Unwin. 2006. "Renal tubular acidosis." *J. Nephrol.* 19 Suppl 9S46–S52.

Rodriguez-Soriano, J. and A. Vallo. 1990. "Renal tubular acidosis." *Pediatr. Nephrol.* 4268–75.

McSherry, E. 1978. "Acidosis and growth in nonuremic renal disease." *Kidney Int.* 14349–54.

Vesicoureteral Reflux

Katherine Wesseling Perry

Vesicoureteral Reflux is a congenital condition of retrograde flow of urine from the bladder and ureters to the kidneys. Reflux is graded based on the following classification system:

- Grade 1: Reflux from the bladder into the distal ureters.
- Grade 2: Reflux to the level of the renal pelvis.
- Grade 3: Reflux into the renal pelvis with some dilation of the renal pelvis.
- Grade 4: Distortion of the renal pelvis and blunting of the calyces.
- Grade 5: Severe distortion of the renal pelvis and calyces with intra-renal reflux.

Etiology

Reflux occurs due to abnormal insertion of the ureters into the bladder or to ureteral obstruction. Renal scarring accompanies reflux and may be congenital or develop due to episodes of pyelonephritis.

Clinical Presentation and Prognosis

Demographics: Reflux is more common in boys than in girls. There is an increased incidence in other family members, particularly younger male siblings (reflux decreases with age, thus is more likely to be detected in younger children).

Presenting signs and symptoms: Reflux is the most common abnormality identified in pediatric patients with pyelonephritis/urinary tract infection. Renin-mediated hypertension may also be a presenting sign; this may develop years after the reflux has resolved and signal reflux that occurred earlier in life. Proteinuria and chronic kidney disease (CKD) may occur with severe kidney damage from reflux.

Clinical course: Reflux decreases with time, resolving by age 7 in the majority of cases. Renal scarring, whether congenital or due to pyelonephritis, does not resolve and may lead to hypertension or (if severe) renal insufficiency.

Prognosis: Prognosis depends on the severity of the reflux and the degree of renal failure at presentation. Patients with lower grades of reflux (1 and 2) tend to completely resolve with time; no surgical intervention is usually necessary in these patients. Higher grades (4 and 5) of reflux also improve with time; however, surgical intervention is often required in these patients to decrease the frequency of pyelonephritis and to preserve renal function. Patients with increased serum creatinine levels and proteinuria due to reflux nephropathy are at risk for progressing to end stage renal disease. Patients with hypertension due to renal scarring often need life-time anti-hypertensive therapy.

Diagnosis

A voiding cystourethrogram (VCUG) is needed to diagnose reflux. High grades of reflux may be seen in real time on renal ultrasound. However, ultrasound is not a sensitive test for reflux and is used primarily to evaluate structural abnormalities of the kidney.

Renal scarring can be identified on radionuclide scans, such as the technetium-99m-labeled dimercaptosuccinic acid (DMSA) scan. In older patients, the reflux itself may have resolved, yet scarring on the DMSA suggests a prior history of reflux and/or pyelonephritis.

Management

Medications: Antibiotic prophylaxis has been traditionally prescribed for patients with reflux in order to prevent future urinary tract infections and renal scarring. However, there is little evidence that this strategy is effective in preventing scars and current guidelines recommend prompt treatment of infections, rather than prophylactic antibiotics.

Angiotensin Converting Enzyme Inhibitor (ACEI) therapy controls hypertension, reduces proteinuria and protects kidney function. ACEI may prolong the time until dialysis in patients with chronic kidney disease and should be administered in anyone with proteinuria and/or hypertension.

Pearls and Precautions

Consultations: Patients with stages IV and V reflux should be referred to Urology for evaluation as ureteric reimplantation may be indicated.

Nephrology consultation should be obtained for patients with renal failure, hypertension, or proteinuria.

Monitoring: Blood pressure, serum creatinine, and urine protein excretion should be monitored at least yearly in all patients with a history of reflux nephropathy. Closer follow-up is warranted in patients with renal failure and those with severe hypertension.

References

Cendron, M. 2008b. "Antibiotic prophylaxis in the management of vesicoureteral reflux." *Adv. Urol.* 825475.
Cendron, M. 2008a. "Reflux nephropathy." *J. Pediatr. Urol.* 4414-21.
Estrada, C. R., Jr. 2008. "Prenatal hydronephrosis: early evaluation." *Curr. Opin. Urol.* 18401–3.

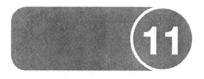

Neurological Disorders

Table of Contents

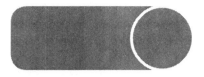

Epilepsy and Seizures

General Introduction to the Management of Seizure Disorders

Raman Sankar, Shaun Hussain, Christopher C. Giza

Seizures result from a state of hyperexcitability and hypersynchrony of the neuronal population. Such a state can result from intrinsic misfunction of neurons where no gross structural or biochemical problems exist—these were once called the "primary" or "idiopathic" epilepsies. Now we know that the basis for many of these can be mutations in ion channels that govern the excitability of neurons. Seizures can also result in response to discernible structural pathology or biochemical derangements—these are generally referred to varyingly as "secondary" or "symptomatic" epilepsies.

Both idiopathic and primary epilepsies can also be classified on the basis of whether there is a "focus" of neuronal dysfunction where the seizures begin and subsequently spread sometimes (localization-related epilepsies, formerly called partial epilepsies) versus the entire brain enters the seizure all at once (generalized epilepsies).

Depending on the semiology (manifestations) of the disease, its electroencephalographic markers, and other clinical aspects, many "epilepsy syndromes" have been defined, and this classification is particularly useful in estimating the prognosis of the condition and in counseling families. Some of the benign syndromes with a favorable prognosis include febrile seizures, childhood absence epilepsy, rolandic epilepsy, et cetera. On the other hand, infantile spasms, the Lennox-Gastaut syndrome, and the various progressive myoclonic epilepsies carry a poor prognosis for the child to return to a "normal" condition.

Diagnostic approach

EEG: The electroencephalogram (EEG) is an especially useful test in assisting the neurologist to classify the type of epilepsy. Arriving at a specific diagnosis typically requires correlating the EEG with other clinical information. Under certain circumstances, the brain may continue to experience seizures even though overt clinical manifestations are lacking. The EEG becomes a critical tool to understand such "subclinical" seizure activity. Conditions that increase the probability for such activity include inadequately treated status epilepticus, neonatal seizures, and sometimes, treating certain epilepsies with the wrong antiepileptic drug (AED).

Neuroimaging: An MRI is the standard in working up a child with suspected "symptomatic" seizures. However, your neurology consultant may choose not to proceed with imaging in cases where a syndromic diagnosis can be made based on the clinical circumstances and the EEG. Thus, a child with absence epilepsy or rolandic epilepsy may not be routinely imaged. Hence, it is reasonable to obtain an EEG before the decision to obtain an MRI in some special circumstances.

Even though biochemical derangements such as electrolyte abnormalities or hypoglycemia typically produce "acute" seizures, some children with chronic epilepsy may still be vulnerable to breakthrough seizures caused by such derangements, especially during a bout of acute infectious illness.

Extensive genetic and metabolic testing for the etiology of the seizure disorder and accompanying neurodevelopmental issues is not within the scope of this volume.

Therapeutic considerations

The choice of an AED for a particular child is influenced by many considerations, beginning with the precise understanding of the epilepsy syndrome. For instance, medications such as phenytoin, carbamazepine, and oxcarbazepine may exacerbate certain generalized epilepsies.

Understanding of age-specific and/or chronic toxicities associated with specific AEDs is also important. Thus, long-term use of phenytoin poses a much greater risk of gingival hyperplasia and coarsening of facial features in a pediatric patient. The hepatotoxic potential of valproic acid is greater in children under age two, especially when used in the context of polypharmacy. The potential for serious cutaneous reactions such as Stevens-Johnson syndrome associated with lamotrigine has been estimated to be greater in children, and is also exacerbated when used in combination with valproic acid.

Other factors that influence selection include effects on appetite and body weight. Valproic acid, pregabalin, gabapentin, and to a lesser extent carbamazepine, are known to contribute to weight gain and increased body mass index. With some AEDs, especially felbamate, topiramate, and zonisamide, decrease in appetite and/or nausea at higher doses can contribute to weight loss, creating a special problem for the child with chronic nutritional and thriving issues. The effect can be worse when such drugs are used in combination.

Some AEDs such as felbamate and lamotrigine when used in high doses or in combination may produce insomnia. Sleep deprivation can result in worsening of the seizure disorder as well as the behavioral comorbidities of epilepsy. While on this topic, it is important to stress asking the care provider about the patient's sleep characteristics. Sometimes, identification of obstructive sleep apnea and referring a loud snorer with frequent awakenings for surgical removal of tonsils and/or adenoids may lead to decreased AED burden from improved seizure control as well as improved behavior. On the other hand, use of sleep aids such as benzodiazepines may further contribute to obstructive apnea from laxity of pharyngeal muscles as well as poor clearance of secretions in neurologically impaired children.

Many children with chronic epilepsy also experience behavioral comorbidities that include effects on attention, learning, and behavior. Behavioral concerns can range from mood disorders to thought disorders and mental retardation. It is important to differentiate between depression as a comorbidity of epilepsy from depression resulting from barbiturate therapy. Some AEDs, such as lamotrigine, carbamazepine, and valproic acid may have some beneficial effects on mood. Thus, it should be recognized that barbiturates and benzodiazepines may contribute to attention and learning problems. Highly specific problems with word fluency and frontal lobe executive functioning have been associated with topiramate. On the other hand, some AEDs, especially topiramate and valproate, are effective in the prophylactic treatment of migraine, another comorbidity of epilepsy—especially some childhood epilepsies.

In some adolescent girls, puberty may bring on fluctuating control of seizures with their hormonal cycles. Seizure threshold is elevated by progesterone and lowered by estrogen. Thus, some patients do poorly during midcycle when estrogen peaks, while others respond adversely to the sharp decline in progesterone levels in the beginning of menses. The clearance of some medications (e.g., lamotrigine) can be affected by hormonal fluctuations as well. Thus, we often consider progestational therapy (Depo-Provera) for some patients as an adjunct to seizure management. This could also protect from undesirable pregnancy in a mentally retarded adolescent with seizures.

Some children with medically refractory epilepsy may be candidates for therapeutic or palliative surgical procedures. Other children may benefit from non-pharmacologic approaches such as vagus nerve stimulation, which requires the implantation of a pacemaker-like device that delivers programmable regular afferent input to the brain to increase the seizure threshold. There is also an "on demand" feature for rescue therapy, and some beneficial effects on mood and attention have been noted. The vagus nerve stimulation approach is adjunctive to the use of AEDs.

The ketogenic diet is now a well-established and efficacious approach to the treatment of epilepsies in children. Variations such as the modified Atkins diet and the low glycemic index dietary therapy are expanding the scope of patients who may benefit from these approaches. In the majority of patients, the diet is employed adjunctively with medications, but a good response in many patients leads to decreased medication burden.

Thus, optimum therapy of seizure disorders requires balancing the antiseizure effect of AEDs with other effects that may benefit or detract from the overall physical and mental health of the patient—indeed, the quality of life. Table 11.1 is a compilation of AED therapies.

References

Sankar R. Initial treatment of epilepsy with antiepileptic drugs: pediatric issues. *Neurology* 2004;63(10 Suppl 4):S30–9.

Alexopoulos AV, Kotagal P, Loddenkemper T, Hammel J, Bingaman WE. Long-term results with vagus nerve stimulation in children with pharmacoresistant epilepsy. *Seizure* 2006;15(7):491–503.

T Neal EG, Chaffe H, Schwartz RH, Lawson MS, Edwards N, Fitzsimmons G, Whitney A, Cross JH. The ketogenic diet for the treatment of childhood epilepsy: a randomised controlled trial. *Lancet Neurol* 2008;7(6):500–6.

Table 11.1: Treatment and Dosages for Seizure Disorders

Drug	Forms	Starting Dose	Maintenance Dose	Pharmacology	Notable Side Effects
ACTH Acthar®	gel 80 IU/mL, 5 mL vial	150 IU/m2/day IM ÷ QD/ BID x 14 days; taper over 14 days	n/a	t½ 15 min	Immunosuppression, irritability, increased appetite, hypertension, hyperglycemia, hypokalemia
Carbamazepine Tegretol® Tegretol XR® Carbatrol® Equitro® (XR)	tab 100, 200, 400 chew 100 elixir 100/5 mL XR 100, 200, 300 Carbatrol 100, 200, 300	5–10 mg/kg/day; titrate 5–10 mg/kg/day, ~q7d.	10–30 mg/kg/day ÷TID Adult: 600–2400 mg/day	t½ 20–60 h 4–12 μg/mL H (3A4), Inducer (3A4, 1A2, 2C9) 70% protein bound	Rash, SJS (assoc w/ HLA B1502) sedation, pancreatitis, hepatitis, GI upset, leukopenia, aplastic anemia, hyponatremia, diplopia, ataxia, impaired cardiac conduction
Clobazam Frisium®	tab 10	0.25 mg/kg/day; titrate weekly	0.5–1.25 mg/kg/day ÷BID Adult 30–60 mg/day	t½ 20 h H (3A4, 2C19)	Sedation, GI upset
Clonazepam Klonopin®	tab 0.5, 1, 2 wafer 0.125, 0.25, 0.5, 1, 2	<30 kg: 0.01–0.03 mg/kg/ day ÷ BID/TID >30 kg: 0.5 mg TID, titrate ~q3 days	0.1–0.3 mg/kg/day; Adult: 1.5–20 mg/day	t½ 30 h H (3A4)	Sedation, hyperactivity, increased secretions, GI upset
Clorazepate Tranxene®	tab 3.75, 7.5, 15	0.3 mg/kg/day ÷ BID-QID	0.3–1.0 mg/kg/day ÷BID-QID Adult: 21.5–90 mg/day	t½ 40 h H (unknown CYP)	Sedation, rash, ataxia, dizziness, head- ache, hyperkinesia, rhinitis, asthma
Diazepam Diastat®	Supp 2.5,5, 10, 15, 20 tab 2, 5, 10 sol 5/1, 5/5 mL IM, IV	<6y: 0.5 mg/kg PR x1 6-12y: 0.3 mg/kg >12y: 0.2 mg/kg IV: 0.1–0.3 mg/kg x1 (max 5–10 mg/dose)	n/a ESES: 1 mg/kg PO qhs x1, then 0.5/kg PO qhs, then taper over several weeks.	t½ 20–100 h H (3A4, 2C19)	Sedation, hypotension, hypoventila- tion
Ethosuximide Zarontin®	cap 250 syrup 250/5 mL	<6y: 10 mg/kg/day >6y: 250 mg/day, titrate q4–7 days	12–40 mg/kg/day ÷TID (usually 15–20 mg/kg/ day) Adult: 1000–2000 mg/day	t½ 60 h 40–100 μg/mL H (3A4) 5% protein bound	Rash, leucopenia, pancytopenia, lupus-like reaction, sedation
Felbamate Felbatol®	tab 400, 600 susp 600/5 mL	15 mg/kg/day; titrate in 10 mg/kg incre- ments (blood tests q2wks)	40–100 mg/kg/day ÷TID Adult: 1200–4800 mg/day	t½ 20 h H (2E1>3A4) Induces (3A4) Inhibits (2C19) 30% protein bound	Aplastic anemia, hepatotoxicity, GI upset, ataxia, anorexia, insomnia

Drug	Formulations				Side effects
Gabapentin Neurontin®	cap 100, 300, 400, 600, 800 susp 250/5 mL	10 mg/kg/day; titrate ~q3-7d, ~5 mg/kg increments	30–60 mg/kg/day ÷ TID Adult 900–4800 mg/day	t½ 6 h U (unchanged) 0% protein bound	Rash, behavioral changes, sedation, dizziness, ataxia, constipation, pruritis, hostility, hyperkinesia, dry mouth
Lacosamide Vimpat®	tab 50, 100, 150, 200 IV	Adult: start 50 bid, titrate weekly by 50 bid	Adult: 200–400 mg/day ÷ BID	t½ 13 h H (2C19) but minimal 15% protein bound	Headache, fatigue, nystagmus, diplopia, GI upset, apoptosis in rat pups
Lamotrigine Lamictal® Lamictal XR®	tab 25, 100, 150, 200 chew 5, 25 XR 25, 50, 100, 200	Mono: 0.5–0.8 mg/kg/day +inducer: 1–1.5 mg/kg/day +VPA: 0.15 mg/kg/day incr q1–2wks!	10 mg/kg/day ÷ BID + VPA: 5 mg/kg/day + inducer: 15 mg/kg/day Adult: 200–700 mg/day	t½ 25 h 3–15 µg/mL H (unknown CYP) 60% protein bound	Rash (esp. with VPA), SJS, hepatotoxicity, diplopia, tremor, flu-like sx, sedation, headache, GI upset, irritability
Levetiracetam Keppra® Keppra XR®	tab 250, 500, 750, 1000 susp 100/1 mL XR 500, 750 IV	10–20 mg/kg/day ÷ BID; titrate q3–7d by 10 mg/kg	20–60 mg/kg/day ÷ BID Adult 1000–4000 mg/day	t½ 7 h U (unchanged) 5% protein bound	Somnolence, ataxia, behavioral changes, hyperactivity, abnormal gait
Lorazepam Ativan®	tab 0.5, 1, 2 sol 2/1 mL IV, IM	Status: 0.1 mg/kg/dose (≤2 mg/dose)	n/a	t½ 14 h hepatic	Sedation, hypotension, hypoventilation
Oxcarbazepine Trileptal®	tab 150, 300, 600 susp 300/5 mL	10–20 mg/kg/day	50 mg/kg/day ÷ BID Adult: 1200–1400 mg/day	t½ 2 h H Induces (3A4, 3A5) Inhibits (2C19) 40% protein bound	Hyponatremia, sedation, vision disturbance, rash, headache; (no hepatic/bone marrow toxicity c/w CBZ)
Phenobarbital	elixir 20/5 mL tab 15, 30, 60, 100	Status: 20 mg/kg x1	<1y: 5–8 mg/kg/day ÷BID >1y: 3–5 mg/kg/day Adult: 2–3 mg/kg/day	t½ ~100 h 15–40 µg/mL H (2C9>2C19, 2E1) 50% protein bound	Rash, lethargy, hyperactivity, behavioral changes, irritability, lethargy
Phenytoin Dilantin® Phenytek®	chew 50 (infatab) ER 30, 100, 200, 300 susp 125/5 mL IV	Status: Fosphenytoin 20 mg/ kg x1	5–10 mg/kg/day ÷ BID Adult: 200–600 mg/day	t½ 20 h 10–20 µg/mL H (2C9>2C19) Induces (2C9,2C19,3A4) 90% protein bound	Rash, hepatitis/transaminitis, ataxia, aplastic anemia, lethargy, coarse facies, gingival hyperplasia, serum sickness, lupus-like syndrome, neuropathy, arrhythmia

Table 11.1 (Continued)

Table 11.1: Treatment and Dosages for Seizure Disorders

Drug	Forms	Starting Dose	Maintenance Dose	Pharmacology	Notable Side Effects
Pregabalin Lyrica®	tab 25, 50, 75, 100, 150, 200, 225, 300	Adult: start 75 bid, titrate over several weeks	Adult: 150–600 mg/day ÷BID	t½ 6 h U (unchanged)	Rash, behavioral changes, sedation, dizziness, ataxia, constipation, pruritis, hostility, hyperkinesia, dry mouth
Primidone Mysoline®	susp 250/5 tab 50, 250	2–5 mg/kg/day	12–25 mg/kg/day ÷TID Adult: 750–2000 mg/day	t½ 10 h 5–12 µg/mL (+PHB) H (3A4 inducer) 20% protein bound	Rash, hyperactivity, behavioral changes, irritability, lethargy
Rufinamide Banzel®	tab 200, 400	10 mg/kg/day, increase weekly by 10/kg	40 mg/kg/day ÷ BID Adult 3200 mg/day	t½ 8 h H (hydrolysis) Weak inducer (3A4) Weak inhibitor (2E1) 30% protein bound	Leukopenia, QT shortening, SJS
Tiagabine Gabitril®	tab 4, 12, 16	0.1 mg/kg/dy; incr q wk 0.1 mg/kg	0.5–1.0 mg/kg/day ÷BID + inducer: 0.7–1.5 mg/kg/day Adult: 32–56 mg/day	t½ 8 h H (3A4) 95% protein bound	Lethargy, confusion, cognitive problems, NCSE, GI upset, rash, asthenia, dizziness
Topiramate Topamax®	sprinkle 15, 25 tab 25, 100, 200	1–2 mg/kg/day; incr q3-5d by 1 mg/kg/dy	5–10 mg/kg/day ÷BID Spasms: 15–25 mg/kg/day Adult: 200–800 mg/day	t½ 20 h 5–20 µg/mL U (H minimal) 15% protein bound	Weight loss, hyperactivity mental dullness, irritable, anhydrosis/ hyperthermia, sedation, renal stones, diplopia, parasthesias
Valproic Acid Depakote® Depakene® (syrup) Depacon® (IV)	syrup 250/5 mL sprinkle 125 mg cap 125, 250, 500 ER 250, 500 IV	15 mg/kg/day; increase by 10–15 mg/kg q 3–5 days	30–80 mg/kg/day ÷TID (÷ BID if ER) Adult: 1000–4000 mg/day	t½ 15 h 50–150 µg/mL H (inhibits 2C9) 20% protein bound	Rash, SJS, hepatotoxicity, anemia, thrombocytopenia, weight gain, tremor, pancreatitis, abdominal pain, GI upset, sedation, osteopenia, PCO, alopecia, hyperammonemia, Fanconi syn
Vigabatrin Sabril®	tab 500 sachet 500	25–50 mg/kg/day ÷BID titrate ~q2 days, to 100 mg/kg/day	Max 200 mg/kg/day ÷BID Adult: 3 g/day	t½ 5 h U 0% protein bound	Retinotoxicity (peripheral visual field loss), mood changes, sedation
Zonisamide Zonegran®	caps 25, 50, 100	2–4 mg/kg/dy titrate ~q7d by 1/kg Spasms: may start at 5–10 mg/kg/day	8–12 mg/kg/day ÷BID Spams: 15–25 mg/kg/day Adult: 100–600 mg/day	t½ 60 h 10–40 µg/mL H (3A4) 55% protein bound	Somnolence, ataxia, behavioral changes, nephrolithiasis, rash, GI upset, diarrhea, hypohydrosis/hyper-thermia, insomnia, depression

Compiled by Shaun Hussain, M.D.

Common Pediatric Epilepsy Syndromes

Raman Sankar, Christopher C. Giza

This chapter will describe a number of well-defined syndromes that can be recognized by the clinical presentation, confirmed with appropriately selected diagnostic tests, and treated effectively with anticonvulsant medications. Familiarity with these syndromes improves the confidence of the pediatrician in managing these seizure disorders, especially in terms of counseling the family regarding prognosis and the need for dealing with the comorbidities.

Etiology

The syndromes described under this heading generally fit the classification criteria for idiopathic epilepsies. The basis for these syndromes is not due to congenital malformations of the brain or insults to the brain. They are considered inheritable types of epilepsy, often with a dominant-like picture, but with incomplete penetrance. Modern studies are revealing a number of mutations in genes coding for ion-channel proteins associated with these epilepsies. It should be appreciated that these disorders display considerable genetic heterogeneity and are not monogenic disorders with a truly Mendelian inheritance.

A. Childhood Absence Epilepsy (CAE) and Juvenile Absence Epilepsy (JAE)

Clinical presentation and prognosis: The classic presentation of these syndromes involves staring spells, often fleeting, that end abruptly without postictal phenomena. The spells are often only a few seconds in duration, and are significantly briefer than those associated with complex partial seizures. Frequent absence spells may first be reported by a teacher before the parents in some circumstances, and may be inadvertently described as a lack of attention in class. Absence spells are sometimes accompanied by minor automatisms like eye lid myoclonia (a frequent and rhythmical blinking or fluttering of the eyelids), but are never as complex as in complex partial seizures; the latter typically end gradually and the patient displays postictal confusion and/or lethargy. There is no loss of postural reflexes or sphincter control. The typical age of presentation of CAE is between 5 and 9 years while JAE is considered to start beyond the age of 9 years. Patients with JAE may develop other seizure types such as generalized tonic-clonic seizures, and are best treated with broad spectrum AEDs.

The prognosis for remission is very good in CAE, but less so in JAE. Some patients with JAE may evolve into juvenile myoclonic epilepsy, discussed further downstream in this chapter. Recent studies have identified increased incidence of neurocognitive and behavioral abnormalities in CAE.

Diagnosis

In the clinic, an absence paroxysm can be readily elicited by having the child hyperventilate for up to 3 minutes. Indeed, hyperventilation is routinely undertaken during an electroencephalogram (EEG) recording and results in a 3–4 Hz generalized spike-wave discharge. Unless there are other neurological findings in the history or examination, we do not routinely undertake neuroimaging in these patients.

The staring spells associated with CAE are easily differentiated from those seen in patients with complex partial seizures by the fact that absence spells occur daily and at numerous times, which is very uncommon in the latter. The staring spells in CAE do not evolve into other focal seizure manifestations.

Management

Children with CAE have been traditionally treated with ethosuximide, an AED that is quite specific for absence paroxysms. Subsequently, valproic acid became a popular choice. Among the new generation AEDs, lamotrigine has documented efficacy for this seizure type. Preliminary results from a recent NIH-sponsored study suggest that ethosuximide and valproic acid were more effective in a larger fraction of patients than lamotrigine. However, lamotrigine appeared to be the best tolerated. The major adverse effects with ethosuximide involved gastrointestinal complaints, while valproic acid had a negative effect on attention and behavior in some children. While no rigorous studies have been undertaken with levetiracetam, experience suggests that it could be an option for some children.

Several AEDs can exacerbate the spells associated with CAE. These include medications like phenytoin, carbamazepine, oxcarbazepine, gabapentin, pregabalin, and vigabatrin.

If a child is seizure free for two years and the EEG is normal (no spike-wave paroxysms during hyperventilation), an attempt can be made to taper and discontinue medication. Appropriate referrals for neurocognitive and behavioral concerns should be made.

B. Benign Epilepsy of Childhood with Central-Temporal Spikes (BECTS, Rolandic Epilepsy)

Clinical presentation: Most cases have their inception between 7 and 10 years. These seizures typically occur shortly after the youngster has fallen asleep or before wakening (during non-REM sleep). The most obvious manifestations involve oropharyngeal and sensory and motor symptoms and hemifacial twitching which may spread to arms. The youngster may describe tingling or numbness accompanied by speech arrest in the early phase of the seizures. Grunting and gurgling noises as well as hypersalivation may be witnessed. The youngsters recall the events and can generally describe them well to the physician. The physical examination is normal, as a rule. There is a significant association between rolandic epilepsy and migraines.

Most children experience only a few seizures and enjoy remission by pubertal years. Many may not require ongoing AED prophylaxis. But a few will have frequent seizures, and may benefit from AED therapy for a couple of years. Rare, and atypical evolution of rolandic epilepsy into the Landau-Kleffner syndrome has been described.

Diagnosis

EEG is the most valuable diagnostic tool for this syndrome. The background is typically normal. Characteristic centro-temporal spikes appear in trains during drowsiness. Thus, it is important to ensure that the recording includes drowsiness and sleep. Experienced encephalographers discern an electrical anomaly that may be reported as a surface (tangential) dipole.

Management

Among AEDs available in the U.S., gabapentin has been demonstrated to be effective in a randomized, double blind, placebo-controlled study. Because of the potential for irritability, it is not commonly used. It is more common to see carbamazepine, oxcarbazepine, or levetiracetam used to treat this syndrome. Levetiracetam is unlikely to produce organ toxicity, but some children may experience irritability and mood problems.

C. Other Benign Localization-Related Epilepsies of Childhood

Syndromes that are somewhat related to rolandic epilepsy include the occipital epilepsies. The variant known as Panayiotopoulos syndrome typically has its inception between 3 and 6 years of age. Distinctive features include an association with sleep, autonomic symptoms, and the ictus begins with emetic symptoms such as nausea, retching, and vomiting. Pallor (most common) or cyanosis and flushing (less common) may be seen. Ictal deviation of the eyes and head are also common. Interictal EEG shows a normal background, but variously located spike foci, becoming more abundant in sleep, may be seen. Occipital spike-waves are commonly seen. Despite a high incidence of status epilepticus, the long-term prognosis is highly favorable. Treatment is similar to that in rolandic epilepsy.

A later onset (peak age of onset: 8 years) variant, sometimes referred to as the Gastaut type, shows a more consistent pattern of occipital spike-waves, and photosensitivity. The EEG paroxysms are abolished by fixation and central vision, clinically produced by asking the child to open his/her eyes. The semiology of the seizures includes visual hallucinations, and the seizures often end with a migraine. Sometimes this epilepsy is confused with migraine, although experts distinguish these two conditions by their forms of visual phenomena. In true migraine, they are black and white and have sharp, jagged contours. In Gastaut type occipital epilepsy, these forms can be colored and rounded. Occasionally, there could be an evolution to a generalized tonic-clonic seizure (GTC). Because of this possibility, and the photoparoxysmal features in the EEG, valproic acid or levetiracetam probably represent the best choices. The majority of patients enjoy a remission after 2–3 years, although seizures may continue in a significant minority.

D. Juvenile Myoclonic Epilepsy (JME)

Clinical presentation: Juvenile myoclonic epilepsy is one of the most common forms of epilepsy seen in the adolescent population. In early stages of the appearance of this syndrome, brief bursts of myoclonus appear. Often, these are not recognized as seizures by the patient or the family, although queries will confirm "clumsiness" and a tendency to drop objects and/or fall down, especially upon wakening. Evolution to a GTC is typically what prompts the patient and the family to seek medical attention. Seizures are sensitive to sleep deprivation, stress, fatigue or alcohol consumption. Some of the patients experience absences as well.

Common teaching is that JME does not remit and is a life-long disorder. Nevertheless, many patients seem to enjoy substantial improvement over the years, and discontinue taking medications.

Diagnosis

Obtaining a good history is the most important aspect of the diagnosis. EEG background is typically normal, but high amplitude, 4–6 Hz, generalized polyspike-wave complexes may be elicited by photic stimulation.

Management

The classic or legacy therapy for JME has involved valproic acid. However, valproic acid can produce weight gain and associated endocrine abnormalities. It is also associated with rare instances of pancreatitis, hepatic failure, thrombocytopenia, and sometimes a bleeding diathesis without thrombocytopenia. Hence, many new AEDs have been tried. The GTCs can be effectively controlled with lamotrigine or topiramate, but neither of them control the morning myoclonia well. In a few patients, lamotrigine may exacerbate the myoclonus, although it is highly effective against absences. Levetiracetam has gained FDA approval for its use for controlling both myoclonic seizures and GTCs associated with JME—the language of the regulatory approval suggests adjunctive use, even though no AED has been specifically approved as initial therapy of JME.

Several AEDs can exacerbate the myoclonus and absences associated with JME. These include medications like phenytoin, carbamazepine, oxcarbazepine, gabapentin, pregabalin, and vigabatrin.

Especially as this syndrome affects adolescents, management of JME requires considerable effort at stressing compliance and counseling regarding the impact of lack of sleep, alcohol use, and stress on seizures— and hence on the patient's future ability to obtain and keep a driver's license. Female patients will also require counseling regarding birth control because of the potential for AEDs to produce birth defects. We place all female JME patients on a folic acid supplement regimen.

References

Sankar R. Initial treatment of epilepsy with antiepileptic drugs: pediatric issues. Neurology 2004;63(10 Supp; 4):S30–39.

Panayiotopoulos CP. A Clinical Guide to Epileptic Syndromes and their Treatment. Bladon Medical Publishing, Oxford, UK, 2002 (various chapters).

Pellock JM, Bourgeois BFD, Dodson WE, Nordli DRJr, Sankar R (Eds). Pediatric Epilepsy: Diagnosis and Therapy, Third Edition, Demos Publishing, New York, NY, 2008 (various chapters).

Infantile Spasms (West Syndrome)

Christopher C. Giza, Raman Sankar

Infantile spasms is a development-specific catastrophic epilepsy syndrome of infancy associated with clusters of sudden extensor or flexor muscular contractions. It may have multiple etiologies.

Etiology

Understanding the etiology of infantile spasms is important to determine optimal treatment approach and prognosis. Focal cerebral etiologies may be amenable to surgical treatment as well as medical treatment. Metabolic disorders may also have disease-specific treatment interventions.

Focal etiologies include

- **Cortical dysplasia/cerebral dysgenesis** [overall 30%+] including focal cortical dysplasia, hemimegalencephaly, lissencephaly, schizencephaly, polymicrogyria, brain tumor, arteriovenous malformation, distant cerebral infarction.

Diffuse or multifocal etiologies include

- **Pre- or Perinatal insults** [up to 25%] including chorioamonitis, intraventricular/periventricular hemorrhage, hypoxic ischemic encephalopathy, perinatal hypoglycemia, prematurity;
- **Neurocutaneous syndromes** including tuberous sclerosis [up to 20%], neurofibromatosis, Sturge-Weber syndrome [often lateralized and thus amenable to surgical therapy], incontinentia pigmenti;
- **pyridoxine deficiency/dependency,** Metabolic disorders including PKU, MSUD, mitochondrial encephalomyopathy, hyperammonemia, traumatic brain injury / nonaccidental trauma / birth trauma, congenital infection (CMV, toxoplasmosis, rubella, syphilis); and
- **chromosomal disorders** (Trisomy 21, Duplication of 15q).

Clinical Presentation and Prognosis

Demographics: Age of onset is typically between 3–8 months. Eighty-five percent of cases present under 1 year of age; 93% present at <2 years. Incidence has been estimated at 20–25/100,000.

Presenting signs and symptoms: The most important step in the diagnosis of infantile spasms is to recognize the clinical history and appearance of seizures. When infantile spasms are suspected, then initiate diagnostic workup and referral to a specialist.

- Sudden muscular contractions, flexor or extensor, head/neck may flex, legs may be drawn up.

- Occur in clusters, usually upon awakening.
- Classified as either:
  CRYPTOGENIC—occurring in previously normal infant, in whom no obvious cause can be elicited; or
  SYMPTOMATIC—associated with known etiology and often with developmental delay/regression.
- *West syndrome:* (1) Infantile spasms; (2) hypsarrhythmia; and (3) developmental delay/regression.
- *Aicardi syndrome:* (1) Infantile spasms; (2) agenesis of the corpus callosum; and (3) optic atrophy.

Differential diagnosis includes benign myoclonus of infancy (normal EEG), severe myoclonic epilepsy of infancy, Sandifer syndrome—gastroesophageal reflux, hyperactive Moro response (normally gone by 5 months), and colic.

Clinical course: Spasms may occur multiple times per day. Developmental progress generally slows or even regresses; many symptomatic patients have pre-existing developmental delay. Clinical course is influenced by the underlying etiological diagnosis. However, the clinical spasms may persist, spontaneously remit and/or evolve into other seizure types. A proportion of patients with infantile spasms will either recur or transform into Lennox-Gastaut syndrome.

Prognosis: These patients have variable prognosis, but the symptomatic group does poorly—only 5% are normal or with mild delay. Cryptogenic/idiopathic group does better—up to 30–40% are normal or with mild delay only.

Poor prognostic factors include: Symptomatic etiology with pre-spasms developmental or neurological abnormality; onset <5 months of age; post-spasms regression; poor response to medications; and, recurrence after initial medical response.

Good prognostic factors include: Cryptogenic with normal pre-spasms development; focal abnormality with early surgical intervention; and, good response to initial medical (or surgical, when appropriate) treatment.

Diagnosis

The single most important diagnostic test to evaluate a clinical suspicion of infantile spasms is the EEG. The diagnostic EEG pattern is termed *hypsarrhythmia* with a chaotic, high-voltage multifocal spikes, polyspikes, and slow-wave pattern. This EEG pattern changes over time and may include periods of suppression, pseudo-normalization or paroxysmal fast activity (PFA) and may evolve into multifocal independent spike discharges (MISD) or slow spike and wave (indicating a transition to the Lennox-Gastaut syndrome). MRI is always indicated to determine whether there is an underlying structural abnormality such as cortical dysplasia, tuberous sclerosis, infarction, etc. In the absence of a structural etiology, laboratory studies should be sent for serum amino acids, urine organic acids, ammonia, lactate, pyruvate, and CO_2. Cerebrospinal fluid studies may be helpful in intractable cases without etiological diagnosis. This includes low CSF glucose (GLUT1 glucose transporter deficiency) and elevated CSF Glycine (hyperglycinemia), to give a couple of examples.

Management

Medications: The following medications are typically administered by a pediatric neurologist in an attempt to control infantile spasms.

1. *Prednisolone* 2–4 mg/kg/day for 2 weeks, then taper; perhaps less effective than ACTH.
2. *ACTH:* (150 U/m²/day) intramuscularly (IM) or 40–120 Units IM daily or divided twice a day for 2 weeks, then taper. ACTH is the traditional drug of choice, although extreme cost and relative difficulty in obtaining it may make a trial of prednisolone more readily available.

Side effects of hormonal therapy include hyperglycemia, hypertension, hypokalemia, behavior change/ irritability, weight gain, and insomnia. It is generally recommended that infants receiving these therapies be seen once or twice weekly by their pediatricians to monitor for developing hypertension and/or hyperglycemia.

1. *Vitamin B6 (pyridoxine):* It is always worth a trial of 100 mg IV while on EEG if etiology is not apparent. An alternative means of administration is to give up to 15–30 mg/kg/day orally for 5 days as a trial.
2. *Vigabatrin:* 50–200 mg/kg/day twice daily. This is a drug of choice for patients with tuberous sclerosis, having a 70–90% response rate. Prolonged use may be associated with irreversible constriction of visual fields. Transient white matter signal changes have been noted on the MRI, and treatment with vigabatrin is not recommended for a prolonged period.
3. *Zonisamide:* Up to 10–25 mg/kg/day divided twice daily, with 26–40% response rate. Side effects include rare renal stones, diminished sweating/heat intolerance, weight loss and metabolic acidosis.
4. *Topiramate:* 1–10 mg/kg/day divided twice daily; up to 25 mg/kg/day has been used. Patients have a 17–21% response; up to 50% improved. Side effects are similar to zonisamide.
5. *Valproic acid:* Previously used more widely for this diagnosis. However, fatal hepatotoxicity in this age group approaches 1 in 700, reducing enthusiasm for its use as a first-line agent. Clonazepam was also more popular in years past.

Surgery: In patients with well-defined focal structural cerebral lesions, epilepsy surgery may be a treatment option. Those with single lesions limited to one hemisphere, with a normal or nearly normal contralateral hemisphere are the best candidates. Patients with multifocal disease are unlikely to be surgical candidates. Evaluation for surgery includes video/EEG monitoring to capture seizure/spasm events. High resolution structural MRI is also essential. Positron emission tomography (PET) may show focal hypometabolism in the region of cortical dysplasia. In surgical candidates, resection may range from a focal lobar to multilobar resection to hemispherectomy.

Diet: In intractable patients, the use of a ketogenic diet has been reported to improve seizure/spasm control by some centers.

Therapy: All patients with infantile spasms should be carefully evaluated for developmental delay. Physical therapy, occupational therapy and/or infant stimulation programs should be initiated as early as possible.

Social: Families undergoing evaluation for epilepsy surgery often benefit from meeting/contacting other families who have gone through the experience.

Pearls and Precautions

Phenobarbital is not an effective treatment for this diagnosis.

References

Korinthenberg R, Schreiner A. Topiramate in children with west syndrome: a retrospective multicenter evaluation of 100 patients. J Child Neurol. 2007, Mar;22(3):302-6.

Riikonen R. The latest on infantile spasms. Curr Opin Neurol. 2005, Apr;18(2):91-5.

Yanagaki S, Oguni H, Yoshii K, Hayashi K, Imai K, Funatsuka M, Osawa M. Zonisamide for West syndrome: a comparison of clinical responses among different titration rate. Brain Dev. 2005 Jun;27(4):286-90.

The Lennox-Gastaut Syndrome (LGS)

Raman Sankar, Christopher C. Giza

Lennox-Gastaut syndrome (LGS) represents a severe, development-specific epileptic encephalopathy characterized by multiple seizure types that are refractory to treatment, and associated mental decline. LGS is generally symptomatic of diffuse or multifocal brain dysfunction and presents as a generalized epilepsy syndrome. A fraction of the cases are considered cryptogenic.

It is also considered an "epileptic encephalopathy of childhood" along with the Landau-Kleffner syndrome and epilepsy with continuous spike and waves during slow wave sleep (CSWS). It is readily differentiated from myoclonic-astatic epilepsy, also known as Doose syndrome (see below under differential diagnosis).

The classic triad of LGS include multiple seizure types (prominently tonic, atonic, myoclonic, and atypical absences), mental compromise, and a classic electroencephalogram (EEG) pattern referred to as "diffuse slow spike and waves."

Etiology

The etiology of LGS can be varied. Approximately a third of these patients are considered cryptogenic, while in the remaining patients LGS may be a reflection of a genetic disorder (many associated with cerebral maldevelopment) or a remote brain injury, such as perinatal asphyxia. Interestingly, many children who initially present with infantile spasms (West syndrome) may go on to develop LGS at a later time. Up to 30% of the patients with LGS may evolve from West syndrome.

Clinical Presentation and Prognosis

Demographics: This syndrome has a low overall incidence of approximately 3 per 10,000. It can start anywhere between one and 7 years of age, with a peak between 3–5 years. A slight preponderance (60%) of boys are affected. However, because of its highly refractory nature, its prevalence may be as high as between 5 and 10% of children with epilepsy.

Presenting signs and symptoms: There is no single classic presentation, although a generalized tonic clonic seizure (GTC) may bring the patient in. As the syndrome evolves, the most disabling seizures are the tonic or atonic seizures that are collectively called "drop" attacks. Frequent spells of atypical absences differ from classic absences in lacking a crisply identifiable onset or termination, and in occurring in the setting of mental subnormality. The evolution from West syndrome can be gradual or after a period of no seizures.

Clinical course and prognosis: The very definition of this syndrome incorporates medical refractoriness. Available treatments rarely lead to complete seizure cessation. Episodes of both non-convulsive and convulsive status epilepticus are not uncommon. Some patients who have had a history of infantile spasms may go through a phase of "juvenile spasms" with a transitional EEG before evolving into LGS. Remission is not expected, and as the child grows, worsening cognitive, behavioral and educational problems are not uncommon.

Differential diagnosis: Due to multiple seizure types and age of onset, LGS may be confused with Doose syndrome, but is distinguishable on clinical grounds and there are distinctive characteristics separating one from the other. In Doose, there is normal development at seizure onset and tonic seizures are atypical. The EEG pattern shows generalized polyspikes and there is a better prognosis in Doose syndrome. In LGS, the patient is already developmentally delayed. The EEG pattern shows a slow spike wave and there is an earlier onset of severe myoclonic epilepsy. Landau-Kleffner Syndrome is primarily associated with language delay/regression, a mild seizure disorder (or no seizures) and a different EEG pattern (electrical status epilepticus during sleep). CSWS shows a similar seizure and EEG pattern to LKS, but in a setting of more global developmental impairment.

Diagnosis

The most important components of the diagnostic work-up are integration of the clinical history and evaluation of the *EEG*. An *overnight video-EEG study* may be especially useful in documenting different seizure types and in the assessment of different EEG features. Background slowing is typical. The generalized slow spike-wave complexes (1.5–2.5 Hz) are pathognomonic and may accompany atypical absences. Paroxysms of fast activity may accompany tonic spells. During sleep, EEG discharges tend to increase. Evolution to multifocal spike discharges is common.

In most symptomatic cases, the etiology is already obvious (HIE, neonatal stroke, cerebral malformations, etc.). Those with a cryptogenic presentation will undergo a diagnostic work-up that will include neuroimaging with *MRI*, and other tests as indicated by the specific constellation of findings.

Management

Successful therapy often requires multimodal treatment approaches which may evolve and change over time. The overall goal should be optimum seizure control keeping in mind the overall quality of life for the patient as well as the family. Complete seizure control may not be possible for all LGS patients.

Medications: The pharmacological options for the treatment of LGS have expanded considerably in recent times. Although there has been no randomized controlled trial (RCT) demonstrating efficacy, the classic broad spectrum AED, which is still an important medication for this syndrome, was valproic acid. The first AED to be subjected to an RCT for LGS was felbamate (as adjunctive therapy), which is highly effective against drop seizures, myoclonic seizures, partial seizures, and to a reasonable degree, atypical absences. Interestingly, no medication has achieved regulatory sanction as initial or monotherapy. Since regulatory acceptance requires placebo-controlled trials, LGS does not lend itself to such trials due to seizure severity. Felbamate is not used as an early choice due to concerns about serious idiosyncratic reactions that include aplastic anemia and liver failure. In some patients, the anorexia produced by felbamate may complicate nutritional issues. Others may be sensitive to its potential to cause insomnia, which in turn can exacerbate seizures as well as behavior. Other medications with an indication for LGS based on RCTs include topiramate and lamotrigine. As a general rule, topiramate is best used in the lower dose range (up to 5 mg/kg/d), as higher doses may not bring about additional seizure control without producing anorexia, weight loss, and in some cases, acidosis. Lamotrigine has to be titrated very carefully to minimize the possibility of Stevens-Johnson syndrome. Rufinamide is the most recently approved AED with a specific indication for seizures associated with the LGS. Another AED that will likely be approved for use in LGS is clobazam. The clinical trials have been concluded, but many families already obtain it from other countries and the pediatrician may very well encounter patients already on it. Clobazam belongs to the benzodiazepine class of AEDs, but its modified structure seems to render it less sedating and patients are less likely to become refractory to it compared to AEDs like clonazepam. Limited experience suggests modest efficacy with levetiracetam in some patients. Please consult the attached tables for typical dosing regimens and available dosage forms.

Drop attacks (tonic-atonic seizures), atypical absences, and myoclonic seizures can be exacerbated by phenytoin, carbamazepine, oxcarbazepine, gabapentin and pregabalin.

Because of the tenuous nature of seizure control in many patients with LGS, and the expected exacerbation with common illnesses, the availability of rescue medications can minimize the cost of visits to the emergency department while also avoiding disruptions to family life and work. Commonly used approaches include oral benzodiazepines such as lorazepam or clonazepam, as well as rectal diazepam gel when the patient's condition is more severe.

Many children and adults with LGS have significant behavioral problems, and are sometimes treated with risperidone or aripiprazole. Parents often complain about sleep-related problems. Not addressing sleep problems effectively can lead to a cycle of seizure and behavioral exacerbation, followed by increase in antiseizure and antipsychotic medication, ultimately worsening the encephalopathy. Effective approaches (after ruling out obstructive sleep apnea either from lymphoid hyperplasia, or overly sedating medication combination) include therapy with melatonin, or in some patients, a bedtime dose of clonidine. When benzodiazepines are used in high doses for seizure control, one can expect increased secretions (especially with clonazepam) as well as laxity of pharyngeal muscles, contributing to sleep disturbance.

Many children with LGS may also have a need for medical management of spasticity—please see details under separate heading. Another sometimes serious problem is drooling. It is exacerbated by overmedication. Limited benefit is seen with glycopyrrolate. Rarely, patients may require a referral for special procedures by a head and neck surgeon.

Surgery: Patients with LGS may present with a focal lesion amenable to surgical resection, but this is very uncommon. Drop seizures can sometimes respond to a corpus callosotomy, but we consider this a procedure of last resort. At our center, and many others, a trial with vagus nerve stimulation (VNS) typically precedes a decision to subject the patient to a corpus callosum resection. Drop seizures, which are the most disabling of the seizures comprising LGS, seem to be especially responsive to VNS therapy. Corpus callosum sectioning provides modest relief from drop seizures, but may produce deterioration in partial seizures. In some patients, the procedure may also result in perceptible cognitive deterioration. In many patients, VNS appears to reduce injuries, limit AED toxicity, and produce some improvements in mood and attention.

Diet: Dietary therapy may be especially of benefit to patients with LGS. Responders often experience significant seizure reduction as well as increased alertness and improved behavior (likely due to diminished AED burden as well as seizure reduction). The most stringent form of dietary therapy, the ketogenic diet, has the best evidence for efficacy, but requires considerable effort on the part of the family. Recent literature indicates some benefit also from a modified Atkins' diet as well as a low-glycemic index therapy. Dietary therapy should only be undertaken in collaboration with a center experienced in its implementation, and requires careful medical and laboratory follow-up.

Therapy: Young children with LGS may benefit from physical, occupational, and speech therapy. There are usually state supported centers for providing such services until the child enters the school system. Some of these agencies also provide respite assistance with visiting personnel for the family.

Social: Caring for a child with LGS imposes a considerable burden on the family. They may require social services such as respite care, and may benefit from referrals to support groups such as the Epilepsy Foundation. They may also require advocacy with the school system. Transporting the child becomes more challenging as the patient grows to a larger physical proportion, and the physician can assist with the obtaining of a handicapped permit from the Department of Motor Vehicles.

Pearls and Precautions

1. Very difficult to achieve total seizure freedom. Titrate therapy to maximize quality of life.
2. Patients are susceptible to injury from falls—provide for helmets and counsel family about configuring household for maximal safety.
3. Nutrition can be challenging in some, and AED selection may contribute to decreased appetite and an iatrogenic "failure to thrive" problem.
4. Identify and manage sleep problems. This can include iatrogenic contributions as discussed above.
5. Since common illnesses produce seizure exacerbation, maintain immunization status.
6. Recognize the need for rescue therapy and implement.
7. Support, support, support – remember respite care.

References

Sankar R. Initial treatment of epilepsy with antiepileptic drugs: pediatric issues. *Neurology* 2004;63(10 Supp; 4):S30–39.

Panayiotopoulos CP. *A Clinical Guide to Epileptic Syndromes and their Treatment.* Bladon Medical Publishing, Oxford, UK, 2002 (various chapters).

Pellock JM, Bourgeois BFD, Dodson WE, Nordli DR Jr, Sankar R (Eds). *Pediatric Epilepsy: Diagnosis and Therapy,* Third Edition, Demos Publishing, New York, NY, 2008 (various chapters).

Frost M, Gates J, Helmers SL, Wheless JW, Levisohn P, Tardo C, Conry JA. Vagus nerve stimulation in children with refractory seizures associated with Lennox-Gastaut syndrome. *Epilepsia* 2001;42:1148–52.

Kostov K, Kostov H, Taubøll E. Long-term vagus nerve stimulation in the treatment of Lennox-Gastaut syndrome. *Epilepsy Behav* 2009;16:321-4.

Vining EP. Tonic and atonic seizures: medical therapy and ketogenic diet. *Epilepsia* 2009;50 Suppl 8:21–4.

Muzykewicz DA, Lyczkowski DA, Memon N, Conant KD, Pfeifer HH, Thiele EA. Efficacy, safety, and tolerability of the low glycemic index treatment in pediatric epilepsy. *Epilepsia* 2009;50:1118–26.

Kossoff EH, McGrogan JR, Bluml RM, Pillas DJ, Rubenstein JE, Vining EP. A modified Atkins diet is effective for the treatment of intractable pediatric epilepsy. *Epilepsia* 2006;47:421–4.

Arzimanoglou A, French J, Blume WT, Cross JH, Ernst JP, Feucht M, Genton P, Guerrini R, Kluger G, Pellock JM, Perucca E, Wheless JW. Lennox-Gastaut syndrome: a consensus approach on diagnosis, assessment, management, and trial methodology. *Lancet Neurol* 2009;8:82–93.

Landau-Kleffner Syndrome (LKS)

Christopher C. Giza, Raman Sankar

Landau-Kleffner syndrome (LKS) or acquired epileptiform aphasia is a syndrome characterized by regression of previously acquired language, beginning typically with receptive language, and associated with electrical status epilepticus during slow-wave sleep (ESES) seen on EEG. ESES refers to the EEG pattern showing sleep activated epileptiform activity in >85% of slow-wave sleep. Continuous spike waves during slow-wave sleep (CSWS) refers to a syndrome (sometimes called Tassinari syndrome) of broader neurocognitive impairment occurring with an EEG showing ESES. In this latter syndrome, typically there is global developmental delay and seizures even prior to the onset of ESES.

Etiology

The etiology of Landau-Kleffner is unknown. Rare cases have been associated with structural brain lesions.

Clinical Presentation and Prognosis

Demographics: The age of onset ranges between 3–10 yrs. No gender predisposition has been reported.

Presenting signs and symptoms: Onset is heralded by a language regression characterized by auditory verbal agnosia in a previously normal child—i.e., the child begins having difficulty understanding the spoken word, decreases spontaneous speech, and eventually develops word deafness. Clinical seizures occur, but 30–40% will not have seizures. Problems such as hyperactivity, impulsivity, behavior disorder and/or personality change occur fairly commonly (50–70%).

Clinical course: After onset of language difficulties, seizures, cognitive dysfunction and/or behavioral problems occur. When seizures occur, they may be partial, generalized or atypical absence but are not generally frequent or hard to control.

Prognosis: The prognosis is variable for LKS with fairly benign seizure outcomes, but less favorable language outcomes. In fact, seizures usually cease by the age of 10 years, and almost always by 15 years. Long-term language and neurobehavioral abnormalities occur in 50–80%, and tend to be the most debilitating component of this syndrome.

In some cases, improved prognosis has been reported after treatment with corticosteroids/ACTH. However, relapse may occur in those who do show an initial successful treatment response requiring subsequent long-term or repeated treatments. In general, CSWS patients tend to have a worse prognosis than do LKS.

LKS is generally idiopathic while CSWS more often is symptomatic of some underlying etiology. The differential diagnosis of these syndromes includes autism or pervasive developmental delay (PDD) with seizures, hearing loss, other focal and mixed epilepsies, a dominant hemisphere cerebral infarct/ischemia—and, very rarely—temporal lobe tumor, vasculitis, neurocysticercosis or encephalitis.

Diagnosis

A clinical diagnosis of LKS requires normal language and cognitive development prior to the onset of symptoms, and a *hearing test* must be normal. Overnight *EEG* showing spike and slow waves making up 80–85% of slow-wave sleep meets the strict definition for ESES. There is some suggestion that the ESES in LKS is more focal and more generalized in CSWS. *MRI* is performed to rule out a structural lesion and is normal. *Neuropsychological testing* may be helpful to characterize the level of cognitive impairment.

Management

Medications

1. *Diazepam* can be given 1 mg/kg orally after the overnight EEG; then 0.5 mg/kg daily for 3–4 weeks, at which time a repeat overnight EEG is done. If EEG is improved, then use a slow 2.5 mg/month taper, and if there is no change, then taper rapidly (Riviello 2001).
2. *Corticosteroids (or ACTH): Prednisone:* 2 mg/kg/d (max 60 mg) for 1 month, followed by a slow taper. If given early in the course, it has been reported to normalize the EEG as well as improve seizures and speech (Marescaux 1990). Prior to initiating this therapy, make sure immunizations are up to date.
3. Valproate, ethosuximide and other benzodiazepines may improve EEG and language.
4. Carbamazepine and phenytoin may control seizures, but do not appear to affect speech. Because these medications may theoretically worsen seizures/EEG, they are infrequently used. There is also an impression that carbamazepine or oxcarbazepine may sometimes induce the progression of a benign childhood epileptic syndrome like rolandic epilepsy to LKS, and many epileptologists avoid those medications. Phenobarbital is ineffective.
5. Intravenous immune globulin has been reported to be effective in isolated case reports.
6. There are also recent reports describing the beneficial effects of levetiracetam in some cases.

Surgery: Multiple subpial transections were reported to recover speech in 11/14 children (Morrell 1995), although subsequent series have not shown this dramatic effect.

Therapy: Speech therapy and sign language training may be helpful in managing these patients.

Psych: Formal neuropsychological testing to monitor cognitive status and educational/developmental progress can be helpful. Psychiatric consultation is also warranted to help with the management of behavioral co-morbidities such as ADHD (which may be managed with stimulants) and autism (which may be managed with SSRIs).

Social: Additional information about epilepsy in general, including information about this rare (LKS) condition is available at http://www.epilepsyfoundation.org/. A website/organization that specifically focuses on LKS is located at http://www.friendsoflks.com/Home_Page.htm.

Pearls and Precautions

Likely complications: Be sure to rule out hearing impairment. Proper diagnosis of this syndrome requires consultation with a child neurologist and availability of prolonged EEG capable of capturing slow-wave sleep (which usually means an overnight hospital stay, rather than a routine outpatient EEG).

School/education: These children will need careful educational assessment, speech therapy and an integrated educational plan. The severity of the language impairment does not correlate with the severity of clinical seizures (often there are none or few), but there appears to be developmental potential, particularly if the ESES pattern can be effectively suppressed.

References

Landau WM, Kleffner FR. Syndrome of acquired aphasia with convulsive disorder in children. Neurology. 1957 Aug;7(8):523-30.

Marescaux C, Hirsch E, Finck S, Maquet P, Schlumberger E, Sellal F, Metz-Lutz MN, Alembik Y, Salmon E, Franck G. Landau-Kleffner syndrome: a pharmacologic study of five cases. Epilepsia. 1990 Nov-Dec;31(6):768-77.

McVicar KA, Shinnar S. Landau-Kleffner syndrome, electrical status epilepticus in slow wave sleep, and language regression in children. Ment Retard Dev Disabil Res Rev. 2004;10(2):144-9.

Morrell F, Whisler WW, Smith MC, Hoeppner TJ, de Toledo-Morrell L, Pierre-Louis SJ, Kanner AM, Buelow JM, Ristanovic R, Bergen D, et al. Landau-Kleffner syndrome. Treatment with subpial intracortical transection. Brain. 1995 Dec;118 (Pt 6):1529-46.

Progressive Myoclonus Epilepsy (PME)

Christopher C. Giza, Raman Sankar

The progressive myoclonus epilepsies are a group of epileptic disorders characterized by myoclonic seizures, generalized tonic-clonic seizures and progressive neurological deterioration. The diagnoses often included in this group include Unverricht-Lundborg (Baltic myoclonus) disease, Lafora disease, myoclonic epilepsy with ragged red fibers (MERRF), neuronal ceroid lipofuscinoses (NCL) and sialidosis. Each of these disorders has distinct clinical characteristics, while the general management of the worsening seizures and neurological deterioration in this group of disorders also has elements in common.

General management of PMEs

Outpatient supportive care is the main mode of management for these patients. Accommodations for the patient and caregivers to meet the increasing challenges of everyday tasks should be planned and coordinated in an organized fashion. Many of these patients will progress to a debilitated state where they need tracheal suctioning, mobility assistance, assistance with feeding by mouth or via G-tube, and diapers for incontinence. Given the degenerative nature of these diseases, advanced care directives discussed with the family in advance may be helpful to minimize late-stage aggressive surgical or respiratory interventions.

Medication: Antiepileptics are intended to control seizures. Outpatient management, including rescue medications for seizure exacerbations, can be important to help the family avoid frequent emergency department visits and hospitalizations.

1. Medications particularly valuable for myoclonic seizures include valproate, levetiracetam, clonazepam (or other benzodiazepines), zonisamide and felbamate. Although not readily available in the U.S., piracetam may also be effective for myoclonus/myoclonic seizures.
2. Other broad spectrum anticonvulsants that may be effective for other seizure types include topiramate and phenobarbital. Lamotrigine is another broad spectrum agent, but should be used with caution as it may exacerbate myoclonic seizures.
3. Rescue medications may include diazepam rectal gel that is dosed by weight. Side effects include sedation and respiratory compromise if overdosed. However, this agent is particularly effective at controlling seizure flare-ups and is very rapidly absorbed in an urgent situation, without requiring intravenous access. Other rescue medications may include lorazepam orally or midazolam delivered intrabuccally.
4. Medications known to exacerbate myoclonus and therefore to be avoided include phenytoin, carbamazepine, gabapentin, vigabatrin and tiagabine.

Surgery: G-tube or tracheostomy placement may be considered as the disease advances. See above, though, regarding palliative care and keeping with parental and patient's wishes regarding aggressive management in the late stages of some of these diseases.

Feeding and aspiration: Swallowing and handling of secretions are important functions that become compromised as the diseases progress. Aspiration precautions should be in place.

Sleep: Melatonin, diphenhydramine and lorazepam may be used symptomatically.

Toilet: Diapers will often be required in advanced stages of these diseases.

Skin: These patients can get skin infections or tissue breakdown.

A. Unverricht-Lundborg (Baltic myoclonus) disease

Etiology

This PME is an autosomal recessive disorder caused by mutations in the CSTB gene (also named EPM1), which codes for cystatin B, a cysteine protease inhibitor.

Clinical Presentation and Prognosis

Demographics: Unverricht-Lundborg is the most common PME, with a prevalence of 1:20,000 in the Baltic regions. Age of onset is typically between 6–15 years.

Clinical signs and symptoms: In half the cases, stimulus-sensitive myoclonus is the presenting symptom. Other seizures include generalized tonic clonic and absence. Neurological exam is initially normal. Over time, there is gradual development of ataxia, dysarthria, tremor and incoordination. Cognitive impairment is insidious and may be mild. After a period of adolescent worsening, some patients will show clinical stabilization. With adequate treatment of myoclonic seizures and supportive care, the patients may live into their 50–60s.

Diagnosis

Electroencephalogram (EEG) findings are nonspecific and show generalized high voltage spike wave discharges, ranging from 2–3 Hz up to 4–6 Hz. Photoparoxysmal responses are common. MRI is often normal and not diagnostic. *Genetic testing* for a mutation in the cystatin B gene can be done, but is not readily commercially available.

Management

For anticonvulsant/anti-myoclonus therapy, see above under general medical management. Levetiracetam may be particularly effective. Phenytoin should be avoided as it exacerbates myoclonus and cerebellar signs. Vagal nerve stimulation has shown promise in improving myoclonic seizures.

B. Lafora disease

Etiology

Autosomal recessive disease that in 80% of the cases is due to a detectable mutation in the EPM2A and EPM2B locus located in chromosome 6q. The neurodegenerative process and epilepsy seem to be related to accumulation of small polyglucosans called Lafora bodies, but it is not clear how Lafora bodies cause this disease.

Clinical Presentation and Prognosis

Demographics: Age of onset is usually in the second decade of life, but could be as early as 6 years of age.

Clinical signs and symptoms: The clinical presentation is usually seizures/epilepsy. Many types occur including myoclonic, occipital (with transient blindness or visual hallucinations), photoconvulsive, atypical absence, atonic and complex partial seizures. One or all of these seizure types could be present in a single patient; photosensitivity is common; and, status epilepticus is seen as the disease progresses. Other clinical findings are a rapid decline in cognitive function, ataxia, cortical blindness, bulbar dysfunction, hypertonia, hyporeflexia (and rarely), cardiac dysfunction. The clinical course is a relentlessly progressive seizure disorder that evolves into almost continuous myoclonus, spastic quadriparesis and dementia. Most patients die within 10 years from the time of diagnosis due to complications such as respiratory failure.

Diagnosis

EEG and MRI are nondiagnostic. *Skin biopsy* and PAS staining demonstrate Lafora bodies, being the least invasive and perhaps the most definitive diagnostic test. Biopsy of the liver and muscle tissue can also demonstrate the presence of Lafora bodies. The *genetic testing* for known mutations (EPM2A and EPM2B DNA tests) can be done at Athena Diagnostics Testing www.athenadiagnostics.com.

Management

For seizure medications, see above under general management. Seizures and myoclonus in Lafora tend to be very difficult to control. Supportive/palliative care is also important (see above under general management).

C. Myoclonic epilepsy with ragged red fibers (MERRF)

Etiology

MERRF is caused by a mutation of mitochondrial tRNA gene (MTTK) found in 90% of patients, and may be maternally inherited or sporadic.

Clinical Presentation and Prognosis

Demographics: Age of onset and clinical severity can be quite variable, even within a family. There is some overlap between MERRF and mitochondrial encephalomyopathy, lactic acidosis and stroke-like episodes (MELAS), with MERRF having a longer course and generally milder cognitive impairment.

Clinical signs and symptoms: Onset can be gradual, with progressive myopathy, neuropathy and hearing loss as major features. Optic atrophy, dementia, short stature, pigmentary retinopathy, cardiomyopathy, pyramidal tract signs, ophthalmoparesis, cutaneous lipomas and diabetes mellitus can occur and worsen over time.

Diagnosis

Genetic defect can be confirmed through *mitochondrial DNA blood testing. Muscle biopsy* is more invasive, but may also be diagnostic.

Management

See above for general anticonvulsant management, with the caveat that valproate therapy may inhibit carnitine uptake. Thus, valproate should be used cautiously and in conjunction with carnitine supplementation. Due to the underlying mitochondrial defect, these patients may also be empirically treated with combinations of vitamins and antioxidants, including coenzyme Q10 and L-carnitine.

D. Neuronal ceroid lipofuscinoses (NCL)

Etiology

Autosomal recessive disorders characterized by lysosomal accumulation of lipopigments. Multiple genetic types have been identified, at least 6 of which may present with PME. These include type CLN1 (infantile), CLN2 (late infantile), CLN3 (juvenile), CLN4 (adult), CLN5 (variant late infantile, Finnish) and CLN6 (variant late infantile, Costa Rican/Portuguese). The genetic defect and inheritance pattern for the adult-onset (Kufs) variant remains unclear. The general term 'Batten disease' is sometimes used to refer to CLN3 specifically and sometimes to the NCLs as a group.

Clinical presentation and prognosis: The NCLs generally present with seizures (often myoclonic or GTCs), ataxia, visual impairment and developmental regression. However, the timing, severity and age-of-onset of these signs varies by the specific genetic defect and the type (Table 11.2).

Diagnosis

Diagnosis is initially based upon clinical suspicion in the setting of the appropriate clinical constellation of findings. Pathological diagnosis is supported by the presence of distinct lysosomal inclusion bodies identified by electron microscopy on *conjunctival/skin biopsy* (although other tissue biopsies may also show these findings). *EEG* will show epileptiform abnormalities (spikes, spike waves, photoparoxysmal responses), but is generally not specific. Some patients with CLN2 will have giant occipital spike-waves in conjunction with low frequency photic stimulation. *Electroretinograms (ERGs)* may show abnormalities in the types where visual impairment occurs (CLN1, 2, 3, 5 and 6). *Brain MRI* is nonspecific showing cerebral and cerebellar atrophy, cortical thinning and occasionally T2 hyperintensity in lobar white matter. Commercially available gene tests are not yet available for these diseases, and the specific gene for CLN4 has not yet been identified. However, there are specialty laboratories throughout the world that provide diagnostic services for the NCLs by measuring either enzyme activity or DNA-based testing for known mutations. A listing of many of these centers (by country) is found at http://www.ucl.ac.uk/ncl/diaglabs.shtml.

Table 11.2: Neuronal ceroid lipofuscinosis Clinical Presentations

Gene	Name	Age of Onset	Clinical Signs/Symptoms	Diagnostic Findings	Life Expectancy
CLN1	Infantile; Santavuori	<2y	Early irritability, seizures (myoclonic) and visual failure, then ataxia and developmental regression	Granular osmiophilic inclusions	4–8 years of age
CLN2	Late infantile; Jansky-Biels-chowsky	2–4y	Early seizures (myoclonic, GTCs), then marked ataxia, visual failure (retinopathy) & cognitive regression	Reduced TPP1 enzyme in fibroblasts or leukocytes; Curvilinear lysosomal inclusions	6–20 years
CLN3	Juvenile; Spielmeier-Vogt; Batten	4–10y	Early visual failure (optic atrophy, pigmentary retinopathy), then dementia, ataxia and extrapyramidal features. Seizures (GTC, myoclonus) are milder.	Fingerprint lysosomal inclusions	15–30 years
CLN4	Adult; Kufs	Adult	Dementia, ataxia, extrapyramidal signs, later myoclonus. No visual failure.	Fingerprint inclusions	Variable; 10 years after onset
CLN5	Variant late infantile; Finnish	5–7y	Ataxia, hypotonia, visual impairment, then seizures (myoclonic, GTCs) and cognitive regression	Fingerprint or curvilinear inclusions	13–35 years
CLN6	Variant late infantile; Costa Rican/ Portuguese	3–7y	Early gait and speech disturbances, seizures, visual impairment and cognitive regression	Fingerprint, curvilinear and rectilinear inclusions	20–40 years

Management

No disease specific therapy yet exists. Symptomatic treatment of seizures/myoclonus is indicated as discussed above. Antioxidant therapy (vitamins E, C and methionine) has proven inconclusive for CLN3. Flupirtine is an analgesic available in Europe that has been proposed as treatment for CLN2, possibly through an anti-apoptotic effect and effects on potassium channels. For NCLs where the molecular defect is known (CLN2), molecular therapy is theoretically possible and future interventions are being investigated such as enzyme replacement, gene transfer or stem cell transplantation.

Supportive care becomes increasingly important as the disease progresses. The Batten Disease Support and Research Association (http://bdsra.org/) provides opportunities for family networking and information about ongoing research trials.

References

Ramachandran N, Girard JM, Turnbull J, Minassian BA. The autosomal recessively inherited progressive myoclonus epilepsies and their genes. Epilepsia. 2009 May;50 Suppl 5:29-36.

Shahwan A, Farrell M, Delanty N. Progressive myoclonic epilepsies: a review of genetic and therapeutic aspects. Lancet Neurol. 2005 Apr;4(4):239-48.

E. Sialidosis

Etiology

There are two forms of sialidosis. Type I is caused by alpha-neuraminidase deficiency. Type II is caused by a deficiency of both N-acetyl neuraminidase and beta-galactosialidase. Both are autosomal recessive.

Clinical Presentation and Prognosis

Demographics: Juvenile or adult onset occurs with type I. Type II has even more variable onset ranging from the neonatal period to young adult. Both forms are rare causes of PME.

Clinical signs and symptoms: Type I may present with isolated intention or action myoclonus. Progression is very slow and without concomitant dementia. Neurological deterioration includes visual impairment, GTC seizures and ataxia. A cherry-red spot is classic (hence 'cherry-red spot myoclonus'). In addition to myoclonus, type II patients develop coarsened facial features, corneal clouding, hepatomegaly, skeletal dysplasia and learning disabilities reminiscent of other storage disorders.

Diagnosis

Urine testing reveals elevated sialyloligosaccharides. Diagnosis is confirmed by demonstration of *lysosomal enzyme deficiency in WBCs or fibroblasts.*

Management

General anticonvulsant management (see above) is needed for myoclonus and seizures. Given the molecular defect, enzyme replacement is a potential therapeutic strategy being investigated.

References

Ramachandran N, et al., The autosomal recessively inherited progressive myoclonus epilepsies and their genes, Epilepsia 2009

Shahwan A, et al., Progressive myoclonus epilepsies : a review of genetic and therapeutic aspects, Lancet Neurol 2005.

Rasmussen Encephalitis

Christopher C. Giza, Raman Sankar

Rasmussen encephalitis is a catastrophic childhood epilepsy syndrome that is characterized by focal motor seizures generally involving a single hemisphere. Focal motor status epilepticus (SE) or *epilepsia partialis continua* (EPC) is a hallmark of this syndrome. It is generally progressive and leads to hemispheric degeneration, ultimately resulting in hemiparesis. Early recognition and hemispherectomy may result in seizure control and improved long-term neurocognitive outcome, but at the price of early hemiparesis.

Etiology

The etiology of Rasmussen encephalitis is unknown. Several theories have been promoted including a viral origin due to herpesvirus or CMV. However, no viral particles have been consistently found on pathologic specimens. An alternative hypothesis is that it has an autoimmune etiology. In some cases, autoantibodies to glutamate receptors (GluR3) have been reported in CSF.

Clinical Presentation and Prognosis

Demographics: Onset of this disease is typically in childhood (median age 5–6 years), in a previously normal child. In 85% the onset is before age 10, but adult cases have been reported. A history of infection or inflammation within 1 month of onset has been mentioned in 38% of cases.

Presenting signs and symptoms: Rasmussen encephalopathy typically presents as intractable focal seizures, often epilepsia partialis continua (persistent focal clonic motor activity that occurs without alteration in mental status). Focal neurologic deficit/hemparesis may occur in conjunction with early EPC, but typically develops over time. Progressive epileptic encephalopathy/dementia occurs later. This condition is very resistant to anticonvulsant medications.

There is a substantial differential diagnosis of etiologies that can cause EPC or intractable partial epilepsy that must be ruled out during the diagnostic process. The differential diagnosis of Epilepsia partialis continua (EPC) includes tumor, cerebrovascular disease, focal cortical dysplasia, tick-born encephalitis, systemic lupus erythematosis, hepatic encephalopathy, mitochondrial encephalomyopathy with lactic acidosis and stroke-like episodes (MELAS), and measles encephalitis. The differential diagnosis of intractable partial epilepsy includes tumor, degenerative cortical disease, focal cortical dysplasia, tuberous sclerosis and Sturge-Weber syndrome.

Clinical course: Focal seizures may occur tens or even hundreds of times per day. Patients may present with intact mental status and focal motor status epilepticus. Seizures tend to be resistant to anticonvulsants. As the syndrome advances, multiple partial seizure types may emerge (simple partial, complex partial, secondarily generalized). Progressive hemispheric atrophy and signal changes marking gliosis may be discerned on MRI. Worsening hemiparesis contralateral to the seizure focus develops over months to years after the onset of epilepsy (average 2.8 years). For left brain Rasmussen syndrome, progressive aphasia can be a major problem. Mental deterioration and dementia also occur—on average about 5 years after onset—but usually after the seizures have become intractable.

Prognosis: Untreated, most result in relentlessly progressive hemiparesis and cognitive decline until they "burn out" after years. Individuals may be left wheelchair bound and demented. Rare cases of spontaneous remission have been reported. Very rare cases have involved bilateral involvement.

Diagnosis

The diagnosis of Rasmussen syndrome/encephalitis is a diagnosis of exclusion (see above for differential diagnosis). *EEG* shows unilateral epileptiform activity, and often simple partial or complex partial status epilepticus. Early in the course, *MRI* can be normal. Later, neuroimaging most often shows hemispheric atrophy with unilateral ventriculomegaly. Areas of increased T2/PD/ADC or FLAIR signal and hyperintense DWI in predominantly one hemisphere are typical. Lumbar Puncture can be used to rule out CNS infection; may consider checking CSF IgG synthesis, oligoclonal bands and anti-GluR3 autoantibodies. *SPECT/PET/MRS* may show hemispheric metabolic abnormality(ies).

Brain biopsy: Acutely: Perivascular cuffing, scattered glial nodules, diffuse microglial proliferation, and fibrotic meninges may be seen. Chronically: Atrophy, gliosis, spongy degeneration, and neuronal loss without inflammation may be observed. No viral particles are typically seen. However, some report finding viral nucleic acids by PCR.

Management

The definitive therapy for Rasmussen encephalitis is hemispherectomy.

Medical: These interventions have sometimes been used to temporize, but are not definitive. If undertaken, these therapies should not delay evaluation for hemispherectomy at a comprehensive pediatric epilepsy center.

1. *Intravenous immune globulin (IVIg):* 8 out of 9 patients had short term seizure reduction with IVIG therapy. Suggested dosage is 1000 mg/kg/d for 2 days or 400 mg/kg/d for 5 days.
2. *Methylprednisolone:* Administered intravenously. Suggested dosage is 400 mg/m^2 IV, daily, times 3 doses. There are some reports of good response.
3. *Prednisolone or ACTH:* 10 out of 17 patients had reported short term seizure reduction. However, the response is not as good as methylprednisolone.
4. *Plasmapheresis:* Has led to short term benefits and may be repeated in responders.
5. *Cytoxan:* Has also been reported to be beneficial.
6. Standard anticonvulsants are often used. However, they are generally NOT adequate to control seizures.

Surgical: If surgery is done, hemispherectomy is the procedure of choice. Focal resections generally lead to recurrence of seizures. The timing of this procedure may be problematic as the diagnosis is being confirmed, particularly in cases involving the language-dominant (usually left) hemisphere. Later surgery (>10 yrs.) has a theoretical risk of being less likely to show good language recovery/plasticity. Earlier hemispherectomy may be optimal for best developmental outcome.

Therapy: Prior to surgery involving the language-dominant hemisphere, it is advisable to have speech therapy consultation to provide training with possible language assistive devices that may be used post-hemispherectomy. Learning sign language is also easier preoperatively. Post-operatively, intensive neurorehabilitation is necessary for gait retraining and to optimize upper extremity function, as well as language/speech. Assistive braces are helpful in hemiparetic patients to minimize contractures.

Psych: Patients may require psychiatric consultation for behavioral problems and/or situational coping/depression.

Social: The Hemispherectomy Foundation (http://hemifoundation.intuitwebsites.com/welcome.html) is a recently created support group for patients/families undergoing this procedure. The Epilepsy Foundation of America (EFA; http://www.epilepsyfoundation.org/) is an established national organization with useful information and local support groups.

Pearls and Precautions

School/education: Patients with language-dominant hemisphere involvement will require additional educational resources in order to continue in school.

Be sure to rule out a structural lesion as the underlying cause of focal status epilepticus or focal intractable seizures.

Prior to definitive surgical intervention, anticonvulsant therapy is only palliative. It may prove impossible to control every single partial seizure. It may be preferable to have some ongoing simple partial seizures than to be so sedated from medication that the patient is unable to function.

References

Bien CG, Granata T, Antozzi C, Cross JH, Dulac O, Kurthen M, Lassmann H, Mantegazza R, Villemure JG, Spreafico R, Elger CE. Pathogenesis, diagnosis and treatment of Rasmussen encephalitis: a European consensus statement. Brain. 2005 Mar;128(Pt 3):454-71. Epub 2005 Feb 2.

Hart Y. Rasmussen's encephalitis. Epileptic Disord. 2004 Sep;6(3):133-44.

Migraine

Christopher C. Giza, Raman Sankar

Migraine is a relatively common episodic neurological disorder characterized by headache, nausea, vomiting and other intermittent neurological symptoms. Symptomatic episodes are separated by symptom-free intervals. The accurate diagnosis of pediatric migraine is complicated by several factors including the presence of migraine syndromes in which headache is less prominent, limited ability of the child to articulate their symptoms, and variations in parental interpretation of symptoms. In addition, the differential diagnosis of episodic neurological symptoms in childhood can include a large number of rarer conditions that may mimic aspects of pediatric migraine.

Etiology

The exact etiology of migraine is unknown, although neurovascular mechanisms implicated include: (1) vasodilation; (2) meningeal inflammation; (3) spreading depression; and (4) neurotransmitter changes (reduced serotonin turnover during attack). There appears to be some genetic contribution to migraine disorders, and some genetic syndromes associated with ion channelopathies (see below) have migraine as a clinical manifestation. In addition, migraine has comorbidity with some types of childhood epilepsy and psychiatric disorders such as depression. In some individuals, migraine attacks can be specifically triggered by hormonal changes (menses, etc.), ingestions (foods, caffeine, medications, etc.), head injury/TBI, seizures and other physiological stressors (fever, lack of sleep, etc.).

Clinical Presentation and Prognosis

Demographics: The prevalence of migraine increases with age, tending to peak in adolescence (up to 8–23% during high school). Prior to the onset of puberty, more boys are affected than girls, but in adolescence and after, the incidence of migraine shows a clear female predominance. Migraine without aura is the most common form of migraine in the pediatric population (up to 85%).

Presenting signs and symptoms: Headaches tend to be shorter in children (<2 hrs.) than in adults. Also, non-headache and complicated migraine variants more common in children.

International Headache Society (IHS) Criteria
Migraine headache has the following characteristics and is not attributed to some other underlying disorder. Migraine without aura (most common type in children - presenting in 60–85% of cases)

a. ≥ 5 attacks fulfilling features B–D.

b. Duration 1–72 hrs

c. ≥ 2 of 4 features: Bilateral or unilateral (frontotemporal) location; pulsating; moderate to severe intensity; aggravated by routine physical activity

d. ≥ 1 of 2 features: Nausea±vomiting, photo and phonophobia (inferred from behavior).

Migraine with aura (less common - presenting in 15–30% of cases)

a. ≥ 2 attacks fulfilling criteria B.

b. ≥ 3 of 4 features: ≥ 1 fully reversible aura symptoms indicating focal cerebral or brainstem dysfunction; ≥1 aura symptoms developing gradually over ≥ 4 min OR ≥ 2 symptoms in succession; no individual symptoms ≥ 60 min duration; headache follows aura <60 min OR may begin before or during aura.

For migraine with aura, the most common transient neurological symptoms include binocular or monocular visual impairment or scotoma, visual distortions or even visual hallucinations. Hemisensory disturbances, aphasia, ataxia and even hemiparesis can occur.

Complicated migraine types and migraine variants—not uncommon in pediatrics (all may have headache but it is not required):

a. *Basilar (3–19% of pediatric cases):* This variant is characterized by brainstem symptoms such as vertigo, ataxia, drop attack, visual disturbance, diplopia and/or obtundation. May be familial.

b. *Hemiplegic:* This subtype has autosomal dominant inheritance and the predominant subtype (familial hemiplegic migraine 1 FHM1) is caused by a missense mutation in a calcium channel gene (CACNA1A). The aura for FHM is typically a stroke-like onset of hemiplegia or hemiparesis occuring 30–60 minutes prior to the headache but often extended thereafter for hours or days. The headache occurs contralateral to the hemiparesis. Other subtypes (FHM2, FHM3) are caused by mutations in a sodium-potassium pump (ATP1A2) or sodium channel (SCN1A), respectively.

c. *Confusional migraine:* Is characterized by aphasia, confusion, combativeness and agitation. Sometimes triggered by mild traumatic brain injury (mTBI).

d. *Alice-in-Wonderland:* This is a migraine variant with profound visual perceptual distortion and vivid visual hallucinations.

e. *Ophthalmoplegic migraine:* Is no longer considered a migraine variant but more likely a cranial neuralgia with diplopia, periorbital pain and CN III palsy. The pain and ophthalmoparesis may occur well into the headache and persist long after, distinguishing it from a true aura.

f. *Benign paroxysmal vertigo:* Presenting signs and symptoms are sudden attacks of vertigo, nystagmus and gait disturbance.

g. *Cyclic vomiting syndrome (CVS):* Occurs with episodic severe GI disturbance, nausea and vomiting and in-between periods of normalcy.

h. *Abdominal migraine:* This syndrome has more vague or dull abdominal discomfort associated with other migraine symptoms and lasting for hours.

i. *Benign paroxysmal torticollis:* This is an intermittent dyskinesia with attacks of head tilt but may also have vomiting and ataxia. Usual onset of these attacks is during infancy, and may be an early manifestation of basilar migraine.

j. *Ocular migraine:* Is associated with monocular visual loss with or without eye pain.

Clinical course: Very early manifestations of migraine may present with nonheadache migraine variants including vertigo, dizziness or intermittent vomiting. Typically, more conventional symptoms of pulsatile headache with or without associated aura will occur more regularly in adolescence. Onset of attacks may be associated with selective triggers such as psychological stress, sleep deprivation, hunger, specific foods (cheeses, nuts, citrus, chocolate, caffeine, wine/alcohol, etc.), exercise/exertion, medications, perfume, motion sickness, menstruation, head trauma and/or environmental extremes.

Prognosis: Frequency of headaches can be greatest during the teenage and young adult years with a gradual decrease in number and severity of headaches as the patient ages. Long term prognosis studies (over 5–20 years) suggest that 20–38% showed headache remission, 42–60% continued to have migraines, and 25–33% developed tension-type headaches. Of those with persistent headaches, approximately two-thirds indicated that the headaches improved. Intractable migraines may 'transform' into chronic daily headache or 'transformed migraine' which tend to be difficult to treat and often require preventative pharmacotherapy as well as non-pharmacological management to achieve an optimal result.

Diagnosis

Diagnosis of migraine is generally made on clinical grounds, following the clinical characteristics described by the IHS (see above). Diagnostic testing is generally reserved for situations where an underlying cause to the headache is suspected or where the presenting headache is atypical for migraine. Central nervous system imaging (*CT/MRI*) is not routinely indicated for classic migraine, but may be considered for complicated migraine or migraine with aura. In this case, it is used to rule out a focal structural cerebral lesion. Electroencephalograms (*EEG*) are also not routinely indicated but can be ordered to help rule out seizure with/without focal features and ictal/postictal headache, including benign occipital epilepsy. Lumbar puncture (*LP*) is necessary in cases where it is necessary to rule out central nervous system (CNS) infection or possible subarachnoid hemorrhage.

The acute classic clinical picture is characteristic. However, the differential diagnosis may include the following: (1) Intracranial hemorrhage (including arteriovenous malformation [AVM]); (2) brain tumor; (3) meningitis; (4) traumatic brain injury; (5) gastrointestinal disturbance/gastroesophageal reflux disease (GERD); (6) ischemia/infarction; (7) intoxication; (8) idiopathic intracranial hypertension; (9) other primary headache syndrome; and (10) benign occipital epilepsy—associated with complex visual distortions, headache, autonomic symptoms and seizures.

Management

Headache monitoring: For intermittent and infrequent migraines, rigorous monitoring is generally not necessary. However, it is still helpful to have parents be looking for triggers that may be avoidable if a consistent pattern emerges. For patients with chronic, frequent migraines, a headache calendar or diary can be very helpful to identify patterns and monitor for gradual changes in frequency and severity. Care should be taken not to overly focus on documenting headache details, but the child and parents can be instructed to mark down each day whether a headache occurred, how severe it was (scale of 1–3 mild, moderate, severe or 1–10), time of day, how long it lasted and whether there was an associated trigger (see above under etiology and clinical course).

Trigger avoidance: It is important not to be unduly restrictive in the types of food or activities in which the patient may partake. However, if a particular stimulus is clearly associated with migraine onset in more than a couple of well documented instances, efforts should be made to avoid that stimulus while continuing the headache calendar/diary. Trigger avoidance is most effective if the identified trigger is something fairly specific and readily avoidable. For example, 'lemons' or 'chocolate' can be identified as triggers and avoided (at least for a test period to determine if it is causing headaches) far more readily than 'stress,' which is hard to objectively quantify and generally difficult to avoid. Overly restrictive diets are not recommended as they add stress to the parent-child relationship and tend to be difficult to maintain.

Nonpharmacological approaches: Biobehavioral strategies should be emphasized as much as pharmacological treatments. These include trigger avoidance, good nutrition, adequate sleep and regular moderate exercise. In addition, stress management, relaxation therapy, meditation and biofeedback can be important measures, particularly for older adolescents and those with more chronic headaches. Other types of nonpharmacological intervention include acupuncture, aromatherapy and hypnosis.

Medications: Pharmacotherapy for migraine is generally divided into 2 types. The first is abortive or "stop" medication, taken acutely at the time of headache onset in an attempt to terminate an acute headache. The second is prophylactic or "prevent" medicine, which is taken every day, headache or not, in an effort to prevent headaches and/or reduce the frequency and severity of headaches. In general, abortive or "stop" medication alone is warranted for infrequent attacks with little chronic functional impairment; this is the main type of migraine pharmacotherapy for the majority of sufferers. If attacks occur more frequently than 3–4 per month and/or are associated with missing school or other important activities, then prophylactic "prevent" medication should be emphasized.

It is extremely important that the family and patient understand the distinctions between these two different treatment strategies, lest they prematurely determine that one or the other is ineffective. A common misconception by the family is that all medications only need to be taken when a headache occurs—obviously, preventive medications are not effective in this context. Another important point is that abortive medications are generally most effective at the onset of the migraine. Abortive medications should not be taken more than twice for a given headache, and if taken too frequently or in too high of a dose, may predispose to the development of rebound headaches.

Abortive "STOP" medications: The main considerations for effective abortive medication therapy are to take an adequate dose and take it as soon as possible. This medication may need to be made available at school or afterschool activities.

1. *Over the counters* (OTCs): Acetaminophen 15 mg/kg, ibuprofen 7.5–10 mg/kg. These agents are effective in 50–80% of migraines and have proven efficacy in pediatric clinical trials, even for those <12 years old. Care should be taken to avoid overly frequent administration (no more than 3–5 per week) due to association with analgesic rebound headache.
2. *Triptans* (serotonin receptor 1B/1D agonists)
    a. Sumatriptan: 5–20 mg nasal spray effective in clinical trials in adolescents. Off label use includes 50–100 mg orally and 3–6 mg OR 0.06 mg/kg subcutaneous injection.
    b. Rizatriptan: 5–10 mg orally disintegrating tablet is effective in adolescents.
    c. Zolmitriptan: 5 mg nasal spray is effective in adolescents.
    d. Almotriptan: 6.25, 12.5, 25 mg tablets are effective in adolescents.
3. *Midrin* (isometheptene/dichloralphenazone/acetaminophen): 1 capsule orally at onset of headache.
4. *Antiemetics* (chlorpromazine, prochlorperazine, metoclopramide, ondansetron): For severe nausea associated with acute migraine attacks.
5. *Other:* (Indomethacin po; naprosyn po; ketorolac IV/po; valproate IV; dihydroergotamine (DHE) 0.15-0.5 mg IV OR nasal spray).

Prophylactic "PREVENT" medications: Generally considered if migraine attacks occur more than 3 times per month and/or are causing functional impairment (school absenteeism, etc.). Each medication should have an adequate treatment trial (2–3 months) so as to avoid prematurely eliminating effective agents. Preventive medications are not intended for life-long treatment, and may be weaned after several months of good control. Weaning over the summer school break is one strategy favored by many families.

1. *Antidepressants*
   a. Amitriptyline: 1 mg/kg OR 5–10 mg po nightly. Titrate weekly up to effective dose (10–50 mg/d). Electrocardiogram (ECG) may be considered for those with history of cardiac problems or on higher doses. Main side effects include sedation, dry mouth, urinary retention and weight gain.
   b. Nortriptyline: Same dosing as amitriptyline with fewer anticholinergic side effects, but potentially slightly higher risk for cardiac adverse effects.
   c. Trazodone: And selective serotonin reuptake inhibitors (SSRIs: fluoxetine, sertaline, etc.) have also been used, but efficacy has not been demonstrated in controlled trials.
2. *Anticonvulsants*
   a. Topiramate: 12.5–200 mg orally daily or divided twice daily. Start low and once nightly and titrate upward as needed. Side effects include weight loss, cognitive slowing, word finding difficulties.
   b. Valproate: 15–45 mg/kg/day; has proven effectiveness in adults and open label efficacy results in children.
   c. Levetiracetam: 250–500 mg orally divided twice daily; has shown efficacy in open label trials in children.
   d. Others (gabapentin; zonisamide; lamotrigine)
3. *Antihistamines* (cyproheptadine 2–4 mg orally daily). The main side effects are sedation and weight gain.
4. *Antihypertensives* (propranolol 80 mg OR 2–4 mg/kg/d orally daily or divided twice daily). Clonidine did not show efficacy.
5. *Calcium channel blockers* (flunarizine has proven effectiveness in pediatrics, but is not available in the United States). Other possibilities include verapamil or nifedipine. Nimodipine has not been proven as an effective agent.

Homeopathic treatments: Vitamin supplements and herbal remedies have been tried with varying degrees of success in migraine, although not necessarily in pediatric/adolescent migraine. Some of these are listed here:

1. Magnesium (400–800 mg/d): Effective in adults.
2. Riboflavin (400 mg/d): Effective in adults
3. Butterbur root: Uncertain efficacy in trials, although showed improvement in one trial when used in conjunction with music therapy.
4. Coenzyme Q10 (1–3 mg/kg/d): Possibly effective in children with documented low CoQ10 levels.

Therapy: In some cases, where migraines have become chronic, are associated with bad posture, and are triggered by neck or muscle spasms, use of physical therapy and massage may offer anecdotal improvement.

Psychiatric: Most cases of migraine are readily managed with education and appropriate pharmacotherapy. In cases associated with chronic pain intractable to standard medications, incorporation of a psychologist or other regular counselor is often helpful. Identification and treatment of underlying psychiatric diagnoses (depression, anxiety, etc.) is important.

Social: Social supports are important, both within the family and within the peer group. Students whose migraines have resulted in them staying home from school may benefit from partial days at school with reduced work loads, at least to ensure some peer-related social interaction, as well as to alleviate some of the stress from returning back to school full-time after a prolonged absence.

Pearls and Precautions

Status migrainosus: This represents a rare but severe type of migraine, described as >72 hours of continuous migraine headache symptoms. In these circumstances, patients may be admitted to the hospital for more intensive treatment, generally in conjunction with a neurologist or pain specialist.

1. *Dihydroergotamine protocol:* In adults—DHE 0.5-1 mg IV q8h + metoclopramide 10 mg IV q8h. May substitute *prochlorperazine* or *ondansetron.*
2. *Chlorpromazine:* 2 mg/kg/d orally (po) divided every 4–6 hours OR 4 mg/kg/d per rectum divided every 6–8h for 5–6 days.
3. *Prochlorperazine:* 0.13–0.15 mg/kg IV acutely.
4. *Prednisone:* Up to 1–2 mg/kg/d po or perhaps even IV methylprednisolone or dexamethasone in severe cases.

Catamenial migraines: Migraines consistently associated with a particular phase of the menstrual cycle may also respond to low dose oral contraceptives or acetazolamide.

Nutrition: Eating regular and balanced meals is generally encouraged. Avoiding food triggers is important in cases where such have been identified.

Sleep: Getting regular and adequate sleep is also important. Particularly for teenagers, inadequate sleep and 'stress' may be associated with periods of worsened migraine control.

Possible complications: In the short term, neurological symptoms with migraine are generally completely reversible. However, across the lifetime, migraine is associated with a slightly increased risk of ischemic stroke. Treatment with vasoconstrictive agents such as ergots and triptans should be avoided in patients with ischemic heart disease or other vasculopathies. Such agents should also be used with caution in patients with basilar migraine.

School/education: School attendance should be encouraged in all but the most severe cases, as the psychological effects of lost peer socialization and the anxiety of returning to school after a prolonged absence can create additional obstacles to recovery. Partial school days and gradual catching up on school assignments should be attempted for those with severe or frequent headache absences. Even for patients whose migraines readily respond to abortive therapy, some communication with the school is desirable, particularly to allow the administration of the abortive agents as close to the onset as possible and to provide a quiet and/or dark place for the migraineur to rest until the headache is over.

Things to be avoided (medications, situations, herbs, etc.): (See listings of potential triggers in categories of Etiology and Clinical course above.)

References

Lewis DW. Pediatric migraine. Neurol Clin. 2009 May;27(2):481-501.

Walker DM, Teach SJ. Emergency department treatment of primary headaches in children and adolescents. Curr Opin Pediatr. 2008 Jun;20(3):248-54.

Winner P. Pediatric headache. Curr Opin Neurol. 2008 Jun;21(3):316-22.

Pseudotumor Cerebri (PTC)

Christopher C. Giza, Raman Sankar

Pseudotumor cerebri is a syndrome of intracranial hypertension in the absence of a structural lesion or cerebrospinal fluid (CSF) flow abnormality. Historically, it was also referred to as benign intracranial hypertension (BIH). However, the severity of the headaches and the potential for visual field loss do not qualify as benign. It has also been referred to as idiopathic intracranial hypertension (IIH), although in some cases an associated and treatable risk factor can be identified.

Etiology

PTC may be classified as either idiopathic or symptomatic. Symptomatic etiologies include: anemia, cerebral venous occlusion, mastoiditis, radical neck dissection, hypoparathryoidism, hypervitaminosis A, lupus, renal disease, polycythemia, medication (tetracycline, minocycline, nalidixic acid, nitrofurantoin, isotretinoin, oral contraceptives, corticosteroids [withdrawal]). It is important to consider treatable symptomatic etiologies when working up for PTC. Obesity, menarche and pregnancy may be contributing factors. Treatment with levothyroxine or growth hormone has been implicated in the onset of PTC in some pediatric cases.

Clinical Presentation and Prognosis

Demographics: The stereotypical patient is a young, overweight female. This syndrome is rare in males, thin patients and prepubescent children.

Presenting signs and symptoms: Predominant symptom is a dull to severe headache (usually bilateral). There can be associated visual loss, transient visual obscurations, pulsatile tinnitus, diplopia, retro-orbital pain, and (rarely) shoulder/arm pain. Neurological examination may show visual field defects, loss of contrast sensitivity, papilledema, and uni- or bilateral cranial nerve 6 palsy.

Proposed diagnostic criteria for idiopathic PTC (Friedman & Jacobson, 2002):

1. Signs and symptoms due to elevated intracranial pressure (ICP) or papilledema.
2. Elevated CSF pressure by lumbar puncture (LP) in lateral decubitus position (>200 mm H_2O).
3. Normal CSF profile.
4. No structural abnormality on neuroimaging.
5. No alternative etiology (including medication).

Differential diagnosis: It is essential to rule out a structural lesion (such as hydrocephalus, mass lesion or tumor), and to rule out other symptomatic etiologies (which may be amenable to therapy). Differential diagnosis for PTC includes: (1) Chronic daily headache/transformed migraine; (2) chronic meningitis (infectious or neoplastic); (3) cerebral venous thrombosis; (4) hypertension; (5) gliomatosis cerebri; and (6) optic nerve head anomalies

Clinical course: Presentation with intractable headache without localizing signs may elude initial diagnostic suspicion. Development of visual field defects, papilledema, cranial nerve 6 palsy should suggest elevated intracranial pressure. Untreated, PTC may result in permanent visual loss and intractable headaches. Fortunately, following diagnostic lumbar puncture, symptoms often abate or are at least transiently mitigated. Most cases respond to lumbar puncture or medical therapy, or to identification and treatment of a secondary etiology. Only a few require ongoing escalation of medical therapy or potential surgical intervention.

Prognosis: PTC generally improves and does not require chronic medical management. However, with malignant papilledema and progressive visual loss, aggressive medical management and surgery may be necessary.

Predictors of visual loss include recent weight gain, high-grade or atrophic papilledema, subretinal hemorrhage, significant visual loss at presentation, and hypertension.

Nonpredictors of visual loss include symptom duration, transient visual obscurations, diplopia, headache severity, LP opening pressure, or pregnancy.

The most concerning signs and symptoms—"red flags"—include atypical demographics, cranial nerve palsies (other than 6), altered mentation, focal neurologic signs, abnormal CSF profile, rapid/explosive onset of signs and symptoms, intranuclear ophthalmoplegia, and vertical gaze disturbance.

Diagnosis

Lumbar puncture: Is the cornerstone of proper diagnosis. Opening pressure should be measured in the lateral decubitus position. Thresholds of above 250 mm water in adults and more than 200 mm in children have been proposed. Normal cell count and chemistry are required to make this diagnosis. It is often beneficial to remove enough CSF so that the closing pressure is under 200 mm of water.

By definition, neuroimaging (*CT / MRI*) should be normal with no structural lesion identified. In some cases, an empty sella is seen. *Ophthalmologic exam* is also required for all patients with suspected PTC. Relevant findings include papilledema, diminished visual fields and, although less likely, reduced visual acuity.

Magnetic Resonance Venography (MRV): May be added to the imaging sequences to definitively rule out venous thrombosis. Laboratory studies are helpful to rule out associated conditions including calcium, ionized calcium, complete blood count (CBC), alkaline phosphatase, parathyroid hormone (PTH) [low], and phosphorus [high]. See above under etiology for a list of commonly associated conditions.

Management

Identification and treatment of associated conditions is simple and often warranted. More definitive treatment is required for those with visual loss and sometimes for intractable headaches. Frequent ophthalmological examinations may be necessary early in the treatment to monitor for progressive visual compromise.

Lumbar puncture: Initially diagnostic, and upon identification of elevated CSF opening pressure in a likely patient, it is imperative to collect CSF to rule out abnormalities in CSF chemistry or cell counts. Enough CSF should be drawn off such that the closing pressure is reduced below 200 mm water. Often this therapeutic drainage is enough to alleviate symptoms, at least temporarily. On occasion, serial LPs may eventually provide lasting relief. Permanent drainage is often not required, but see surgery (below).

Medications: After treatment of underlying conditions and the initial lumbar puncture, use of medications is a common therapeutic intervention. The goal is reduction of CSF production so carbonic anhydrase inhibitors are the first line therapies including:

- *Acetazolamide*: From 250–1000 mg orally twice daily. Side effects include mild diuresis and distal paresthesias. Other options include methazolamide and topiramate.
- *Furosemide or other diuretics*: Can be tried if acetazolamide doesn't work.
- *Corticosteroids*: Have some limited use for intractable cases or those awaiting surgical intervention. Problems with corticosteroids include the possibility of causing rebound headaches or worsening of symptoms. Also, weaning from corticosteroids could exacerbate headaches.

Surgery: Surgical intervention is generally reserved for those with rapid/progressive visual loss and/or severe papilledema. Optic nerve sheath decompression may be done by ophthalmological surgeons retro-orbitally, and in cases with visual compromise (preferred by some).

CSF diversion may be initially undertaken by serial LPs. However, at some point more permanent drainage may be required. This is usually via an LP shunt, although some have used VP shunts. Patients without visual compromise, but intractable headaches may be candidates for this shunting rather than optic nerve fenestration, although this has not been proven.

Bariatric surgery for weight control may be a consideration in morbidly obese patients.

Diet: Weight loss may be beneficial, and for obese patients, consultation with dietary/nutrition may be valuable.

Pearls and Precautions

Avoid use of opiates or excessive analgesics, which can set the stage for rebound headaches that will invariably complicate headache management.

References

Friedman DI, Jacobson DM. Idiopathic intracranial hypertension. J Neuroophthalmol. 2004 Jun;24(2):138-45.
Friedman DI, Jacobson DM. Diagnostic criteria for idiopathic intracranial hypertension. Neurology. 2002 Nov 26;59(10):1492-5.

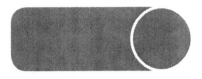

Neurocutaneous Syndromes

Neurofibromatosis

Raman Sankar, Christopher C. Giza

Neurofibromatosis (NF) is no longer considered a single disorder. The two genetically distinct forms have been named NF1 and NF2. Neurofibromatosis1 is much more common and is a classic disorder among the neurophakomatoses, involving tumors of the skin, nervous system, and other organs. Despite the prominent cerebral involvement, seizures and mental retardation constitute less of a problem in NF than in tuberous sclerosis. The range of problems in NF2 are more restricted and the clinical picture is dominated by bilateral vestibular schwannomas (acoustic neuromas). The genes involved in both NF1 and NF2 code for tumor suppressor proteins.

Etiology

The gene for NF1 resides on the 17q11.2 locus and is rather large, consisting as it does of 60 exons spread over 350 kb of genomic DNA. This size accounts for the very high mutation rate. The protein product, *neurofibromin*, inactivates the tumor gene *p21ras,* thus subserving a tumor suppressor function. The majority of mutations result in truncated and nonfunctioning neurofibromin.

The gene for NF2 has been mapped to 22q11, and codes for *merlin* (formerly schwannomin) which also serves as a tumor suppressor. It shares homology with actin-associated cytoskeletal proteins and plays a role in regulating cell-cell adhesion. It is completely absent in schwannomas, meningiomas, and ependymomas.

Clinical Presentation and Prognosis

Demographics: The more common of these disorders, NF1, is estimated to occur at a rate of 2–3 per 10,000 live births. Inheritance mode is autosomal dominant with a variable, but very high, penetrance rate. The gene mutation rate of 1 in 10,000 is among the highest in humans, and one-half of the cases appear to be sporadic.

A much lower incidence rate of one in 33,000–40,000 is estimated for NF2. Inheritance is autosomal dominant, but roughly half the cases represent spontaneous mutations.

Presenting signs and symptoms: Clinical suspicion for NF1 is often initiated by the presence of café-au-lait spots since they are present at birth (see diagnostic criteria below). The number of spots does not correlate with disease severity. Macrocephaly is often present early in children. Learning disabilities, variable degree of mental retardation, and seizures can be part of the presentation.

Skin lesions are extremely uncommon in NF2. The tumors, most commonly vestibular schwannomas (acoustic neuromas), become symptomatic around puberty or later. The most common presenting complaint is hearing loss. Dizziness or vertigo may also occur. In one series, seizures were a presenting complaint in only 8% of patients with NF2.

Clinical course and prognosis : The clinical course of NF1 can be relentlessly progressive, presenting many management challenges. Progressive cutaneous tumors, plexiform neurofibromas including those that produce exophthalmos, can be quite disfiguring and the youngster will likely need emotional support. The neurofibromas carry a 5–10% lifetime risk for malignant transformation. Skull deformities and suprasellar lesions can compromise growth hormone release and produce short stature. Even without intracranial lesions, many children experience migraine-like headaches. Intracranial tumors include optic gliomas (sometimes bilateral), and the presentation may be subtle with slight change in visual acuity and an afferent pupillary defect, or with more severe visual compromise accompanied by strabismus, papilledema, and proptosis. One study suggests that if magnetic resonance imaging (MRI) does not demonstrate optic glioma by one year of age, future studies are likely to remain negative for these tumors. However, there is an increased risk for ependymomas, meningiomas, primitive neuroectodermal tumors (PNETs), as well as malignant schwannomas of cranial nerves. Brain stem gliomas associated with NF1 are significantly more benign than in those without NF1, more likely to occur in the medulla than the pons, and are seldom treated with chemotherapy or radiotherapy. Intraspinal tumors and syringomyelia can occur. NF1 can lead to vascular problems, including a relationship with moyamoya disease, an increased risk for renovascular hypertension and a higher rate of cerebral infarction. Pheochromocytomas resulting in hypertension are not uncommon.

Bony dysplasias of long bones (especially tibia) are common, as is scoliosis. The presence of dural ectasias results in a characteristic convexity to the shape of vertebral bodies in X-rays.

Cognitive difficulties are common, although the rate of mental retardation is not particularly increased over the general population. Learning disabilities are common, and deficits in attention, performance, reading and short term memory can be encountered. Prevalence of epilepsy in this disorder is low, despite the preponderance of cerebral lesions. Seizure disorders associated with NF1 are relatively easier to manage than those encountered in patients with the tuberous sclerosis complex.

The course of NF2 is dominated by the occurrence of vestibular schwannomas, and similar tumors can occur in other cranial nerves. Cataracts are common, and ophthalmologic evaluation is recommended. Seizure and cognitive difficulties are uncommon in NF2.

Diagnosis

Diagnostic criteria for NF1

Two or more of the following:

- Six or more café-au-lait spots 1.5 cm or larger in post-pubertal individuals, 0.5 cm or larger in pre-pubertal individuals.
- Two or more neurofibromas of any type or one or more plexiform neurofibroma.
- Freckling in the axilla or groin.
- Optic glioma (tumor of the optic pathway).
- Two or more Lisch nodules (benign iris hamartomas).
- A distinctive bony lesion: Dysplasia of the sphenoid bone or dysplasia or thinning of long bone cortex.
- A first-degree relative with NF1.

Diagnostic criteria for NF2

Confirmed (definite) NF2:

- Bilateral vestibular schwannomas (VS) (also known as acoustic neuroma).

Presumptive (probable) NF2:

- Family history of NF2 (first degree family relative) plus:
- Unilateral VS or any two of the following:
- Meningioma, glioma, schwannoma, juvenile posterior subcapsular lenticular opacity, juvenile cortical cataract

Individuals with the following clinical features should be evaluated for NF2:

- Unilateral VS plus at least two of any of the following: Meningioma, glioma, schwannoma, juvenile posterior subcapsular lenticular opacities/juvenile cortical cataract
- Multiple meningiomas (2 or more) plus unilateral VS or any two of the following: Glioma, schwannoma, juvenile posterior subcapsular lenticular opacities/juvenile cortical cataract.

Management

Management of patients with NF1 as well as NF2 is symptomatic and involves the surgical specialties much more than neurologists. Neurosurgeons and orthopedic surgeons are more likely to be involved in the care of the evolving problems of the patient with NF1 while head and neck surgeons may play a more prominent role in managing NF2 patients.

Seizure management will require the customary work-up involving electroencephalography (EEG), while imaging (MRI) typically is undertaken regardless of seizures because of the other concerns described. Depending on the seizure type or epilepsy syndrome encountered, a wide choice of anticonvulsant drugs (AEDs) exists. Please see the separate tables listing available AEDs.

Coordinating the services to assist with the patient's neurocognitive function is especially important. Depending on the extent of physical disabilities, appropriate referrals need to be made.

Pearls and Precautions

1. Recognize the need for multidisciplinary approach.
2. Referral to an NF clinic in the region.
3. Depending on the extent of problems related to scoliosis, pulmonary function may be suboptimal, and regular immunization against influenzas and pneumococcal disease can be recommended.
4. Routine pediatric care should include blood pressure check (risk for renovascular hypertension).
5. Support, advocacy, social work referral regarding eligibility for social security.

References

Maria BL and Menkes JH. Neurocutaneous Syndromes, in Menkes JH, Sarnat HB, Maria BL: *Child Neurology*, Seventh Edition, Lippincott Williams & Wilkins, Philadelphia, 2006, pp.803–828.

Cross JH. Neurocutaneous syndromes and epilepsy-issues in diagnosis and management. *Epilepsia* 2005;46 Suppl 10:17–23.

Sturge-Weber Syndrome (SWS)

Raman Sankar, Christopher C. Giza

Sturge-Weber syndrome (SWS) is one of the neurophakomatoses that occurs sporadically. This condition is characterized by the triad of vascular malformations of the skin, the eye, and the central nervous system. The facial port-wine nevus and the associated localization-related epilepsy and contralateral hemiparesis and are easily recognized. It should be remembered that port-wine stains are relatively common in infants and that only about 5–15% of infants with such a dermatological finding actually have SWS.

Etiology

No genetic association has been discerned for SWS. It is an embryonic developmental anomaly involving mesodermal and ectodermal development. The underlying pathologic substrate for seizures and mental retardation is leptomeningeal angiomatosis. The vascular disturbance has its inception early in gestation (approximately 5–8 weeks) and affects poor venous drainage of the superficial cortical vessels. Vascular stasis produces chronic hypoxia of the cortex and underlying white matter, leading to atrophy and calcification. Recurrent venous thromboses may produce transient neurologic dysfunction, which may become progressive. The leptomeningeal lesion is predominantly seen in the parietal and occipital lobes, although any part of the brain can be involved. One series found 25% of the patients to have bilateral cerebral involvement. Over time, cerebral atrophy and calcification ensue, along with refractory seizures and hemiparesis.

Clinical Presentation and Prognosis

Demographics: SWS has no clear genetic pattern, and two affected individuals almost never arise in the same family. The syndrome presents in all races and with equal frequency in both sexes. Port wine stain birthmarks occur in 3 of 1000 newborns. In a patient with a facial port wine stain, the overall risk of having SWS is only about 8%–15%. The risk of having SWS increases to 25% when half of the face, including the ophthalmic division of the trigeminal nerve is involved and rises to 33% when both sides of the face, including the ophthalmic division of the trigeminal nerve are involved. See http://www.sturge-weber.org/frintro.asp.

Presenting signs and symptoms: The cutaneous port-wine stain is what alerts the clinicians to the possibility of SWS. As stated earlier, only a small minority of babies born with such a cutaneous marking actually represent patients with SWS. Glaucoma is sometimes seen in the newborn, and eventually develops in an estimated 60% of the patients. Magnetic resonance imaging can confirm cerebal involvement.

Clinical course and prognosis : Seizures develop in up to 90% of the patients and often become refractory to medical therapy. In one series, the average age of onset of seizures was around 4 months of age. Prognosis seems to vary widely, which is not surprising since the extent of the lesion as well as the inception of refractory seizures can both influence the prognosis. Ongoing ophthalmologic care can help preserve the optic nerve. Hemiparesis and hemianopsia are common, with or without hemispherectomy.

Diagnosis

The diagnosis of SWS is made on the basis of the presence of ophthalmologic or neurologic disease. The port wine nevus by itself does not constitute SWS. However, the likelihood increases when the cutaneous nevus involves the ophthalmic division of the trigeminal nerve. The preferred diagnostic modality is MRI, including a contrast study with gadolinium.

Management

Primary management aspects involve three major systems.

1. *Dermatologic:* The skin lesions respond best to very early therapy with pulsed dye laser and several treatments may be necessary. This will minimize evolving hyperpigmentation, hypertrophy, and nodularity. There is also a psychological benefit to early therapy in order to minimize the cosmetic consequences.
2. *Ophthalmologic:* Glaucoma is common, and the patient should receive periodic assessments. Many are treated with carbonic anhydrase inhibitors (to decrease aqueous humor production), and beta-blockers and/or adrenergic agonists to promote drainage) as eye drops. Trabeculotomy and/or goniotomy may also be performed to improve the drainage of aqueous humor.
3. *Neurologic: Seizures:* Develop in most patients with SWS, but not everyone develops highly refractory seizures in the first year of life. The choice of anticonvulsant medicine will depend on the various considerations mentioned in the introductory chapter on seizure management. No data exists to suggest superiority of one medication over another. One study suggested that for best results in terms of neurocognitive development, hemispherectomy should be performed early. A retrospective survey of families cast some doubt, but the methodology did not include formal testing of intellect. At our center, we are more persuaded to offer hemispherectomy early to those with medically refractory epilepsy.

In some children, transient neurologic deficits may be seen which are unrelated to epilepsy (i.e., not post-ictal phenomena), but are attributed to recurrent venous thromboses. Some clinicians advocate aspirin prophylaxis for these patients. No data are available to support or argue against this approach.

Other aspects of care that are not specific to the pathology, but require attention include management of hemiparesis—weakness, spasticity, requiring physical therapy, supportive items like ankle-foot orthotics, braces etc.

Pediatricians should weigh the need for circumstantial use of medications like diphenhydramine for either sleep or for the treatment of allergies, since the antimuscarinic effect of this medication may adversely impact the management of intraocular pressure.

Psychosocial: The facial disfigurement, spasticity, seizures, and the overall disability contribute to the need for psychosocial support and appropriate referrals.

Pearls and Precautions

1. Only a small minority of babies born with a port-wine nevus actually have Sturge-Weber syndrome.
2. Referral to a qualified dermatologist with appropriate experience improves cosmetic outcome.
3. Prompt and regular ophthalmologic care minimizes optic nerve damage.
4. Aggressive therapy, including hemispherectomy for patients with refractory seizures may help cognitive outcome.
5. It is important to address the psychosocial needs of the patient and the family.

References:

Bodensteiner JB, Roach ES. Sturge-Weber Syndrome, The Sturge-Weber Foundation, Mt Freedom, New Jersey, 1999. (various chapters)

Maria BL and Menkes JH. Neurocutaneous Syndromes, in Menkes JH, Sarnat HB, Maria BL: *Child Neurology*, Seventh Edition, Lippincott Williams & Wilkins, Philadelphia, 2006, pp.803–828.

Cross JH. Neurocutaneous syndromes and epilepsy-issues in diagnosis and management. *Epilepsia* 2005;46 Suppl 10:17–23.

Tuberous Sclerosis Complex (TSC)

Raman Sankar, Christopher C. Giza

Tuberous sclerosis complex (TSC) is a genetic disorder that is readily identified by the characteristic skin lesions and one that produces tumors in multiple organs, especially the brain, eyes, heart, kidney, skin and lungs. Major manifestations include severe, medically refractory seizures and mental retardation, especially autism spectrum disorders. Even though a multidisciplinary team is required to care for these patients, the role of the neurologist and that of the psychiatrist typically seem paramount.

Etiology

The genetic basis of TSC has been attributed to mutations in two genes whose products function together as a protein complex. Thus, the phenotypic expressions of these two defects appear to be similar. The TSC1 gene (9q34.3) codes for *hamartin*, while the TSC2 gene (16p13.3) codes for *tuberin*. The two proteins form a complex that regulates growth and proliferation by inhibiting the mammalian target of rapamycin (mTOR). A mutation in either gene results in ineffective inhibition of mTOR and exuberant, unregulated cell growth. Understanding these mechanisms may provide insight into potential therapeutic targets (see below).

Clinical Presentation and Prognosis

Demographics: Birth incidence has been estimated to be one in 6,000–9,000. The inheritance of TSC is generally autosomal dominant with variable penetrance, although more than half the cases (est. 60–70%) represent spontaneous mutations.

Presenting signs and symptoms: Two types of clinical presentations are especially common. One is a neonatal presentation due to a cardiac tumor, a rhabdomyoma. These can produce heart failure. However, if the acute situation is managed successfully, its importance diminishes over time, as the heart chamber enlarges with growth and development, while the tumor tends to regress. The other common presentation is between 4 and 8 months, with the onset of infantile spasms. Work-up at this time typically reveals characteristic skin lesions, and the MRI is quite diagnostic. Those that present with seizures well past the first year of life seem to have better prognosis for neurocognitive development. Retinal hamartomas are relatively common, while renal angiomyolipomas tend to occur later. Pulmonary lesions, typically lymphangiomatsis of the lung, are seen much more commonly in women. Other common lesions include dental pits in the enamel, periungual neurofibromas, and angiokeratomas (also known as adenoma sebaceum) of the skin, especially on the face. The last mentioned lesion can be quite disfiguring and care by an experienced dermatologist can minimize the complications of this lesion.

Clinical course and prognosis: While the cardiac lesions tend to diminish in their importance with time, the brain lesions tend to produce extremely difficult to treat seizures, neurodevelopmental (including autism spectrum disorders) problems, mental retardation of varying severity, and neuropsychiatric manifestations.

Diagnosis

The clinical criteria for diagnosis are presented in Table 11.3. The brain lesions are highly characteristic, making the diagnosis during a work-up for the seizure disorder and/or developmental delay relatively straightforward. Confirmation with the *gene tests* for TSC1 and TSC2 is commonly undertaken now, and are also sought in the parents, to facilitate genetic counseling.

The MRI diagnosis is based on the detection of (1) cortical tubers; (2) subependymal glial nodules; and (3) subependymal giant cell astrocytomas (SEGA). The last mentioned is not invariably present, but can evolve, often near the foramina of Monro, obstructing CSF drainage and producing hydrocephalus. They are treated promptly with surgery since malignant transformation is possible.

The diagnostic work-up of a patient includes initial screening with *ultrasound* interrogation of the viscera, a *consultation* with the *ophthalmologist, cardiologist,* and when indicated (as problems evolve) other specialists.

Management

Successful therapy often requires multimodal treatment approaches which may evolve and change over time. The neurologist—and when available—the psychiatrist tend to be involved in routine medical management of the patient with TSC.

Medications: The pharmacological options for the treatment of seizures associated with TSC are already covered elsewhere, since they depend on the type of seizures that are encountered (infantile spasms, Lennox-Gastaut syndrome, etc.). Special mention must be made of the utility of vigabatrin in TSC patients with infantile spasms. The efficacy of vigabatrin in this particular instance has approached 95% in some studies, and is generally excellent in all studies. Therapy with ACTH in this particular circumstance seems to often result

Table 11.3: Revised Diagnostic Criteria for Tuberous Sclerosis

Major Features	Minor Features
• Facial angiofibromas or forehead plaque	• Multiple randomly distributed pits in dental enamel
• Non-traumatic ungual or periungual fibroma	• Hamartomatous rectal polyps
• Hypomelanotic macules ('Ash-leaf spots'; more than three)	• Bone cysts
• Shagreen patch (connective tissue nevus)	• Cerebral white matter migration lines
• Multiple retinal nodular hamartomas	• Gingival fibromas
• Cortical tuber	• Non-renal hamartoma
• Subependymal nodule	• Retinal achromic patch
• Subependymal giant cell astrocytoma	• "Confetti" skin lesions
• Cardiac rhabdomyoma, single or multiple	• Multiple renal cysts
• Lymphangiomyomatosis	
• Renal angiomyolipoma	

Definite TSC: Either 2 major features or 1 major feature with 2 minor features
Probable TSC: One major feature and one minor feature
Possible TSC: Either 1 major feature or 2 or more minor features

in spasm recurrence, and there is also some concern about the effect of ACTH on cardiac rhabdomyomas. Because of the concern for retinal toxicity associated with vigabatrin, it is usually deployed only for a limited period to treat the infantile spasms, and ophthalmologic follow-up has been recommended by the FDA. The ability to prescribe vigabatrin has been restricted to registered physicians who agree to comply with the careful suggested follow-up regimen.

Because of the tenuous nature of seizure control in many patients with TSC, and the expected exacerbation with common illnesses, the availability of rescue medications can minimize the cost of visits to the emergency department while also avoiding disruptions to family life and work. Commonly used approaches include oral benzodiazepines such as lorazepam or clonazepam, as well as rectal diazepam gel when the patient's condition is more severe.

Many children and adults with TSC have significant behavioral problems, and are sometimes treated with risperidone or aripiprazole. Others may require treatment for attention or mood problems. The need for interventions to assist with learning disabilities should also be evaluated. Children who display autistic traits should be referred for behavioral intervention as early as possible. Screening for autism should be especially important as part of primary care in any patient who carries the diagnosis of TSC.

Please see sections under Infantile Spasms, Lennox-Gastaut syndrome, and Management of Spasticity for the management of other common problems.

An important emerging area of therapeutic investigations pertains to mTOR inhibitors (rapamycin) to treat SEGAs, and if early treatment with mTOR inhibitors may ameliorate the development of epilepsy.

Dietary therapy: Dietary therapy may be especially of benefit to patients with TSC. Responders often experience significant seizure reduction as well as increased alertness and improved behavior (likely due to diminished AED burden as well as seizure reduction). The most stringent form of dietary therapy, the ketogenic diet, has the best evidence for efficacy, but requires considerable effort on the part of the family. Recent literature indicates some benefit also from a modified Atkins' diet, as well as a low-glycemic index therapy. Dietary therapy should only be undertaken in collaboration with a center experienced in its implementation, and requires careful physical and laboratory follow-up.

Surgery: Neurosurgical intervention commonly involves resection of SEGAs, and of ventriculo-peritoneal shunt placement for hydrocephalus when indicated. Despite the presence of multiple cerebral lesions capable of producing seizures, select patients may be eligible for resective therapy. The evaluation process for determining that seizures are not of substantially multifocal origin, and weighing the risk of potential neurologic deficits versus benefit of improved seizure control—and, sometimes, associated behavioral problems, secondary to the reduction in seizure and medication burden—is a highly specialized one and is not in the scope of primary care practice. Those who are not candidates for a focal resection may benefit from the vagus nerve stimulation. But, most patients with TSC will benefit from referral to a comprehensive epilepsy center, where the various options for management of complex seizure disorders may be explored.

In the United States, there are also regional centers of excellence for TSC which operate multidisciplinary TSC clinics. These centers benefit from coordination by the *Tuberous Sclerosis Alliance* (http://www.tsalliance.org/), which is dedicated to advocacy for the patient and family as well as to fostering research.

Therapy: Young children with TSC may benefit from physical, occupational, and speech therapy. There are usually state supported centers for providing such services until the child enters the school system. Some of these agencies also provide respite assistance with visiting personnel for the family. It is especially important to be alert and recognize signs of autism early and make appropriate referrals.

Social: Caring for a child with TSC imposes considerable burden on the family. They may require social services such as respite care, and may benefit from referrals to support groups such as the Epilepsy Foundation and the Tuberous Sclerosis Alliance. They may also require advocacy with the school system. Transporting the child becomes more challenging as the patient grows to a larger physical proportion, and the physician can assist with the obtaining of a handicapped permit from the Department of Motor Vehicles.

Pearls and Precautions

1. Recognize the need for multidisciplinary approach.
2. Early referral to a TS clinic if available within reach.
3. Comprehensive Epilepsy Centers may be of great help in defining options for seizure management.
4. Important referrals, almost always: neurology, psychiatry, ophthalmology, cardiology, nephrology, dermatology.
5. Since common illnesses produce seizure exacerbation, maintain immunization status.
6. Recognize the need for rescue therapy and implement.
7. Support, support, support, do not forget advocating for respite care.

References:

Maria BL and Menkes JH. Neurocutaneous Syndromes, in Menkes JH, Sarnat HB, Maria BL: *Child Neurology*, Seventh Edition, Lippincott Williams & Wilkins, Philadelphia, 2006, pp.803–828.

Chiron C, Dumas C, Jambaqué I, Mumford J, Dulac O. Randomized trial comparing vigabatrin and hydrocortisone in infantile spasms due to tuberous sclerosis. *Epilepsy Res* 1997;26:389–95.

Curatolo P, Bombardieri R, Cerminara C. Current management for epilepsy in tuberous sclerosis complex. *Curr Opin Neurol* 2006;19:119–23.

Kossoff EH, Thiele EA, Pfeifer HH, McGrogan JR, Freeman JM. Tuberous sclerosis complex and the ketogenic diet. *Epilepsia* 2005;46:1684–6.

Elliott RE, Carlson C, Kalhorn SP, Moshel YA, Weiner HL, Devinsky O, Doyle WK. Refractory epilepsy in tuberous sclerosis: Vagus nerve stimulation with or without subsequent resective surgery. *Epilepsy Behav* 2009;16:454–60.

Franz DN, Leonard J, Tudor C, Chuck G, Care M, Sethuraman G, Dinopoulos A, Thomas G, Crone KR. Rapamycin causes regression of astrocytomas in tuberous sclerosis complex. *Ann Neurol* 2006;59:490–8.

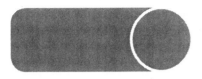

Neurodevelopmental Disorders

Cerebral Palsy (CP)

Christopher C. Giza, Raman Sankar

Cerebral palsy (CP) is a disorder of movement and posture resulting from NONPROGRESSIVE damage/ injury to the developing brain. It is a syndrome, a constellation of clinical signs and symptoms, rather than a specific diagnosis with a specific etiology.

Etiology

The *definite cause of CP is not known for MOST cases.* However, there are many potential causes that have been implicated in the development of CP. Awareness of these potential etiologies sheds some insight into the subtype of CP and its prognosis. Such etiologies include the following: (1) Pre- / Perinatal infection; (2) Pre- / Perinatal stroke or cerebral infarction; (3) Perinatal asphyxia; (4) Cerebral malformations; (5) Metabolic disorders; and (6) Kernicterus.

Clinical Presentation and Prognosis

Demographics: It is estimated that 1.2–2.5 out of 1000 children are diagnosed with CP by early school age. This amounts to 5000 new cases per year in the U.S. Due to increased survival of very low birth weight infants and the higher risk for a neurological insult during the neonatal care of these premature babies, there is an increased incidence of CP in this group.

Presenting signs and symptoms: There are 3 early clinical presentations and 3 chronic presentations of CP. In addition, there is clinical classification of CP based upon the major motor impairment. Understanding these classifications and their interaction give the care provider an understanding of the etiology, the likely problems and the prognosis, for any individual patient.

Clinical Syndromes / Early Presentations: There are 3 main early clinical settings that can be associated with later diagnosis of CP. Two of these will occur in the hospital in the neonatal period. The first is low birth weight / premature infants. The typical presentation includes delayed respiration, neonatal resuscitation, low Apgars (though low Apgar scores alone do NOT necessarily lead to CP), seizures and hypotonia. The patients may experience significant hypoxia, acidosis, intracranial/intraventricular hemorrhage and/or sepsis in the neonatal period, and often require extensive care in the neonatal ICU. The second clinical setting includes sick full term infants. These patients may also present with difficult deliveries and require neonatal resuscitation. They may have seizures, jitteriness/myoclonus, birth hypoxia/asphyxia, hypotonia and sepsis. Intraventricular hemorrhage is less common in full term infants. The third setting for CP is actually in otherwise well full term infants who present with a delayed onset of signs and symptoms. These babies may have a distant in utero event like a stroke or may have cerebral malformations, but are born relatively healthy. The immaturity of the newborn nervous system results in a normal newborn neurological examination and deficits only become apparent as the child develops.

Clinical Syndromes/Late Presentations: There are also 3 clinical scenarios for late presentation for CP, and these correspond to the late outcomes from the 3 early syndromes discussed above. These would typically be seen in a clinic setting. The low birth weight / premature infants who go on to show signs of CP often show spastic diplegia and/or a hemideficit. These outcomes are due to either periventricular leukomalacia (PVL) or a focal ischemic event in the perinatal period. Sick full term infants more often experience a global insult such as hypoxia, infection or a metabolic disturbance. These etiologies can lead to a later spastic quadriparesis or extrapyramidal signs. Well full term infants who present with later signs have CP that is etiology-dependent (post-natally acquired brain injury, in utero ischemic injury, cerebral malformation). These patients may show hemideficits, dyskinesias or athetosis.

Classification: Classification of CP subtype is often based upon the predominant chronic motor deficit. This classification suggests an underlying clinical syndrome, that has concomitant associations with particular etiologies and with specific long-term prognostic implications. The most common subtype of CP is SPASTIC: Simply put, this means CP characterized by pathologically increased muscle tone in the trunk and/or limbs. Spastic diplegia primarily affects patients' lower extremities. This is often associated with PVL (above) as a late consequence of prematurity, birth asphyxia (in a premie), and intraventricular/germinal matrix hemorrhage. The hallmark of spastic hemiplegia is that both extremities on one side are primarily affected. Spastic hemiplegia is due to an underlying focal etiology that can occur any time through gestation and into the neonatal period. Early in utero insults may present as a delayed onset of signs in a previously well infant, whereas perinatal cerebral infarction may present as an acutely ill neonate, often with a superimposed global insult. Spastic quadriplegia typically is seen after a diffuse hypoxic or metabolic injury and results in having all four extremities affected. The next most common form of CP is Dyskinetic/extraphramidal: The primary motor manifestations of this form of CP include dystonia, athetosis and chorea. ATAXIC CP is fairly rare and can be associated with cerebellar malformations. Another rarer form of CP is HYPOTONIC; this may evolve over time into other forms of CP, particularly dyskinetic/extrapyramidal CP, and the persistence of neurological abnormality distinguishes them from those with benign hypotonia of infancy.

Clinical course: The clinical course for CP is one of stable, nonprogressive motor impairment, often with concomitant cognitive and functional deficits. The specifics of clinical course for each CP syndrome are described above. It should be noted that some infants who appear normal may later develop clinical signs of CP such as spasticity. Infants with hypotonic CP may evolve into spastic or dyskinetic forms as their nervous systems mature. These changes do not represent neurodegeneration, but rather reflect ongoing cerebral development in the setting of a fixed neurological lesion. Common sequelae associated with CP include cognitive impairment, delayed development of locomotion, and onset of epilepsy.

Prognosis: First and foremost, CP is nonprogressive!! However, the outward signs and symptoms of CP may change with ongoing brain development (see above). There are 3 main areas where parents and care providers have concern for long-term prognosis, and the outcome is related to the subtype of CP. First is ambulation. Up to 95–99% of hemiplegic CP patients eventually ambulate, with or without assistive devices. Among spastic diplegics, this proportion remains above 50%. Conversely, very few quadriplegics achieve ambulation. Those with extrapyramidal CP have variable ambulatory outcomes. Second is cognition. By far, pure hemiplegics show the highest rates of normal intelligence quotient (IQ), and extrapyramidal CP patients also show relative cognitive sparing. In fact, dyskinetic/extrapyramidal CP patients are often misjudged as to their intelligence, particularly if their movement disorder is very prominent. About half of spastic diplegics can show normal or low normal cognition. Quadriplegics show the greatest cognitive impairments, and rarely demonstrate normal IQs. Epileptic seizures must be distinguished from tremors, clonus and other abnormal movements. Over half of quadriplegics will develop epilepsy at some point. Seizures occur in around 50% of hemiplegics and maybe a slightly lower percentage of spastic diplegics. Extrapyramidal CP patients have variable rates of epilepsy, but seizures are generally rarest in this group.

Management

The mainstay of medical management for CP centers on treatment of spasticity and prevention of seizures.

Medications: Antispasticity treatment consists of systemic medications (baclofen, tizanidine, dantrolene, benzodiazepines), focal medications (botulinum toxin), intrathecal medications (intrathecal baclofen). These, along with nonpharmacological management of spasticity are discussed in the separate section of the same title.

Treatment of seizures is also summarized in the separate treatment section. In short, it consists primarily of anticonvulsants chosen based on seizure type and side effect profile. For individuals with focal lesions, surgical resection may be considered in selected cases. Vagal nerve stimulation can be palliative for intractable seizures. In addition, the ketogenic diet provides improvement in up to 20–30% of those with medically intractable seizures.

Surgery: Surgical intervention involves one of the three following procedures.

1. Release of contractures/tendon lengthening.
2. Dorsal rhizotomy: Surgical section of posterior roots.
3. Vagal nerve stimulation or surgical resection may be used for some individuals with intractable seizures.

Therapy: Supportive care is an important part of the management of CP patients.

1. Vision assessment, correction of misalignment.
2. Hearing assessment, hearing aids.
3. Motor assessment, PT/OT, range of motion, assistive devices for locomotion, orthotics.
4. Language assessment, speech therapy, assistive communication devices.

Social: There are several national organizations and support groups for CP patients such as United Cerebral Palsy (www.ucp.org), which also has many local chapters.

Pearls and Precautions

Nutrition: Patients with CP should have balanced nutrition and adequate calories. In severe cases, gastrojejunostomy (G/J)-tube may be necessary to provide sufficient intake. Also, osteoporosis can be a problem chronically, particularly for CP patients who are not weight-bearing. Calcium supplementation and monitoring of bone density may be helpful. New devices that support patients in weight bearing postures and vibrate rapidly are being investigated as potentially helpful for maintaining bone density.

Aspiration precautions: Patients with uncoordinated swallowing require careful aspiration precautions, foods of certain consistencies, speech/swallowing therapy and may ultimately require tracheostomy, Nissen fundoplication and/or G/J-tube to prevent recurrent aspiration pneumonia. They may be evaluated with a barium swallowing study.

Toilet: Bowel and bladder care are important to avoid UTI and skin breakdown in more debilitated patients.

Likely complications: CP patients can live for many years. Due to the nonprogressive nature of their neurological injury, good medical care can result in a much improved quality of life for these patients and their families. Coordination of care by a primary physician often contributes substantially to this quality of life.

School/education: CP patients may have relatively spared cognitive abilities in comparison to their motor impairments, particularly those with hemiplegic and extrapyramidal CP. All should have careful cognitive assessments and individualized education plans to maximize their potential. Assistive devices and communication boards may be particularly important.

References

Dodge NN. Cerebral Palsy: medical aspects. Pediatr Clin N Am. 2008 Oct;55(5):1189-207.

Shankaran S. Prevention, diagnosis, and treatment of cerebral palsy in near-term and term infants. Clin Obstet Gynecol. 2008 Dec;51(4):829-39.

Management of Spasticity

Christopher C. Giza, Raman Sankar

Spasticity refers to a state of increased muscle tone that increases with the speed of movement, generally indicative of chronic damage or injury to upper motor neurons. Spasticity is a final common outcome after many types of pediatric neurological conditions, both congenital (cerebral dysgenesis, cerebral palsy, etc.); and acquired (traumatic brain injury, post-encephalitic, post-anoxic, etc.). It can be clinically distinguished from two other movement disorders associated with increased muscle tone, namely rigidity and dystonia. Rigidity is characterized by a uniform increase in muscle tone across the full range of motion regardless of the speed of movement. Dystonia is generally an abnormal motor position due to forced contraction of a muscle or muscles that may distort the limb or body part.

All forms of abnormally increased tone may result in motor impairment, delayed motor milestones, impaired coordination, skin breakdown, orthopedic problems, and chronic pain. The aim of antispasticity treatment is to identify the etiology (fixed problem vs. progressive problem), provide pharmacotherapy aimed at improving muscle tone and reducing pain, correct orthopedic misalignments and optimize the patient's functional state.

Etiology

There are many causes of spasticity. These may be characterized as nonprogressive or progressive. Nonprogressive causes are usually due to an injury to the developing nervous system and may be classified as congenital or acquired. Congenital etiologies are generally secondary to cerebral malformations (Chiari malformations, schizencephaly, lissencephaly, cortical dysplasia, etc.); or, other in utero neurological insults (cerebral infarction, congenital infection, congenital hydrocephalus). Acquired etiologies are due to an injury or insult to a previously normally developing central nervous system (hypoxic-ischemic encephalopathy, meningoencephalitis, traumatic brain or spinal cord injury, brain tumor, transverse myelitis). Most spastic types of cerebral palsy would fit into this category.

Progressive etiologies of spasticity are generally due to an underlying ongoing disease process. This would include progressive degenerative or metabolic disorders. Leukodystrophies (white matter disorders) often overlap between degenerative and metabolic etiologies, and typically result in intermittent or progressive spasticity and motor impairment. Examples of degenerative diseases that have prominent progressive spasticity include Rett syndrome, Friedriech ataxia and multiple sclerosis. Many primary metabolic disorders may also show progressive spasticity as the disease advances. Some examples of these include adrenoleukodystrophy, Krabbe disease and subacute combined degeneration/vitamin B12 deficiency. Some progressive etiologies may be mixed, such as the gradual spinal cord compression that can occur in patients with mucopolysaccharidoses.

Determining the etiology of spasticity can be important in case there is a specific treatment for the underlying disease, such as decompressive procedures for Chiari malformations. Beyond that, the management of the spasticity itself, and the potential complications that arise from this abnormal muscle tone should also be important considerations in the proper care of these patients.

Clinical Presentation and Prognosis

Associated signs and symptoms: While the evolution of spasticity may take place over months or even years, the signs and symptoms associated with spasticity include increased muscle tone, hyperactive deep tendon reflexes, muscle spasms, clonus and upgoing Babinski responses. Weakness and incoordination may occur in paretic or paralyzed limbs, and joint contractures and discomfort are also common. In infants, early signs associated with spasticity can include persistent or asymmetric cortical thumbs/fisting, asymmetries of neonatal/infantile reflexes and scissoring of the lower extremities on vertical suspension. On the other hand, an upgoing Babinski response may be normal up to 9–12 months of age, particularly if symmetric.

Clinical course: Even in patients with nonprogressive etiologies, the clinical manifestations of spasticity may still change over time. For infants with in utero or early postnatal acquired central nervous system (CNS) injuries, the initial motor manifestations of the insult may be undetectable or may be subtle, such as development of a clear hand preference or an asymmetric Moro response in an infant (this would suggest that the nonpreferred hand is paretic). As motor development proceeds, an increase in motor tone and a delay in motor development in the affected limbs may be noted. Asymmetries in upper extremity motor function become more apparent with the onset of voluntary reaching, grasping and rolling over at the ages of 3–6 months and after. Abnormalities in lower extremity tone and motor function may become apparent slightly later, from 6–12 months as the infant begins learning to sit, crawl and stand. During this stage of development, asymmetries may be discerned in the emergence of protective reflexes, such as the buttressing and parachuting responses. These changes in motor function, when secondary to a fixed neurological insult, do not represent worsening of the condition, but merely superimposition of ongoing development onto the nonprogressive injury.

For nonprogressive spasticity acquired later in childhood, the acute onset of a CNS injury may occur secondary to trauma, hemorrhage, infarction, etc., and the initial tone manifestation may be one of hypotonia in the affected limb/limbs. For example, a patient with an acute spinal cord injury may initially present with spinal shock and flaccid hypotonia and paralysis in all muscles below the level of the injury. Over time (days-weeks), however, there is gradually increasing muscle tone. Again, these changes in motor function do not generally represent progression of the initial lesion, but the natural evolution of the injury and the recovery process.

Progressive cases of spasticity tend to vary in their course depending upon the underlying cause. Degenerative diseases such as Rett syndrome have gradually worsening of spasticity, but also may show particular problems with spasticity during particular stages of the underlying disorder. Metabolic diseases that present with intermittent attacks may show stepwise progression of increasing spasticity with each attack. Storage disorders that can cause spinal cord compression may show gradually worsening paraparesis with delay or even regression of motor skills.

Management

General rules for spasticity management include the following: (1) Interventions for spasticity should be undertaken only when spasticity is results in problems (impaired function, pain, poor hygiene and/or cosmesis); (2) benefits of reducing spasticity should be balanced with the potential loss of 'useful' spasticity (increased tone that may aid function in certain circumstances); (3) goals should be realistic but be set jointly by the patient/parent and medical caregiver; and (4) medical or surgical interventions aid but do not substitute for regular individualized physical and/or occupational therapy.

Medications: Oral medications are best when spasticity is mild and/or widespread. They are generally simpler to administer, but have the potential for systemic side effects. Medication-induced tone reductions can, on occasion, result in diminished function. If, for example, lower extremity stiffness functionally compensates for concomitant lower extremity weakness, then reduction of this spasticity/stiffness might result in impaired transfers, standing or ambulating.

1. *Baclofen:* The recommended starting dose is 2.5–5 mg orally daily or up to three times daily (qd-tid). Titrate upward to the following maximums: 2–7 years of age—40 mg/day; 8–11 years—60 mg/day; and, >12 years—80 mg/day. Adverse effects include weakness and sedation. Rarely, seizure exacerbation may occur, but this should not discourage a careful trial. Discontinuation must be performed gradually to avoid withdrawal.

2. *Tizanidine:* The starting dose for tizanidine is 1–2 mg orally at bedtime. It may be titrated up to 4–8 mg/day divided three times daily. Side effects include potential hepatotoxicity, sedation and weakness. This agent may be particularly effective for spasticity causing discomfort during sleep. Clonidine has a similar mechanism of action as tizanidine, and is used in pediatrics for other indications; however, its efficacy as an antispasticity agent is unproven.

3. *Diazepam:* Diazepam has been shown efficacious in children, either alone or in combination with dantrolene. Daily dosage ranges from 0.12–0.8 mg/kg divided into 3 or 4 doses. Sedation is often a limiting side effect, although this agent may be used similarly to tizanidine, above. Longer acting benzodiazepines such as clonazepam or clorazapate may also be tried.

4. *Dantrolene:* This agent works systemically at the level of muscle and thus has less sedation and CNS problems as side effects. Shown to be effective at reducing spasticity in pediatric populations. Starting dose may begin at 0.5 mg/kg/day and be titrated up to 2 mg po tid. Hepatotoxicity is a concern and occurs in about 1% of those taking it.

5. *Other muscle relaxants (cyclobenzaprine, methocarbamol, carisoprodol):* These agents are unproven for spasticity but have been used for muscle spasms in adults and may be second- or third-line considerations for older adolescents in selected cases.

6. *Botulinum toxin:* Botulinum toxin (BoNT) works by preventing presynaptic neurotransmitter release, and thus selectively paralyzing/weakening the injected muscle. One of the major advantages of BoNT is the absence of CNS side effects. Dosing of BoNT varies substantially with both serotype (types A and B are currently available), as well as with brand. The beneficial effects of BoNT include reduction in spasticity, improved function and pain relief. These improvements may last approximately 3 months, requiring repeated injections to maintain efficacy. Over time, immunoresistance to the toxin may develop, and has been reported in about 3% of adult recipients.

Surgery

1. *Orthopedic surgery/release of contractures/tendon lengthening:* As a general rule, orthopedic surgery should be delayed until the gait is mature (after 6–10 years of age), and PT/medical therapy is helpful while waiting. Common orthopedic problems requiring intervention in this patient population include hip subluxation/dislocation and equinovarus foot. Some advocate for staged procedures, although simultaneous multilevel surgical intervention has been proposed to minimize recovery times and accelerate mobilization.

2. *Dorsal rhizotomy:* This is a selective surgical section of posterior (sensory) spinal nerve roots with the goal of interrupting the hyperactive afferent component of spasticity. This procedure is sometimes done with intraoperative EMG, although it is unclear whether this additional monitoring definitively improves outcomes. Most studies indicate obvious reductions in spasticity, although objective improvements in global function are more difficult to demonstrate definitively. Complications include back pain (approximately 10%), sensory changes and neurogenic bladder or bowel disturbances. Weakness is a theoretical concern but is not prominently reported. Dorsal rhizotomy may be particularly helpful for young children (ages 4–8 years old) with predominantly lower extremity spasticity and relatively preserved lower extremity strength. Most will eventually require orthopedic surgical correction of spasticity-induced deformities. Post-operative PT/medical therapy is essential to long-term recovery.

3. *Intrathecal Baclofen:* Direct delivery of baclofen intrathecally reduces the overall dosage to about 1% of the oral dose, and greatly decreases problems with sedation and CNS side effects. Evaluation may begin with a screening dose administered via lumbar puncture; if effective, then a catheter trial may be implemented with gradual titration of the intrathecal (IT) baclofen dosage up to a maintenance level. Baclofen pumps are programmable with a telemetry wand, and contain a transdermal drug reservoir that is typically refilled every 2–3 months. Complications of intrathecal baclofen include infection, accidental overdosing (which can cause coma and respiratory complications) or abrupt withdrawal (due to running out of drug, or catheter or pump malfunction).

Baclofen withdrawal can be a serious syndrome and deaths have been reported. Clinical signs of baclofen withdrawal include increased spasticity, dysautonomia (tachycardia, hypo- or hypertension, and, in males, priapism), encephalopathy, paresthesia/pruritis and reduced seizure threshold. Recognition of withdrawal and restoration of baclofen therapy is the intervention of choice, while general supportive measures and intravenous benzodiazepines may be helpful and/or necessary during the acute phase.

Therapy: Stretching and PT are useful to address range of motion, particularly while the child is developing. These interventions may temporize the need for definitive surgery until the child reaches the appropriate age. Ongoing physical and occupational therapy will likely be necessary to maintain the gains from any surgical corrections.

Intensive PT (1 hour/day, 5 days/week) did not appear to provide any long-term additional benefit when compared to regular amounts of PT in several studies. One study showed greater compliance with PT when it was administered on an intermittent rather than a continuous schedule.

Constraint-induced therapy involves using a brace or splint to immobilize the child's better functioning upper limb, and has been suggested to improve function in the more impaired limb. Initially studied after strokes, this type of therapy also appears to have benefits for children with hemiparetic upper extremities due to cerebral palsy.

Ankle-foot orthoses (AFOs) are helpful to prevent excessive plantar flexion due to increased lower extremity spasticity. This may improve standing and gait.

Social: It is important to discuss the practical aspects of spasticity management with the patient/parent. Sometimes, the main issue is difficulty getting dressed or changing a diaper. Discussing these objectives makes developing a management plan more collaborative and realistic.

Pearls and Precautions

Nutrition: Feeding may pose particular problems for individuals with clinically significant spasticity. Severely affected quadriparetic patients may also have brainstem involvement and be at risk for aspiration. Upper extremity spasticity and weakness may require occupational therapy and assistive devices to allow the patient to effectively feed him/herself.

Sleep: Painful spasms may interfere with sleep. The sedation side effect of most oral antispasticity agents may be beneficial in these patients when dosed before bedtime.

Skin care: Decreased mobility and abnormal resting postures may create pressure points and increase potential for skin breakdown and decubitus ulcers. Careful range-of-motion and turning of severely spastic patients, as well as careful and regular skin inspections are necessary to avoid these complications. Proper fitting of orthotics and ambulatory assistive devices is also important.

Toileting: Patients with spasticity may also have concomitant difficulties with bowel and bladder function. Sometimes, this is due to relative immobility (causing increased risk for constipation and/or difficulty with hygiene), and sometimes the cause of the spasticity may cause neurogenic bowel/bladder problems (e.g., after spinal cord injury). Proper evaluation and treatment should be coordinated. This may include urological consultation, intermittent catheterization or anticholinergic medications to help with bladder function.

References

Tilton A. Management of spasticity in children with cerebral palsy. Semin Pediatr Neurol. 2009 Jun;16(2):82-9.

Wusthoff CJ, Shellhaas RA, Licht DJ. Management of common neurologic symptoms in pediatric palliative care: seizures, agitation, and spasticity. Pediatr Clin North Am. 2007 Oct;54(5):709-33.

Autism

Christopher C. Giza, Raman Sankar

Autism is a developmental syndrome of disordered brain function characterized by a triad of: (1) Impaired social interaction; (2) verbal/nonverbal communication problems; and (3) unusual or severely limited behaviors or interests. Autism and autistic spectrum disorders (ASDs) refer to a group of developmental disorders that generally includes classic autism, Asperger syndrome, and pervasive developmental disorder-not otherwise specified (NOS). Childhood disintegrative disorder and Rett syndrome represent distinct disorders that can have prominent autistic features, but are generally not included under the umbrella of ASDs.

Etiology

Autism and ASDs are a clinical syndrome that probably represents many different etiologies that have a common behavioral and developmental phenotype. There is a genetic risk, with a high concordance in twin studies (>70%). With one autistic child, the estimated risk of having a 2nd child with autism has been reported to be approximately 5%. Advanced paternal age may also be a risk factor. It is important to note that NO causal relationship was identified between vaccines/thimerosal and autism in many high-quality epidemiological studies.

Less than 10% of cases of autism are associated with an underlying medical condition or known genetic syndrome.

Clinical Presentation and Prognosis

Demographics: There has been an apparent increase in the incidence of autism over the last few decades. The cause of this has been much debated, but it does not appear to be solely due to broader diagnostic criteria. The theory that increased rates of autism are due to increases in vaccinations has effectively been disproven by multiple, well-done investigations.

The reported incidence of autism depends to some extent upon the diagnostic criteria applied: It is estimated to be about 1/150–200 persons for ASD, while substantially rarer (1/500) for strict autism. The male:female ratio is about 4:1.

Presenting signs and symptoms: Symptoms usually appear within the first 1–3 years of life. Severity varies widely from very unusual, repetitive, aggressive and self-injurious behavior, to relatively mild personality disturbances with some developmental delay. There is a classic triad of symptoms that is seen to varying degrees in the ASDs and are listed here:

1. *Impaired socialization (ASD):* ASD children are nonresponsive to name, demonstrate poor eye contact and inappropriate response to facial expression or tone of voice, and are unaware of feelings of others.
2. *Delayed/impaired language skills:* Language development is one of the most noticeable issues in these children. They are slow to start speaking, and have limited range of topics. More severely affected children may not gain useful language abilities.
3. *Repetitive, restricted movements, behaviors or interests:* Rocking, spinning, and hair twirling are some of the typical repetitive motions noted in these children.

The relative severity and timing of the neurobehavioral deficits differs among several variations of autism. There are at least 5 clinical diagnoses listed in the DSM-IV, each with a slightly different combination of signs and symptoms. Numbers 1, 2 and 3 are often collectively referred to as the autistic spectrum disorders (ASDs, see above). These diagnostic categories of the ASDs are eliminated in the proposed revisions to the DSM-5.

1. *Autistic disorder:* 'Classic' autism; triad listed above.
2. *Pervasive developmental disorder-NOS:* 'Atypical' autism; some autistic symptoms, but not enough to be diagnosed with classical form.
3. *Asperger syndrome:* Autistic behavior with better developed language function.
4. *Rett syndrome:* Females, acquired microcephaly, seizures, autistic behavior.
5. *Childhood disintegrative disorder:* Normal development thru 2–4 years of age, then severe deterioration and regression.

Other areas of impairment include motor delay, sleep disturbances, gastrointestinal disturbances, epilepsy, developmental regression, sensory abnormalities (insensitive or overly sensitive), self-injurious behavior and psychiatric diagnoses (ADHD, conduct, aggression, mood disorders).

Clinical course: Signs and symptoms may be detectable early in infancy in some cases, but many do not become clear until after the age of 12 months or later. There may then be a notable delay or regression in language and communication skills, increasing concern for abnormal socialization, and/or more obvious restriction of interests or behaviors. Rett syndrome has a well-described course (see chapter on Rett), and childhood disintegrative disorders tend to have a later onset but a more fulminant course.

Most autistic children will demonstrate signs and symptoms as a toddler, and while regression can occur, challenges also arise from delayed development of higher social and communication skills that become more and more obvious as the affected child falls rapidly behind developing peers. Asperger children will often have very functional language, but still demonstrate deficits in the other 2 parts of the triad. The behavioral impairments associated with ASDs may show signs of improvement with maturation, but these children are also not immune to the sometimes abrupt social and developmental problems that arise with adolescence, and may have fewer resources with which to meet them.

Prognosis: Most individuals with ASDs will demonstrate some degree of social and communicative impairment lifelong, although outcomes can vary across a broad range. About 50% of children with ASDs will have an intelligent quotient (IQ) above 70, and, while facing social or behavioral challenges, would not be considered cognitively disabled. Those with Asperger syndrome may often be able to live independently, and can even excel in particular tasks/jobs that require attention to details and less social interaction. Patients with Rett and childhood disintegrative disorder invariably have regression and require increasing levels of care and support.

Diagnosis

The diagnoses of autistic disorder and Asperger syndrome are based upon clinical criteria, parental report and observation, without any definitive diagnostic test.

For autistic disorder, patients will demonstrate at least 6 items from the following 3 behavioral categories.

1. *Impaired social interaction (≥2 of the following):* Impaired nonverbal behaviors (eye contact, facial expression, body gestures, etc.); lack of age-appropriate peer relationships; lack of spontaneous sharing of interests or enjoyment with others; lack of social/emotional reciprocity.

2. *Impaired communication (≥1 of the following):* Delay or total lack of language; inability to initiate or sustain a conversation; stereotyped language use, lack of age-appropriate make-believe or imitative play.

3. *Restricted or stereotyped behavior or interests (≥1 of the following):* Preoccupation with one or more narrow areas of interest, inflexible adherence to routines/rituals; stereotyped motor mannerisms (hand flapping, twisting, spinning, etc.); persistent preoccupation with parts of objects.

In addition, delayed or abnormal function in social interaction, social language and/or symbolic play will be noted before 3 years of age, and the individual's impairments are not due to Rett or childhood disintegrative disorder.

For Asperger syndrome, affected individuals will show impairments in the following 2 behavioral categories.

1. *Impaired social interaction (≥2 of the following):* Impaired nonverbal behaviors (eye contact, facial expression, body gestures, etc.); lack of age-appropriate peer relationships; lack of spontaneous sharing of interests or enjoyment with others; lack of social/emotional reciprocity.

2. *Restricted or stereotyped behavior or interests (≥1 of the following):* Preoccupation with one or more narrow areas of interest; inflexible adherence to routines/rituals; stereotyped motor mannerisms (hand flapping, twisting, spinning, etc.); persistent preoccupation with parts of objects.

In addition, there will be clinical significant impairment in social or occupational functioning and yet no clinically significant delay in language and no clinically significant delay in cognition. Criteria for other pervasive developmental disorders or schizophrenia are not met.

Early screening for language problems should be prompted by the following "RED FLAGS" shown in Table 11.4.

Differential diagnosis: Autism may be confused with hearing loss, speech problems, mental retardation, and other types of developmental delay. However, the majority of cases are of unknown etiology and unassociated

Table 11.4: Red Flags for Early Language Screening

Age	Problem or Presenting Sign/Symptom
6 months	No vocalization
12 months	No multisyllable babbling sounds
18 months	No single words (mimicked or echoed words don't count)
24 months	No spontaneous phrases
36 months	No spontaneous sentences
Any time	Any loss of babbling, single words or phrases
Any time	Any loss of understanding/comprehension, including response to name

with another disorder. Autistic behavior can be a manifestation of Angelman syndrome, congenital rubella, fragile X syndrome, tuberous sclerosis, PKU, fetal alcohol syndrome, Rett syndrome and Smith-Lemli-Opitz syndrome. While schizophrenics may have autistic-like behavior, other hallmarks of schizophrenia, such as hallucinations and delusions, are not typically autistic.

Autism may coexist with Tourette syndrome, learning disabilities, epilepsy, ADHD and other psychiatric diagnoses.

Diagnostic testing can be targeted to detect underlying etiology or comorbid conditions in selected patients. Careful cutaneous exam including *Wood's lamp* exam will help identify neurocutaneous syndromes. *Hearing testing* is essential in cases of language delay. *Serum lead testing* may be used to monitor for toxicity in patients with pica. *Fragile X genetic testing* and *microarray comparative genomic hybridization* may be indicated.

MRI is the imaging study of choice if structural neurological abnormalities are suspected, such as those with focal neurological deficits or neurocutaneous syndromes. *EEG* is helpful for determining the type of seizure in ASD patients with epilepsy, but routine screening of those with ASDs is not indicated. This is due to a high rate of interictal epileptiform abnormalities in asymptomatic children with ASDs. So while it is helpful to treat seizures, there is no clear evidence that treating these types of EEG abnormalities in the absence of seizures results in any behavioral improvements. *Metabolic workup* is generally not recommended as a screening test in those with ASDs, but may be indicated in settings of intermittent encephalopathy, cycling vomiting, early seizures, dysmorphic or coarsened features and/or ongoing developmental regression. See below for unproven diagnostic tests that should generally be avoided.

Management

There are no curative interventions. Treatments are supportive and targeted to the specific problems demonstrated by the individual.

Medications: Targeted to underlying medical/behavioral conditions or diagnoses.

1. *Epilepsy:* Anywhere from 11–39% of individuals with ASDs will also have epilepsy. Anticonvulsants should be administered when epilepsy/seizures are diagnosed, based upon the proper therapy for that particular type of epilepsy.
2. Repetitive behaviors and Obsessive Compulsive Disorder symptoms: SSRIs (fluoxetine, fluvoxamine, citalprolam, escitalprolam, paroxetine, sertraline), antitypical antipsychotics (risperdone, aripiprazole, olanzapine, quetiapine, ziprasidone), valproate.
3. Hyperactivity/attention problems, ADHD: Stimulants (methylphenidate, dextroamphetamine), $\alpha2$-agonists (clonidine, guanfacine), atomoxetine, atypical antipsychotics, opiate antagonists (naltrexone).
4. Aggression, self-injury: Atypical antipsychotics, $\alpha2$-agonists, anticonvulsants (topiramate, valproate), SSRIs, β-blockers (propranolol, nadolol, metoprolol, pindolol).
5. Sleep dysfunction: Melatonin, ramelteon, antihistamines (diphenhydramine, hydroxyzine), $\alpha2$-agonists, mirtazapine.
6. Anxiety: SSRIs, buspirone, mirtazapine.
7. Depressive symptoms: SSRIs, mitrazapine.
8. Bipolar phenotype: Anticonvulsants (carbamazepine, lamotrigine, oxcarbazepine, valproate, topiramate), atypical antipsychotics, lithium.
9. Constipation: Fiber, stool softeners.

Therapy: Appropriate early educational interventions (speech therapy, social skills instruction, occupational therapy, sensory integration therapy) may improve socialization/development.

1. *Educational interventions:* There are several schools of thought as to the optimal means of applying these interventions, which may be divided into the following 3 categories:
   a. Behavior analytic techniques are based upon experimental psychology approaches to systematically direct behavior towards a desired goal. There are multiple studies indicating the effectiveness of this approach, although it has been criticized for not being generalizable and for providing mostly modest educational gains without substantial benefits in social/emotional domains.
   b. Developmental approaches target the core ASD impairments in social reciprocity using play and interpersonal relationships to individually tailor the therapy to the child. The efficacy of this strategy has been demonstrated in a recent study.
   c. Structured teaching relies on an educational environment that is organized and predictable. Schedules and routines are used, although some flexibility is built into the system.
2. *Speech and language therapy:* Typical systems where the child is removed from the classroom for a short period are generally less effective. Greater benefits are suggested when speech therapists interact closely with teachers, families and the children's peers throughout the school day. Alternative communication methods and devices may also be helpful.
3. *Social skills instruction:* These interventions target social responsiveness, initiation of interactive behaviors and reduction of repetitive or perseverative behaviors.
4. *Occupational therapy and sensory integration therapy:* Traditional occupational therapy may help in improving function and self-care. Sensory integration theory is aimed at helping abnormalities in the interpretation of incoming sensory information, although definitive studies remain to be done.

Psychological: Involvement of a child psychiatrist in the comprehensive care plan is optimal. In addition to more in depth assessment of the individual's behavioral interactions, child psychiatrists may be able to recommend more definitive behavioral therapy and also are most familiar with using psychopharmaceuticals to modulate behaviors.

Social: Most of the therapies suggested above are best implemented with considerations for the child's peers and family groups in mind. Support groups may be helpful for families and for higher functioning, older children with ASDs.

Complementary and alternative medicine (CAM): This category refers to medical and health care practices and products that are not currently part of conventional medical management. Up to 90% of parents of children with ASDs have tried CAM therapies, and, although many indicate they would like advice or information, only 36–62% of these parents specifically told the primary care physician. It is therefore worthwhile to ask, and to work with families to evaluate which CAM avenues may be helpful, or at least not harmful (medically or financially).

While most CAM treatments have simply not been thoroughly tested, some types of CAM have shown promising albeit preliminary efficacy. These include vitamin C supplementation and music therapy. For therapies that have actually been studied and disproven, see below (section Things to avoid).

Pearls and Precautions

GI/Nutrition: Many individuals with ASDs may have GI complaints, and a balanced diet and proper evaluation and management of complications such as constipation should be provided; there is no indication for an extensive GI screening for those with ASDs. This includes excessive allergy testing and overly restrictive diets (see below).

Sleep: It is important to diagnose and treat underlying medical problems that may contribute to sleep disturbances, such as obstructive sleep apnea and gastroesophageal reflux. There is some evidence that melatonin secretion is altered in children with ASDs, and that melatonin may be effective in improving onset of sleep in this patient population. Other pharmacological agents have also been used for insomnia, and/or selection of medications needed for behavior management may be tempered by their effectiveness for treating comorbid problems like sleep disturbances.

School/education: See above for educational therapies and other interventions. While some of these may be implemented earlier in those where ASD is diagnosed at an early age, many of these treatments will continue for years and be most readily implemented through the school system.

Things to be avoided or approached with caution: Unproven diagnostic modalities for ASD screening include skin/hair testing for heavy metals, serum for celiac antibodies, allergy screening tests, immunological screening, vitamin levels, stool analysis, urinary peptides and thyroid function tests. These tests may be avoided except in select clinical situations where a specific medical diagnosis is suspected and must be ruled out. They are not indicated in the routine workup for autism.

While it is important not to summarily dismiss parents' interests in CAM, there are several treatment modalities that have effectively been disproven. These include administration of secretin (proven ineffective for ASDs in multiple randomized, placebo-controlled studies) and the use of facilitated communication (where the communication produced has actually been shown to arise from the facilitator, rather than the patient).

Some general guidelines by which to critically evaluate claims of effective treatments include looking for the following characteristics: (1) Overly simplified explanations/mechanisms; (2) broad ranging efficacy of a given treatment for many, mechanistically unrelated disorders; (3) claims of cure or dramatic and rapid improvement; (4) evidence is based upon individual cases and anecdotes; (5) absence or paucity of peer-reviewed references (be cautious for 'publications' in 'open-source' journals, blogs or websites that do not require traditional scientific review); and (6) treatments with no side effects or reported problems. The adage "If something sounds too good to be true, it usually is" should be remembered.

References

Geschwind DH, Advances in Autism, *Annual Rev Med,* 2009, 60:367-80; Greenspan SI, et al., Guidelines for Early Identification, Screening and Clinical Management of Children with Autism Spectrum Disorders, commentary, *Pediatrics,* 2008, 121(4): 828–830.

Johnson CP, et al., Identification and Evaluation of Children with Autism Spectrum Disorders, *Pediatrics,* 2007, 120(5):1183-1215; Myers SM, et al., Management of Children with Autism Spectrum Disorders, *Pediatrics,* 2007, 120(5): 1162–1182.

Rett Syndrome

Christopher C. Giza, Raman Sankar

Rett syndrome (RTT) is a female predominant developmental regression occurring after age of 6–18 months, characterized by acquired microcephaly, hand-wringing, seizures, altered respiratory patterns, bruxism, and severe dementia. It is classified as a specific subtype of autistic spectrum disorder.

Etiology

Rett syndrome is caused by mutations (>99% sporadic) in the methyl–CpG-binding protein 2 (MeCP-2) located on chromosome Xq28. Some female carriers are asymptomatic due to selective inactivation of mutated X chromosome. Among patients with classic RTT, 65–90+% have MeCP-2 mutation. Atypical RTT has lower rates (32%) of MeCP-2 mutation. Over 75 different mutations have been described. 7–8 "common" mutations account for 64–77% of mutation-positive cases. Other genes that have been identified with an RTT-like phenotype include CDKL5 (Xp22, presents with early onset seizures) and FOXG1 (14q12, presents as congenital RTT).

Clinical Presentation and Prognosis

Demographics: Generally occurs only in girls and is extremely rare in boys. Prevalence is 1:10,000-22,000 in girls, making it the number two cause of mental retardation in females.

Presenting signs and symptoms: Developmental arrest begins at age twelve months on average, but can begin as early as six- or as late as eighteen months. It is followed by severe developmental regression, loss of language, and autistic behavior.

Other cardinal features include, deceleration of head growth (eventual microcephaly), seizures (tend to be generalized tonic clonic, complex partial or myoclonic seizures with onset between 1–3 years), respiratory irregularities (hyperventilation and apnea, often in response to stimulation), scoliosis/hypotonia, and gait apraxia.

Other important features include, loss of useful hand movements (sometimes/classically with repetitive hand-wringing by age 3 years), bruxism, and a choreoathetoid movement disorder.

Atypical Rett syndrome patients may have preserved language, some hand use, higher cognition, normal head circumference and preserved ambulation.

Clinical Course: These children appear normal at birth (clinical stage 1). Early signs of involvement include slowing/arrest of neurological and cognitive development, followed by period of rapid regression within a year or two of symptom onset (clinical stage 2). Autistic features develop, along with loss of hand skills, loss of language and regression of social abilities. Fully developed Rett may show hand-wringing stereotypies, mental retardation, respiratory abnormalities, seizures and motor problems (clinical stage 3). After 2–3 years, there is some stabilization, but problems with scoliosis, autonomic dysfunction and anxiety may develop. After 10 years or more, there can be late motor regression with spasticity, complete loss of mobility and parkinsonian features (clinical stage 4).

Prognosis: Typical Rett patients ultimately develop catastrophic developmental outcomes. Late manifestations include spastic para/quadriparesis and severe dementia. Atypical cases have slightly milder phenotype and slower course. Seizures, which can range from easily controlled to intractable, tend to become less problematic in adolescence and young adulthood.

Diagnosis

Originally RTT was diagnosed by clinical presentation including deceleration of head growth and developmental arrest around 1 year of age in a girl. Now, clinical suspicion should lead to gene testing for mutations in MeCP-2. Since testing for CDKL5 is expensive, we suggest testing for it only if MECP2 testing is negative. Other diagnostic tests (serum amino acids, urine organic acids, lysosomal enzyme screen, thyroid studies, lactate, pyruvate, ammonia) may be useful to help rule out other causes of regression, seizures or movement disorder, depending upon presentation.

Secondary diagnostic tests that can be useful in management include EEG to help distinguish abnormal movements/behaviors from epileptic seizures. Neuroimaging is generally less helpful, particularly in genetically proven Rett.

Management

Much of the management of Rett syndrome consists of providing information and supportive care to the family and patient. Constipation can occur and should be treated. Loss of ambulation generally occurs during the teenage years and a wheelchair will be required. Osteopenia is not uncommon, resulting in increased risk of fractures. With increasing immobility in adulthood, bowel and bladder care and skin care become increasingly important. In later stages, autonomic dysfunction may manifest as tachycardia, prolonged QT intervals and/or sinus bradycardia.

Medications

1. Anticonvulsants may be necessary for seizure prevention once epilepsy occurs. In general, broad spectrum anticonvulsants (lamotrigine, topiramate, valproic acid, levetiracetam) are preferred, but selection of specific medication may be guided by clinical and EEG characterization of seizure type, as well as by the clinical manifestations exhibited by the patient (for example, a patient with very disruptive autistic behaviors may have worsened behavior on levetiracetam).
2. Behavioral outbursts, autistic-like behaviors and anxiety may require pharmacological intervention, although by teenage years, increasing motor impairment makes these symptoms generally less of an issue.
3. Naloxone has been tried for respiratory irregularities and proven ineffective.

Therapy: Physical and occupational therapy can be important to maintain function for as long as possible. Due to language impairment/regression, administering these therapies can be challenging. Educating the family with regards to regular application of some of the therapies is also important. A wheelchair will eventually become necessary for patients, usually during adolescence.

There have been reports of beneficial effects from therapies using multisensory environments. Music therapy facilitated learning and communication skills in a study of 7 patients, although there was no control group.

Social: Anticipatory guidance regarding clinical progression is important for families to have appropriate expectations and to prepare for future needs.

Pearls and Precautions

Respiratory: Patients will typically develop abnormal respiratory patterns (hyperventilation), particularly when stimulated or anxious.

Nutrition: Weight loss is common, even with adequate appetite. Maintaining a nutritionally adequate diet is important. Some studies suggest calcium absorption is increased, even in the setting of osteopenia. The effectiveness of calcium supplementation has not yet been determined.

Skin and dental care: In late stages, good skin care and decubitus prophylaxis are helpful. Adequate dental care needs to be provided, both to prevent caries but also to monitor and treat bruxism.

Toileting: May need assistance, and eventually will require diaper and/or urinary catheter.

School/education: Potential for learning is limited, but having school/day care activities is important, as most of these patients will survive until adulthood.

References

Chahrour M & Zoghbi HY. The story of Rett syndrome: from clinic to neurobiology. Neuron 2007, Nov 8;56(3):422-37.

Percy AK. Rett syndrome: recent research progress. J. Child Neurol 2008, May;23(5):543-9.

PercyAK & Lane JB. Rett syndrome: clinical and molecular update. Curr Opin Pediatr 2004 Dec;16(6):670-7.

Spina Bifida (SB)

Christopher C. Giza, Raman Sankar

Spina bifida cystica (SBC) is a relatively common neural developmental defect characterized by failure to close the caudal end of neural tube and is associated with Chiari II malformation (over 95%). It can include meningoceles and myelomeningoceles. Meningocele is a neural tube defect with herniation of meninges without neural tissue, and myelomeningocele is where all underlying structures (spinal cord, nerve roots, vertebrae, meninges and skin) are involved. Spina bifida occulta is a defect in the posterior bony elements of the spine without cord or meningeal involvement. Meningocele and myelomeningocele are generally visible at birth, while spina bifida occulta may have only subtle abnormalities visible on the surface.

SBC is almost always associated with a Chiari II malformation, an extensive constellation of intracranial neurodevelopmental anomalies. These may include multiple posterior fossa malformations—such as extension of brainstem and cerebellar tonsils into the upper cervical canal—and aqueductal abnormalities, midbrain compression, cerebellar dysplasia, cerviomedullary kink, cranial nerve nuclei hypoplasia and syringohydromyelia. However, supratentorial malformations are also seen including corpus callosum abnormalities, absent cingulate gyrus, colpocephaly (enlarged occipital horns of the lateral ventricles), large massa intermedia, polymicrogyria and heterotopias.

Etiology

Risk factors for developing spina bifida include: Pregestational maternal diabetes or hyperthermia as well as inadequate maternal folic acid or possible excessive maternal levels of retinoic acid. Other factors may include anticonvulsants (such as valproic acid or carbamazepine); neural tube defect (NTD) in an earlier child is associated with a 1.5-2% risk; this rises to 6% if two prior offspring have a NTD. Other family members with NTD may also increase the chance for SB.

Clinical Presentation and Prognosis

Demographics: Neural tube defects detected at birth have a slight female predominance. Prevalence rates of spina bifida range from 0.26–2.9/100 live births, although rates have declined as routine folate supplementation has become more widespread. Family history and other risk factors have already been discussed above.

Presenting signs and symptoms: Spina bifida cystica (SBC) is generally obvious at birth, with a visible spine defect, most commonly in lumbar or lumbosacral area (80%). The physical appearance may range from a saclike structure to actual exposure of neural contents. The defect may involve bone, meninges, spinal cord and/or nerve roots. Motor findings include a flaccid, areflexic paraparesis and sphincteric dysfunction. Distal sensory deficits are also seen along with lower limb joint deformities, contractures, hip dislocations and kyphoscoliosis.

Spina bifida occulta (SBO) is more subtle, occurring in up to 5% of the general population but usually being asymptomatic. It may be an incidental finding on a spine or abdominal X-ray. A subtle physical examination finding such as a sacral tuft of hair, cutaneous angioma/lipoma or a sacral dimple with a sinus tract may provide a clue as to the underlying abnormality. The underlying lesion may be a fibrous band, lipoma, dermoid, epidermoid, tethered cord or diastematomyelia. SBO may be asymptomatic or have only subtle symptoms, including slowly progressive weakness, spasticity, sensory loss, bowel/bladder dysfunction, recurrent urinary tract infections, recurrent meningitis, foot deformity, gait abnormality, accelerated Babinski signs and trophic ulcers.

Clinical course: SBC is diagnosed prenatally or at birth. SBC is frequently associated with underlying intracranial abnormalities including the Chiari II malformation (95%) and/or hydrocephalus. Main concerns acutely include meningitis. There is some debate as to the benefits of Cesarean delivery versus vaginal. After perinatal surgical repair, children with SBC need to be followed carefully for development of complications. Enlarging head size, bulging fontanelle, unexplained vomiting and presence of a 'sunset' sign (limited upgaze with pupils resembling a setting sun) indicate development of hydrocephalus. Brainstem dysfunction (poor feeding, vomiting, apnea, respiratory abnormalities) may occur due to physical compression of brainstem structures or development of syringobulbia. These children will have a flaccid paraparesis and sensory deficits below the level of the lesion, which may result in orthopedic problems and deformities over time. Sphincter impairment is also common, resulting in urinary tract/renal dysfunction (incontinence, hydronephrosis, repeated urinary tract infections) that ultimately becomes the major cause of long term morbidity.

SBO may be detected incidentally or have very slowly progressive symptoms at any time. Progressive neurological symptoms in a setting of SBO should warrant a workup for tethered cord syndrome and if indicated, surgical intervention. Symptoms of tethered cord include stable or slowly progressive paraparesis/myelopathy, foot deformities, sphincter dysfunction, sensory loss and kyphoscoliosis. Upper extremity symptoms are rarer but can occur.

Prognosis: Early mortality for SBC may be up to 10–15%, due primarily to meningitis. Later (>2–3 years of age) urinary tract problems (infection or other complications) are the major causes of mortality/morbidity. Up to 66% of patients are incontinent. Despite these challenges, up to 60–70% may have normal intelligence (IQ>80), although they are at increased risk of learning disorders and epilepsy (25%). Some (25%) will develop precocious puberty.

Visual problems are also common (66%), including strabismus, corneal scarring, or blindness.

For walking, the location of the lesion is important. Patients with lesions above L3 are generally unable to ambulate; for those below S1, unassisted ambulation is likely, and if between L3–S1, assistive devices may be necessary to ambulate. Overall, up to 66% of patients with myelomeningocele will be in a wheelchair by adolescence.

Due to early exposures and frequent procedures, patients with SBC/myelomeningocele have higher rates for developing latex allergies.

SBO may be asymptomatic, stable or progressive. Worsening symptoms in a patient known to have SBO warrants imaging workup for tethered cord.

Diagnosis

Prenatal: Elevated maternal serum alpha fetoprotein (AFP) detects 79% of cases and elevated amniotic fluid AFP, 98%. Prenatal ultrasound detects up to 99%. Folic acid supplementation (early in pregnancy) reduces NTD risk, even to some degree in those with a family history.

SBC: No test is necessary to diagnose, as these are directly visible at time of birth. However, brain MRI may be useful to diagnose Chiari malformation, hydrocephalus and other associated intracranial abnormalities.

SBO: X-ray is often the way an incidental SBO is detected. Spine MRI is helpful in cases of occult spinal dysraphism and to rule out tethered cord (also for patients with repaired SBC but progressive symptoms). Associated syrinx has been reported in up to 70–80%. Spine ultrasound may also be helpful to diagnose low spinal cord lipomas or other lesions associated with tethering of the conus meduallaris.

Management

Medical

1. *Mode of delivery:* For cases of SBC diagnosed in utero, some studies suggest that labor and vaginal delivery may increase the risk for additional neurological deficit or infection, but others showed no difference between vaginal and Cesarean delivery. Currently, there is no clear evidence to favor Cesarean delivery in the absence of frank hydrocephalus, breech presentation or other obstetrical indications.

2. *Presurgical, post-delivery management:* For SBC, the exposed neural tissue should be covered with a sterile dressing. Prophylactic antibiotics are often administered, although the evidence supporting this practice is scant. While it used to be considered a neurosurgical emergency, most current practice allows for stabilization of the infant and some maternal contact, so long as closure occurs within 48–72 hours.

3. Medical management for urinary tract problems depends upon type of dysfunction, which is best evaluated using urodynamics in conjunction with urology and nephrology.

    a. Intermittent cathertization is a mainstay of medical urological management. Sometimes the crede maneuver is helpful, but this generally is not effective in the long term.

    b. Reduced sphincter tone may be treated with **ephedrine** or **imipramine.**

    c. Increased sphincter tone may respond to agents like **phenoxybenzamine** or **diazepam.**

    d. Increased bladder tone has been treated with anticholinergics (**oxybutynin, propantheline, hyoscyamine**) or tricyclics (**imipramine**).

    e. Prevention and treatment of infections with **antibiotics** is important, however, treatment of asymptomatic bacteriuria is not always required.

4. Epilepsy/seizures occur in 15–20% of patients with SBC/myelomeningocele and are more common in those who have required shunting for hydrocephalus. Proper treatment of seizures includes **anticonvulsants**, as well as monitoring for shunt malfunction and/or infection in situations of seizure exacerbation.

5. Medical management is needed for optimal bowel care and includes dietary modifications, laxatives and manual evacuation. Retrograde (and occasionally, anterograde) enemas may also play a role.

6. Awareness of the increased risk of latex allergy and attempts to minimize exposure are important considerations.

Surgery:

1 *In utero SBC repair:* There is some evidence that the exposed neural tissue may suffer additional injury due to pressure and trauma during late pregnancy. Uncontrolled studies of in utero surgical repair have shown better neurological function and a lower rate of shunt dependent hydrocephalus after repair than in historical controls. This has led to a randomized trial of predelivery surgical repair with longer followup, but the results of this study are still several years away.

2. All delivered cases of SBC will require presurgical care (below) and early surgical closure within 24–72 hrs. This is intended to reduce the subsequent risk of meningitis.

3. Monitoring for hydrocephalus is important, but the decision to place a shunt should be made on clinical and radiographic grounds rather than automatically. Past series demonstrate shunt rates of up to 90% in patients with myelomeningoele, however shunt placement does not come without its complications. Shunt dependency, multiple shunt revisions, infection, cognitive impairment and shorter life expectancy have all been associated with shunt placement in patients with myelomeningocele. For patients with clear clinical or imaging signs of hydrocephalus, shunting is necessary, but some advocate tolerating a degree of stable mild-moderate ventriculomegaly and avoiding shunt placement when possible.

4. Monitoring for signs and symptoms of brainstem dysfunction is also part of the early and long-term care for patients with SB. SBC patients may require surgical decompression for Chiari II, brainstem/C-spine syrinx (20%).

5. A tethered cord can present with progressive myelopathy and paraparesis. Patients with repaired SBC and also those with known SBO should be monitored regularly for any progressive neurological dysfunction, which may require surgical untethering.

6. Patients with spina bifida have a higher risk for lower extremity contractures, foot deformities and kyphoscoliosis. They should be monitored for these problems and may require orthopedic surgical correction.

7. Urinary tract complications ultimately become the major cause of mortality and morbidity in these children, thus warranting regular urological consultation and testing. This serves to evaluate for malformations and abnormalities. Urodynamic testing is crucial to delineate the physiological type of sphincter dysfunction, as is being alert to signs and symptoms of urinary tract infection. Sometimes surgical interventions are necessary, including vesicostomy, enterocystoplasty, bladder neck repair, placement of an artificial urinary spincter or creation of a continent catherizable channel. For medical management of bladder dysfunction, see below.

8. Bowel care occasionally requires a cecal channel through which to administer full antegrade colonic enemas.

Therapy: Orthotics, leg braces and hip stabilization may be important non-operative orthopedic interventions. Physical, and occasionally, occupational therapy are important to enhance and maintain function. Other assistive devices such as walkers and wheelchairs are often necessary, particularly for patients with spinal lesions above the sacral levels.

Psych: Psychological counseling and/or psychiatric care are helpful to allow children to accept and manage their condition. Early in life, counseling is important for the parents to ensure that they understand the long-term implications of their child's disorder and to help them to cope with the many challenges that follow.

Social: Adolescent years are associated with a gradual transition of routine urological management from parents/caregivers to the actual patients themselves. This will require education and monitored opportunities for increasing independence.

Pearls and Precautions

Respiratory: Significant respiratory symptoms may indicate lower brainstem involvement, including compression and/or syringobulbia. These may be evaluated by brain MRI and occasionally require surgical decompression.

Skin and dental care: Due to reduced mobility and diminished sensation, good skin care is essential to prevent decubitus ulcers, burns and other cutaneous damage.

Toileting: See extensive management discussion above for both medical and surgical interventions.

Likely complications: After the infant period, renal complications become the main cause of morbidity/mortality.

School/education: For patients with SBC and Chiari II malformations, supratentorial involvement invariably occurs and developmental/cognitive challenges should be anticipated. However, many children with spina bifida (particularly with SBO, but also with SBC) will have normal or low normal intelligence, so educational and psychological settings should be arranged appropriately.

References

Joseph DB. Current approaches to the urological care of children with spina bifida. Current Urology Reports, 2008 Mar;9(2):151-7.

Thompson DN. Postnatal management and outcome for neural tube defects including spina bifida and encephalocoeles. Prenatal Diagn. 2009 Apr;29(4):412-9.

Muscular Dystrophies

Raman Sankar, Christopher C. Giza

The muscular dystrophies are distinguished from other disorders of muscle by the overt evidence of active muscle destruction, best seen histologically. Elevation of muscle enzymes such as creatine kinase (CK) or aldolase are prominent in disorders like *Duchenne* muscular dystrophy (DMD), but may not be seen consistently in other slowly progressive dystrophies such as *facioscapulohumeral* (FSHD) or *limb-girdle* (LGMD) dystrophies. There is genetic heterogeneity in the various dystrophic syndromes. The congenital muscular dystrophies (CMD) (*merosin deficiency, Fukuyama muscular dystrophy, Walker-Warburg disease, muscle-eye-brain disease*) present catastrophically in the neonatal period and are considered beyond the scope of this section and are only alluded to briefly. Primary care physicians should also appreciate that the family of muscular dystrophies does *not* include *congenital myotonic dystrophy* (covered separately), congenital myopathies such as *nemaline myopathy, central core disease*, etc., nor disorders of the spinal motor neuron such as *Werdnig-Hoffman disease,* covered separately under the section on *spinal muscular atrophy*.

Etiology

The muscular dystrophies are distinguished from other neuromuscular disorders by the fact that they are primary muscle disorders and involve myofiber degeneration. They are genetically determined and are progressive, some very rapidly so. Despite the involvement of distinct genes coding for different proteins (with the exception of *Duchenne* and *Becker* (BMD) dystrophies in which mutations of the same gene, dystrophin, are involved), the pathologic findings in all muscular dystrophies are similar. There is plasma membrane breakdown, resulting in calcium influx, activation of endogenous proteases, and breakdown of myofibrils. Muscle fibers appear hyalinized, atrophied, and there is interstitial fibrosis.

In DMD and BMD, the gene involved (Xq21.2) is very large at over 2 million base pairs. The gene product (mol wt 427,000) is a cytoskeletal protein located just below the inner surface of the cell membrane (sarcolemma) and is anchored by a number of dystrophin-associated glycoproteins. Mutations in the genes for the latter are also associated with muscular dystrophies. In simple terms, in DMD the mutations result in premature truncation, while in BMD, a much milder disease, the entire reading frame may be shifted such that there is shortening of the rod domain of dystrophin only.

Emery-Dreifuss dystrophy (EDMD) involves laminin genes, and can be either X-linked, autosomal dominant or recessive. What has been clinically known as Limb-Girdle muscular dystrophy (LGMD), now appears to be a number of distinct disorders involving a large number of dystrophin-associated glycoproteins. The defect in the clinically distinctive facioscapulohumeral dystrophy (FSHD) seems to involve the double homeobox protein 4 (DUX4) which controls the fragment length at telomere of chromosome 4 (4q35). A major form of congenital muscular dystrophy which presents dramatically in the newborn period involves the gene for merosin (a subunit of laminin in the extracellular matrix), responsible for anchoring the dystrophin-glycoprotein complex to the basal lamina.

Clinical Presentation and Prognosis: Our discussion will focus much more on DMD, the one most likely to involve partnering in chronic care by the pediatrician. Becker dystrophy is a mild disorder, while the CMDs are quite catastrophic.

Demographics: The most common of these disorders is DMD, affecting 1 in 3000 boys. The incidence of BMD is an order of magnitude lower at about 1 in 30,000 boys. Because of the early demise of patients afflicted with DMD, the prevalence of DMD and BMD are similar. The incidence of FSHD is estimated to be up to 5 per 100,000. Genetic analysis of LGMD reveals a very extensive molecular heterogeneity. Likewise, there are several subtypes of congenital muscular dystrophies, most of which also involve severe involvement of the brain and eye. They are rare, and accurate data on incidence is not readily available.

Presenting signs and symptoms: We will stress DMD in this section. The typical age of onset is 3 – 5 years of age. The child presents with parental observations about difficulty in climbing stairs and getting up from the floor. The Gowers' sign may be observed by asking the child to rise from the floor. The affected child will get up on all fours (hands and feet on the ground), and then 'walk' their hands up their legs to push themselves in to an upright position. Striking pseudohypertrophy of the calf muscles (from extensive fibrosis) may be seen. Mental subnormality and gastric hypomotility are often present but tend to be either overlooked by the family or not felt to be related to the motor concerns.

Becker dystrophy presents typically in the second decade with signs and symptoms of proximal muscle weakness, but much less dramatically compared to DMD. There is much less impressive calf hypertrophy, but there could be loss of ankle reflexes and *pes cavus.*

Emery-Dreifuss dystrophy is quite rare, presents between 5 and 15 years, and in addition to weakness, flexion contractures of the elbows and posterior cervical muscles give the patient a distinctive appearance.

Weakness in facial muscles, shoulder and upper arm characterize FSHD. Lips can not be pursed, and the patient may exhibit a transverse smile. Shoulder muscle wasting and scapular winging may be seen. There is tremendous molecular diversity in the etiology of the family of disorders that present as LGMD. Presenting signs and symptoms point to shoulder girdle weakness, and pelvic girdle weakness with ambulatory difficulties.

Clinical course and Prognosis: The clinical course of DMD is relentless, and typically ambulation is lost before the end of the first decade. Significant gastrointestinal disturbances can be attributable to smooth muscle dysfunction. Weakness of the rectus abdominus can add to that problem, producing fecal retention and distention. Severe scoliosis and respiratory muscle weakness can contribute to respiratory complications. Dilated cardiomyopathy, tachycardia and cardiac failure may eventually occur in up to 50–80% of individuals affected with DMD.

Cardiomyopathy is also associated with some cases of LGMD and EDMD. In EDMD, conduction problems have been described as well.

The course of BMD is much less dramatic. Generally speaking, FSHD and LGMD progress much more slowly.

Diagnosis

The diagnosis is made from a combination of clinical observations, routine *laboratory testing for muscle enzymes,* electrodiagnostics (*electromyography and nerve conduction studies*), molecular testing (often using muscle tissue), and histopathological examination of the tissue. The most dramatic increases in CK are seen in DMD and certain subtypes of LGMD (those involving defects in dysferlin or caveolin-3). In the latter, the CK elevations are very disproportionate to the mild weakness.

Because of the extreme complexity and ever evolving nature of the *molecular diagnostics*, the clinics most qualified for directing the diagnostic work-up tend to be the regional neuromuscular clinics sponsored by the Muscular Dystrophy Association (MDA), often located in academic centers.

Suspected cases of CMD will require cerebral MRI and *ophthalmologic consultation*, as well as an EEG. Molecular diagnosis can follow. The prognosis for these children is poor.

Management

No specific treatment is available for effective management of the muscular dystrophies. A few investigational approaches may delay disability, especially in DMD. These are also best directed by a specialized neuromuscular clinic.

In DMD, there is some evidence that early treatment with glucocorticoids (prednisone, deflazacort) may extend walking (by 2–5 years), reduce falls, and improve pulmonary function. Treatment has to be undertaken early. Prednisone given in doses of 2.5–5 mg/kg/d on Fridays and Saturdays has been suggested. However, the Cochrane review points to a daily prednisone dose of 0.75 mg/kg/d. Deflazacort may produce less weight gain. There is less experience with oxandrolone. There is some promise that β-2 agonist (albuterol) therapy may offer some benefit by increasing muscle mass and improving exercise performance, but dosing regimens may be critical and are not fully worked out. The stuttering course of attempts at gene therapy has not progressed to benefit today's patient with DMD. A promising novel approach utilizes anti-sense technology to 'skip" the involved exon to produce a reasonable approximation of dystrophin that is shorter, but has partial functionality.

Many DMD patients with cardiomyopathy seem to benefit from therapy with angiotensin converting enzyme inhibitors or β-adrenorecptor blockers.

Currently, the mainstay of primary care relies on supportive care and involves many systems.

1. *Motor disability:* Referral to appropriate physical and occupational therapies—best to coordinate through an MDA clinic, or at least use a regional MDA clinic as a resource for consultation. Monitor for complications of corticosteroid therapy, if the patient is enrolled.
2. *Respiratory care*: Patients may need chest braces to minimize respiratory complications of scoliosis.
3. *Respiratory infection avoidance*: Meticulous schedule of immunizations, especially against influenzae and pneumococcal infections.
4. *Cardiac function monitoring*: Regular assessments with a cardiologist experienced in the muscular dystrophies. This expertise is typically available in the MDA-sponsored muscle clinics.
5. *Nutritional issues:* Should take into account the gastrointestinal issues pertaining to hypomotility and constipation. Common sense dictates that counseling patients to add generous portions of fruits and vegetables may help not only with gastrointestinal complaints, but may ameliorate the sodium-retaining, potassium-wasting effects of glucocorticoid therapy, and assist in maximizing muscle function. This intervention provides the family with a meaningful role in therapeutics and may be of psychological benefit.
6. Psychosocial support and genetic counseling.

Infants who present with congenital muscular dystrophy (CMD with merosin deficiency, Walker-Warburg, Fukuyama myopathy, muscle-eye-brain disease) will require seizure management (covered in detail in other chapters on epilepsy) and follow-up with ophthalmology.

Pearls and Precautions

- Our understanding of muscle diseases continues to expand very rapidly—have the patient connected to an MDA clinic or a comparable resource.
- Effective management of cardiac and respiratory risks minimizes early morbidity and prolongs life.
- Dietary approach to accommodate medical needs and, at the same, time involve the parents by providing them a role for positive intervention.

References:

One of the most comprehensive resources for the neuromuscular disorders: http://neuromuscular.wustl.edu/

Sarnat HB and Menkes JH. Disorders of the Motor Unit, in Menkes JH, Sarnat HB, Maria BL: *Child Neurology*, Seventh Edition, Lippincott Williams & Wilkins, Philadelphia, 2006, pp.969–1024.

Muntoni F. Cardiomyopathy in muscular dystrophies. *Curr Opin Neurol* 2003;16:577–83.

Moxley RT 3rd, Ashwal S, Pandya S, Connolly A, Florence J, Mathews K, Baumbach L, McDonald C, Sussman M, Wade C; Quality Standards Subcommittee of the American Academy of Neurology; Practice Committee of the Child Neurology Society. Practice parameter: corticosteroid treatment of Duchenne dystrophy: report of the Quality Standards Subcommittee of the American Academy of Neurology and the Practice Committee of the Child Neurology Society. *Neurology* 2005;64:13–20.

Angelini C. The role of corticosteroids in muscular dystrophy: a critical appraisal. *Muscle Nerve* 2007;36:424–35.

Manzur AY, Kuntzer T, Pike M, Swan A. Glucocorticoids corticosteroids for Duchenne muscular dystrophy. *Cochrane Database Syst Rev* 2008 Jan 23;(1):CD003725.

Markham LW, Kinnett K, Wong BL, Woodrow Benson D, Cripe LH. Corticosteroid treatment retards development of ventricular dysfunction in Duchenne muscular dystrophy. *Neuromuscl Disord* 2008;18:365–70.

Fenichel GM, Griggs RC, Kissel J, Kramer TI, Mendell JR, Moxley RT, Pestronk A, Sheng K, Florence J, King WM, Pandya S, Robison VD, Wang H. A randomized efficacy and safety trial of oxandrolone in the treatment of Duchenne dystrophy. *Neurology* 2001;56:1075–9.

Skura CL, Fowler EG, Wetzel GT, Graves M, Spencer MJ. Albuterol increases lean body mass in ambulatory boys with Duchenne or Becker muscular dystrophy. *Neurology* 2008;70:137–43.

Heemskerk H, de Winter CL, van Ommen GJ, van Deutekom JC, Aartsma-Rus A. Development of antisense-mediated exon skipping as a treatment for duchenne muscular dystrophy. *Ann N Y Acad Sci* 2009;1175:71–9.

Myotonic Dystrophy

Raman Sankar, Christopher C. Giza

Myotonic dystrophy is an autosomal dominant multisystem disorder characterized by myotonia, muscular dystrophy, cardiac involvement, cataracts and endocrine disorders. Myotonia is a condition of impaired relaxation after muscular contraction.

Etiology

Myotonic dystrophy type 1 (DM1) is inherited in an autosomal dominant fashion and shows the phenomenon of genetic anticipation—namely, that successive generations are more severely affected. It is caused by a trinucleotide (CTG) repeat in the 3' untranslated region of the DMPK gene (dystrophin myotonin-protein kinase) at the locus Chr. 19q13.3. However, current thoughts are that the manifestation of this disease is not necessarily due to a specific problem in this DMPK protein, but actually through induction of an RNA processing defect that has wide-ranging impact on multiple cellular pathways in many different tissues, thus accounting for its broad clinical manifestations. There is also a type 2 (DM2), but the onset occurs only in adulthood. The myotonic disorders include different types of myotonia that are associated with mutations in chloride or sodium channels, and may resemble the clinical presentation of DM1.

Clinical Presentation and Prognosis

Demographics: Incidence has been reported to be 13.5/100,000 births, with congenital and juvenile cases comprising 20% of total number of individuals affected with myotonic dystrophy. There are 3 subtypes of DM1: A severe congenital/neonatal form, a milder childhood form, and an adult form.

Presenting signs and symptoms: The neonatal form is the most severe and can occur in the offspring of affected mothers. The mother's weakness and myotonia may worsen during preganancy and labor may be prolonged. Affected neonates may have the following: (1) respiratory difficulties; (2) facial diplegia with upper lip shaped like an inverted V; (3) generalized hypotonia, with proximal weakness and reduced/absent DTRs; (4) joint deformities (including arthrogryposis); and (5) gastrointestinal dysfunction with regurgitation, aspiration, dysphagia and/or gastroparesis. Cardiomyopathy can occur in neonates, while congenital cataract is very rare.

Classic signs and symptoms of *childhood onset* myotonic dystrophy include normal early development with subsequent slowly appearing weakness in face and distal limb muscles, clinical myotonia (impaired muscle relaxation after contraction), and mental handicaps (in learning and speech).

Clinical course: Those with the neonatal form may have postnatal difficulties in respiration and feeding, and may present with perinatal asphyxia. Neonates do not initially demonstrate clinical myotonia. Over time, facial features become more dysmorphic and speech impairment, motor delays and myotonia become more evident.

Over years, multisystem problems appear such as cataracts, endocrinopathies (insulin-resistant DM before adolescence), frontal baldness and testicular atrophy (in males), temporal wasting, and cardiac problems (arrhythmias, cardiomyopathy). Cognitive impairment, neuropsychological abnormalities and hypersomnolence also become more prominent with time. Gastrointestinal involvement can include irritable bowel, gallstones and elevations of hepatic transaminases.

Prognosis: For neonatal DM1, mortality can be high, particularly when associated with perinatal asphyxia and respiratory insufficiency. However, with onset after the neonatal period, prognosis is a little better, with most attaining ambulation. In fact, mental impairment rather than motor delays is more often the limiting factor in patients presenting post-neonatally. Cardiac abnormalities such as arrhythmias or cardiomyopathy present in the second decade and most individuals with the neonatal variant will die before age 30 years. Myotonia becomes prominent, as do audiological problems, gastrointestinal distress and infertility. For childhood DM1, life expectancy is not necessarily shorter, but symptoms of adult DM1 become more noticeable over time. Cardiac problems are again a cause of sudden death. Adult onset DM1 patients become disabled late in life, and are at higher risk for respiratory aspiration and sudden cardiac death.

Subsequent generations of an affected family show more severe phenotype due to expansion of genetic triplet repeats (anticipation). This information should be included in genetic counseling.

Diagnosis

Definitive diagnosis can be made using genetic testing; the DNA probe for the expansion of the trinucleotide repeats is specific for >96% of patients. Electromyogram (EMG) may show myotonia in the mother, but this result is less likely in an affected infant with DM1. Myotonia is characterized by repetitive firing of very short potentials, or a "dive-bomber" sound on EMG. Muscle enzymes (creatine kinase) are usually normal. Slit lamp exam may identify a spoke-like posterior capsular cataract. In most cases, a diagnosis can be made using clinical exam, genetic testing and examination of the patient's mother. Muscle biopsy is generally not necessary to make the diagnosis, although it may help to rule out alternative diagnoses.

For neonatal presentations, the differential diagnosis is broad and may include the following: (1) Cerebral hypotonia due to cerebral malformations, chromosomal disorders, or metabolic disorders; (2) spinal cord injury (rarely) resulting from excessive neck traction during delivery; (3) spinal muscular atrophy—Werdnig-Hoffman, etc., (4) neuromuscular junction disorders (such as infantile botulism, myasthenia); (5) congenital myopathy or muscular dystrophy; and (6) hereditary sensory-motor neuropathies.

Childhood onset and adult onset DM1 may present with only mild weakness. The main clinical problems may be cognitive and intellectual impairments.

Management

Medications

1. Pharmacotherapy for myotonia includes sodium channel blockers (carbamazepine, phentyoin, mexilitene). Procaine, corticosteroids, antihistamines and calcium channel blockers (nifedipine) have also been tried. These agents may minimize myotonia, but not affect weakness.

2. Metoclopramide or other motility agents for gastroparesis.
3. Anti-arrhythmics (mexilitene, others) may be used when needed if arrhythmias develop.

Surgery: Orthopedic interventions may include surgery if more conservative bracing and physical therapy are ineffective, or may be needed to correct congenital joint deformities. Placement of G-tube is beneficial for some patients. Also, these patients may show decompensation even hours following general anesthesia and so should be watched in a monitored unit post-operatively.

Therapy: Physical and occupational therapy are often indicated. Proper splinting and bracing, including plastic foot orthoses, may help with the common joint/foot deformities.

Pearls and Precautions

Nutrition: In general, nutritional issues will center on difficulty swallowing in more severely affected individuals. These may require G-tube feedings and/or caloric supplementation. Watching for development of diabetes is also important.

Respiratory: Severely affected infants may require intubation, ventilation and/or aspiration precautions.

Toilet: Chronic constipation and intermittent urinary tract symptoms are fairly common.

Likely complications

- Cardiology consultation and followup, including regular ECG monitoring, are helpful to identify and treat any potential arrhythmias as early as possible.
- Endocrinology consultation and followup is helpful to identify predisposition for diabetes/insulin resistance and hypogonadism.

School/education: It is important to ensure that children with DM1 are in the appropriate educational setting to maximize developmental potential. It is also important to realize that the childhood presentation of this disorder is most commonly characterized by cognitive delay +/- myotonia, but with relatively mild weakness.

Things to be avoided (medications, situations, etc.): Children with DM1 may be sensitive to sedation or anesthesia (barbiturates, opiates). They need to be monitored closely for decompensation at these times, including for several hours after the conclusion of any general anesthesia, as delayed decompensation has been reported.

References

Schara U, Schoser BG. Myotonic dystrophies type 1 and 2: a summary on current aspects. *Semin Pediatr Neurol* 2006;13(2):71–9.

Wheeler TM, Thornton CA. Myotonic dystrophy: RNA-mediated muscle disease. *Curr Opin Neurol* 2007;20(5):572–6.

Spinal Muscular Atrophy (SMA)

Raman Sankar, Christopher C. Giza

Spinal muscular atrophy (SMA) is a progressive neuromuscular disease that usually presents in childhood with hypotonia, motor delay or loss of motor milestones and bulbar symptoms.

Etiology

SMA is a genetic disorder with autosomal recessive inheritance. 95% of SMA patients have a homozygous deletion/absence of exon 7 and 8 for the survival motor neuron 1 gene (SMN1). SMN2 copy number and gene expression may modify the phenotype, with higher levels of SMN2 showing milder clinical phenotypes.

Clinical Presentation and Prognosis

Demographics: The incidence of SMA is 1:10,000–25,000 with a carrier frequency of 1:50–80. SMA represents the 2nd most common hereditary neuromuscular disorder after Duchenne muscular dystrophy.

Presenting signs and symptoms: There are three (to five) clinical forms of the disease that range across a spectrum, without sharp demarcation between each phenotype. The most severe form presents in utero and is sometimes termed type 0. Presenting signs include prenatal reduced fetal movements and postnatal findings of profound hypotonia and respiratory distress. Type 1 is known as acute infantile (or Werdnig-Hoffman) which also presents with profound infantile weakness and hypotonia, frog-leg posture, a sharp distinction between social awareness and motor function, bulbar signs, respiratory difficulties, pectus excavatum, tongue fasciculations and reduced to absent deep tendon reflexes. Type 2 is intermediate. These individuals may have an onset of weakness and motor delay that becomes evident only after 6 months. Type 2 SMAs have less prominent bulbar symptoms and a less malignant course. Other signs and symptoms include upper extremity tremor, gastrocnemius hypertrophy and variable deep tendon reflexes. Type 3 SMAs present as juveniles (also known as Kugelberg-Welander) with milder weakness, more gradual progression and hypotonia. Adult onset variants (sometimes known as type 4) may show only mild development of diffuse weakness.

Clinical course: The clinical course is related to the type. Neonatal and infantile forms typically present with severe problems very early, although the regression is a little slower for those with postnatal presentation. Some infants may even show a temporary period of stabilization or apparent improvement, followed by worsening. Those with the intermediate form (SMA 2) may initially appear normal around 6 months but then show gradually progressive weakness and motor delays by 18 months. Nonetheless, type 2 SMA children may learn to sit. Type 3 SMA symptoms may not present until after 18 months, often in later childhood or adolescence. Progression is very slow. SMA 4 is typically characterized by onset in adulthood and has the mildest course. Ambulation can be achieved by those with SMA type 3 and 4.

Clinical course and prognosis are obviously worse in children with SMA who also experience a significant hypoxic-ischemic event.

Prognosis: Those with prenatal or neonatal SMA rarely survive the first year of life. Infants with type 1 SMA develop worsening respiratory complications (aspiration, infection, respiratory insufficiency) and generally succumb before age 2–3 years. SMA 2 children have a slower clinical course and with excellent care may survive into adolescence or beyond. SMA 3 and 4 show milder symptoms and survive well into adulthood.

Diagnosis

The diagnosis of SMA should be suspected in a hypotonic infant with little extremity movement, but appears alert and not encephalopathic. Eye movements are preserved, but reflexes are reduced or absent and tongue fasciculations may be present. In these cases, the *SMN1 gene deletion test* should be performed, which, if present, indicates a diagnosis of SMA.

If the *SMN1 test* shows no deletion, or if the clinical presentation is atypical, then additional diagnostic testing may be of value. Electromyography *EMG* can demonstrate changes consistent with denervation (SMA, motor neuropathy) or problems at the neuromuscular junction (myasthenia). Slowing of *nerve conduction* would suggest a demyelinating neuropathy. Laboratory studies may also be helpful. While *creatine kinase (CK)* levels may be elevated up to 5-fold normal in SMA, larger elevations would point towards muscular dystrophies. Other laboratory tests that may be used in the diagnosis of progressive hypotonia and weakness include *aldolase* (chronic muscle breakdown), *ESR* (inflammatory disorders, myositis), *carnitine* (deficiencies), *TSH* (hypothyroidism), *lactate/pyruvate* (mitochondrial disorders) and *serum amino acids/urine organic acids* (inborn errors of metabolism). Infantile botulism should be considered in those with new onset hypotonia and oculomotor weakness. *Muscle/nerve biopsy* is not generally indicated for the diagnosis of SMA, but may be necessary to definitively diagnose other types of myopathy or metabolic disease that resemble SMA.

In older children, clinical suspicion may be lower because of more gradual onset of symptoms. However, workup would still follow the general guidelines above, including laboratory studies where appropriate, as well as *EMG/NCV* (nerve conduction velocity).

Management

Consensus guidelines suggest that supportive management be based on functional level, rather than SMA type. Functional levels are divided into 3 groups: Nonsitters, sitters, and walkers.

Pulmonary: Pulmonary complications are one of the major causes of mortality and morbidity in SMA patients. Proper pulmonary care involves regular assessment every 3–6 months, depending upon the functional status of the child. Ancillary tests that will aide assessments (beyond history, observation and physical examination), include polysomnography, intermittent pulse oximetry, blood gases, chest X-rays, swallowing studies and pulmonary function testing.

- *Nonsitters:* Evaluate cough effectiveness, observe breathing and monitor gas exchange. Most nonsitters will not be able to perform standard pulmonary function testing (PFTs) due to young age and degree of muscle weakness. Polysomnography and pulse oximetry may be helpful in assessment, but the effectiveness of continuous pulse oximetry is unproven.

- *Sitters:* Same as nonsitters plus monitoring for scoliosis. These patients will be more likely to perform formal PFTs.
- *Walkers:* This group of patients generally has preserved respiratory function until late in their course. Assessments may include PFTs and monitoring for scoliosis. Specific ancillary testing should be directed by signs and symptoms.

Treatment interventions should be preferentially discussed in an anticipatory fashion rather than waiting until some respiratory crisis. Anticipatory care includes management of secretions, consideration of noninvasive ventilation, routine immunizations, maintaining mobility and careful discussion of advanced care directives.

Chronic pulmonary management may be divided into several categories, including airway clearance, respiratory support/ventilation, perioperative planning and other supportive care. Strategies to assist airway clearance include assisted coughing, chest PT, postural drainage and suctioning. Respiratory support is important, particularly in children with daytime hypercapnia. Noninvasive ventilation is the mainstay for providing this support and should be administered in consultation with pulmonary specialists. The use of tracheostomy is controversial and should be undertaken only after careful consideration of long-term goals, noninvasive options including palliative care, and patient comfort. Perioperative care should be planned well in advance, with the goal of optimizing the child's respiratory status before and after surgery to avoided prolonged ventilation. Other supportive care includes nutrition, hydration, reflux management (see below) and asthma treatment where necessary. Chronic mucolytic use is not supported.

Medications: Pharmacological management includes both experimental therapies directed at the underlying genetic defect, as well as supportive interventions for systemic complications.

1. Pulmonary problems may be addressed medically through judicious use of bronchodilators (for asthma/bronchospasm), antibiotics (for aspiration/pneumonia) and routine immunization.
2. Gastroesophageal reflux may be managed medically using antacids (magnesium or calcium carbonate), acid inhibitors (famotidine, ranitidine, omeprazole) and prokinetics (metoclopramide, erythromycin).
3. There is some evidence to support carnitine supplementation (particularly in those with carnitine depletion or who are being concomitantly treated with valproic acid).
4. Other medications being utilized experimentally include 4-phenylbutyrate (with variable results reported), valproic acid (with some suggestion of benefits for SMA types 2–4), and riluzole (possible benefit in SMA1).

Surgery: For patients with reflux and/or impaired swallowing, gastrostomy and fundoplication should be considered earlier, when their respiratory status is more tolerant of anesthesia and surgery. Correction of scoliosis, if necessary, should likewise be performed early. Orthopedic surgical interventions are aimed at maximizing function. For respiratory support, noninvasive ventilation is much preferred to tracheostomy.

Diet: Feeding and swallowing problems are common in nonsitters and sitters, but not often in walkers. Signs and symptoms related to this should be evaluated formally with a swallowing/feeding consultation, including a swallowing study where indicated. Changes in food consistency, proper positioning during mealtimes and aspiration precautions may all be helpful. Monitoring and treating gastroesophageal reflux and constipation are important. When determining nutritional needs, body fat may be underestimated because these children have diminished lean body mass. Nutritional supplementation may thus focus more on high protein/low fat diets. Nonsitters (and some sitters) are more likely to present with growth failure, while most sitters and walkers are actually at higher risk for obesity.

Therapy: The goals of therapy are to maintain joint mobility, maximize function and minimize discomfort. Sometimes braces and orthotics may be helpful, but care should be taken not to correct postural deviations at the price of lost function. Sitters and walkers should be monitored for scoliosis. Appropriate devices to assist with mobility should be provided (wheelchairs, standers, walkers).

Social/counseling: Psychosocial considerations are important for both the patient and family. Respite care should be provided. In late stages, palliative care and advance directives should be addressed before acute decompensation, so as to provide optimum comfort and dignity. In addition, genetic counseling is needed to discuss reproductive risks (for parents and for more mildly affected older patients), as well as consideration for testing of presymptomatic siblings.

Pearls and Precautions

Respiratory: See above.

Nutrition: See above.

Skin care: Good skin care is necessary for SMA patients with reduced mobility, particularly severely affected phenotypes (SMA 1 and 2) but also including later stages of those with milder phenotypes.

Toileting: May need assistance, and some may eventually require diaper and/or urinary catheter.

School/education: Potential for learning is normal. Primary limitations are due to motor impairment. Cognition is generally intact and devices to assist in communication are valuable. Instructors should be reminded not to presume children with SMA are cognitively delayed.

Research: Several ongoing clinical trials or trial registries are available for interested families, including the following:

1. *AmSMART (American Spinal Muscular Atrophy Randomized Trials, www.amsmart.org).*
2. Project Cure SMA (www.projectcuresma.org).
3. Pediatric Neuromuscular Clinical Research Network, in the Northeast U.S. (http://www.unmc.edu/sma/; http://www.columbiasma.org/research.htm)

References

Darras BT, Kang PB. Clinical trials in spinal muscular atrophy. *Curr Opin Pediatr* 2007;19(6):675–9.

Wang CH, Finkel RS, Bertini ES, Schroth M, Simonds A, Wong B, Aloysius A, Morrison L, Main M, Crawford TO, Trela A; Participants of the International Conference on SMA Standard of Care. Consensus statement for standard of care in spinal muscular atrophy. *J Child Neurol* 2007;22(8):1027–49.

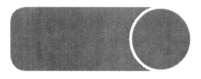

Other Neurological Diseases

Adrenoleukodystrophy

Christopher C. Giza, Raman Sankar

Adrenoleukodystrophy is a genetic disorder associated with accumulation of very long chain fatty acids and characterized clinically by progressive dysfunction of the adrenal cortex and the cerebral white matter.

Etiology

The gene locus for ALD is Xq28. The gene product is a peroxisomal membrane protein named ABCD1. Ultimately, this defect causes dysfunction of peroxisomal enzymes, with accumulation of unbranched, saturated C24+ fatty acids.

Clinical Presentation and Prognosis

Demographics: X-linked, incidence 1:20,000 in boys. Incidence in boys and heterozygote girls is 1:17,000. Phenotypes vary within the same kindred. Male hemizygotes may present with classic ALD or a more chronic variant, adrenomyeloneuropathy.

Presenting signs and symptoms: There are 5–6 distinct phenotypes. Childhood onset is usually greater than 3–4 years of age with the average age of onset being 7 years.

1. Childhood cerebral (CCALD): Onset is around 4–8 years of age. Initial symptoms include hyperactivity, worsening school performance, visual disturbances, ataxia, seizures and strabismus. Mild hyperpigmentation may be seen.
2. Adolescent-adult cerebral: Onset is 10–21 years of age. It is similar to childhood variant, but slower progression. 10% present acutely with status epilepticus, encephalopathy, adrenal crisis, and coma.
3. Adrenomyeloneuropathy (AMN): Onset is during late adolescence or adulthood. Main sign/symptom is a progressive paraparesis. AMN may occur with cerebral white matter (WM) involvement (20% of AMN).
4. "Addison only": This variant may constitute up to 25% of male Addison patients, many of whom have subtle/no neurological signs. Many go on to get AMN in adulthood.
5. Asymptomatic: Biochemical ALD defect without neurological or endocrine dysfunction. Eventually, patients have some neurological symptoms, but they may be delayed or subtle.

The initial clinical differential diagnosis is primarily behavioral and includes ADHD, a psychiatric disorder, dementia, epilepsy or other developmental regression/learning disability.

Clinical course: After presentation for childhood cerebral ALD, there can be a rapid progression to spasticity and paralysis; visual and hearing loss; dysarthria, dysphagia, and dementia. Adrenal symptoms are usually not recognized, but present in 50–90% of ALD patients. The mean interval to severe impairment is <2 years, but then survival can last up to 10+ years. Adolescent onset cerebral ALD progresses more slowly. AMN and its variant AMN with cerebral WM involvement start later and generally advance more slowly.

Prognosis: Patients experience relentlessly progressive initial cerebral symptoms. The average time to reach a persistent vegetative/minimally responsive state after initial onset is less than two years. If untreated, the 5-year survival rate in CCALD boys is less than 40%. The survival rate increases to as much as 56% after hematopoietic stem cell transplant.

Diagnosis

Plasma very long chain fatty acids (VLCFA) are elevated in 100% of males and 85% of female heterozygotes. Should be performed in all males with Addison disease, men with progressive paraparesis and all at-risk family members of known individuals with XL-ALD. DNA-based genetic testing is the test of choice to detect female carriers. Prenatal diagnosis may be possible by measuring VLCFA from cultured amniocytes, but should be confirmed with genetic testing.

Brain CT/MRI shows symmetric, periventricular posterior parieto-occipital white matter lesions. Rarely, the white matter involvement is more frontal or focal. Cortrosyn stimulation test can demonstrate subnormal cortisol in response to ACTH; and, plasma ACTH is elevated. Somatosensory, brainstem auditory and visual evoked potentials may be normal in early stages of the disease, but invariably show abnormalities as the disorder progresses.

Management

Medical

1. Corticosteroid replacement for adrenal insufficiency helps in general, but doesn't change neurological symptoms.
2. Glyceryl trioleate:glyceryl trierucate 4:1 (Lorenzo's oil) taken in combination with a low fat diet normalizes VCLFA, but is not effective in treating symptomatic patients. May be most effective in asymptomatic <6–8 year old boys with normal MRIs and should be used in conjunction with adrenal replacement therapy.
3. Hematopoeitic stem cell transplantation (HSCT) carries a high risk, but is effective at arresting the disease process if undertaken before significant neurological deterioration occurs. However, HSCT itself can cause disease acceleration (GVHD).
   Generally NOT recommended if
   - performance IQ <80 (too much neurological damage has been done); OR
   - for asymptomatic individuals with completely normal MRIs (as half of them will never progress).

As cerebral ALD progresses at a rapid pace, the benefit of HSCT is minimized becase in over 50% of these patients, significant neurological damage has been done, thus eliminating them as HSCT candidates. However, in those patients that do qualify for HSCT, benefits can clearly be seen. The overall 3-year transplant survival rate is 85% (overall 3-year ALD mortality with no HCST is 78%). As previously mentioned, the five-year post-transplant survival rate is 56% (overall untreated ALD survival is less than 40%.) The five-year survival rate increases to 92% in boys with no more than one neurological defect and an MRI rating of less than nine.

The window for HSCT is narrow. Screening for ALD should be liberal in suspected or at-risk individuals in hopes of identifying them before the disease has progressed beyond this window.

4. Ineffective: Interferon-b, other immunosuppression.
5. Proposed: Lovastatin, 4-phenylbutyrate, gene therapy.
6. Spasticity can be symptomatically treated using baclofen, tizanidine, benzodiazepines.
7. Seizures should be treated with standard anticonvulsants.

Surgery: The main surgical interventions are supportive as the disease advances, including tracheostomy and/or gastrostomy.

Therapy: Physical and occupational therapy may be helpful in maintaining function to some degree, although the disease itself is generally rapidly progressive if untreated.

Psychiatric: Presenting symptoms are often behavioral, but treatment of the behavioral syndromes does not alter long term disease progression. Psychiatric and psychological care may be helpful in the early phases, but rapid progression eventually leaves the affected individuals significantly impaired.

Social: Supportive care is extremely important, with a need for support groups and family counseling. Genetic counseling is beneficial to discuss extended family screening and the importance of identifying asymptomatic males and female carriers. Prenatal diagnosis is available via amniocentesis.

Pearls and Precautions

Screening using VLCFA and/or, where indicated, genetic testing should be used liberally in young males with Addison disease and in adult males with progressive myelopathy. In addition—and based upon family history—any suspected carriers or at-risk individuals should be screened. As the two main ALD treatments are Lorenzo's oil and HSCT and since they must be administered before major neurological damage has occurred, it is imperative to acquire ALD diagnoses as early as possible.

Monitor boys <10 years old with a diagnosis of ALD every 6 months with Brain MRI, neurological examination, neuropsychological assessment & adrenal function testing.

Nutrition: Progressive dysphagia may require a soft diet and eventually a G-tube. For carriers and asymptomatic males, a combination of 'Lorenzo's oil' and a low fat diet may slow/arrest disease progression.

Sleep: Early on, sleep wake changes may respond to mild nighttime chloral hydrate, or diphenhydramine.

References

Moser HW, Raymond DV, Dubey P. Adrenoleukodystrophy: new approaches to a degenerative disease. JAMA 2005 Dec 28;294(24):3131-4.

Moser HW & Barker PB. Magnetic resonance spectroscopy: a new guide for the therapy of adrenoleukodystrophy. Neurol 2005 Feb 8;64(3):406-7.

Peters C, Charnas LR, Tan Y, Ziegler RS, Shapiro EG, DeFor T, Grewal SS, Orchard PJ, Abel SL, Goldman AI, Ramsay NK, Dusenbery KE, Loes DJ, Lockman LA, Kato S, Aubourg PR, Moser HW, Krivit W. Cerebral X-linked adrenoleukodystrophy: the international hematopoietic cell transplantation experience from 1982 to 1999. Blood. 2004 Aug 1;104(3):881-8.

Friedreich Ataxia

Christopher C. Giza, Raman Sankar

Friedreich ataxia is a progressive, genetic ataxia with corticospinal tract involvement.

Etiology

Friedreich ataxia is inherited in an autosomal recessive pattern. It is a trinucleotide repeat disease involving Chr 9q13-21–frataxin gene. Trinucleotide repeat disorders show genetic anticipation, namely an increase in disease severity with successive generations. Abnormal frataxin may be deposited in the mitochondrial membrane, resulting in impairment of energy metabolism and intramitochondrial iron accumulation, hence some of the therapies being investigated focus on improving mitochondrial dysfunction.

Clinical Presentation and Prognosis

Demographics: This is the most common hereditary ataxia with an incidence of 1–4:100,000 in the general population. The disorder seems to be limited to those of European, Middle Eastern, North African and Indian descent. East Asians and Native American Indians do not seem to be at risk for this disease. Subsaharan Africans also appear not to be affected.

Presenting signs and symptoms:

Neurological: Progressive gait and limb ataxia – onset usually between 5–15 years, with nystagmus, explosive dysarthria, Romberg positive, absent deep tendon reflexes, extensor plantar response, distal weakness—especially in the hands, impaired vibratory and proprioceptive sense (may be normal at presentation), light touch and pain impairment. Intelligence is generally preserved. Flexor spasms in advanced cases may be painful.

Non-neurological: Kyphoscoliosis and pes cavus may precede onset of neurological symptoms by years. Visual and hearing loss can occur. Hypertrophic cardiomyopathy and diabetes mellitus are other important systemic complications.

Differential diagnosis is extensive and includes cerebellar tumor, congenital brainstem/cerebellar malformations, autosomal dominant spinocerebellar ataxias (SCAs), autosomal recessive ataxias/metabolic diseases (abetalipoproteinemia, ataxia-telangiectasia, ataxia with vitamin E deficiency, Hartnup disease, juvenile GM2 gangliosidosis, juvenile sulfatide lipidosis, maple syrup urine disease, Marinesco-Sjogren syndrome, mitochondrial disease, Ramsay-Hunt syndrome, Refsum disease) and X-linked ataxias (adrenoleukodystrophy, Leber optic atrophy, others).

Clinical course: The course of Friedreich ataxia is one of chronic progressive neurological deficits. Muscle strength is generally preserved but gait and limb ataxia gradually limit ambulation. Vibratory and proprioceptive sensation impairment is usually overt, and even pain and light touch can be affected. Despite some slow progression of neuropathic symptoms, peripheral nerve electrophysiology suggests a relatively stable peripheral neuropathy. Painful nocturnal muscle spasms become more common as the disease progresses. Cranial nerve functions also show progressive involvement (hearing and vision loss, impaired eye movements, dysarthria and dysphagia).

Other system involvement includes the development of cataracts, skeletal abnormalities, pes cavus (55%), hammer toes, kyphoscoliosis (79%, 5% at presentation), diabetes mellitus—insulin resistance (10% onset 3rd decade), hypertrophic cardiomyopathy (40%)—frequent EKG abnormalities are seen. Cardiac arrhythmias and congestive heart failure are leading causes of mortality.

Prognosis: Most patients will require a wheelchair in 10–15 years. Cardiomyopathy and heart failure are associated with worse prognosis. Importantly, intelligence is generally preserved, although some slowing of processing has been described. Life expectancy is 40–50 years.

Diagnosis

A definitive diagnosis is made by the specific *genetic test (PCR or Southern blot)* which will show an unstable triplet repeat expansion at the frataxin gene. Presymptomatic testing is generally not recommended, although this may change if new neuroprotective strategies are proven effective.

As patients with Friedreich ataxia often have cardiac involvement, electrocardiograms may show abnormalities such as deep Q waves, low QRS complexes, S-T wave changes or T wave inversion. Echocardiography can reveal a reduced ejection fraction. Ophthalmological examination is recommended upon diagnosis, as is testing for blood count, electrolytes and serum glucose. Brain MRI may also help distinguish between progressive cerebellar degenerations which show significant atrophy over time, and Friedreich ataxia which typically shows no or only mild cerebellar atrophy. Spine MRI may show thinning of the cervical cord and abnormal signal intensity in the posterior columns.

Nerve conduction studies are generally abnormal, showing sensory > motor neuropathic changes. Sural nerve biopsy generally shows loss of myelinated fibers. Somatosensory evoked potentials are either absent or severely delayed. Brainstem auditory and visual evoked potentials are also often abnormal.

Management

Medications

1. Coenzyme Q (400 mg qd), vitamin E (2100 IU/qd): Antioxidant targeted therapy that improved cardiac and muscle metabolism in an open-label pilot study.
2. Idebenone (5 mg/kg/d): Free radical scavenger, reduces cardiomyopathy in pilot studies. Higher doses 10–45 mg/kg/d may provide additional benefit, may halt disease progression.
3. L-carnitine (3 g/d) or L-acetylcarnitine (2 g/d): Improves metabolic parameters but did not improve ataxia or cardiomyopathy.
4. Antispasticity medications: Baclofen and tizanidine may be used for more global spasticity; botulinum toxin injections may be helpful in the management of spastic foot deformities.

5. Pain management.
6. Other investigational medications: Deferiprone (iron chelator); erythropoietin or histone deacetylase inhibitors (increase frataxin expression).

Surgery: Orthopedic interventions including surgical correction of scoliosis and/or limb deformities (i.e., pes cavus). Progressive kyphoscoliosis is more common in earlier onset cases.

Consultations: Given that Friedreich ataxia is really a multisystem disease, other specialty consultations should be obtained as needed.

Therapy: Supportive care includes physical and occupational therapy. Assistive devices such as braces, splints or a wheelchair will likely be needed for locomotion. Exercise may be helpful in maintaining aerobic fitness in early stages of the cardiomyopathy.

Patients should be monitored for hearing loss and provided hearing aids when necessary. Speech therapy with special voice treatments can be helpful for ataxic dysarthria. In later stages, the use of communication devices such as an alphabet chart.

Psych: Psychiatric support is helpful for social isolation, anxiety and depression. Selective serotonin reuptake inhibitors (fluoxetine, sertraline, paroxetine, citalprolam, escitalprolam) may be better than tricyclics. Family support is important.

Social: Genetic counseling is recommended to answer patient's/families' questions about the disorder and its heritability. Support groups and family involvement may be important. The National Ataxia Foundation website (http://www.ataxia.org/) provides information, chat rooms, a list of clinics and a listing of ongoing research studies.

Monitoring: Recommended annual check-up should include general medical evaluation (including vision and hearing screening), blood count, electrolytes, glucose, neurology and cardiology evaluations.

Pearls and Precautions

Nutrition: Monitor nutritional state, pay careful attention to development of diabetes. Progressive dysphagia will require dietary modifications, and eventually nasogastric or gastrostomy feeding.

Toilet: Sphincter disturbances may occur in up to 40% of affected patients. Urological consultation may be required. Oxybutinin may help with bladder overactivity. Sexual dysfunction may occur and be medically treatable.

Likely complications

- Electrocardiogram should be checked periodically. Cardiology follow-up and intervention for cardiomyopathy and congestive heart failure. May require regular medical management of heart failure related complications.
- Endocrine follow-up and monitoring for diabetes mellitus. Weight monitoring, diet and oral hypoglycemics may be necessary.
- Ophthalmological follow-up for cataracts, retinitis, optic atrophy.

Medication interactions: Since iron toxicity is part of the presumed pathogenesis, the use of iron supplementation (even in the setting of microcytic anemia) is controversial.

Caution with sedation due to theoretical risks of mitochondrial toxicity with propofol. In surgery or childbearing, care should be taken to monitor for fluid overload to avoid acute heart failure. Pregnant Friedreich patients have been reported to be unusually sensitive to the use of magnesium sulfate.

Reference

Alper G & Narayanan V. Friedreich's ataxia. Ped Neurol, 2003 May;28(5):335-41.

Schulz JB, Boesch S, Bürk K, Dürr A, Giunti P, Mariotti C, Pousset F, Schöls L, Vankan P, Pandolfo M. Diagnosis and treatment of Friedreich ataxia: a European perspective. Nat Rev Neurol. 2009 Apr;5(4):222-34.

Moyamoya Syndrome

Christopher C. Giza, Raman Sankar

Moyamoya syndrome is a syndrome of progressive occlusion of intracranial internal carotid arteries (ICAs) and formation of collaterals. Moyamoya means "puff of smoke" for its appearance on conventional arteriography.

Etiology

Primary moyamoya disease shows a strong hereditary disposition and has been associated with Chr. 3p24.2-p26. Secondary moyamoya syndrome has been associated with neurofibromatosis, sickle cell disease, other hemoglobinopathies, tuberous sclerosis, Down syndrome, congenital heart disease, Williams syndrome, fibromuscular dysplasia, young females (esp. cigarette smoking and OCPs) and post cranial irradiation. It has been reported post-CNS infection if associated with vasculitis. Up to 40% have an underlying hypercoagulable state.

Clinical Presentation and Prognosis

Moyamoya presents with different symptoms depending upon the age of the patient.

Demographics: Moyamoya occurs mostly in Japanese and has been associated with loci on Chr. 3, 6, 8 and 17. It occurs more often in females of less than 5 years of age. While originally described in Asians, it has since been reported in many ethnic populations. Both pediatric and adult presentations can occur.

Presenting signs and symptoms: Pediatric presentation of this disease occurs at approximately 5 years of age, with episodic hemiparesis, headache, seizures or other focal deficits and may be precipitated by exercise, exertion, hyperventilation or crying. However, adult presentation occurs in the mid-40s and presents with brain hemorrhage, usually in deep gray structures.

Four different "clinical" types include:

1. *Transient Ischemic Attack (50–75%):* This is the most common presentation form in children and appears as stroke-like event lasting less than 24 hours.
2. *Infarction (50-75%):* These are stroke-like presentations that persist.
3. *Hemorrhagic (10–40%):* This form is more commonly seen in adults and in Asian populations, presenting with abrupt onset of focal neurological deficit, headache, and alteration in mental status.
4. *Other:* Patients may also present with epilepsy (focal seizure), headache (often migraine-like), chorea, or cognitive or behavioral changes.

The differential diagnosis for the acute stroke-like presentation is very large and includes bacterial/viral infection, trauma, cardiac abnormalities, sickle cell disease, arteritis/vasculitis, AVMs, intracranial hemorrhage, Mitochondrial Encephalomyopathy, Lactic Acidosis, and Stroke-like episodes (MELAS), demyelinating disease and homocystinuria. Other considerations include seizure with subsequent Todd's paralysis (temporary paralysis following a seizure), or hemiplegic migraine.

Clinical course: Symptoms may occur abruptly and result in completed cerebral infarction. More common are episodic transient neurological deficits resembling transient ischemic attacks. Over time, there is progressive hemispheric or bihemispheric ischemia that can result in both focal and global neurological impairment.

Prognosis: In general, pediatric patients in better clinical neurological condition had better long-term post-surgical outcomes. Symptom progression occurs in 2/3 of patients over a 5 year period and medical therapy alone may not halt progression. A meta-analysis showed only 2.6% reported symptomatic progression after surgical intervention, but follow-up was variable ranging from 1 month to 19.5 years.

Untreated, mental impairment becomes more prominent over time (65% after 5 years). Hemorrhagic or epileptic presentations may have worse outcome/recovery.

Diagnosis

Neuroimaging is the most important diagnostic modality for diagnosis of moyamoya. Conventional angiography or magnetic resonance angiography *(MRA)* show bilateral internal carotid artery (ICA) occlusion. Middle cerebral and anterior cerebral arteries are also frequently involved. Collaterals appear as a "puff of smoke" on conventional angiography. *MRI* may reveal multiple areas of cerebral infarction. May see prominent signal voids in basal ganglia due to enlarged perforators/collaterals. *Diffusion weighted MRI* can demonstrate areas of acute ischemia, and *perfusion MRI* may show areas of impaired perfusion.

Labs to rule out underlying etiological diagnoses or hypercoagulable states include *CBC/platelets, anticardiolipin antibody, factor V Leiden, antithrombin III, protein C and protein S activity and levels, serum lipids, urine homocysteine. Echocardiography* may be ordered to look for structural cardiac disease or an embolic source.

Management

Surgical revascularization:

Direct surgical approach involves anastomosing the superficial temporal or occipital artery to the middle cerebral artery (MCA). This approach is less often used in children but provides immediate revascularization.

An indirect approach is more often used in children and takes time to fully develop collaterals from implanted bypass tissue to cortex. These include:

a. Encephalo-duro-arteriosynangiosis (EDAS): Dural graft.
b. Encephalo-arteriosynangiosis (EAS): Scalp artery bypass.
c. Encephalo-myo-synangiosis (EMS): Temporalis muscle flap graft.

Pediatric patients with EDAS have an excellent outcome (70%) of the time and an additional 17% have good function with some deficit. Patients have decreased risk of subsequent symptoms or stroke after a revascularization procedure.

Medications for stroke prevention (temporizing while waiting for surgery)

1. Aspirin: 81 mg qD, possibly other antiplatelet agents (clopidogrel)
2. Low molecular weight heparin
3. Verapamil: Use has been reported in case reports with moyamoya, but be careful not to cause hypotension.

Medications for acute ischemia (not necessarily Moyamoya in particular):

1. Aspirin: 81 mg qD, possibly other antiplatelet agents (clopidogrel).
2. Acute tPA: Effective within 4.5 hrs after thrombosis in adults. Use and risk in children has not been definitively studied.
3. Anticoagulation with heparin or low molecular weight heparin: May be used for gradually worsening strokes, recurrent emboli and hypercoagulable states. Anticoagulation with warfarin rarely used for strokes in children.
4. Negative trials: Hemodilution, nimodipine, steroids, naloxone.

Therapy: Physical, occupational and speech therapy are indicated for rehabilitation from completed strokes.

Social: There currently is no specific national foundation for moyamoya. However, there is a website and chatroom for those seeking information about this disease at www.moyamoya.com.

Pearls and Precautions

Likely complications: Completed strokes will require neurorehabilitation, depending upon the type of residual neurological deficit.

School/education: Education should be followed closely. In children who do not suffered repeated ischemic events, cognitive outcome may be relatively preserved. Children who present later or after completed ischemic events may have cognitive or developmental impairments and require appropriate educational assessment and intervention.

References

Bonduel M, Hepner M, Sciuccati G, Torres AF, Tenembaum S. Prothrombotic disorders in children with moyamoya syndrome. Stroke. 2001 Aug;32(8):1786-92.

Hoffman HJ. Moyamoya disease and syndrome. Clin Neurol Neurosurg. 1997 Oct;99 Suppl 2:S39-44.

McLean MJ, Gebarski SS, van der Spek AF, Goldstein GW. Response of moyamoya disease to verapamil. Lancet. 1985 Jan 19;1(8421):163-4.

Scott RM, Smith ER. Moyamoya disease and moyamoya syndrome. N Engl J Med. 2009 Mar 19;360(12): 1226-37.

Tic Disorder / Tourette Syndrome

Christopher C. Giza, Raman Sankar

A tic is a sudden, stereotyped, repetitive but nonrhythmic involuntary movement or sound. Motor tics typically involve movements in the face, head, neck or upper extremity but can occur anywhere in the body. Vocal (or phonic) tics are due to involuntary motor activity of the mouth, tongue or throat and result in sounds or even words being uttered. Tourette syndrome (TS) is a chronic neurobehavioral syndrome characterized by both motor and vocal tics, which represents the severe extreme of the spectrum of tic disorders. The vast majority of children with tics will not have Tourette syndrome but rather a tic disorder (transient, chronic or secondary).

Echolalia is a phenomenon of imitating words/sounds of others. Echopraxia is imitating actions of others. These reportedly occur in 11–44% of patients. Palilalia occurs when one repeats one's own last syllable or phrase and occurs in 6–15%. Coprolalia is a vocal tic characterized by utterance of obscenities, but is much rarer in real life than most laypersons would expect (10% of those with TS, 1% of all those with tic disorders). Copropraxia can be a tic consisting of obscene gestures (1–2%).

Etiology

Tic disorders and Tourette syndrome are believed to have a strong genetic component and may exist along a spectrum or continuum of severity. However, multiple genetic analyses have failed to identify any single locus for tics, which are most likely polygenic in origin. It has also been proposed that there is a neuroimmunological mechanism, although definitive evidence for this is lacking. By definition, the diagnoses of tic disorder and Tourette syndrome must not be associated with an underlying primary etiology. An interaction between environmental causes (brain injury, prenatal or perinatal difficulties, CNS infection, etc.) and underlying genetic predisposition has been proposed.

Secondary tic disorders are associated with an underlying etiology, including but not limited to Huntington chorea, post-encephalitis, lupus, medication-related (stimulants, neuroleptics, lamotrigine, carbamazepine, β-adrenoreceptor agonists used as bronchodilators, etc.), Wilson disease, traumatic brain injury, post-anoxia, Sydenham chorea, stroke and carbon monoxide poisoning. In general, the various etiologies represent an alteration in the functioning of the circuits involving the basal ganglia.

Clinical Presentation and Prognosis

Demographics: Tics are very common in childhood, with a prevalence of 4–19% (average 5%). Tourette syndrome is much rarer, with prevalence reported at 0.5–3.8% (average 1%). Tics of all sorts are more common in boys, with a gender preference of up to 5:1. Age of onset is typically early school years.

Presenting signs and symptoms: The most common presenting tics involve face and neck such as eye blinking, eye rolling, shoulder shrugging and facial grimacing, but virtually any type of abrupt involuntary motor activity can be a tic. Initial tics are frequently simple motor tics, that is, they involve only a single muscle. However, it is not possible to predict how many simple tics will remain stable versus which ones will go on to involve more muscles or also develop phonic tics.

Many patients describe a premonitory sensation or 'urge' usually referable to an anatomical region, that is relieved after the tics occurs. This is reported more commonly in adults and older adolescents than in younger children. Tics are often suppressible, at least for short periods of time. Many patients describe a buildup when suppressing tics that eventually needs to be 'released.' Tics often occur in clusters, and may be precipitated by many stimuli, varying between individuals but frequently remaining consistent within an individual. Stimuli or exacerbating factors include stress, fatigue, boredom, anxiety and caffeine/stimulants. Tics may persist in sleep.

Clinical course: After onset in early childhood, tics generally show a peak of severity in the preadolescent age range. Most tics decline in frequency and severity in the later teenage/early adult years. Most tics start as simple motor tics. They may then progress to more complex motor tics and/or include vocal/phonic tics. It is important to recognize exacerbating factors, and also to be aware that all tic disorders typically wax and wane over time. Therefore, just because a child is having a problem with tics at a given moment does not necessarily mean that the tics will be a persistent severe problem.

Prognosis: As indicated above, the prognosis for most chronic tics is a waxing and waning course with gradual improvement as the child matures. The major factors for long-term prognosis generally center more on behavioral comorbidities associated with tic disorder and TS than with the tics themselves. As a general rule, about 1/3 will resolve, 1/3 get better and 1/3 will have ongoing symptoms. A video study in adults demonstrated that even though tics persisted, the individuals were often unaware of and untroubled by them. Behavioral comorbidities that impact long term outcome include concomitant attention deficit hyperactivity disorder (ADHD) and obsessive compulsive disorder (OCD).

Diagnosis

The diagnosis of tics is generally done through clinical observation and history. For typically appearing or typically described tics in the setting of an otherwise normal neurological examination, extensive ancillary diagnostic workup is generally unfruitful. MRI and EEG are not indicated in a typical clinical presentation.

Clinical diagnosis of primary tic disorders separates them into 3 categories, all of which require that there be no underlying primary etiology secondarily resulting in the tics.

1. *Transient tic disorder.* This diagnosis is associated with single or multiple motor or vocal tics (but not motor and vocal), that may occur many times per day, occurring before the age of 18 years. The duration of tics is longer than 4 weeks but less than 12 months.
2. *Chronic tic disorder.* The diagnostic criteria for this are the same as transient tic disorder, with the exception that the symptoms must last >12 months, and that there was never a tic-free period of >3 months.
3. *Tourette syndrome.* Tourette syndrome is characterized by both motor and vocal tics at some time (although not necessarily concurrent), occurring for >12 months and never showing a tic free period >3 months. Again, the onset should be under the age of 18 years.

Tics that have onset outside the typical age range, or show atypical features or clinical course, should be worked up to rule out whether they may be due to some secondary cause (see etiology above).

Management

A general rule for the management of tic disorders and Tourette syndrome is to identify and target the most disabling symptoms for treatment. Sometimes this is the tics, but often it may be the behavioral comorbidities. Educating parents, children as well as teachers and peers is important, as many misperceptions about tics abound. For mild tics, education and reassurance are often all that is required, and medications may be kept in reserve for exacerbations that interfere with school or daily activities.

Medications: There is a broad range of medications with effectiveness in controlling tics. Often the best choice pharmacologically is an anti-tic medication that also addresses one of the comorbid conditions. Use of medications to suppress tics should be directed towards tics that are disabling due to social reasons, pain or self-injury. Parental concern in the absence of any tic-related distress in the child should not be an indication for medications. Since tics naturally wax and wane, some tics may spontaneously resolve, and even when treatment with drugs is initiated, periodic attempts at weaning may be successful after a period of good control.

1. Alpha-2-adrenergic agonists may be helpful for both tics and ADHD.
   a. Clonidine is effective in 50% of patients. Main side effects are sedation. It is available as a weekly patch, although some develop cutaneous hypersensitivity reactions.
   b. Guanfacine is potentially superior to clonidine, as it is less sedating and has a longer duration of action. Syncope has been reported as a side effect in rare cases.
2. Dopamine (D2) receptor antagonists.
   a. Risperidone is as effective as older neuroleptics, but is better tolerated. Its main side effects are weight gain and sedation.
   b. Pimozide is effective in 70% of cases, with fewer adverse effects than haloperidol. One potentially serious adverse effect is that it can cause cardiac arrhythmias.
   c. Haloperidol is similar in efficacy to pimozide. It has a higher rate of side effects (sedation, weight gain, tardive movements) than other agents in this class.
3. Dopamine receptor agonists that can be used for tics include low doses of pergolide and ropirinol.
4. Tetrabenazine is effective for hypekinetic movement disorders including tics; however, it is not readily available in the U.S. One advantage of this agent is the absence of associated tardive dyskinesia, but it can cause depression and/or parkinsonism in some individuals.
5. Benzodiazepines may be useful acutely for tic exacerbations, but due to sedation they are less well tolerated as a maintenance therapy.
6. Other agents have been used anecdotally and may have efficacy, including ondansetron, verapamil, levetiracetam and others. For very focal tics, some have successfully used botulinum toxin injections.

Surgery: Deep brain stimulation is an interesting new treatment for intractable tics/Tourette syndrome and potentially also shows benefits for intractable OCD. Regions stimulated and showing efficacy in recent reports include anterior limb of the internal capsule, intralaminar thalamic nuclei and globus pallidus pars interna. Ablations, including unilateral pallidotomy and bilateral anterior capsulotomy have also been reported to be effective.

Psychiatric therapy: Psychiatric consultation and management is extremely valuable for the comorbid behavioral complications seen in children with tics and Tourette syndrome. Three major categories of comorbid behavioral disturbance that may require intervention are ADHD, OCD and rage attacks. Other behavioral issues include anxiety and depression. There is benefit from the primary physician being aware of these therapies, even though they are best managed in consultation with a child psychiatrist.

1. *ADHD:* Use of stimulants has a theoretical risk of exacerbating underlying tics. However, this risk appears to be modest, and the benefits of effectively treating ADHD are substantial. Use of alpha-2-adrenergic agonists may be effective for both tics and ADHD. There is some evidence to suggest that combined therapy with methylphenidate and clonidine is more effective than either alone. Atomoxetine may also be effective for both tics and ADHD.

2. *OCD/OCB:* First line pharmacotherapy for obsessive compulsive symptoms are the selective serotonin reuptake inhibitors (SSRIs), such as fluvoxamine, sertraline, fluoxetine and paroxetine. There is a slightly increased risk of suicidality reported with these agents, particularly in patients with existing depression.

3. *Rage:* There is a paucity of data from controlled trials for management of rage/emotional lability in kids with Tourette syndrome. If there is concomitant ADHD, a trial of a stimulant +/- clonidine may be considered. Mood stabilizing drugs such as valproate, carbamazepine and lithium have shown some efficacy. Other drugs that have been anecdotally effective include the atypical neuroleptics, such as risperidone, ziprasidone and olanzapine.

Therapy: Cognitive behavioral therapy is of limited effectiveness in controlling tics, although in the hands of an experienced therapist, can be quite helpful for OCD. For single tics that are disabling, the use of habit reversal therapy (HRT) has shown evidence of sustained improvement in some cases.

Transcranial magnetic stimulation: Open label use of this modality over the supplementary motor area has been reported to reduce tics. This treatment is still in the research stage.

Social: The mainstay of therapy for mild tics is education and reassurance to the family and child. Often the presence of tics is more troubling to the parent than the young child. Older children and adolescents may face some social stigma, depending upon the type of tic(s) they have. Support groups also exist and may be beneficial. Helpful websites with valuable information include www.tsa-usa.org (U.S.) and www.tourette.ca (Canada).

Pearls and Precautions

Sleep: Sleep disturbances are fairly common in children with Tourette syndrome (20–50%), and less so in children with tic disorders. If hyperactivity or obsessive thoughts are contributing, then management of those comorbid conditions may be helpful.

School/education: Learning difficulties occur in up to 25% of children with Tourette syndrome and may be due to the tics themselves, ADHD, OCB/OCD or as adverse effects from medications. Identifying and treating the underlying condition(s) is likely beneficial, as is proper assessment and educational placement/intervention for identified learning disabilities.

References

Dooley JM. Tic disorders in childhood. Semin Pediatr Neurol. 2006 Dec;13(4):231-42.
Shprecher D, Kurlan R. The management of tics. Mov Disord. 2009 Jan 15;24(1):15-24.

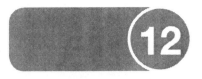

12 Oncologic Disorders

Table of Contents

Acute Lymphoblastic Leukemia (ALL)

Pamela Kempert, Theodore B. Moore

Acute Lymphoblastic Leukemia (ALL) is a clonal expansion or arrest at a specific stage of normal lymphoid development. It results from a clonal transformation of hematopoietic precursors through the acquisition of chromosomal rearrangements and multiple gene mutations. ALL comprises 75% of all the childhood leukemias and the peak incidence occurs between 2–5 years of age.

Etiology

The etiology of ALL is unclear although there appears to be both a genetic predisposition as well as an environmental or infectious trigger.

Clinical Presentation and Prognosis:

Demographics: The incidence is approximately 40 cases per million with approximately 7000 new cases diagnosed each year in the United States. ALL accounts for more than 80% of childhood leukemia with acute myelogenous leukemia and chronic myelogenous leukemia accounting for most of the rest. The majority of ALL are precursor B-cell leukemias, with approximately 15% of the cases T-cell, and less than 5% mature B-cell.

Presenting signs and symptoms: Onset of clinical symptoms is typically insidious and related to leukemic proliferation in the reticuloendothelial system. Replacement of the marrow results in thrombocytopenia, anemia and neutropenia. This may be manifest by petechiae, pallor and fevers. There is often the complaint of bone pain. Extramedullary proliferation may be appreciated as lymphadenopathy, splenomegaly or a mediastinal mass.

Clinical Course: Without intervention, the patient's disease will progress leading to death from primarily either bleeding or infection. With induction chemotherapy, resolution of signs and symptoms should occur after 2–4 weeks.

Prognosis/survival: Patients with standard risk ALL have long-term remission in more than 85% of cases, with the vast majority cured of their disease. There are certain prognostic factors at diagnosis that affect their outcome. Treatment is modified based on these factors. Favorable factors include: Initial white blood cell count (WBC) of <50,000/L and age 1–9 years; pre-B subtype, hyperploidy, lack of organomegaly, low bone marrow blasts on day 8 or 15 of induction therapy; and less than .01% at day 29; trisomy of chromosomes 4 and 10; and, t(4:11) or Tel/AML1 translocations. Poor prognostic factors include: WBC >50,000/L; age of less than 1 year or more than 10 years; organomegaly, central nervous sytem (CNS) involvement at diagnosis; the presence of a mediastinal mass; lymphoma-like features; failure to achieve remission by day 15 or 29; and, certain chromosomal translocations—especially the Philadelphia chromosome and the MLL gene rearrangements (11q23) in infants.

Diagnosis

A high index of suspicion for ALL should be maintained when a patient presents with the above signs and symptoms. A complete blood count with a full differential should be obtained for screening and provide evidence with the presence of blasts on the peripheral blood smear. Confirmation of the diagnosis is made based on a bone marrow aspiration or flow cytometry on the peripheral blood if there is a high leukemic blast count. Examination by flow cytometry typically demonstrates CD-10 (common acute lymphoblastic leukemia antigen-CALLA), CD-19, and terminal deoxynucleotidyl transferase (TDT) positive markers in the majority of the precursor B-cell leukemias. Cytogenetic examination of the blast cells should be ordered as well, as these results may have significant prognostic implications. A chest X-ray must be performed to evaluate for a mediastinal mass which is often found in T-cell ALL and may represent an oncologic emergency.

Management

In the initial management of ALL, there are four most urgent issues that must be dealt with: (1) Tumor lysis syndrome; (2) hyperleukocytosis; (3) transfusion needs; and (4) evaluation for a mediastinal mass.

Tumor Lysis: Tumor lysis syndrome may be present at diagnosis and may be manifest as hyperkalemia, hyperuricemia and hyperphosphatemia. These may lead to renal failure and cardiac arrest. Intravenous fluids (without potassium added) should be started at 1.5–2 times maintenance and sodium bicarbonate or sodium acetate added to the fluids to keep the urine pH neutral. Low pH may result in crystallization of uric acid in the kidneys and high pH may result in calcium phosphate crystals formation, both of which may lead to renal failure. Tumor lysis labs (potassium, uric acid, phosphorous, creatinine) should be followed every 6–8 hours until normalized. Allopurinol or rasburicase should be administered to treat hyperuricemia. Phosphate binders should be given and, if necessary, measures to reduce potassium levels. The nephrology service should be alerted regarding the patient in case the need for dialysis arises from renal shut down. Prompt referral to a pediatric hematologist should be made for the initiation of therapy.

Hyperleukocytosis: High presenting white blood cell counts (WBCs) may represent an oncologic emergency from the significant amount of tumor lysis as well as from the effects of hyperviscosity of the blood. Symptoms of hyperviscosity may manifest as headache, neurologic defects, priapism and others. Prompt referral to a pediatric hematologist should be made to begin either apheresis, chemotherapy or both.

Transfusion: Correction of thrombocytopenia and anemia must be done judiciously. Platelet transfusions should be considered for symptomatic patients or those with a platelet count less than 20. Patients with anemia should be considered for red cell transfusion if they are symptomatic or have a hemoglobin level less than 6. This must be done slowly as to not put the patient into pulmonary edema. A useful rule of thumb would be to transfuse an initial volume in milliliters equal to the product of the hemoglobin times the weight in kilograms (cc=hgb x Kg) over a 2–4 hour period of time and reassess prior to each subsequent transfusion. If possible, transfusion of patients with hyperleukocytosis should be deferred until reduction of the white blood cell count as this may exacerbate the hyperviscosity. All blood products must be irradiated.

Mediastinal Mass: All patients suspected of having ALL should have a screening chest X-ray to evaluate for a mediastinal mass.

Chemotherapy: Induction chemotherapy should be started promptly by a qualified practitioner initiating therapy with a diagnostic and therapeutic lumbar puncture with intrathecal chemotherapy administration, followed by systemic chemotherapy. Therapy is given over a 3 ¼ year period for boys and 2 ¼ year period for girls and is primarily outpatient in nature. Therapy begins with Induction consisting of vincristine, prednisone, and peg-asparaginase, CNS prophylaxis and the addition of daunomycin, depending on risk stratification. This is followed by additional therapy consisting of the following phases: Consolidation, interim maintenance; delayed intensification; 2ⁿᵈ interim maintenance; and, maintenance.

Surgery: Central venous access should be placed, preferably with a "port-a-cath," so as to minimize the trauma to the patient of frequent blood draws and chemotherapy infusions.

Psychologic: Counseling should be recommended for the patient, parents and siblings. As many as 25% of parents may develop post-traumatic-stress-syndrome. Siblings may "act-out" for attention as a greater portion of parents time will focus on the patient. Child Life should provide therapy to children and their siblings.

Social: It is crucial that a social worker assess and provide assistance to these families. Often, one parent must take a leave of absence from their employment to facilitate getting their child to their treatments. Many states have a family leave act and other such programs that the social worker can access for the family. In addition, resources from the leukemia society, Make-a-Wish, college scholarship fund and other such programs can be facilitated through the social worker. Parents can find additional information and support at: www.leukemia-lymphoma.org, www.rmhc.org/, www.wish.org, and www.candlelighters.org/.

Survival and monitoring: The 5-year survival rate is >85% in children with "good-prognosis" ALL following standard therapy. Even children with high risk factors who receive intensive therapy may have an overall long-term survival of at least 70%. However, patients with very high risk disease (e.g., Ph + disease) may require aggressive therapy which could include a hematopoietic stem cell transplant. Sites of relapse include the CNS, testes, and bone marrow. The risk for relapse after 3 years of therapy is very low. Patients are followed monthly for disease recurrence and organ dysfunction with complete blood counts and complete metabolic panels for the first year; every 3 months for the second year; every 6 months for the third year; and, then yearly thereafter.

ALL patients should be followed lifelong for any long term complications from the disease or its treatment. This should be coordinated within a clinic that has experience in following these patients and should include education for the patient of their disease and its therapy, evaluations for growth and development, organ function, fertility issues, cognitive/school issues as well as counseling regarding future health insurance and peer networks.

Pearls and Precautions

Immunization: Immunizations are generally held during the chemotherapy treatment due to poor vaccine response. No live viral vaccines can be safely given. Inactivated or "killed" Influenzae vaccines are recommended.

School/education: Patients will miss a significant amount of school. A qualified school reintegration specialist is an integral part of the team, bridging the gap between the patient and his school work, school mates and teacher.

Herbs and nutrition: Many herbs and high dose vitamins can interfere with the activity of chemotherapy or interfere with platelet function. All herbs and nutritional supplements must be approved by the treating physician. Survivors of Childhood ALL have a higher rate of obesity than age matched siblings. Careful counseling about a healthy diet and exercise is essential while on- as well as off of therapy. Additional information regarding the use of herbal medications and cancer can be obtained at:

NCI website for herbal medicines: www.cancer.gov/cam/health_camaz.html.

Memorial Sloan Kettering Cancer Center website: www.mskcc.org/html/58481.cfm.

Likely complications: Patients may have frequent admissions for fever and neutropenia while on therapy. Any fever represents an emergency because of the patients' immunodeficient state as well as the presence of an indwelling central venous catheter in most of the patients. Patients must emergently seek medical assistance which should include at minimum an evaluation of the blood counts, blood cultures and consideration of the initiation of intravenous antibiotic therapy to cover both gram negative and positive microganisms depending on local sensitivities. Patients may develop several common toxicities from their medication in addition to neutropenia including pancytopenia, constipation, alopecia, foot drop, mouth sores and others.

Miscellaneous

- Monitor closely for tumor lysis and administer IV fluid hydration in children suspected of having ALL.
- CHEST X-RAY should be performed to evaluate for a mediastinal mass as can be found in T-cell ALL.
- Long term outcome is excellent for most of the patients.

References

Pui CH, Robison LL, Look AT. Acute lymphoblastic leukaemia. Lancet. 2008 Mar 22;371(9617):1030–43.

Pui CH, Campana D, Pei D, et al. Treating childhood acute lymphoblastic leukemia without cranial irradiation. N Engl J Med. 2009 Jun 25;360(26):2730–41.

Revised Long Term Follow-up Guidelines from the Children's Oncology Group at www.curesearch.org.

Acute Myelogenous Leukemia (AML)

(Acute nonlymphocytic leukemia (ANLL))

Pamela Kempert, Theodore B. Moore

Acute Myelogenous Leukemia is a clonal expansion or arrest at a specific stage of normal myeloid development. It also results from a clonal transformation of hematopoietic precursors through the acquisition of chromosomal rearrangements and multiple gene mutations.

Etiology

AML is only 15–20% of all new leukemia in children.

It is a clonal transformation of hematopoietic precursors through the acquisition of chromosomal rearrangements and multiple gene mutations.

In most children, no identifiable cause can be found. However, AML has been associated with exposure to chemotherapy, radiation therapy, herbicides, petroleum products, organic solvents, and pesticides (organophosphates).

A large number of inherited conditions predispose children to the development of AML. These include Down's syndrome, Fanconi anemia, severe congenital neutropenia (Kostmann), Schwachmann Diamond, Diamond Blackfan (pure red cell aplasia), Neurofibromatosis type I, Noonan syndrome, Dyskeratosis Congenital (BM failure syndrome), congential amegakaryocytic thrombocytopenia, ataxia-telangiectasia, Kleinfelter syndrome, Li Fraumeni syndrome and Bloom syndrome. In addition, AML has been associated with acquired aplastic anemia, myelodysplastic syndrome, acquired amegakaryocytic thrombocytopenia and paroxysmal nocturnal hemoglobinuria.

Mutations in genes that confer a proliferative and/or survival advantage underlie most cases, but the changes do not affect differentiation. These include Flt3, ALM, Ras, PTPN11 and BCR/ABL and TEL/PDGFβR gene fusion. Other mutations impair differentiation and apoptosis. AML/ETO PML/RARα, MLL rearrangements, and mutations of CEBPA, CBF, HOX and CBP/P300. AML results when the cells acquire both types of mutations. Favorable karyotypes t(8;21), t(15;17), inv 16 have survival of 72%

Unfavorable karyotypes monosomy 5, monosomy 7, del (5q) and (3q) or other complex karyotypes have a very poor survival.

Clinical Presentation and Prognosis:

Demographics: The incidence is 5–7 cases per million people per year with a peak of 11 cases at 2 years of age. The incidence reaches a low point at 9 years and then increases during adolescence. The incidence is the same in the white and black population as it is in males and females. There is some evidence that the incidence is highest in Hispanic children. All subtypes of AML are equal across ethnic backgrounds and racial groups with the exception of Acute Promyelocytic Leukemia which has a higher incidence in the Hispanic population.

Presenting signs and symptoms: The normal bone marrow cells are replaced; therefore, many patients present with pancytopenia or neutrophilia with anemia and thrombocytopenia. Children usually have fatigue, pallor, fever, bleeding and petechiae, bone pain, and possibly infection. Patients may present with disseminated intravascular coagulation especially in acute promyelocytic leukemia (APML). Infiltration of lymph nodes with enlargement as well as liver and spleen occurs in greater than 50%. Some patients have chloromas (infiltration of the blasts into the orbit, ear canal or the central nervous system). Infiltration of the skin known as leukemia cutis is especially seen in infants with the monocytic M5 leukemia. Disease in the orbit, epidural space or testes is very rare. Disease occurs in the central nervous system 15% of the time especially in infants. Patients who present with extremely high white counts may show signs of leukostasis, most often affecting the lungs and the brain.

Clinical course: Patients who present with leukostasis will most likely need pharesis and immediate diagnosis and treatment. They may develop tumor lysis with renal failure, hyperuricemia, hyperkalemia, hypocalcemia and hyperphosphatemia. They will require hydration, rasburicase and correction of hyperkalemia and hyperphosphatemia. Please see ALL management of tumor lysis for specific management issues.

Chemotherapy to most patients is given in several dose intensive induction courses. After the second induction course the patient may remain pancytopenic with high risk of infection for 3–4 weeks. Patients need to receive a minimum of 4 induction courses. This is usually followed by several intensification courses. None of the patients except APML receive maintenance chemotherapy courses.

Prognosis: The rate of complete remission is as high as 80–90% and overall survival rates of 60% are now reported. In a recent study of 13 treatment studies, the relapse rates were 30–40%; event free survival rate was 50%; and, overall survival at 5 years was 60%.

Diagnosis

Physical Exam: The exam may show pallor, petechiae, lymphadenopathy, hepatosplenomegaly. Careful exam of the eyes and ears for signs of chloromas is required. All patients need a careful Neurologic assessment to rule out signs of central nervous system (CNS) disease, epidural compression or increased intracranial pressure from CNS chloromas.

Laboratory: A complete blood count will often show anemia thrombocytopenia and variably low or high WBC. A complete metabolic profile including calcium, phosphorous, uric acid and Lactate Dehydrogenase (LDH) which is likely to show elevated uric acid and elevated LDH. In addition, coagulation studies prothrombin time, partial thromboplastin time, fibrinogen and fibrin split products need to be checked which are likely to show disseminated intravascular coagulation, particularly in patients with APML as well as renal and hepatic function panels. CMV titers as a baseline are important to check for exposure and need for CMV negative blood products. Varicella titers are needed to check for exposure and immunity respectively.

Radiology studies: A chest X-ray needs to be done to look for leukemic infiltrate in the lungs and (rarely) mediastinal mass. A CT or brain and orbit MRI should be considered both to look for any CNS symptoms as well as any evidence of chloramas, meningeal, or cranial nerve enhancement.

Invasive procedures: These include a bone marrow aspirate and biopsy with flow cytometry and cytogenetics (exception is extremely high WBC which can provide cells for diagnostic studies); and, a lumbar puncture for cytology to determine the presence of blasts in the CSF.

Classification: M0 undifferentiated: M1 myeloblastic, M2 myeloblastic with differentiation, M3 acute promyelocytic, M4 both monocytic and myelocytic differentiation, M5 monocytic, M6 erythroleukemia, and M7 megakaryoblastic leukemia.

Prognosis: Factors associated with poor prognosis include WBC > 100,000, Monosomy 7, Secondary AML, Flt3 ITD, and residual disease after induction.

Management

Chemotherapy: The treatment is based on anthracyclines either daunomycin or idarubicin, cytarabine and etoposide with several cycles of induction chemotherapy. This is followed by additional post remission chemotherapy or bone marrow transplant. Studies in Europe and the U.S. have shown no benefit to maintenance therapy for ANLL except for all trans retinoic acid therapy for APML.

Transplant: Chemotherapy in some patients may be followed by bone marrow transplant. Patients with Down's syndrome, APML, t 8;21 and inversion 16 are not candidates for bone marrow transplant since they have a favorable prognosis without it.

Surgery: Placement of central line or PIC line for the administration of chemotherapy.

Therapy: Physical and occupational therapy to maintain developmental milestones and muscle tone may be very beneficial during long hospitalizations and isolation due to severe neutropenia.

Psychological: Psychological counseling should be recommended for the patient, parents and siblings. Siblings may "act-out" for attention as a greater portion of parents time will focus on the patient. Child life should provide therapy to children and their siblings.

Social: It is crucial that a social worker assess and provide assistance to these families. Often one parent must take a leave of absence from their employment to facilitate getting their child to their treatments. Many states have a family leave act and other such programs that the social worker can access for the family. In addition, resources from the leukemia society, Make-a-Wish, college scholarship fund and other such programs can be facilitated through the social worker. Parents can get additional support and information at the following websites:

- Most up to date treatment summary at (NCI PDQ summary) www.cancer.gov/cancertopics/pdq/treatment/childhodgkins/healthprofessional/
- Listing of all open clinical trials in the U.S. www.cancer.gov/clinicaltrials
- Revised Long Term Follow-up Guidelines from the Children's Oncology Group at www.curesearch.org.

Pearls and Precautions

Immunization: Same as ALL.

Likely complications: Short term complications include anemia, thrombocytopenia and neutropenia that leads to an increased risk of infection is one of the most common and serious side effects. Patients are especially at risk of Streptococcus Viridans due to the administration of cytosine arabinoside and require Vancomycin as well as broad spectrum antibiotic coverage for gram positive and gram negative micro-organism. If they have signs of typhlitis or acute abdomen, then anaerobic coverage should be added. In addition, if fever persists for

3–5 days despite adequate coverage, then antifungal medication needs to be added. Also, patients have hair loss, nausea and vomiting, diarrhea and/or constipation as well as mucositis. Patients can develop peripheral neuropathy secondary to the vinca alkaloids. For control of nausea, vomiting, and mucositis and pain, please see the section on chemotherapy and radiation therapy.

Until a decision is made regarding the need for bone marrow transplantation and if any of the family is a match, no first or second degree relatives should be blood donors. All blood products need to be irradiated.

Long term complications include, cardiomyopathy, infertility, and secondary malignancy. Doxorubicin with or without radiation therapy to the chest may lead to decreased cardiac mass, which may result in reduced contractility and cardiomyopathy. Infertility due to a high dose of cyclophosphamide and/or radiation therapy to the abdomen can occur in girls. Male fertility can be affected by high doses of alkylator therapy (cyclophosphamide) used with bone marrow transplant. Girls also have a risk of ovarian failure and premature menopause after bone marrow transplantation. The most serious risk is secondary malignancy.

School/education: Patients will miss a significant amount of school. A qualified school reintegration specialist is an integral part of the team, bridging the gap between the patient and his school work, school mates and teacher.

Medications/situations/herbals to be avoided: The patient should not be exposed to anyone with a known infectious illness. Many herbs and high dose vitamins can interfere with the activity of chemotherapy or interfere with platelet function. All herbs and nutritional supplements must be approved by the treating physician. No herbal medications or supplements that are made from roots, bark or plant parts that have not been sterilized should be given due to the possibility of fungal or bacterial contamination of these products. The best reference for the use of specific herbal medicines and their safety are:

- NCI website for herbal medicines: www.cancer.gov/cam/health_camaz.html.
- Memorial Sloan Kettering Cancer Center website: www.mskcc.org/html/58481.cfm.

Miscellaneous

- A large number of inherited conditions predispose children to the development of AML, especially BM failure syndromes, Down's syndrome, Neurofibromatosis I, Noonan's syndrome, Bloom's syndrome and Li Fraumeni syndrome.
- Patients may present with disseminated intravascular coagulation especially in acute promyelocytic leukemia (APML).
- Patients are especially at risk of Streptoccocus Viridans due to the administration of cytosine arabinoside and require Vancomycin as well as broad spectrum antibiotic coverage for gram positive and gram negative micro-organisms for any febrile neutropenic episodes.

References

Ravindranath Y. Balwierz, W Armata, J. et. Al. Pediatric Oncology Group studies of acute myeloid leukemia conducted between 1981 and 2000. Leukemia 2005;19:2101–16.

Rubnitz, Jeffrey, Brenda Gibson and Franklin Smith. Acute Myeloid leukemia. Pediatric Clinics of North America. 2008;55:21–51

S. Shenoy and FO Smith. Review Hematopoietic stem cell transplantation for childhood malignancies of myeloid origin. Bone marrow transplantation. 2008; 41:141–148.

Smith, FO, Alonzo TA and Gerbine RB, et. al. Long Term Results of children with acute myeloid leukemia: a report of three consecutive ANML-BFMM trials. Leukemia 2005; 19:2030–42.

Ewing Family Tumors

(Ewing sarcoma, Primitive neuroectodermal tumor)

Pamela Kempert, Theodore B. Moore

The Ewing family of malignant tumors includes both Ewing sarcoma of bone, extraosseous Ewing Sarcoma and primitive neuroectodermal tumor (PNET). It is one of the pediatric small round blue cell tumors (SRBCT), anaplastic in appearance, and CD99 positive. Greater than 85% carry the translocation involving chromosomes 11 and 22 resulting in the formation of a ews-fli1 chimera. The tumor may also be able to be distinguished from other such SRBCT by the presence of p30/32 MIC2 in some of the tumors.

Etiology

The Ewing family of tumors (EWS) includes both Ewing sarcoma of bone, extraosseous Ewing Sarcoma and primitive neuroectodermal tumor (PNET). The etiology is unclear at this time, although a genetic predisposition cannot be ruled out, as it is more common in certain ethnicities.

Clinical Presentation and Prognosis

Demographics: The incidence is approximately 1.5 cases per 1 million. Seventy percent of cases are in patients 4–16 years of age with a peak incidence at 12 years for girls and 15 years for boys. The male to female ratio is 1.5:1. It's occurrence is rare in children of African descent.

Presenting sign and symptoms: This disease often presents as a painful local swelling or a palpable mass over the site of the tumor. These typically occur mid shaft in the long bones, but can also occur in any bony portion of the body. In addition, they can occur in extraosseous sites. When PNET's occur in the chest wall they are referred to as Askin tumors. Twenty to thirty percent of patients have metastatic disease at the time of presentation. The lungs are the most common site of metastasis. Other sites include lymph nodes, bone, bone marrow and CNS. Patients may also present with fever and a high white count, which may make it difficult clinically to distinguish from acute or chronic osteomyelitis. An MRI may be helpful in making this distinction. Other diseases for which this may be confused include but are not limited to osteosarcoma, neuroblastoma, eosinophilic granuloma and lymphoma.

Clinical course: Treatment involves a multidisciplinary approach in order to optimize outcome. The treatment team should be experienced with treating pediatric oncology patients. Inappropriate therapy has been shown to decrease survival chances.

Prognosis/survival: Patients with localized limb lesions have better prognosis (event free survival 76%) than those with central or metastatic lesions (< 30%). Fever, an elevated Lactate Dehydrogenase (LDH) and a high white blood cell count may also be predictive of a more aggressive disease.

Diagnosis

A biopsy of the suspected lesion should be performed by an experienced surgical oncologist or interventional radiologist. Pretreatment studies include an erythrocyte sedimentation rate, radiograph (frequently demonstrates a lytic lesion; may have classical "onion skin" appearance), MRI of the primary site, CT of chest, bilateral bone marrow biopsies, bone scan and a baseline PET scan to follow for active disease.

Management

An aggressive multimodal approach must be used to affect a cure. Good local control through surgery and/or radiation is crucial.

Chemotherapy: Adjuvant chemotherapy is useful in the treatment of EWS. Active drugs that are commonly utilized include (but are not limited to) vincristine, doxorubicin and cyclophosphamide alternating with ifosfamide and etoposide. Presurgical chemotherapy administration may provide reduction of tumor load improving the chances of obtaining a total surgical resection.

Surgical/radiation therapy: A central venous catheter should be placed so as to minimize the trauma to the patient due to frequent blood draws and chemotherapy infusions. For localized disease, a total surgical resection improves the chance for cure. If the surgical margin of a localized tumor is greater than 1 cm, radiation therapy may not be needed. When radiation therapy is utilized, it is typically fractionated over several weeks delivering a total dose in the range of 3,000–5,400 Gy.

Psychological: Counseling should be recommended for the patient, parents and siblings. Siblings may "act-out" for attention as a greater portion of parents' time will focus on the patient. Child life should provide therapy to children and their siblings. It is crucial for these families to receive social worker assessment and assistance. Often one parent must take a leave of absence from their employment to facilitate getting their child to their treatments. Many states have a family leave act and other such programs that the social worker can access for the family. In addition, resources from the American Cancer Society, Make-a-Wish, college scholarship fund and other such programs can be facilitated through the social worker.

Monitoring: Patients are followed for disease recurrence with repeat CT/MRI every 6 months for the first two years and then annually times two years. The patients should be followed lifelong for any long term complications from the disease or its treatment. This should be coordinated within a clinic that has experience in following these patients and should include education for the patient of their disease and its therapy, evaluations for growth and development, organ function, secondary malignancies, fertility issues, cognitive/school issues as well as counseling regarding future health insurance and peer networks.

Pearls and Precautions:

Immunization: Please see ALL.

Herbs and nutrition: Many herbs and high dose vitamins can interfere with the activity of chemotherapy or interfere with platelet function. All herbs and nutritional supplements must be approved by the treating physician. Careful counseling about a healthy diet and exercise is essential while on therapy as well as off of therapy. Additional information regarding the use of herbal medications and cancer can be obtained at:

- NCI website for herbal medicines: www.cancer.gov/cam/health_camaz.html.
- Memorial Sloan Kettering Cancer Center website: www.mskcc.org/html/58481.cfm

Likely complications: Patients may have frequent admissions for fever and neutropenia while on therapy. Any fever represents an emergency because of the patient's immunodeficient state as well as the presence of an indwelling central venous catheter in most of the patients. Patients must emergently seek medical assistance which should include the minimum of an evaluation of the blood counts, blood cultures and consideration of the initiation of intravenous antibiotic therapy. Patients may develop several common toxicities from their medication in addition to neutropenia, including pancytopenia, constipation, alopecia, foot drop, mouth sores and others.

Miscellaneous

- Periosteal reaction with new bone formation gives an onion peel-like appearance on plain radiogram which is suggestive of EWS.

References

Ludwig JA. Ewing sarcoma: historical perspectives, current state-of-the-art, and opportunities for targeted therapy in the future. Current Opinion in Oncology 2008, 20:412–418

Heare T, Hensley MA, Dell'Orfano S. Bone tumors: osteosarcoma and Ewing's sarcoma. Curr Opin Pediatr. 2009 Jun;21(3):365–72.

Caudill JS, Arndt CA. Diagnosis and management of bone malignancy in adolescence. Adolesc Med State Art Rev. 2007 May;18(1):62–78

Hodgkin Lymphoma

Pamela Kempert, Theodore B. Moore

Hodgkin lymphoma is a malignancy of lymph nodes characterized by a progressive enlargement of one or more lymph nodes. Hodgkin lymphoma is felt to be a tumor of B lymphocyte origin, specifically germinal center B cells with rearranged immunoglobulin genes.

Etiology

Hodgkin lymphoma is a malignancy of lymph nodes characterized by a progressive enlargement of one or more lymph nodes. The worldwide incidence of Hodgkin lymphoma is 2–4 new cases per 100,000 population per year. The childhood form (less than 15 years) is associated with lower socioeconomic status, but the adolescent form is associated with a higher economic status in the industrialized world. The risk decreases with increased family size and higher birth order. There are family clusters and this may be related to specific HLA types. There is concordance in first degree relatives. The incidence is also increased in patients with immunodeficiency disorders, either acquired or congenital.

A prior history of Epstein Barr Virus infection increases the risk fourfold. Although the virus genome is identified in the Reed Sternberg cells, its precise role in the pathogenesis of Hodgkin lymphoma is unknown. The viral genome is more frequently seen in children less than 10 years of age and in cases occurring in developing countries. Hodgkin lymphoma is felt to be a tumor of B lymphocyte origin, specifically germinal center B cells with rearranged immunoglobulin genes.

Clinical Presentation and Prognosis

Demographics: The incidence peaks at 15–25 years of age and again after age 50. It makes up only 5–6% of childhood cancers in children younger than 15 years, but 16% of cancers in adolescents. Thus, it is the most common malignancy in this age group. The male to female ratio is 1.7–2:1.

Presenting signs and symptoms: These include painless lymphadenopathy in 90% of patients with the highest incidence in the cervical (60–80%), and mediastinal area (60%) (bulky disease is determined by measuring the mass at the T 5–6 level with mass/thoracic ratio above 0.33). Patients may present with superior vena cava syndrome. Axillary, inguinal, and retroperitoneal nodes are frequently involved. Nodes or conglomerate of nodes that are greater than 10 cm are considered to be bulky disease. Splenomegaly is frequent. Systemic symptoms consist of intermittent fever, anorexia, fatigue, weakness, night sweats, weight loss, pruritis (15–25%), and alcohol induced pain in lymph node. Neurologic symptoms at diagnosis may be due to epidural compression. Paraneoplastic symptoms include subacute cerebellar ataxia, subacute necrotic myelopathy, limbic encephalitis, subacute motor neuropathy and Guillian Barre syndrome and central pontine myelinolysis. Renal manifestations are present in 13% of cases and include glomerulonephritis or nephrotic syndrome. Hematologic manifestations include anemia (including Coombs positive anemia), immune thrombocytopenia, thrombotic thrombocytopenic purpura, autoimmune neutropenia, and eosinophilia. Other symptoms such as hypercalcemia are present in less than 5% of cases.

Clinical course: Patients with painless lymphadenopathy undergo a biopsy and then are started on chemotherapy. The lymph nodes usually shrink after one to two courses of chemotherapy. Associated symptoms such as nephrotic syndrome, pruritis or "B symptoms" which include, fever, weight loss and night sweats, decrease dramatically after the chemotherapy is started.

Prognosis: Low risk group: The 5 year overall survival is 95%. High risk group with intensified therapy: The 5 year overall survival improved from 85 to almost 100% with the event free survival (EFS) approaching 88–93% in those 16–21 years of age.

The Pediatric Oncology group in the U.S. showed that children less than 13 had improved survival but the German Cooperative Group found no difference in survival between the two age groups.

Diagnosis

PE is likely to show the presence of painless lymphadenopathy as well as splenomegaly. The lymph nodes are firm and almost rubbery in consistency. All enlarged LN should be measured.

Laboratory studies: CBC may show normochromic normocytic anemia, neutrophilia in 50%, eosinophilia in 15%, and lymphocytopenia may be seen in advanced disease. Usually the ESR or C reactive protein is elevated. Renal and hepatic function tests should be checked as well as alkaline phosphatase. Although not required, the ferritin and copper levels are also elevated.

Radiographic studies: CHEST X-RAY for mediastinal mass and a PET/CT to include neck, chest, abdomen and pelvis should be performed. An MRI may be substituted for CT.

Biopsy: Lymph node and bone marrow aspirates and biopsies bilaterally except for stage I and II A.

Management

Staging: Stage I has involvement of single lymph node region or single extralymphatic organ or site. Stage II involves two or more lymph node regions on the same side of the diaphragm, or one region with one extralymphatic site. Stage III has involvement of lymph node regions on both sides of the diaphragm, which may be accompanied by involvement of the spleen or extralymphatic site. Stage IV has disseminated involvement of extralymphatic tissues.

If the disease is accompanied by no systemic symptoms, then the stage number is followed by A, and if there are symptoms, then the letter B is used for fever, night sweats or weight loss of more than 10% of body weight.

All treatments need to be decided by a multidisciplinary team including the oncologist, the radiation therapist and the patient and family, and preferably according to a study protocol. All current active protocols can be found at the National Cancer Institute (NCI) website (http://www.cancer.govwww.cancer.gov); PDQ summary (http://www.cancer.gov/cancertopics/pdq).

Medications: There are many multiagent chemotherapy regimens that have been reported to be successful in treating Hodgkin lymphoma. Most include prednisone, vinca alkaloid, an alkylating agent, usually cyclophosphamide, and an anthracycline. Some regimens also include etoposide or bleomycin. Advanced stage disease such as IIB, III A and IV A and especially IIIB and IVB require more aggressive regimens than the adult standard adriamycin, bleomycin, vinblastine and DTIC (ABVD).

Surgery: Surgery is only performed to obtain diagnostic material. In addition, a central venous access device is usually required for the administration of the chemotherapy.

Radiation therapy: Several studies have shown the efficacy of chemotherapy alone in the treatment of childhood Hodgkin lymphoma. The results of controlled randomized trials in the U.S. have shown that the addition of radiation therapy may improve the event free survival, but not overall survival of unfavorable and advanced stage Hodgkin lymphoma. However, the German Cooperative Group has shown efficacy of chemotherapy alone. Therefore, patients treated for advanced staged Hodgkin lymphoma should be treated according to randomized cooperative group trials until studies have shown equivalent event free and overall survival to chemotherapy without adjuvant radiation therapy in patients with rapid response of their disease. Those patients who do not show rapid response of their disease with chemotherapy will continue to require involved-field low dose radiation therapy.

Psychological: Every family needs the support of a social worker and school reintegration specialist. In many cases, some patients may need the help of a child psychologist. Please see the recommendations under ALL and AML.

Social: Please see the recommendations under ALL and AML.

Monitoring: Institutional and protocol follow-up guidelines may vary. Patients are generally followed with PET- CT of the involved lymph node regions every 3 months for 2 years; then every 6 months for one year. Lab work follow-up includes complete blood counts, chemistry panels every 3 months for one year, every 6 months for one year, and then yearly. If involved at diagnosis, bone marrow biopsies and bone scans may also need to be followed. In addition, yearly thyroid function levels with TSH need to be followed if the patient received radiation therapy to the thyroid area. An echocardiogram should be performed at therapy completion.

The patients should be followed lifelong for any long term complications from the disease or its treatment. This should be coordinated within a clinic that has experience in following these patients and should include education for the patient of their disease and its therapy, evaluations for growth and development, organ function, secondary malignancies, fertility issues, cognitive/school issues as well as counseling regarding future health insurance and peer networks.

Pearls and Precautions

Immunization: Please see the recommendations under ALL and AML.

Likely complications:

Short term: Complications include anemia, thrombocytopenia and neutropenia leading to an increase risk of infection is one of the most common and serious side effects. In addition, patients have hair loss, nausea and vomiting, diarrhea and/or constipation as well as mucositis. Patients treated with Prednisone may experience weight gain, stria and hyperglycemia, mood swings, and (rarely) psychosis.

Long term: Doxorubicin with or without radiation therapy to the chest may lead to decreased cardiac mass which may result in reduced contractility and cardiomyopathy. There is an increased risk of hypothyroidism and thyroid carcinoma after radiation to the neck and mediastinum. Infertility due to a high dose of cyclophosphamide and/or radiation therapy to the abdomen can occur in girls. Male fertility can be affected by high doses of alkylator therapy (cyclophosphamide). In addition, patients who do become pregnant have an increased risk of prematurity after abdominal radiation. They also have a risk of ovarian failure and premature menopause. The most serious risk is secondary malignancy due to the combination of chemotherapy and radiation therapy. Adolescents are at greater risk than younger children. There is an increased risk of non Hodgkin lymphoma, leukemia, gastrointestinal cancers, melanoma, thyroid cancer and breast cancer. The risk of secondary malignancy is higher in Hodgkin lymphoma than any other childhood malignancy.

Medications/situations/herbals to be avoided: See AML for guidelines

Miscellaneous

- Presentation of the disease consists of painless lymph nodes swelling.
- B symptoms consist of night sweats, fevers and weight loss greater than 10% of body weight.
- A chest X-ray should be done to rule out airway compression by a mediastinal mass.
- Accurate diagnosis requires a tissue biopsy.

References:

Useful websites: See AML.

References

Bradley MB, Cairo MS. Stem cell transplantation for pediatric lymphoma: past, present and future. Bone Marrow Transplant. 2008 Jan;41(2):149–58. Epub 2007 Dec 17.

Hochberg, Jessica, Ian Waxman, Kara Kelly, Erin Morris and Mitchell Cairo,

Adolescent non-Hodgkin lymphoma and Hodgkin lymphoma: state of the science. British Journal of Hematology. 2008: 144:24–40.

Olson MR, Donaldson SS. Treatment of pediatric hodgkin lymphoma. Curr Treat Options Oncol. 2008 Feb;9(1):81–94. Epub 2008 May 7.

Medulloblastoma (MB)

Pamela Kempert, Theodore B. Moore

Medulloblastoma is a malignant neuroepithelial tumor of the cerebellum. It is the second most common CNS tumor in children. The pathology of MB includes various types including Medulloblastoma, Medullomyoblastoma (striated muscle present, poorer prognosis), Melanotic Medulloblastoma (melanin-forming neuroepithelial cells present, poorer prognosis), Desmoplastic Medulloblastoma (lies near the edge of the cerebellar hemisphere, more often in adolescents and young adults), Large Cell Medulloblastoma (4% of MB, bulky spinal mets, aggressive disease, OS = 10% at 5 years).

Etiology

Although it is not known what causes the development of MB tumors, there are some genetic and environmental clues to potential contributing factors. In a small number of children, there is a genetic predisposition to the development of MB including those with the following syndromes: Gorlin's, Turcot's, Li-Fraumeni, ataxia telangiectasia, Coffin-Siris. There are several infectious and environmental factors that have been speculated to contribute to tumor development including specific viral infections, high voltage power lines, and cured meats to name a few. However, there is no substantive evidence to base any conclusions on these exposures.

Clinical Presentation and Prognosis

Demographics: MB has an incidence of seven cases per one million children with a peak incidence at age of four years (although more than twenty percent occur in those greater than fifteen years). The ratio of males to females is 1.5:1.

Presenting signs and symptoms: Signs and symptoms of MB are primarily related to the location of the tumor with impact on cerebellar function and cerebrospinal fluid (CSF) flow and may develop over the course of several months. These may include obstructive hydrocephalus with frontal or occipital headache, morning emesis, double vision, papilledema, ataxia, motor weakness and macrocephaly with bulging fontanelle in infants. They may also be more subtle and include mood and behavioral changes, poor academics and clumsiness.

Clinical course: Without proper intervention, the disease will progress leading to herniation and death. Treatment involves a multidisciplinary approach involving primarily surgery and radiation with or without the use of chemotherapy. In high risk cases, disease median time to recurrence is 14 months (6 months for infants).

Prognosis/Survival: The overall survival for all MB at 5 years is approximately 60%; at 10 years, it is approximately 40–50%. Histologic subtype, cytogenetics and molecular markers play an important role in determining survival as well as extent of initial surgical resection. Improved outcome is expected in tumors with low proliferative index (low Ki-67/MIB-1) and high apoptosis rate. Other determinants of improved outcome include hyperdiploidy which is superior to diploidy which is better than aneuploidy. The presence of trkC also is supportive of a better prognosis. A somewhat poor prognosis is expected with loss of heterozygosity of 17p (associated with Large Cell MB), elevated erbB2, c-myc, and calbindin-D28k.

Diagnosis and staging: Initially a CT is often performed because of the ease of obtaining it rapidly after consideration of the signs and symptoms previously described, and then a mass is recognized. However, an MRI provides superior information, especially for visualization of the posterior fossa. It is typically obtained as an MRI of the Brain and Spine (with and w/o Gadolinium). This is followed by an attempt at gross total resection by the neurosurgeon. Following surgery, a post-operative brain MRI (within 48–72 hours post-operation), spine imaging if not already done (delay 10–14 days following surgery), lumbar puncture for cerebrospinal fluid cytology (delay 10–14 days following surgery) and a Bone Scan should be performed. A bone marrow biopsy is no longer recommended unless there is clinical evidence of marrow involvement. All medulloblastoma by histology are considered aggressive and staging is determined by the successful surgical removal of the tumor. Patients of 3 years or more are considered "Average Risk" if there is less than 1.5 cm^2 residual tumor or Stage M0. Patients are "High Risk" if there is greater than 1.5 cm^2 residual or Stage M1-4.

Management: Surgical resection remains the mainstay of therapy with the goal of obtaining a gross total resection. It is followed by radiotherapy, typically started three to four weeks after surgery to allow healing. Baseline neurocognitive and endocrine testing should be performed before therapy is initiated and after its completion. Chemotherapy may be useful in allowing a reduction (or, in the case of infants/small children, a delay or elimination of radiation) in the dose of radiation administered, thus reducing sequelae. In high risk disease, it may improve survival when added to radiotherapy. Typical regimens may be similar to the following:

- *Average Risk:* Craniospinal 36 Gy. Posterior Fossa (PF) boost totaling 50–55.2 Gy (70% 5 year EFS). Alternative 23.4 Gy craniospinal irradiation (CSI) with 55.2 to PF with weekly Vincristine and 8 courses of lomustine, cisplatinum and vincristine= 78% 5 year EFS. Can develop darkened skin pigmentation and hypersensitivity reaction. Patients can develop peripheral neuropathy secondary to the vinca alkaloids.
- *High Risk:* Craniospinal 36 Gy + VCR, then Post-irradiation lomustine, cisplatinum and vincristine. x 8. Posterior Fossa boost totaling 50–55.2 Gy.

Psychological: Every family needs the support of a social worker and school reintegration specialist. In many cases, some patients may need the help of a child psychologist. Please see the recommendations under ALL and AML.

Social: Please see the recommendations under ALL and AML.

Monitoring: Institutional and protocol follow-up guidelines may vary. Patients should be followed with MRI of the brain and spinal cord every 3 months for 2 years, then every 6 months for one year, and then yearly to monitor for disease recurrence as well as the occurrence of secondary malignancies in the area of radiation therapy. Patients who have received chemotherapy need to have blood work every 3 months until normal and then at least yearly to monitor for signs of organ toxicity and secondary malignancy including complete blood counts and chemistries as well as urine samples. As stated above, these patients need formal neuropsychological testing as well as audiological testing after radiation therapy or cisplatinum chemotherapy. Patients who receive spinal radiation therapy also require cardiac and pulmonary screening. Patients who receive cranial radiation therapy should be evaluated by endocrinology when they complete therapy and their growth and developmental milestones should also be monitored carefully.

The patients should be followed lifelong for any long term complications from the disease or its treatment. This should be coordinated within a clinic that has experience in following these patients and should include education for the patient of their disease and its therapy, evaluations for growth and development, organ function, secondary malignancies, fertility issues, cognitive/school issues as well as counseling regarding future health insurance and peer networks.

Pearls and Precautions

Current therapy is aimed at achieving cure, while preserving quality of life.

Immunization: Please see the recommendations under ALL and AML.

School/Education: Patients will miss a significant amount of school. A qualified school reintegration specialist is an integral part of the team, bridging the gap between the patient and his school work, school mates and teacher. Neurocognitive deficits resulting from the tumor and its' treatment may be substantial and lifelong. Formal neurocognitive testing forms an integral part of the treatment of all children with brain tumors. See likely complications below. Special individualized educational programs should be provided for these children.

Herbs and nutrition: Many herbs and high dose vitamins can interfere with the activity of chemotherapy or interfere with platelet function. All herbs and nutritional supplements must be approved by the treating physician. Careful counseling about a healthy diet and exercise is essential while on therapy as well as off of therapy. Additional information regarding the use of herbal medications and cancer can be obtained at:

NCI website for herbal medicines: www.cancer.gov/cam/health_camaz.html

Memorial Sloan Kettering Cancer Center website: www.mskcc.org/html/58481.cfm

Likely complications: Cranial radiotherapy of 36 Gy or more, in children less than 9 years of age is likely to cause a drop in IQ of 15–30 points with the most impact seen the youngest children. This drop may be decreased as much as half by a 33% reduction in the dose of therapy. In addition to cognitive deficit, multiple endocrine deficiencies may be observed including but not limited to, growth hormone deficiency, hypothyroidism, gonadal dysfunction, hearing loss, and renal dysfunction.

Patients may have frequent admissions for fever and neutropenia while on therapy. Any fever represents an emergency because of the patient's immunodeficient state as well as the presence of an indwelling central venous catheter in most of the patients. Patients must emergently seek medical assistance which should include the minimum of an evaluation of the blood counts, blood cultures and consideration of the initiation of intravenous antibiotic therapy. Patients may develop several common toxicities from their medication in addition to neutropenia, including pancytopenia, constipation, alopecia, foot drop, mouth sores and others.

Miscellaneous

- Subtle changes in behavior or school performance may be early signs of a brain tumor and warrant a careful neurological examination.
- Headaches in the night or early morning, especially if accompanied by emesis, warrant a careful neurological examination.
- Neurocognitive testing and individualized education plans are key components to optimizing the quality of life in these patients.

- Medulloblastoma is a malignant neuroepithelial tumor of the cerebellum. It is the second most common CNS tumor in children. Its etiology is not clear, although an aggressive multimodal approach has resulted in increasing survival. Late effects of current therapy remain a significant challenge.

References

Pizer BL, Clifford SC. The potential impact of tumour biology on improved clinical practice for medulloblastoma: progress towards biologically driven clinical trials. Br J Neurosurg. 2009 Aug;23(4):364–75.

RJ, Vezina G. Management of and prognosis with medulloblastoma: therapy at a crossroads. Packer Arch Neurol. 2008 Nov;65(11):1419–24.

Kaderali Z, Lamberti-Pasculli M, Rutka JT. The changing epidemiology of paediatric brain tumours: a review from the Hospital for Sick Children. Childs Nerv Syst. 2009 Jul;25(7):787–93. Epub 2008 Dec 11.

Neuroblastoma

Pamela Kempert, Theodore B. Moore

Neuroblastoma is a tumor of the neural crest cells. The tumor arises from the adrenal medulla or the sympathetic ganglion. It is the most common extracranial solid tumor of childhood.

Etiology

No environmental causes have been proven to be associated, but there have been familiar clusters associated with multifocal disease. The following disorders have been associated with neuroblastoma: Neurofibromatosis, Hirschsprung disease with aganglionic colon, Pheochromocytoma in a family member, and possibly fetal hydantoin syndrome, fetal alcohol syndrome and Nesideroblastosis.

The most common site is the adrenal gland, but the tumor can occur anywhere along the sympathetic neural pathway. Amplification of the NMYC gene on chromosome 2 is related to poor prognosis, as is unfavorable histology per the Shimada classification system.

Clinical Presentation and Prognosis

Demographics: It is the most common extracranial solid tumor of childhood with an incidence of 8–10% of all childhood cancers. In the U.S., the incidence is 10.4 per million per year in white children and 8.4 in blacks. There is a 1.1:1 male to female ratio. Forty percent of patients are diagnosed under one year of age and 90% by age 10. It is the most common congenital tumor and occurs in 1 of 7000 live births

Presenting signs and symptoms: Most neuroblastoma tumors occur in the abdomen (65%), and most commonly present as an asymptomatic abdominal mass. Almost 75% present with metastasis. Infants have higher incidence of chest and neck primary tumors. Presentation depends on the site:

Head and neck: Horner's syndrome (miosis, ptosis, anhydrosis, enophthalmos)

Orbit and eye: Orbital metastasis with hemorrhage ("*raccoon eyes*"), exophthalmus, surpraorbital mass, edema of eyelids and ptosis. Cerebral involvement: papilledema, retinal hemorrhage, optic atrophy, paresis of the external rectus muscle, and strabismus may be present at presentation. With cervical involvement: Heterochromia Iridis, anisocoria, Horner's syndrome and opsoclonus ("*dancing eyes*") may be seen.

Chest Presentations include: Upper thoracic dyspnea, pneumonia, dysphagia, lymphatic compression and Horner's syndrome. Lower thoracic usually have no symptoms.

Abdominal: Abdominal masses lead to anorexia and vomiting, abdominal pain and a palpable mass. Massive involvement of the liver due to metastatic disease may cause respiratory distress in a newborn (Stage 4S). Pelvic primary tumors may lead to constipation, urinary retention and presacral mass felt on rectal exam. Remember a rectal exam.

Paraspinal mass (dumbbell shaped): Presents with back pain and localized tenderness, weakness of lower extremities, hypotonia, muscle atrophy, paraplegia, scoliosis, bladder and sphincter dysfunction.

Lymph node metastatic disease presents as painless enlargement, while many patients with bone marrow and bone disease have pain, irritability and limp. In addition, they may have painless skin nodules that are "bluish" in color in stage 4S in infants.

They may also have pancytopenia due to bone marrow involvement as well as fever and failure to thrive.

Paraneoplastic Syndromes: Include Vasoactive intestinal peptide (VIP) secretion which leads to intractable diarrhea, hypokalemia and dehydration. VIP may also be secreted by benign ganglioneuroma. Opsoclonus myoclonus ("dancing eyes") and myoclonus motor incoordination due to frequent irregular jerking movements are caused by anti-neuronal antibodies and occur in 2–4% of cases. There is a good prognosis for tumor outcome, but 70–80% of patients have long-term neurological deficits including cognitive behavioral, motor and language delays. All children who present with OMS need to be evaluated for neuroblastoma (30% of them will have occult tumor). Excessive catecholamine (Vanillylmandelic Acid (VMA)/Homovanillic Acid (HVA)) may cause intermittent sweating, flushing, pallor, headaches, palpitation, and hypertension. Hypertension is usually due to renin that is induced by neurovascular compromise by the tumor mass.

Clinical course:

Most low-risk patients (stage I completely resected and II (microscopic and/or LN ipsilateral +)) are treated with surgical excision alone and more than 90% of them are cured. Intermediate risk patients are treated with chemotherapy and have a high rate of cure and a 75–95% 3-year disease-free survival. These patients include: Stage 3 patients less than 1, non NMYC amplified stage 3 or 4 tumors in 1–21 yrs.; and, stage 4S less than 1 yr. with non amplification of NMYC. High-risk patients are, in general, those with NMYC amplification, higher stage and/or unfavorable histology, but they generally respond well to chemotherapy, radiation therapy and autologous transplant. However, they have a high rate of relapse with only an approximately 45% 3-year disease-free survival.

Prognosis/survival: Survival is excellent for patients with low or moderate risk disease and the newest studies try to minimalize therapy. Three-year disease-free survival for low risk patients is more than 90%, and for intermediate risk patients is more than 75%–90%. By contrast, high risk disease (in general stage 3 or 4 with NMYC amplification) have shown only a small increase in survival—with only approximately 45% of patients with three-year disease-free survival—despite an intensification of treatment, including autologous bone marrow transplant.

Diagnosis

Physical exam: With special attention to evidence for Horner's syndrome, opsoclonus myoclonus, hypertension, cranial nerve deficits, motor or sensory deficits especially in the lower extremities, decreased rectal tone on exam as well as any evidence of masses in the orbit, neck or abdomen.

Laboratory studies: Should include a complete blood count to detect pancytopenia from bone marrow involvement, full chemistry panel with special attention to the electrolytes and renal function as well as liver function panel with total protein and albumin. Disease specific diagnostic tests include urine for catehclamines VMA and HVA. Most labs can do this on a spot sample, but this needs to be delivered to the lab in a timely manner. Note that if possible, patients should avoid aspirin, disulfiram, reserpine, and pyridoxine at least 48 hours prior to collection of the specimen. Levodopa should be avoided for 2 weeks before collection. Foods that can increase urinary catecholamines include coffee, tea, bananas, chocolate, cocoa, citrus fruits, and vanilla. Avoid these for several days prior to the test.

Radiological exams should consist of CT or MRI of the primary site; CT or MRI of the abdomen and pelvis; chest CT if the chest X-ray is abnormal or the abdominal mass extends into the chest; bone scan to look for bone metastasis and, if available, a Meta-Iodo-Benzyl-Guanidine (MIBG) scan which will detect not only bony metastasis, but also bone marrow involvement. In addition, bilateral bone marrow aspirates and biopsies should be performed as well as biopsy of the primary tumor.

Management

Stage I and II requires only surgical resection for above 95% survival rate. Stage 4S in infants with liver, skin and bone marrow metastases undergoes spontaneous regression in the majority of cases. Chemotherapy or low dose radiation is reserved for those that have massive hepatomegaly which causes respiratory compromise or liver dysfunction. Intermediate risk neuroblastoma that includes stage III disease or stage IV in infants with no high risk features responds to surgical resection and moderate dose chemotherapy with a greater than 95% survival. High risk disease however, is treated with intensive induction chemotherapy, second look surgical resection, and autologous stem cell transplant. Then, local control with radiation therapy is followed by biologic therapy with retinoic acid, all for a maximum survival rate of 45–50%. New data has shown that the addition of Interleukin 2, Granulocyte stimulating factor and monoclonal antibody therapy to a surface marker on the tumor cell may further improve survival rates.

Medications: Chemotherapy agents such as cytoxan, adriamycin, etoposide, cisplatinum or carboplatinum, topotecan, vincristine, biologic therapy and maturational agent retinoic acid have all been used in the treatment. In addition, patients must receive adequate pain control at diagnosis.

Surgery: Surgical interventions are for excision or biopsy of the tumor at diagnosis, or as a second look procedure, as well as placement of a central venous access device for the administration of chemotherapy and nutrition.

Radiation therapy: This is usually delivered to the primary site of disease and any residual MIBG positive metastatic disease after auto stem cell transplant.

Therapy: Many children will require extensive physical and occupational therapy due to lower extremity weakness and resulting developmental delay. See discussion under ALL and AML. In addition, many children require speech therapy secondary to hearing loss caused by the chemotherapy.

Social: Please see the recommendations under ALL and AML.nbhope.org/, www.nant.org/acor.org/ped-onc/diseases/neuro.html.

Monitoring: Institutional and protocol follow-up guidelines may vary. Patients are generally followed with Tumor imaging = CT/MRI and MIBG scan for visualization of all areas of prior or persistent bulk tumor (primary and metastases) every 3 months for one year off therapy; then, every 6 months for two years. Lab work follow-up includes complete blood counts, chemistry panels every 3 months for one year; every 6 months for one year; then yearly. If involved at diagnosis, bone marrow biopsies and bone scans may also need to be followed. An echocardiogram should be performed at therapy completion.

Patients should be followed lifelong for any long term complications from the disease or its treatment. This should be coordinated within a clinic that has experience in following these patients and should include education for the patient of their disease and its therapy, evaluations for growth and development, organ function, secondary malignancies, fertility issues, cognitive/school issues as well as counseling regarding future health insurance and peer networks.

Pearls and Precautions

Immunization: Please see the recommendations under ALL and AML.

Likely complications

Short term: Anemia, thrombocytopenia and neutropenia that leads to an increase risk of infection is one of the most common and serious side effects. See full discussion under ALL and AML. In addition, patients have hair loss, nausea and vomiting, diarrhea and/or constipation as well as mucositis. Patients can develop peripheral neuropathy secondary to the vinca alkaloids and cisplatinum.

Long term: Doxorubicin with or without radiation therapy to the chest may lead to damage to cardiac myocytes which may result in reduced contractility and cardiomyopathy. There is an increased risk of hypothyroidism and thyroid carcinoma after radiation to the neck and mediastinum. Infertility due to a high dose of cyclophosphamide/ifosfamide and/or radiation therapy to the abdomen can occur in girls. Male fertility can be affected by high doses of alkylator therapy (cyclophosphamide). In addition patients who do become pregnant have an increased risk of prematurity after abdominal radiation. They also have a risk of ovarian failure and premature menopause.

Cisplatinum can lead to long-term hearing deficits as well as renal compromise. The most serious risk is secondary malignancy due to the combination of chemotherapy and radiation therapy.

Medications/situations/herbals to be avoided: See AML report.

Miscellaneous:

- It is the most common congenital tumor and occurs in 1 of 7000 live births.
- Most commonly patients present with asymptomatic abdominal masses. Presentation may include Horner's syndrome (meiosis, ptosis, anhydrosis) enophthalmus or paraneoplastic syndromes which include opsoclonus (*"dancing eyes"*).
- *All children who present with opsoclonus need to be evaluated for neuroblastoma* (30% of them will have occult tumor).
- Infants may present with painless skin nodules which are bluish in color in stage 4S.

Useful websites: See list following AML

References

Fischer M, Spitz R, Oberthür A, Westermann F, Berthold F.Risk estimation of neuroblastoma patients using molecular markers.Klin Padiatr. 2008 May-Jun;220(3):137–46. Review.

Oberthuer A, Theissen J, Westermann F, Hero B, Fischer M.Molecular characterization and classification of neuroblastoma. Future Oncol. 2009 Jun;5(5):625–3. Park JR, Eggert A, Caron H. Neuroblastoma: biology, prognosis, and treatment.Pediatr Clin North Am. 2008 Feb;55(1):97–120,

Park JR, Villablanca JG, London WB, Gerbing RB, Haas-Kogan D, Adkins ES, Attiyeh EF, Maris JM, Seeger RC, Reynolds CP, Matthay KK; Children's Oncology GroupOutcome of high-risk stage 3 neuroblastoma with myeloablative therapy and 13-cis-retinoic acid: a report from the Children's Oncology Group. Pediatr Blood Cancer. 2009 Jan;52(1):44–50.

Non Hodgkin Lymphoma (NHL)

Pamela Kempert, Theodore B. Moore

Non Hodgkin Lymphomas is a malignant proliferation of cells of lymphoid lineage. Rarely, they may present in the bone or central nervous system. There are three main types in children: (1) Lymphoblastic Lymphoma: A precursor B or T cell type; (2) Burkitt or Burkitt like lymphoma/leukemia; and (3) large cell lymphomas: Anaplastic large cell lymphoma or Large B cell lymphoma.

Etiology

Lymphomas are malignant neoplasms of lymphoid lineage. Risk factors for the development of the disease include: Immunologic defects, post transplant immunosuppression, previous radiation and viral infections such as Ebstein-Barr Virus (EBV) and HIV. According to the National Cancer Institute, NHL in children can be classified into 3 major types:

1. Lymphoblastic Lymphoma: A precursor B or T cell type.
2. Burkitt lymphoma/leukemia (B ALL) and Burkitt Like Lymphoma (BLL).
3. Large cell lymphomas: Anaplastic large cell lymphoma predominate and Large B cell lymphoma (DLBCL) with increasing incidence as age increases.

Large Cell Lymphomas include anaplastic large cell lymphoma (ALCL) which comprises 30–40% of pediatric large cell lymphomas and 10% of all childhood lymphomas. It is characterized by expression of CD 30 antigen and over-expression of chimeric oncogene nucleophosmin anaplastic lymphoma kinase (NPM-ALK) in 75% of cases. This is felt to be the causative oncogene. In addition, activation of the c myc oncogene or other translocations are necessary to cause tumor development. Large B cell lymphoma occurs in more females (59%) than males. The median age of onset is 14.1 years. It is caused by somatic hypermutation of proto-oncogene BCL-6 on chromosome 3q27.

Burkitt (BL) and Burkitt Like (BLL) comprise 40% of all childhood lymphomas. At least 90% of the B cell lymphomas in childhood are the aggressive subtypes including diffuse large B cell lymphoma (DLBCL). The median age of BL onset is 8 years, while the median age of diagnosis of mediastinal large B cell lymphoma is 13.2 years. The c myc oncogene on chromosome 8 is translocated to the immunoglobin locus on chromosome 14 heavy chain. This maintains the cell in a state of proliferation.

Lymphoblastic Lymphoma (LL) comprises 30% of NHL in children and young adults, and 75% are of T cell origin. Mediastinum masses occur in 50–70% with supraclavicular LN. T cell LL are more likely than B cell origin LL to have CNS and BM involvement. Only 25% are of B cell origin. These present in peripheral nodes and extra nodal sites such as skin, soft tissue and bone, mostly head and neck. The majority present with advanced stage disease. Null Cell LL have a poor prognosis and arise in the retroperitoneal area. T cell LL usually involves T cell receptor rearrangement and may also involve the c myc oncogene. In addition, a variety of other translocations including 10;14, 11;14 and 1;19 are seen.

Clinical Presentation and Prognosis

Demographics: The annual incidence less than 20 years is 1/100,000 with 6.4% of new cancers occurring before age 20. The male to female ratio is 2:1 and peaks at 15–19 years. From 1973–1996, there was a 35% increase in NHL before age 20 years, but only 4.8% increase in those over 14 years of age.

Presenting signs and symptoms: Depends on the location of the tumor. These tumors may present with life-threatening illness at diagnosis due to metabolic abnormalities or airway obstruction. The symptoms depend on tumor location, correlate with histologic subtype and are typically of short duration. The abdomen is the site for 35% of the tumors and usually present in the appendix, ileocecal area or ascending colon. They can present with pain, bleeding, intussusceptions, peritonitis, ascites, obstructive jaundice, hepatosplenomegaly and a right iliac fossa mass. Burkitt lymphoma is the most common in this location. The head and neck region comprises 13% of the lesions. It causes swelling as well as nasal congestion and even cranial nerve palsies. The mediastinal area is the primary site in 26% of patients who can present with superior vena cava syndrome. **The tumor can compress the trachea and the patient can occlude their airway if supine and especially when sedated.** These are usually LL with T cell phenotype. Malignant pleural effusions often occur and they may also have pericardial effusions and cardiac tamponade. T cell lymphoblastic lymphomas are most often associated with bone marrow and central nervous system involvement.

Clinical course: Patients usually show rapid progression of symptoms both in the abdomen and in the mediastinum. Sedation to obtain a biopsy may lead to respiratory arrest and death due to airway compression by the mass. This presenting picture is particularly seen in lymphoblastic, large B cell and anaplastic large cell lymphoma.

Prognosis: Overall, 3-year event-free survival (EFS) of the ALCL patients (based on the results of past studies of both European and U.S. Study Groups) is 92% for localized ALCL, and 80% for disseminated ALCL. Three-year event-free survival in Burkitt and BLL is 98% for localized stage I and II; for stage III, there is an 86–92% EFS; and, for stage IV, the 3-year EFS is 89%. Large B Cell Lymphoma still showed 90% EFS. For localized B cell lymphoblastic lymphoma, the 5 year EFS is 85%; for T cell, the 5 year EFS is 100%. For stage III and IV, the EFS at 6 years is 90–95%.

Diagnosis

Laboratory studies: Complete blood count may show anemia, thrombocytopenia and neutropenia if bone marrow involvement is present. ESR and or C reactive protein are usually elevated, electrolytes may show hyperkalemia, hyperphosphatemia, hyperuricemia or hypocalcemia. It is extremely important to monitor these frequently as well as renal function and to correct any abnormalities before beginning chemotherapy. Rasburicase is frequently used to lower uric acid. Hepatic function test should also be assessed as well as coagulation studies.

Radiographic studies: Chest X-ray with measurement of mediastinal mass should be obtained immediately in the ER. A stat echocardiogram may also be needed for concern of pericardial effusion or tamponade. Diagnostic studies include a PET/CT to include neck, chest, abdomen and pelvis. An MRI may be substituted for CTs particularly if there is decreased renal function.

Biopsy: Lymph node biopsy (if not contraindicated by mediastinal mass); bone marrow aspirates and biopsies bilaterally;and, cerebrospinal fluid for cytology.

Management

Intrathoracic tumors require maintenance of the person in the sitting position and avoidance of sedation. If any procedure is prohibitive to establish the diagnosis, then institution of radiation therapy of the tumor around the airway or the initiation of steroids may be needed. Tumors in the abdomen that lead to bowel obstruction require surgical intervention and then the initiation of chemotherapy. Gastriointestinal bleeding may be treated with endoscopy with or without tumor resection and then the initiation of chemotherapy. Performance of an electrocardiogram and echocardiogram to assess for pericardial effusion and cardiac tamponade is required. When life threatening pericardial tamponade occurs, pericardiocentesis should be performed for cytology examination and then prompt initiation of chemotherapy. Tumor lysis and its metabolic derangements must be handled carefully; occasionally patients require dialysis. Please see management recommendations under ALL. For neurologic emergencies caused by tumor compression, chemotherapy is superior to radiation. Radiation has no routine use in the treatment of NHL.

Lymphobalstic lymphomas are treated in a similar fashion to T cell leukemia with induction and consolidation therapy followed by 2 years of maintenance. Patients with localized BL, BLL or large B cell lymphomas require 2 cycles of intense chemotherapy. Patients with more advanced stages require approximately 6–9 months of intensive chemotherapy. Patients with ALCL are treated with modified BL lymphoma protocols. This usually requires approximately 6 months of intensive chemotherapy courses. Different regimes are used in the U.S. and in Europe.

Medications: There are many multi-agent chemotherapy regimens that have been reported to be successful. Most include prednisone, vinca alkaloid, an alkylating agent usually cyclophosphamide, and an anthracycline. In addition, some protocols to treat BL and BLL use chimeric IgG-1 antibody targeted to CD20 which has been shown to improve EFS and overall survival (OS) when added to CHOP in patients with DLBCL in patients less than 60 years of age.

Surgery: Surgical biopsy is only performed to obtain diagnostic material unless the patient presents with bowel obstruction. In addition, a central venous access device is usually required for the administration of chemotherapy.

Radiation therapy: In most cases, radiation therapy does not improve survival.

Psychological: In many cases, some patients may need the help of a child psychologist. See further recommendations under ALL.

Social: Every family needs the support of a social worker and school reintegration specialist. www.leukemia-lymphoma.org, rmhc.org/, www.wish.org

Monitoring: Institutional and protocol follow-up guidelines may vary. Patients are generally followed with PET- CT of the involved lymph node regions every 3 months for 2 years and then consideration for every 6 months for one year. Lab work follow-up includes complete blood counts, chemistry panels every 3 months for one year, every 6 months for one year and then yearly. If involved at diagnosis, bone marrow biopsies and bone scans may also need to be followed. An echocardiogram should be performed at therapy completion.

The patients should be followed lifelong for any long term complications from the disease or its treatment. This should be coordinated within a clinic that has experience in following these patients and should include education for the patient of their disease and its therapy, evaluations for growth and development, organ function, secondary malignancies, fertility issues, cognitive/school issues as well as counseling regarding future health insurance and peer networks.

Immunization: See further recommendations under ALL.

Likely complications

Short term: Immediate complications include tumor lysis due to rapid lysis of tumor cells especially in Burkitt Lymphoma. Anemia, thrombocytopenia and neutropenia that leads to an increased risk of infection also occurs. In addition, patients have hair loss, nausea and vomiting, diarrhea and/or constipation as well as mucositis. Patients can develop peripheral neuropathy secondary to the vinca alkaloids. Prednisone can cause weight gain, striae, hyperglycemia, mood swings and rarely psychosis.

Long term: Doxorubicin may damage myocytes which may result in reduced contractility and cardiomyopathy. Infertility due to a high doses of cyclophosphamide and (rarely) radiation therapy to the abdomen can occur in girls. Male fertility can be affected by high doses of alkylator therapy (cyclophosphamide). Girls also have a risk of ovarian failure and premature menopause. The most serious risk is secondary malignancy due to chemotherapy.

Medications/situations/herbals to be avoided: See ALL or AML section for information

Miscellaneous

- Large mediastinal tumors may compress the trachea and can occlude the patient's airway if supine, and especially when sedated. Patients with superior vena cava (SVC) syndrome should be maintained in an upright position and should not be sedated for procedures or surgery without careful evaluation of their cardiovascular and pulmonary status.
- Patients with mediastinal tumors also present with malignant pleural effusions and they may have pericardial effusions and cardiac tamponade.
- Patients with large mediastinal or abdominal tumors especially Burkitt B cell lymphoma, have a very high incidence of severe tumor lysis with high uric acid, hyperphosphatemia, hyperklalemia and subsequent renal failure. Hydration and maintenance of adequate urine output is essential.

References

Useful websites: See AML for websites.

Cairo MS, Gerrard M, Sposto R, Auperin A, Pinkerton CR, Michon J, Weston C, Perkins SL, Raphael M, McCarthy K, Patte C; FAB LMB96 International Study Committee Results of a randomized international study of high-risk central nervous system B non-Hodgkin lymphoma and B acute lymphoblastic leukemia in children and adolescents. Blood 2007;109:2736–2743

Hochberg, Jessica, Ian Waxman, Kara Kelly, Erin Morris and Mitchell Cairo, Adolescent non-Hodgkin lymphoma and Hodgkin lymphoma: state of the science. British Journal of Hematology. 2008: 144:24–40.

Patte C, Auperin A, Gerrard M, Michon J, Pinkerton R, Sposto R, Weston C, Raphael M, Perkins SL, McCarthy K, Cairo MS; FAB/LMB96 International Study Committee. Results of the randomized international FAB/LMB96 trial for intermediate risk B-cell non-Hodgkin lymphoma in children and adolescents: it is possible to reduce treatment for the early responding patients. Blood. 2007 Apr 1;109(7):2773–80.

Osteosarcoma (OS)

Pamela Kempert, Theodore B. Moore

Osteosarcoma (OS) is the most frequent malignant bone tumor in children under 20 years of age. It is a tumor in which the malignant spindle cells produce osteoid bone.

Etiology

The etiology of osteosarcoma is unclear although both genetic and environmental factors may play a role in its development. It appears most commonly at a time of rapid bone growth, occurring most frequently adjacent to the growth plate of long bones. Radiation exposure is the only environmental factor known to play a causative role. This is a particularly great risk in those families with a constitutional retinoblastoma (RB) gene mutation. In addition, patients with Li-Fraumeni syndrome (P53 mutation) hereditary multiple exostoses, and fibrous dysplasia are at elevated risk. The most common occurring types of OS include osteoblastic, chondroblastic and fibroblastic.

Clinical Presentation and Prognosis

Demographics: There are approximately 400 new cases of OS diagnosed in the U.S each year with an incidence of approximately 4.8 per million in those under 20 years of age. Its incidence is slightly higher in blacks than in whites, males than in females and is rare in young children.

Presenting signs and symptoms: This tumor typically presents with localized bone pain which is often mistaken as a site of injury. Systemic symptoms are rare. On physical exam, pain may be elicited by direct palpation or by limb movement and may have an overlying warmth and tenderness that may be similar in presentation to osteomyelitis. The most common sites of primary disease are the distal femur (42%), proximal tibia (19%), and proximal humerus (10%), although disease can arise from any bone in the body. Lung metastases rarely are sufficient on initial presentation to cause respiratory symptoms unless disease is advanced. Regional lymph nodes are usually not enlarged.

Clinical course: Without proper therapeutic intervention, disease will progress with both local extension and an increase in metastases especially to the lungs leading to respiratory compromise and death. Treatment involves adjuvant chemotherapy and surgical resection which can effectively alter the course of disease (see management below).

Prognosis/survival: Prior to the use of adjuvant chemotherapy, surgery was the only treatment for OS. Patients without clinically obvious metastatic disease had a 15–25% survival with surgery alone. The use of adjuvant chemotherapy has significantly improved survival. The degree of tumor necrosis following adjuvant chemotherapy and the presence of metastases at diagnosis are two major predictors of outcome. Patients with greater than 95% tumor necrosis at time of definitive surgery have a greater than 80% disease-free 5 year survival. Patients with a less than optimal response have a 40–60% disease-free survival. Patients presenting with metastases at diagnosis only have a 20–30% disease-free survival.

Diagnosis

A biopsy of the suspected lesion must be performed by an experienced surgical oncologist to limit unnecessary spread which may impact prognosis and prevent a successful limb salvage procedure by contaminating the soft tissues. Staging should be performed that includes radiographs and an MRI of the primary site, CT of the chest and lungs to screen for metastases, and a bone scan.

Management

A multidisciplinary approach to the treatment of OS by experienced orthopedic and pediatric oncologists offers the best opportunity for cure.

Chemotherapy: Chemotherapy plays an important role as an adjuvant to surgery. The use of chemotherapy prior to resection allows for a better opportunity at achieving a total surgical resection as well as targeting macro- and micrometastases. Mainstays of chemotherapy include methotrexate, cisplatin and doxorubicin. Other drugs such as ifosfamide are effective in tumor shrinkage. The total course of chemotherapy is typically given over an approximately 9 month period with complete surgical resection performed 10–12 weeks into therapy.

Surgical: Surgery remains the mainstay of therapy for OS. An experienced surgeon should perform both the initial diagnostic biopsy as well as the resection. Limb salvage may be possible in as many as 90% of the patients. However, patient survival should not take second place to heroic attempts to try to spare a limb in circumstances where the local recurrence risk is very high. A central venous catheter should be placed at the beginning of therapy to facilitate chemotherapy administration and minimize venipuncture.

Radiation: Radiation therapy does not play a role in the initial therapy of OS patients. Patients with recurrent disease may receive palliation from radiotherapy.

Therapy: Patients will need referral for physical therapy. It may be helpful for this to be arranged prior to the surgery so that questions may be anticipated and answered for the patient.

Psychological: Counseling should be recommended for the patient, parents and siblings. Siblings may "act-out" for attention as a greater portion of parents' time will focus on the patient. Child life should provide therapy to children and their siblings.

Social: It is crucial that a social worker assess and provide assistance to these families. Often one parent must take a leave of absence from their employment to facilitate getting their child to their treatments. Many states have a family leave act and other such programs that the social worker can access for the family. In addition, resources from the American Cancer Society, Make-a-Wish, college scholarship fund and other such programs can be facilitated through the social worker. In addition, this is a particularly important population for teen support groups and introduction to other patients with the same diagnosis. www.**rmh**c.org/, www.**wish**.org/, www.**sarctrials**.org/ www.**candlelighters**.org/

Monitoring: Patients are followed for disease recurrence with physical examination, repeat radiographs of the chest and primary site every 3 months for the first year, every 6 months for the next 2 years and then yearly for ten years. A CT scan of the chest should be performed every 4–6 months for a minimum of 3 years. These patients should be followed lifelong for any long term complications from the disease or its treatment. This should be coordinated within a clinic that has experience in following these patients and should include education for the patient of their disease and its therapy, evaluations for growth and development, organ function, secondary malignancies, fertility issues, cognitive/school issues as well as counseling regarding future health insurance and peer networks.

Pearls and Precautions

Immunization: For information please see ALL.

School/education: Patients will miss a significant amount of school. A qualified school reintegration specialist is an integral part of the team, bridging the gap between the patient and his school work, school mates and teacher.

Herbs and nutrition: Many herbs and high dose vitamins can interfere with the activity of chemotherapy or interfere with platelet function. All herbs and nutritional supplements must be approved by the treating physician. Careful counseling about a healthy diet and exercise is essential while on therapy as well as off of therapy. Additional information regarding the use of herbal medications and cancer can be obtained at:

- NCI website for herbal medicines: www.cancer.gov/cam/health_camaz.html.
- Memorial Sloan Kettering Cancer Center website: www.mskcc.org/html/58481.cfm.

Likely complications: Patients may have frequent admissions for fever and neutropenia while on therapy. Any fever represents an emergency because of the patient's immunodeficient state as well as the presence of an indwelling central venous catheter in most of the patients. Patients must emergently seek medical assistance which should include the minimum of an evaluation of the blood counts, blood cultures and consideration of the initiation of intravenous antibiotic therapy. Patients may develop several common toxicities from their medication in addition to neutropenia, including pancytopenia, constipation, alopecia, electrolyte alterations, renal abnormalities, mouth sores and others.

Miscellaneous:

- Occurs frequently during periods of rapid growth such as early adolescence.
- Often mistaken for osteomyelitis on initial evaluation.
- Biopsy and surgical resection must be performed by an experienced surgical oncologist to maximize cure and the potential for limb salvage procedure.

Reference

Heare T, Hensley MA, Dell'Orfano S. Bone tumors: osteosarcoma and Ewing's sarcoma. Curr Opin Pediatr. 2009 Jun;21(3):365–72.

O'Day K, Gorlick R. Novel therapeutic agents for osteosarcoma. Expert Rev Anticancer Ther. 2009 Apr;9(4):511–23.

Caudill JS, Arndt CA. Diagnosis and management of bone malignancy in adolescence. Adolesc Med State Art Rev. 2007 May;18(1):62–78

Pheochromocytoma

Pamela Kempert, Theodore B. Moore

Pheochromocytomas are tumors arising from the catecholamine producing chromaffin cells in the adrenal medulla. Closely related tumors that arise in the extra adrenal sympathetic and parasympathetic paraganglia are classified as extra-adrenal paragangliomas. The pheochromocytoma and sympathetic paragangliomas secrete catecholamines, whereas the parasympathetic paragangliomas do not.

Etiology

There is a germ-line mutation in 59% of those less than 18 years, and in 70% of those less than 10 years of age who present with these tumors. The genes responsible are the Von Hippel-Lindau gene, the genes encoding the subunits B and D of succinate dehydrogenase, associated with familial nonsyndromic pheochromocytomas, the RET proto oncogene predisposing to multiple endocrine neoplasia type 2 (MEN 2) or the neurofibromatosis type I (NF1) gene. The most commonly mutated gene is the VHL gene. Familial pheochromocytomas are inherited in an autosomal dominant manner. Some family members may present with a history of sudden death since 50% of catecholamine producing tumors remain undiagnosed until autopsy in adults.

Screening for patients less than 50 years old with a positive family history should include VHL, RET, SDHB and SDHD. Patients with multiple tumors should have SDHB, SDHD and VHL screening, while patients with malignant tumors need to be screened for SDHB and VHL. Additionally, patients with bilateral tumors should be screened for RET, VHL and SDHD.

Clinical Presentation and Prognosis

Demographics: These tumors are responsible for 1% of children's hypertension. Malignant pheochromocytoma occurs in 0.02 per million children. Several studies have quoted 12–56% incidence of malignancy. Bilateral disease occurs in 25–34% and the recurrence risk is 12%. There is a male preponderance in childhood and a female preponderance in the adolescent years.

Presenting signs and symptoms: Patients may present with vague symptoms or very specific conditions such as hypertensive crises. A sudden rise in blood pressure may lead to the following symptoms: Headache (80%), diaphoresis (70%), and palpitations (60%). These symptoms can last minutes to hours and can recur several times each day. In addition, they can have blurred vision, syncope, panic attacks, tremor, parasthesia, gastrointestinal disturbance and weight loss. Hypertension is the most consistent symptom and is sustained and without paroxysms in 29–63% of patients and is associated with norepinephrine secreting tumors. Tumors that secrete epinephrine and norepinephrine have episodic hypertension and those that secrete only epinephrine may have hypotension. About 8% of patients are asymptomatic. The typical clinical signs occur more frequently in benign tumors. Abdominal pain and dorsalgia occurs more frequently in malignant pheochromocytomas. A short history and extra adrenal location are suspicious for malignancy. Patients with high 24 hour urinary dopamine and persistent hypertension are factors that increase the risk of malignancy.

Clinical course: Patients with SDHB mutations present with extra adrenal multifocal disease and they have a high risk of malignant disease. Patients with MEN2 have a low rate of extra adrenal tumor and malignant disease. Pheochromocytomas also secrete PTHrP (hypercalcemia), adrenocorticotropin (Cushing's syndrome), erythropoietin (erythrocytosis) and IL-6 (fever). About 10% of patients present with metastasis at diagnosis.

Other factors can dominate the clinical course such as diabetes mellitus, hypercalcemia or Cushing's syndrome. Cardiovascular episodes and neurologic disorders can dominate the disorder and cause sudden death. Administration of beta blockade alone can precipitate a crisis with hemodynamic collapse. After a prolonged attack shock may occur due to loss of vascular tone, low plasma volume and arrhythmia or cardiac damage. In malignant disease the metastases may secrete neurochemicals after the primary tumor is resected and there is a high rate of recurrence. Patients should be followed indefinitely. Benign tumors have a much lower rate of recurrence.

Prognosis: The percentage of pheochromocytomas that are malignant ranges from 3–36%. Survival rate depends on the location of metastatic lesions. Short term survival is predicted by metastatic lesions in the liver or the lung, and long term survival is correlated with metastasis in the bones. The five year overall survival is 34–60%. Currently except for the SDHB gene mutation, there are no reliable markers to suggest a high probability for the development of metastatic pheochromocytoma, if a primary tumor is found. The survival advantage of debulking resection is not proven. Debulking with surgery may allow smaller radiation fields or make chemotherapy more effective. Radiation palliates symptoms but does not provide a cure. Radiofrequency ablation of lesions may be useful. Chemotherapy may provide tumor regression and relief of symptoms but responses are short lived at best. I labeled MIBG is the most useful treatment modality, but as a single agent there is little chance of cure and no consensus on doses to be used for metastases.

Diagnosis

Physical exam: The physical exam is normal except for hypertension and possibly tachycardia.

Laboratory studies: These include 24-hour urine for catecholamines (epinephrine, norepinephrine) as well as fractionated metanephrines, and plasma concentrations of norepinephrine, epinephrine and free metanephrines. Fractionated metanephrine measurements (normetanephrine and metanephrine) measured separately in the plasma and urine provides superior diagnostic sensitivity to measurement of parent catecholamines. The measurement of the free plasma form can be used in renal failure, but the urinary excretion cannot.

For urine testing, the medications which may interfere with catecholamines and metanephrines include amphetamines and amphetamine-like compounds, appetite suppressants, bromocriptine, buspirone, caffeine, carbidopa-levodopa (Sinemet®), clonidine, dexamethasone, diuretics (in doses sufficient to deplete sodium), methyldopa (Aldomet®), MAO inhibitors, nose drops, propafenone (Rythmol®), tricyclics, and vasodilators. The effects of some drugs on catecholamine results may not be predictable. Levels of NE greater than 170 ug/24 hours, Epinephrine greater than 35 ug per 24 hours, total metanephrines at least 1.8 mg/24 hours and urinary Vanillylmandelic Acid (VMA) at least 11 mg/24 hours makes diagnosis highly probable.

For plasma testing, discontinue epinephrine and epinephrine-like drugs at least one week before obtaining the specimen. The patient must refrain from using acetaminophen for 48 hours before the specimen is drawn and from using caffeine, medications, and tobacco as well as drinking coffee, tea, or alcoholic beverages for at least four hours before the specimen is drawn. Collect the sample after the patient has had 15 minutes of rest in a supine position. An overnight fast prior to sample collection is recommended. Separate plasma immediately within 15 minutes and freeze. Blood pressure must be recorded and if hypertensive, normal values of the fractionated metanephrines make the diagnosis unlikely. Plasma level of normetanephrine less than 112 pg/ml and of metanephrine less than 61 pg/ml make the diagnosis of pheochromocytoma very unlikely. Levels greater than 400 pg/ml and 236 pg/ml make the diagnosis and the need to search for a tumor extremely likely. Basal total plasma catecholamine levels greater than 2000 pg/ml is diagnostic of pheochromocytoma and less than 500 pg/ml rules it out. Levels exceeding 1000 call for more testing, and patients need to be referred for provocative testing.

Radiology studies: CT or MRI of the abdomen and pelvis and if negative, chest and neck should be performed. In addition, functional imaging with MIBG scan may be used to detect the extent of metastases. If doubt remains, venous catheter studies may be done to determine the ratio of epinephrine to norepinephrine in the adrenal veins. PET scan using [18F] flourodopamine, [18F] dihydroxyphenylalanine, and [11C] hydroxyephedrine may be helpful. PET using (2-Deoxy-2-[18F]fluoro-D-Glucose positron emission tomography) [FDP] is nonspecific.

Management

Rapid action is needed in the emergency room to control blood pressure which may require admission for a nitroprusside drip and then referral to follow-up source of care, especially if the patient has a family history of pheochromocytoma or any endocrine multiple cancer syndromes.

Medications: Preoperative alpha adrenergic blockade should be performed. The specific choice of drugs is at the discretion of the treating physician. Selective postsynaptic alpha-1 receptor antagonists such as prazosin, terazosin and doxazosin have been used. For tachyarrythmias, beta adrenergic blockade or calcium channel blockers should be used, but only after alpha adrenergic blockade. Calcium channel blockers have been used to treat blood pressure and cardiovascular symptoms. Hypertensive crises may require nitroprusside, nitroglycerin or phentolamine.

There is no evidence based chemotherapy data and the most widely used protocol is cyclophosphamide, vincristine and dacarbazine. Rapidly progressive and malignant tumors should receive combination chemotherapy at a minimum and consideration for combination with Meta-Iodo-Benzyl-Guanidine (MIBG) which is attached to radioactive iodine therapy. New experimental approaches include inhibition of heat shock protein 90 and human telomerase reverse transcriptase or antiangiogenic drugs.

Surgery: Patients with pheochromocytoma have a high plasma volume requirement during and after surgery. Volume expansion before surgery may be helpful. Tumors less than 10 cm in diameter may be removed with a laparoscopic approach. Biochemical testing should be repeated 14 days after surgery. If the blood pressure remains high after surgery then MIBG scanning for detection of metastasis and investigation into possible trauma to the renal artery should be investigated. Long term periodic follow-up is essential.

Radiation Therapy: For malignant lesions with painful metastases, palliative radiation may be helpful. [131]MIBG may yield partial remission in 24–54% of patients.

Psychosocial support: Please see Neuroblastoma

Monitoring: The risk of recurrence of benign pheochromocytomas was 3.4 fold higher with familial disease, 3.1 fold higher with right rather than left tumors,and 11.2 fold higher with extra adrenal tumors. If the patient has a familial syndrome, then physical examination of the neck and repeated catecholamine assays in combination with plasma calcitonin levels for medullary thyroid carcinoma should be continued for life.

Pearls and Precatuions

Likely complications

Short term: Hypertensive crises and sudden death due to cardiovascular complications.

Long term: Secondary cancer in the area of radiation if this modality is used. Chemotherapy: Please see the chemotherapy chapter.

Medications/situations/herbals to be avoided: See AML report.

Miscellaneous

- High levels of circulating catecholamines during surgery could cause hypertensive crises. Therefore, all patients with biochemically active tumors should receive appropriate preoperative medication to block the release of catecholamines.
- In 59% of tumors, there is a germ-line mutation in those less than 18 years and in 70% of those less than 10 years of age.

References

Useful websites: See list following AML

Armstrong R, Sridhar M, Greenhalgh KL, Howell L, Jones C, Landes C, McPartland JL, Moores C, Losty PD, Didi M. Pheochromocytoma in children. *Arch Dis Child.* 2008 Oct; 93(10):899–904.

Asterios Karagiannis, Dimitri P Mikhailidis, Vasilios G Athyros and Faidon Harsoulis. Pheochromocytoma: an update on genetics and management. *Endocrine related Cancer* (2007) 14:935–956.

Karel Pacak, Graeme Eisenhofer, Håkan Ahlman, Stefan R Bornstein, Anne-Paule Gimenez-Roqueplo, Ashley B Grossman, Noriko Kimura, Massimo Mannelli, Anne Marie McNicol and Arthur S Tischler* Pheochromocytoma: recommendations for clinical practice from the First International Symposium. *Nature Clinical Practice Endocrinology & Metabolism* (2007) 3, 92–102.

Rhabdomyosarcoma (RMS)

Pamela Kempert, Theodore B. Moore

Rhabdomyosarcoma (RMS) is a striated muscle neoplasm. It is the most common soft tissue sarcoma and the third most common extracranial solid tumor in children. There are four major histological types including alveolar, embryonal (including botryoid), mixed and pleomorphic. The majority of the alveolar types have a translocation between chromosomes two and thirteen which results in the fusion of PAX3 and FKHR (forkhead) genes. A translocation between chromosomes one and thirteen involving the PAX7 and FKHR is less commonly seen. Embryonal RMS tumors may demonstrate a loss of heterozygosity for the 11p15 locus. The histologic appearance is that of one of the pediatric small round blue cell tumors and is distinguished from the others by the presence of muscle markers such as MyoD or myogenin as well as cytogenetics. Electron microscopy demonstrates Z-banding.

Etiology

The etiology of the disease is unclear at this time.

Clinical Presentation and Prognosis

Demographics: RMS has an incidence of approximately 8 cases per million.

Presenting signs and symptoms: This tumor typically presents as a painless mass, often brought to attention by trauma to the area. It may occur anywhere in the body where striated muscle is present. Approximately one third typically occur in the head and neck region; another third in the trunk and limbs; and, another third in the genitourinary tract. Genitourinary tumors may present with hematuria or signs of obstruction or as a peritesticular mass.

Clinical course: Without proper intervention, the disease will progress leading to death from disease extension and metastases. Treatment involves a multimodal therapeutic approach utilizing medical, surgical and radiation therapies as described below.

Prognosis/survival: Prognosis is related to disease stage and histological type with the alveolar RMS typically more aggressive than the embryonal. The overall survival rate for RMS is 70% at five years. For localized disease, survival approaches greater than 90%; Stage III disease greater than 60%; and, Stage IV disease approximately 40%.

Diagnosis

A biopsy of the suspected lesion should be performed by an experienced surgical oncologist or interventional radiologist to limit unnecessary disease spread. Staging should be performed and should include plain radiograms and CT or MRI scans of involved regions as well as the chest, abdomen and pelvis. A baseline bone scan should be obtained and a PET scan may be useful for tracking active disease. Bilateral bone marrow biopsies should be obtained to evaluate for marrow involvement.

Management

A multidisciplinary approach offers the best opportunity for cure.

Chemotherapy: Chemotherapy is effective in the treatment of RMS. Vincristine, actinomycin D and cyclophosphamide (VAC) are typically the drugs used in initial treatment. Ifosfamide, etoposide, doxorubicin, irinotecan and others have also shown efficacy, but no survival advantage is recognized over the standard VAC treatment at this time. It is typically used as an adjuvant to surgery in Stage I disease and with radiation in Stage II disease. It is given preoperatively in Stage III and IV disease, both to demonstrate its efficacy and to reduce tumor volume prior to surgical removal. In this case, it is continued postoperatively for a total chemotherapy administrative course that spans 9–10 months, including the preoperative chemotherapy period.

Surgery: An experienced surgeon should be responsible for evaluation at initial presentation as part of the treatment team. A central venous catheter should be placed so as to minimize the trauma to the patient of the frequent blood draws and chemotherapy infusions. A complete excision of the tumor should be performed if it can be done without significant morbidity. This typically includes a regional lymph node sampling for disease evaluation.

Radiation: Radiation therapy is typically given over a course of six weeks. It is usually administered following resection of the tumor or if the tumor is considered inoperable and is administered in fractionated doses for a total of 3600–5040 Gy to the primary tumor site and to areas of metastatic disease as needed.

Psychological: Counseling should be recommended for the patient, parents and siblings. Siblings may "act-out" for attention as a greater portion of parents' time will focus on the patient. Child-life should provide therapy to children and their siblings.

Social It is crucial that a social worker assesses and provides assistance to these families. Often one parent must take a leave of absence from their employment to facilitate getting their child to their treatments. Many states have a family leave act and other such programs that the social worker can access for the family. In addition, resources from the American Cancer Society, Make-a-Wish, college scholarship fund and other such programs can be facilitated through the social worker.

Monitoring: Patients are followed for disease recurrence with repeat CT/MRI every 6 months for the first two years and then annually times two years. The patients should be followed lifelong for any long-term complications from the disease or its treatment. This should be coordinated within a clinic that has experience in following these patients and should include education for the patient of their disease and its therapy, evaluations for growth and development, organ function, secondary malignancies, fertility issues, cognitive/school issues as well as counseling regarding future health insurance and peer networks.

Pearls and Precautions

Immunization: For information please see AML.

School/education: Patients will miss a significant amount of school. A qualified school reintegration specialist is an integral part of the team, bridging the gap between the patient and his school work, school mates and teacher.

Herbs and nutrition: Many herbs and high dose vitamins can interfere with the activity of chemotherapy or interfere with platelet function. All herbs and nutritional supplements must be approved by the treating physician. Careful counseling about a healthy diet and exercise is essential while on therapy as well as off of therapy. Additional information regarding the use of herbal medications and cancer can be obtained at:

- NCI website for herbal medicines: www.cancer.gov/cam/health_camaz.html.
- Memorial Sloan Kettering Cancer Center website: www.mskcc.org/html/58481.cfm.

Likely complications: Patients may have frequent admissions for fever and neutropenia while on therapy. Any fever represents an emergency because of the patient's immunodeficient state as well as the presence of an indwelling central venous catheter in most of the patients. Patients must emergently seek medical assistance which should include the minimum of an evaluation of the blood counts, blood cultures and consideration of the initiation of intravenous antibiotic therapy. Patients may develop several common toxicities from their medication in addition to neutropenia, including pancytopenia, constipation, alopecia, foot drop, mouth sores and others.

Miscellaneous

- The most common soft tissue sarcoma in children.
- Diagnostic biopsy and surgery must be performed by an experienced oncology surgeon.
- Alveolar RMS often has the characteristic t(2;13) or t(1;13) translocation.
- Rhabdomyosarcoma (RMS) is a striated muscle neoplasm. In children, it is the most common soft tissue sarcoma. Treatment with a multimodal approach results in favorable outcome for most stages.

References:

Hayes-Jordan A, Andrassy R. Rhabdomyosarcoma in children. Curr Opin Pediatr. 2009 Jun;21(3):373–8.
Qualman S, Lynch J, Bridge J, Parham D, Teot L, Meyer W, Pappo A. Prevalence and clinical impact of anaplasia in childhood rhabdomyosarcoma : a report from the Soft Tissue Sarcoma Committee of the Children's Oncology Group. Cancer. 2008 Dec 1;113(11):3242–7. Erratum in: Cancer. 2009 Jun 15;115(12):2806.

Wilms' Tumor (Nephroblastoma)

Pamela Kempert, Theodore B. Moore

Wilms' Tumor arises from pluripotent embryonic renal precursors. It is the second most common extracranial solid tumor of childhood and the most common renal malignant tumor.

Etiology

The tumor arises from pluripotent embryonic renal precursors. A tumor suppressor gene WT1 was identified in 1990 that was associated with Wilms' tumor. This gene is located on chromosome 11p13 and is necessary for renal development. The tumor arises due to inactivation of this gene and intralobular nephrogenic rests are associated with this mutation. Germline mutations of WT1 account for the urogenital abnormalities and the development of Wilms' tumor in patients associated with chromosome 11 abnormalities including WAGR, Denys Drash and Beckwith-Wiedemann syndrome. Inactivating point mutations are associated with Denys Drash and LOH of WT2 on 11p15 is associated with Beckwith-Wiedemann. A somatic germline mutation of 11p13 is associated with Wilm's Tumor, aniridia, and growth retardation (WAGR) syndrome. Only 2% of patients have a family history of the disease. In addition, the BRAC2 mutation in Fanconi's anemia group D is associated with Wilms' tumor.

Clinical Presentation and Prognosis

Demographics: Wilms' tumor is the most common pediatric renal tumor in North America accounting for 6% of childhood cancers. About 5% have bilateral disease, 7% multicentric disease, and 5% metastatic disease to the lung primarily, but the tumor also may metastasize to the liver or lymph nodes and (rarely) to bone, bone marrow or brain.

The peak incidence is 2–5 years of age and 95% of patients are diagnosed by age 10. The incidence is greater in black toddlers and lower in Asians.

The ratio is slightly increased for girls 1 : 0.9

Presenting signs and symptoms: Wilms' tumor most often presents as a painless abdominal mass, but hematuria, fever, hypertension due to increased rennin also occurs. In addition, one should look for aniridia, Beckwith-Weidman syndrome (facial dysmorphism, partial or complete hemihypertrophy, genitourinary (GU) anomalies such as hypospadius, cryptorchidism or pseudohermaphroditism.

Paraneoplastic syndromes: Hypertension due to increased rennin production may be seen in all patients. Hypercalcemia occurs in patients with rhabdoid morphology and mesoblastic nephroma. Acquired Von Willebrand's deficiency may also occur in patients with Wilms' tumor.

Clinical Course: In the U.S., most patients undergo surgical resection first, followed by chemotherapy and, depending on the stage at diagnosis, possibly abdominal or chest radiation. In Europe, most patients undergo presurgical chemotherapy.

Prognosis: Currently, greater than 80% of children can look forward to long term survival with less then 20% morbidity at 20 years. Survival has improved from 30% several decades ago, to an almost 90% 5–7 year survival currently.

Diagnosis

Careful abdominal exam as well as blood pressure measurement are the necessary initial steps. In addition, careful exam is necessary to detect the stigmata of Beckwith-Wiedemann syndrome (anorexia, facial dimorphism, hemihypertrophy and genitourinary anomalies), Denys Drash (pseudohermaphrotidism, degenerative renal disease) and WAGR.

Laboratory: Laboratory studies should include a complete blood count to detect anemia or erythrocytosis, electrolytes, blood urea nitrogen (BUN) and creatinine to detect kidney function abnormalities as well as liver function tests and calcium which is increased in rhabdoid tumor and mesoblastic nephroma pathologic subtypes. In addition, a urinalysis to look for hematuria should be performed and consideration given for a Von Willebrand Panel since 8% of new patients have acquired Von Willebrand Disease (VWD).

Radiology studies: These include abdominal ultrasound of the kidney area (can be obtained to determine the organ of origin of the tumor without sedation in young children) as well as a Doppler ultrasound of the inferior vena cava (IVC) to detect tumor thrombus. In addition, a CT scan of the chest and chest X-ray to detect pulmonary metastasis and a CT with contrast of the abdomen or MRI need to be performed. Bone scan is performed for clear cell sarcoma only. Brain MRI is requested for clear cell sarcoma and rhabdoid or renal cell carcinoma of the kidney.

Pathologic subtypes include "Favorable Histology" (FH) and "Unfavorable Histology" (UH) which is made up of Clear Cell sarcoma, Anaplasia focal or diffuse or Rhabdoid sarcoma. Mesoblastic nephroma is a benign pathology that is common in infancy but can be confused with Wilms' tumor

Staging includes the following:

- Stage I: Completely encapsulated and resected;
- Stage II: Extension beyond renal capsule with extension into renal vein and para-aortic nodes with no macroscopic residual;
- Stage III: Macroscopic residual or peritoneal metastasis or tumor spillage;
- Stage IV: Metastatic disease; and
- Stage V: Bilateral disease.

Management

Medications: Stage I and II are usually treated with vincristine and actinomycin D for 11 weeks. The need for additional therapy besides resection for patients who have stage I tumors less than 550 grams is under study. Currently, patients with stage III and IV FH Wilms' tumor receive a three drug regimen including doxorubicin in addition to vincristine and dactinomycin. Patients with anaplastic tumors receive the above three medications plus cyclophosphamide, ifosfamide and etoposide. The same regimen has been found to be successful in the treatment of clear cell sarcoma of the kidney. Metastatic rhabdoid tumor of the kidney is currently under study due to its poor prognosis, but chemotherapy very similar to the therapy used for other soft tissue sarcomas have had some success.

Surgery: Disease control is contingent upon surgical resection whether at the time of presentation (U.S.) or after several cycles of chemotherapy (European). Adequate exploration and biopsy or excision of all suspicious structures is essential. Biopsy of all lymph nodes at the level of the renal vessels has to be completed. Tumor spillage at the time of surgery or preoperatively upstages the disease. Patients with IVC thrombus of tumor should have a planned surgical procedure that removes the entire tumor either at diagnosis or after preoperative chemotherapy or radiation therapy. Minimally invasive surgical techniques are still at this time controversial. In the U.S., bilateral tumors are treated with preoperative chemotherapy following biopsy and staging of both kidney tumors; but, in Europe, preoperative staging only. In about 50% of patients, chemotherapy followed by bilateral kidney sparing surgery is possible after 6–12 weeks.

In summary, parenchyma sparing surgery for patients with unilateral Wilms' tumor is controversial. Therefore, the National Wilms' tumor study currently recommends partial resection only be considered in patients with a solitary kidney, renal insufficiency at diagnosis, bilateral Wilms' tumor and those with genetic syndromes that predispose to Wilms' tumor and renal insufficiency later in life.

Radiation Therapy: No radiation therapy is needed for stage I and II favorable histology disease as demonstrated by National Wilms' Tumor Studies. However, patients with unfavorable histology receive radiation. For stage III disease FH of the abdomen, the recommended dose of X-ray radiation therapy (XRT) is 10 Gy. For UH stage II, the recommended dose is 20 Gy. If the patient presents with stage IV diseases on the chest X-ray, then 12 Gy of pulmonary radiation therapy is indicated. The need for pulmonary radiation for lesions that are only seen on Chest CT is being investigated in current Wilms' tumor study in the U.S. to confirm results obtained in European institutions.

Psychological: In many cases, some patients may need the help of a child psychologist. See recommendations under AML and ALL.

Social: Every family needs the support of a social worker child life and school reintegration specialist.

Monitoring: After therapy, completion will include a history and physical exam every 3 months for 2 years; then, with decreasing frequency until yearly at 5 years. In addition, the patient will need a complete blood count, electrolytes, liver function tests, kidney function tests and urine sample every 6 months for 2 years and then yearly.

Depending on risk group, a chest CT or chest X-ray as well as MRI or CT of the abdomen or abdominal ultrasound should be done every 3 months for 2 years; then, chest X-ray and abdominal ultrasound only every 6 months for 2 years; then, as indicated clinically. Echocardiogram is needed at therapy completion and then according to dose per the long term follow-up guidelines after anthracycline or chest radiation.

Pearls and Precaution

Likely complications

Short term: Anemia, thrombocytopenia and neutropenia that leads to an increase risk of infection is one of the most common and serious side effects. See full recommendations under ALL and AML. In addition patients have hair loss, nausea and vomiting as well as diarrhea and/or constipation and mucositis. Patients who are treated with ifosfamide or carboplatinum may develop decease in renal function, but most of these either have bilateral Wilms' tumor or Denys Drash syndrome know to be associated with a decrease in renal function. Hepatic veno-occlusive disease secondary to radiation and dactinomycin has been described.

Long term: As above, the medications ifosfamide and carboplatinum as well as radiation therapy may lead to a decrease in renal function. Doxorubicin with or without radiation therapy to the chest may lead to cardiac myocytes damage, which may result in reduced contractility and cardiomyopathy. The liver can be damaged by radiation therapy and/or dactinomycin, which is usually temporary. Infertility due to a high doses of cyclophosphamide and/or radiation therapy to the abdomen can occur in girls. Male fertility can be affected by high doses of alkylator therapy (cyclophosphamide and ifosfamide). In addition, patients who do become pregnant have an increased risk of a premature birth after abdominal radiation. Also, they have a risk of ovarian failure. Radiation can lead to scoliosis. The most serious risk is secondary malignancy including secondary leukemia, lymphoma, bone and soft tissue sarcomas due to the combination of chemotherapy and radiation therapy.

Medications/situations/herbals to be avoided: see AML chapter.

Miscellaneous

- Most patients present with a painless abdominal mass.
- Patients may present with hematuria, hypertension, hypercalcemia (rhabdoid or mesoblastic nephromas) or acquired Von willebrand's disease.
- An increased risk of Wilms' tumor is associated with chromosome 11 abnormalities including WAGR, Denys Drash and Beckwith-Wiedemann syndrome.

References

Useful websites: see AML chapter.

Journal Articles:

Ko EY, Ritchey ML Current management of Wilms' tumor in children. J Pediatr Urol. 2009 Feb;5(1):56–65. Epub 2008 Oct 9. Review.

Mitchell C, Pritchard-Jones K, Shannon R, Hutton C, Stevens S, Machin D, Imeson J, Kelsey A, Vujanic GM, Gornall P, Walker J, Taylor R, Sartori P, Hale J, Levitt G, Messahel B, Middleton H, Grundy R, Pritchard J; For the United Kingdom Cancer Study Group. Immediate nephrectomy versus preoperative chemotherapy in the management of non-metastatic Wilms' tumour: results of a randomised trial (UKW3) by the UK Children's Cancer Study Group.Eur J Cancer. 2006 Oct;42(15):2554–62. Epub 2006 Aug 10.

Rao A, Rothman J, Nichols KE Genetic testing and tumor surveillance for children with cancer predisposition syndromes. Curr Opin Pediatr. 2008 Feb;20(1):1–7. Review

Wu HY, Snyder HM 3rd, D'Angio GJ.Wilms' tumor management. Curr Opin Urol. 2005 Jul;15(4):273–6. Review.

Chemotherapy and Radiation Therapy

Pamela Kempert, Theodore B. Moore

Chemotherapy and radiation therapy cause both short and long term toxicities.

Common acute toxicities include myelosuppression, nausea, and vomiting as well as other gastrointestinal (GI) toxicities, mucositis, fatigue, alopecia and possibly infertility.

Transfusion support: Patients with pancytopenia may need platelet transfusion for counts less than 10,000–20,000 and symptomatic anemia. All blood products need to be irradiated to prevent graft versus host disease and should be leukofiltered to decrease the incidence of cytomegalovirus (CMV) transmission. In addition, acute nonlymphocytic leukemia and relapsed lymphoma or ALL patients who are potential transplant candidates should not receive directed donor blood from first and second degree relatives.

Fever and infection: In addition, patients who are neutropenic [Absolute Neutrophil Count (ANC) of < 1000] and have fever of more than 38.4 $^{\circ C}$ times one measurement or more than 38 $^{\circ C}$ for one hour should have bacterial and fungal urine cultures and blood cultures obtained from all central lines and receive broad spectrum antibiotics to cover both gram positive and gram negative microorganisms. Patients with intestinal or perirectal complaints should be given careful consideration for antibiotics that cover anaerobes. Patients who have ANC of less than 500 will almost always require hospitalization. All ANLL and bone marrow transplant patients with fever require hospitalization for fever due to their severely immunosuppressed state. Patients with ANLL, relapsed ALL and some patients with NHL are especially at risk of Streptococcus Viridans sepsis due to the administration of cytosine arabinoside and require Vancomycin as well as broad spectrum antibiotic coverage for gram positive and gram negative micro-organisms and require inpatient admission due to the significant death rate from this infection. If patients have signs of typhlitis or acute abdomen, then anaerobic coverage should be added. In addition, if fever persists for 3–5 days despite adequate coverage, then antifungal medication needs to be added. REMEMBER NEVER TAKE A RECTAL TEMPERATURE OR GIVE RECTAL MEDICATIONS to any oncology or bone marrow transplant (BMT) patients. This may lead to a break in the mucosa and gram negative sepsis.

Antiemetics: Patients may require antiemetics in the emergency room as well as intravenous hydration for uncontrolled nausea and vomiting. Usual medication choices include odansetron, granisetron, or aprepitant for delayed nausea and vomiting as well as diphenhydramine and metachlorpropamide, ativan and (rarely) promethazine as well as the placement of a scopolamine patch. Instructing the patient to take the medications round the clock at home rather than on an as-needed basis.

Constipation: Patients who receive vinca alkaloids may be severely constipated and therefore require stool softeners, osmotic agents like propylene glycol and cathartics likebisacodyl. ENEMAS or SUPPOSITORIES

ARE NEVER SAFE TO DO. Remember to add instruction and medications for constipation for all patients who are prescribed narcotic pain medications.

Mucositis: Patients with severe mucositis may require mouth wash that contains anesthetic medications (a common mixture contains equal proportions of viscous lidocaine and diphenhydramine liquid with/without aluminum hydroxide—therefore, called "2 in 1 or 3 in 1 mouth wash") as well as antibacterial and antifungal agents and intravenous pain medications.

Patients on chemotherapy should not usually receive nonsteroidal anti-inflammatory medications since they can interfere with platelet function. See Table 12.1 for the most common individual chemotherapy agent.

Radiation therapy:

The acute toxicity of radiation therapy is mainly determined not only by the dose, but also by the radiation therapy site. Radiation may result in nausea and vomiting as well as somnolence for several months after completion. See previous subheading "Antiemetics" for care of nausea and vomiting. In addition, patients may develop local erythema of the skin area in the field of radiation. If the radiation field involves any of the digestive systems, then sores as manifested by mycoses or enteritis with pain may result. Local mouth rinses with lidocaine and other components may help relieve local pain. Systemic or oral pain medications may be needed. In addition, the patient may require either enteral or intravenous nutritional support. Gastritis or enteritis with diarrhea and pain may also occur and necessitate IV hydration, and as above, nutritional support.

Chronic toxicity of radiation therapy is dependent on the area of radiation and the dosage. The most serious long term side effect of radiation therapy is the occurrence of second malignant neoplasms such as carcinomas or sarcomas of the soft tissue or bone in the area of radiation as well as second malignant skin cancers. If the radiation involves the central nervous system (CNS), the patient can develop secondary CNS tumors. In addition, patients can develop hormone deficiencies that result in poor growth and delayed or precocious puberty being the most likely rather than adrenal or thyroid deficiencies Significant radiation doses to the CNS may lead to the development of hypopituitarism. Patients also develop varying degrees of academic dysfunction after radiation therapy to the brain. High doses of radiation therapy at an early age may cause a decrease in IQ. High dose radiation can also cause fibrosis in the area of radiation with decrease range of motion of that area i.e., neck or the joint of an extremity. In addition, radiation causes decreased bone growth in the area of radiation therapy. Radiation therapy to the lungs can cause fibrosis and decrease in pulmonary function. Radiation therapy to the cardiac area can cause permanent damage to the myocytes as well as scarring of the pericardium leading to restrictive pericarditis and congestive heart failure years later. In addition, it can lead to scarring of the coronary arteries and early coronary artery disease.

Useful websites:

- The side effects of all chemotherapy medications and radiation therapy are listed at www.cancer.gov.
- Revised Long Term Follow-up Guidelines from the Children's Oncology Group can be found at www.curesearch.org.

Table 12.1: Malignancy, Treatments and Toxicities Associated with Chemotherapy and Radiation

Agent	Malignancy	Mechanism of Action	Serious Acute Toxicities in Addition to Above	Long Term Toxicities	ER Action Needed
Arsenic	APML	DNA fragmentation and apoptosis	– Prolonged QT interval and tachycardia – APML differentiation syndrome treat high dose steroids (fever dyspnea, weight gain, pulmonary infiltrates and pleural effusion)		Medications to treat arrythmias Steroids for APML differentiation syndrome
Asparaginase (Elspar, Peg Asparaginase or Oncaspar)	ALL, NHL and AML	Hydrolysis of asparagine that deprives cancer cells of this amino acid.	– Thrombosis due to depletion of AT III and protein C and S – Anaphylactic reaction – Pancreatitis esp. with steroids and secondary DM – CNS depression fatigue somnolence, confusion, hallucinations and coma.	– DM rare – recurrent pancreatitis – Neurologic secondary to stroke.	– Consider stat FFP to replace AT III,protein C and S if CVA occurs – Check amylase and lipase for abdominal pain even if dose given many months before. – Check blood sugar – Treat anaphylaxis but remember (Peg) must be admitted since half life is at least 5 days and symptoms will recur when anaphylaxis medications effects are gone.
Bleomycin (Blenoxane)	HD, Germ Cell	Binds to DNA causes single and double strand breaks	Anaphylaxis Pulmonary edema	Dose related pnuemonitis with fibrosis esp. if on O2	– Treat anaphylaxis if occurs
Bortezomib (Velcade)	Recurrent lymphoma	A reversible inhibitor of the 26S proteosome which mediates protein degradation	Peripheral neuropathy common and severe in 7% Headache common Hypersensitivity reactions Fever common as well as arthralgias Hypotension occ. and peripheral edema common Rare fatal infiltrative pulmonary disease		– Treat allergic reactions – Consider neurontin for neuropathic pain

Table 12.1 (Continued)

Agent	Malignancy	Mechanism of Action	Serious Acute Toxicities in Addition to Above	Long Term Toxicities	ER Action Needed
Carboplatinum (Paraplatinum CBDCA) Cisplatinum (Cis-Diam-minedichloro-platinum), DDP,CDDP, Platinol) Oxaliplatin (Eloxatin)	Germ Cell Tumors Sarcomas Recurrent lymphomas Liver tumors Neuroblastoma Recurrent solid tumors (Oxaliplati-num) CNS tumors	Heavy metal Binds and cross linking strands of DNA	– Renal tubular damage (Occ irreversible renal failure) Esp cisplatinum – Ototoxocity (greater with cisplatinum) – Severe electrolyte abnormalities – Anaphylaxis – Peripheral neuropathies (oxal-platinum acute neurosensory and neuromotor symptoms may develop Parasthesia and cold induced dyses-thesias chronic sensory neuropathy fine motor disturbance or ataxia)	Decreased renal function Hearing deficit Do follow-up U/A, BP and kidney function as well as Audiogram Secondary leukemia (CBC q year x 10)	– Laryngospasm may develop within 2 hours of the infusion and last up to 5 days. Cold temperatures may induce the spasm. And warm liquids can make it better. (Oxaliplatinum) – Check electrolytes and MG with (Oxaliplatinum) – BUN and Creat due to damage to kidney including Fanconi's renal syndrome. – Treat anaphylaxis
Cortocoste-roids Prednisone, Dexametha-sone Predniso-lone	Leukemia, Lymphoma and Cerebral edema	Halt DNA synthesis Inhibit glucose transport Retard mitosis Inhibit protein synthesis	DM Pancreatitis Immune suppression	Osteoporosis Cataracts f/u bone density at 17–18 Opthamology follow-up at least once off therapy	
Cyclophos-phamide (cytoxan, Neosar, CTX) Ifosfamide (Ifex)	Leukemia, Lymphoma, CNS tumors, all solid tumor Pretransplant preparative regimen	Active alkylating metabolites that effect DNA	– Fluid retention with --hyponatre-mia due to kidney—Hemorrhagic cystitis Interstitial fibrosis CTX Cardiotoxicity rare CTX High dose ie. Pretransplant CNS toxicity somnolemnce hallucinations, depression and seizures IFOS Renal impairment and Fanconi's renal syndrome IFOS Liver dysfunction rare IFOS Peripheral neuropathy (IFOS Phlebitis is rare IFOS	Amenorrhea both azoospermia (both) Secondary neoplasia both esp hematologic	Hydration for hemorrhagic cystitis Electrolyte correction and possible lasix for hyponatremia Antiemetics for N and V Pain medication for peripheral Neuropathy—neurontin Anticonvulsants and neurologic work-up for uncontrolled seizures

Drug	Indication	Mechanism	Side effects		Comments
Cytarabine (Cytosine arabinoside, Ara-C, Cytosar U, Depocyte (liposomal for IT use)	Leukemia and Lymphoma as well as preparative regimen for BMT	Purine analog antimetabolite that when phosphorylated is competitive inhibitor of DNA polymerase	– ARAC syndrome flu like syndrome with fever and arthralgia and sometimes rash – Mild hepatic dysfunction – High dose cereballar ataxia and cerebral dysfunction that may be permanent – Conjunctivitis (steroid drops) – Hepatic toxicity with cholestatic jaundice and sinusoidal obstructive syndrome	Neurologic side effects such as cerebellar ataxia and white matter changes in the brain	May cause serious neurological deficits—consider MRI
Dactinomycin Actinomycin d ACD, Comogen	Wilms' tumor, rhabdomyosarcoma and occ Ewings' sarcoma	Binds to DNA and production of RNA Inhibition of Topoisomerase II prevents	Erythema and increased pigmentation Rarely hepatic sinusoidal obstructive syndrome	Hepatotoxicity especially after radiation. Secondary malignancies	Hydration and antiemetics
Dasaatinib Sprycel Imatinib (Gleevac, STI 571)	CML in chronic accelerated or blast Phase resistant to Imatinib	Inhibitions multiple tyrosine kinases including BCR ABL and the SCR family (Dastinib) Inhibits Plt derived growth factor and c kit tyrosine kinas in GIST tumors as well as BCR ABL (Imagine)	Peripheral neuropathy Do not give with prolonged QTC Fluid retention common and occ. Severe Dyspnea cough URI Fever and fatigue all above Dasatinib Fever and arthralgias are common CHF Elevated LFT and renal compromise are rare (Imatibib)		Hold medicine for prolonged QTC Treat dyspnea due to fluid retention with diuretics. Hold medications for severe liver or kidney dysfunction

Table 12.1 (*Continued*)

Agent	Malignancy	Mechanism of Action	Serious Acute Toxicities in Addition to Above	Long Term Toxicities	ER Action Needed
Daunorubicin (Daunomycin, rubidomycin, DNR, Cerubidinne) Doxorubicin (ADR, Adriamycin, Rubex, Hydfoxyldaunoru-bicin) Liposomal Doxorubicin (daunoXome) Idarubicin (IDA) Idamycin Mitoxantrone (Novantrone)	ALL and AML (daunomycin) (Amyl mitoxantrone) and in addition Sarcoma, Wilms', neuroblastoma, and lymphoma for doxorubicin	DNA strand breakage mediated by effects of topoisomerase II production of RNA Inhibition of Topoisomerase II	CHF and myocarditis Cardiac arrhythmia	Heart failure which is dose dependent and increased in younger children See Cure Search Guidelines for F/U ECHO and EKG Secondary malignancy	For any signs of arrrythmia or CHF do EKG and ECHO and start appropriate medication for arrythmia or CHF.
Docetaxel (Taxotere)	Carcinomas	Stabilization of microtubules	Arrythmia Hypersensitivity reactions Fluid retention syndrome (use steroids to prevent) Mild and reversible parasthesias Reversible hepatoxicity Mild diarrhea Fatigue weakness and myalgia		Steroids for fluid retention syndrome Treat allergic reactions Treat symptomatically
Etoposide (Epipodophyllotoxin VP 16	Germ cell tumors Lymphomas Acute leukemia Neuroblastoma. CNS tumors Sarcomas	Interacts with Topoisomerase II and causes single and double strand breaks in DNA	Severe hypotension Hepatotoxicity is rare Peripheral neuropathy rare. Allergic reaction rare. Congestive heart failure Stevens Johnson rash	Secondary leukemia and MDS So CBC's off therapy at least yearly for 10 years	Treat allergic reactions
Fludarabine	Acute leukemias Transplant preparative regimens	Inhibit DNA polymerase, ribonucleotide reductase and DNA primase	Neurotoxicity uncommon somnolence, twitching, Depression of CD4 and CD 8 counts Allergic pneumonitis Diarrhea		

Gemcitabine	Carcinomas Non Hodgkin's lymphoma Soft tissue sarcoma	cytidine analog inhibits ribonucleotide reductase and competes with deoxycytodine for incorporation into DNA	Mild proteinuria and hematuria common Hemolytic uremic syndrome rare Dyspnea occasional Neurotoxicity rare. Anaphylaxis rare	Pulmonary fibrosis **ARDS** Liver failure
Idarubicin (see Daunomycin) Ifosfamide (see Cyclophosphamide) Imatanib (see Dastinib)				
Irinotecan (Camptosar) CPT 11	Carcinomas Recurrent sarcomas CNS tumors	Inhibitor of topoisomerase I Pretest for UGT1A1 28 allele of uridine diphosphate. Glucuronosyl--transferase gene	Fever Headache Dyspnea cough rhinitis Insomnia or dizziness rare Flushing occ. Anaphylactic reaction is rare.	Note early cholinergic diarrhea may occur early < 24 hours treat with atropine late treat with loperamide. Diarrhea is severe > 7 stools per 24 hours or hypotension occurs add ATB flouroquinolone esp if neutropenic. Also rarely seen sudden thromboembolic events.
Mercaptopurine (6 MP) Purinthol Thioguanine 6TG	Leukemia	Purine antimetabolite	Rare Intrahepatic cholestasis and mild focal centrolobular necrosis with jaundice.	Rare liver toxicity Measure LFT until normal and then yearly off therapy Extremely rarely patients have developed venooccusive disease which is more likely with thioguanine therapy Very carefully administer in renal failure.

Table 12.1 (*Continued*)

Agent	Malignancy	Mechanism of Action	Serious Acute Toxicities in Addition to Above	Long Term Toxicities	ER Action Needed
Methotrexate (MTX)	Leukemia Osteogenic sarcoms Lymphoma Head and neck carcinoma	Inhibit dihydro-folate reductase. Arrest DNA	Acute hepatocellular injury is uncommon Hepatic fibrosis is rare Pneumonitis rare Renal tubular necrosis is rare at standard doses Convulsion and Guillain—Barre like syndrome rare after IT administration.	Short term memory and academic issues as well as seizures Rarely see Leukoencephalopathy after use esp IT and IV together Pulmonary fibrosis rare	Maintain IV hydration and alkaliza-tion to prevent toxicity as well as give leucovorin if vomiting give leucovorin IV at same dose. Avoid ASA, sulfa drugs, phenytoin, and other protein bound drugs that may displace MTX and increase toxicity. Do not give with severe renal insuf-ficiency It is not dialyzable. Do not give with effusion – reservoir effect
Mitoxantrone see daunomycin					
Nelarbine (Aranon)	T cell ALL and T cell NHL	Converted to Ara GTP which causes cell death	Headache Somnolence rare Peripheral neuropathy rare Ataxia occasional Insomnia rare Convulsions and coma rare Leukoencephalopathy and demy-elination and ascending peripheral neuropathy rare. Cough dyspnea and pleural effusion are common Occasional electrolyte abnormalities Edema and MS pain occasional	Rare demyelination of brain pancreatitis	Close monitor for neurologic events consider MRI for changes stop medi-cation CXR for dyspnea Serum lytes Treat pain symptoms with narcotics if needed
Paclitaxel Taxol Onxol	Carcinoma Recurrent solid tumors	Mitotic arrest and see enhance polym-erized microtubules	Anaphylaxis can be minimalized by pretreatment with steroids and antihistamines Sensory neuropathy mild 50% Myalgias and arthralgias Seizures rare Rare significant bradycardia stop drug		Treat anaphylaxis with steroids an antihistannines.

Drug	Indication	Mechanism	Toxicity		Management
Rituximab rituxin	NHL and autoimmune disorders	Monoclonal antibody directed against CD 20	Anaphylaxis with CV collapse rare Abdominal pain and bowel obstruction and perforation with chemotherapy Hepatitis B reactivation Progressive multifocal leukoencephalopathy rare	Prolonged immunosuppression	Treat anaphylaxis with steroids and antihistamines and pressors as needed
Temezolamide Temedor	CNS tumors	CNS tumors Alkylation of the DNA at the O and N positions of guanine	Headache fatigue and fever are common Occ peripheral edema Neurologic symptoms common but may be due to tumor		Provide treatment for fever and neutropenia
Vinblastine VLB Velban Vincristine Oncovin Vincasar	Hodgkins and Non Hodgkin lymphoma Germ cell Histiocytosis (Vincristine Leukemia, NHL, CNS, Germ, Wilms' tumor, neuroblastoma, sarcomas etc. for vincristine Histiocytosis (Velban)	Mitotic inhibition with reversible metaphase arrest due to action on microtubular and spindle contractile proteins.	SIADH Seizures Peripheral neuropathy and jaw pain Abdominal pain and adynamic ileus. Neurotoxicity less frequent with vinblastine.	Peripheral neuropathy Reynaud's phenomena	Pain control Careful abdominal exam Serum electrolytes if decreased urine output to detect hyponatremia.
Vinorelbine Navelbine	Hodgkin	Binds to tubulin and depolymerizes microtubules	Anaphylaxis Myocardial infarction Hepatotoxicity ARDS SIADH Hemorrhagic cystitis Thrombosis Intestinal obstruction		Treat allergic reactions

References

Ben Arush MW, Elhasid R. Effects of radiotherapy on the growth of children with leukemia. Pediatr Endocrinol Rev. 2008 Mar; 5(3):785–8. Review.

Green DM, Sklar CA, Boice JD Jr, Mulvihill JJ, Whitton JA, Stovall M, Yasui Y Ovarian failure and reproductive outcomes after childhood cancer treatment: results from the Childhood Cancer Survivor Study. J Clin Oncol. 2009 May 10;27(14):2374–81. Epub 2009 Apr 13. Review.

Kurt BA, Armstrong GT, Cash DK, Krasin MJ, Morris EB, Spunt SL, Robison LL, Hudson MM. Primary care management of the childhood cancer survivor. J Pediatr. 2008 Apr;152(4):458–66. Review. No abstract available.

Lee C, Gianos M, Klaustermeyer WB. Diagnosis and management of hypersensitivity reactions related to common cancer chemotherapy agents. Ann Allergy Asthma Immunol. 2009 Mar;102(3):179–87; quiz 187–9, 222. Review.

Hammond S, Yasui Y, Inskip PD. Second neoplasms in survivors of childhood cancer: findings from the Childhood Cancer Survivor Study cohort. J Clin Oncol. 2009 May 10;27(14):2356–62. Epub 2009 Meadows AT, Friedman DL, Neglia JP, Mertens AC, Donaldson SS, Stovall M, Mar 2. Review.

Robison LL. Treatment-associated subsequent neoplasms among long-term survivors of childhood cancer: the experience of the Childhood Cancer Survivor Study. Pediatr Radiol. 2009 Feb;39 Suppl 1:S32–7. Epub 2008 Dec 16. Review

Ruggiero A, Ridola V, Puma N, Molinari F, Coccia P, De Rosa G, Riccardi R. Anthracycline cardiotoxicity in childhood. Pediatr Hematol Oncol. 2008 Jun;25(4):261–81. Review.

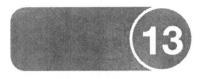 **Pulmonary Disorders**

Table of Contents

Chronic Lung Disease of Infancy (CLDi; Bronchopulmonary Dysplasia)

Roberta M. Kato, Thomas G. Keens

CLDi can be defined as a chronic lung disease following premature birth and/or neonatal lung injury accompanied by chest radiographic changes, and a requirement for supplemental oxygen and/or mechanical assisted ventilation for at least 28-days.

Etiology

Prematurity of less than 32 weeks gestation and/or lung injury during the neonatal period may lead to CLDi. The chronic lung damage has been attributed to the use of supplemental oxygen and/or mechanical assisted ventilation in the neonatal period. However, prematurity alone (air-filled lung which would still be fluid filled in utero) and the acute neonatal lung disease undoubtedly contribute to this disorder. Increased fluid therapy in the neonatal period, and/or a family history of atopy also increases the risk of CLDi.

Clinical Presentation and Prognosis

Age of onset: By definition, CLDi can be diagnosed at 28 days of life, but the pulmonary disease is present at birth or in the neonatal period. Technically, a neonate can not have the diagnosis of CLDi prior to 28-days of age. However, the prognosis can sometimes be ascertained before 28 days in infants with respiratory symptoms and oxygen or ventilator dependence.

Presenting signs and symptoms: Children affected with CLDi present with signs of respiratory distress including tachypnea, nasal flaring, intercostal and subcostal retractions and cyanosis. There may also be poor feeding or oxyhemoglobin desaturation with feeding. Hypoventilation leads to decreased oxygen and CO_2 exchange resulting in hypoxemia and hypercapnia. CLDi also may present as the inability to rapidly wean premature infants from assisted ventilation who were thought to have only neonatal respiratory distress syndrome.

Clinical course: Affected infants may initially demonstrate worsening signs and symptoms that persist from days to months. A chest radiograph may show diffuse infiltrates or a paucity of markings, depending on the etiology of the disease. If respiratory insufficiency or failure develops, the patient may require positive pressure ventilation. In general, if one can avoid further lung damage (such as pneumonia or recurrent aspiration), the lung disease gradually improves over the first few years of life. The clinical sequelae of CLDi in older children may resemble asthma.

Prognosis: Although the long-term prognosis of this condition varies, it is usually good, with minimal lung disease. Most patients are asymptomatic by school-age, while some have asthma. In severe cases, long-term mechanical ventilation may be required though most patients eventually wean after several months to years.

Diagnosis

Since there are no confirmatory tests for this disease, the diagnosis of CLDi is based on both clinical and radiographic findings. Premature infants with a requirement for supplemental oxygen and radiographic findings of hyperlucency, infiltrates, chronic markings, or haziness may be diagnosed with CLDi. Grading of severity depends on the oxygen requirement assessed at 36-weeks postconceptional age for infants born at <32weeks gestation, or at 56 days of life if born >32 weeks gestation:

1. Mild = F_IO_2 of 0.21.
2. Moderate = F_IO_2 of 0.22–0.29.
3. Severe = F_IO_2 of >0.3 or requirement for mechanical ventilatory support.

Management

The goal of managing infants with CLDi is to minimize work of breathing, prevent recurrent lung injury, optimize gas exchange during the time of critical brain growth and development, and prevent complications. CLDi is an inflammatory lung disorder. Systemic corticosteroids were once used frequently to treat exacerbations of CLDi. However, it is now known that their chronic use actually worsens lung hypoplasia, and this should generally be avoided. Inhaled corticosteroids have not been shown to improve CLDi by evidence-based medicine, but research findings of increased inflammatory cytokines in the lung fluids of CLDi patients suggests that they may be useful. Inhaled bronchodilators (short acting beta-2 agonists) improve symptoms of obstruction and may help mucociliary clearance. Diuretics are useful in CLDi, especially in the first few months of life.

Gas exchange should be monitored intermittently by pulse oximetry and by capillary blood gases to assess Pco_2. Hypoxia is a frequent complication of CLDi, which should be treated. Note that hypoxia is worse during feeding and during sleep, and this needs to be specifically assessed during these states. There is little consensus on the goal for minimal S_po_2 in CLDi infants after NICU discharge. There is evidence that more normal S_po_2 values improve neurologic outcome and prevent pulmonary hypertension. Therefore, we aim for S_po_2 values ≥95%, but others accept S_po_2 values ≥92%. Poor growth may be a consequence of hypoxia.

CLDi infants require up to 50% more calories to grow than normal infants. If poor growth persists despite adequate caloric intake, hypoxia should be considered as a cause. CLDi infants with Pco_2 consistently >60–65 torr have a poorer prognosis, and home mechanical ventilation should be considered in these infants.

Nutrition and attention to growth is extremely important. Gastro-esophageal reflux disease (GERD) is common in CLDi infants. This may be due in part to the effect of hyperinflation on the lower esophageal sphincter. GERD can exacerbate lung damage, and it requires treatment. Medical treatment may be sufficient, but anti-reflux surgery is necessary if medications fail.

Pulmonary hypertension can occur from chronic hypoxia and/or lung parenchymal hypoplasia. Ensuring adequate oxygenation with S_po_2 values ≥95% is important in these patients. In addition, diuretics often help. Pharmacologic agents may also be necessary.

Medications: Initial therapy for premature infants in the delivery room or NICU includes exogenous surfactant administration via endotracheal tube and supplemental oxygen. As the disease progresses, inhaled corticosteroids and a short acting beta-2 agonist bronchodilator may be indicated in patients with airways disease. Diuretics may be needed to manage pulmonary edema that result from leaky pulmonary capillaries in CLDi. Electrolytes should be monitored frequently and supplementation provided as needed. Hypochloremia may be treated with potassium or other chloride salts (such as arginine chloride) depending on the patient's needs. Chronic systemic corticosteroids should not be given to treat neonatal pulmonary disease.

Surgery: Surgery has no role in the primary treatment of CLDi. However, anti-reflux surgery (Nissen and fundoplication) may be required for GERD refractory to medical management. Tracheostomy is rarely required for upper airway obstruction or for long-term mechanical ventilation. A gastrostomy may be required if the patient is unable to meet nutritional demands.

Therapy: Physical and occupational therapy and infant stimulation are essential to optimize neurological development. There may be significant delays when the infant has been hospitalized for a prolonged period.

Social: CLDi is a chronic lung disease that can be associated with substantial medical care requirements. Parents often need psychosocial support due to the prolonged nature of this disorder. It is useful to remind parents that most CLDi patients ultimately improve. Respite care may be important depending on the level of care that the infant demands.

Pearls and Precautions

Immunizations: In order to prevent or minimize the morbidity of respiratory synctial virus (RSV) infections which can be devastating, CLDi infants should receive palivizumab monthly during RSV season for the first two-years of life. These infants should receive Prevnar during infancy, and the 23-valent pneumococcal vaccine after two-years of age.

Nutrition: Maintaining adequate nutritional support optimizes the potential for normal lung development.

Miscellaneous: Pco_2 should be monitored and preferably kept near the normal range by the time of NICU discharge. The prognosis is good if care is optimized and infections are avoided or treated immediately.

Reference

Allen J, Zwerdling R, Ehrenkrantz R, et al. Statement on the care of the child with chronic lung disease of infancy and childhood. Am J Respir Crit Care Med, 168 : 356–396, 2003

Congenital Diaphragmatic Hernia (CDH)

Roberta M. Kato, Thomas G. Keens

Congenital diaphragmatic hernia usually presents as a unilateral lung hypoplasia with a defect in the formation of the diaphragm allowing herniation of the abdominal contents into the thorax.

Etiology

The etiology of CDH is unknown. It is a problem with embryological development, causing a defect in the diaphragm. CDH may occur in isolation, but it is commonly associated with other genetic malformations. There is no specific chromosomal abnormality associated with CDH.

Clinical Presentation and Prognosis

Age of onset: CDH is present at birth and is frequently identified on routine prenatal ultrasound. CDH patients are usually born full or near term and present with respiratory distress in the neonatal period.

Presenting signs and symptoms: Affected newborns present with respiratory distress at birth, hypoplastic hemithorax and bowel sounds in the thorax. Herniation of abdominal contents into the thorax may be seen by chest radiograph. There is abnormal gas exchange usually with severe hypoxemia and hypercapnia. However, the degree of respiratory distress depends on the degree of lung hypoplasia, which presumably depends on when the abdominal contents moved into the chest and compressed lung growth. We have seen one 11-year girl, previously asymptomatic, who presented to an Emergency Room with signs of mild respiratory distress. She had a diaphragmatic hernia on chest X-ray, though she had been asymptomatic since birth.

Clinical course: Respiratory insufficiency or failure due to lung hypoplasia, pulmonary hypertension and compression from abdominal contents requires endotracheal intubation and mechanical ventilation. Pulmonary hypertension is frequently present, and this may respond to nitric oxide administration. Extracorporeal membrane oxygenation (ECMO) may be required to stabilize the infant prior to surgical repair of the diaphragmatic defect. While CDH repair was once considered a neonatal surgical emergency, it is now clear that the respiratory distress is due primarily to pulmonary hypoplasia and pulmonary hypertension, and not solely due to compression of the lungs by abdominal contents in the chest. Therefore, surgery should be delayed until the infant has been medically stabilized.

Prognosis: Infants born live with CDH at a single tertiary care facility were reported to have a significantly high (35%) mortality rate. Long-term prognosis is dependent on the severity of pulmonary hypoplasia and associated genetic defects. Those who survive to school age have a relatively good prognosis.

Diagnosis

CDH is best diagnosed through early detection with prenatal ultrasound and postnatal confirmation by chest radiograph.

Management

A majority of CDH patients require intubation and mechanical ventilation upon delivery until surgical correction may be performed. Pulmonary hypertension may necessitate inhaled nitric oxide (iNO), high frequency oscillatory ventilation (HFOV), and ECMO support. The reduction in mass effect from the abdominal contents improves ventilation. However, there is a primary lung parenchymal abnormality that necessitates medical management. Intensive care medical management is usually required for a prolonged period, and corrective surgery is preferably delayed until the infant is medically stable. Due to the diaphragmatic defect, gastroesophageal reflux is common, and it should be managed appropriately. A genetics evaluation is recommended due to the association with other genetic abnormalities.

Medications: Inhaled nitric oxide (NO) may be required initially, and (rarely) a long term use of sildenafil at an initial dosage of 0.25–0.5 mg/kg/dose every 4–8 hours and increased to 1–2 mg/kg/dose every 4–8 hours is used to treat the residual pulmonary hypertension. Diuretics, such as Furosemide (1 mg/kg/dose every 6–12 hours) improve lung compliance. Supplemental oxygen should be provided as needed (see the Medical devices section on "Oxygen").

Anti-reflux medications: Lansoprazole (1.5 mg/kg/dose once daily; or, for children greater than 12 months old, 15 mg once daily under 30 kg; 30 mg once daily for over 30 kg); and, pro-intestinal motility agents (erythromycin ethylsuccinate 10 mg/kg/dose every 8 hours) may be indicated.

Surgery: Operative intervention is performed once the patient is medically stabilized. Surgery is usually approached through the abdomen. The intestines are removed from the thorax, and the diaphragmatic defect is repaired. Repeat repairs may be required if the originally placed diaphragmatic patch fails. In utero repairs do not improve survival or reduce morbidity.

Therapy: Appropriate physical and occupational therapy is required on a case by case need. Commonly patients will require additional physical therapy due to delayed gross motor skills because of prolonged intubation. If there is evidence of swallowing dysfunction, occupational therapy intervention is necessary to ensure adequate skills to prevent long-term aspiration.

Social: Parents who seek support groups for their affected infant, may be referred to The Association of Congenital Diaphragmatic Hernia Research, Advocacy, and Support (CHERUBS) at www.cdhsupport.org

Monitoring: Before school age, patients are monitored by pulse oximetry and blood gases at clinic visits every 2–6 months. When children reach school age, pulmonary function testing provides the most objective measure of lung function, growth, and response to treatment. Older children who are doing well may only require pulmonary visits every 6–12 months.

Medical devices: These patients commonly require supplemental oxygen and the need for it is monitored by pulse oximetry during clinic visits, and sometimes by polysomnography (sleep studies).

Pearls and Precautions

- Lung parenchymal development is abnormal so surgical repair is not a definitive cure.
- In utero procedures have not proven beneficial.
- Reherniation may happen at any point in life and may be life threatening.

References

Langston, C. New concepts in the pathology of congenital lung malformations. Sem Pediatr Surg, 12: 17–37, 2003.

De Buys Roessingh A. Congenital diaphragmatic hernia: current status and review of the literature. Eur J Pediatr. 168: 393–406. 2009.

Congenital Cystic Adenomatoid Malformation (CCAM)

Roberta M. Kato, Thomas G. Keens

This condition is caused by abnormal proliferation of bronchioles leading to cystic dilatation of distal airways.

Etiology

The cause of CCAM is unknown. It is a disorder of embryological development of the lungs. There is no known genetic mutation associated with CCAM. It may be associated with genetic anomalies, but it can also be an isolated finding. There are 5 types (0–4) based on pathologic findings of the size and distribution of the cysts.

Clinical Presentation and Prognosis

Age of onset: This is commonly detected during routine fetal ultrasound.

Presenting signs and symptoms: Neonates may be asymptomatic or have respiratory distress depending on the size and location of the malformation. There may be diminished breath sounds in the region of the lesion. If a thin walled cyst ruptures, there will be sudden onset of tachypnea, respiratory distress and abnormal gas exchange associated with pneumothorax. On the other hand, the CCAM lesion may progressively enlarge with growth in the first year of life, causing later onset respiratory compromise.

Clinical course: There is a range of possible clinical outcomes. The area of malformation may resolve without intervention, or it may affect gas exchange or work of breathing requiring surgical removal. Uncommonly, the malformation may undergo malignant transformation.

Prognosis: Serial fetal ultrasounds may show resolution prior to delivery. Malformations in situ may cause respiratory compromise and have malignant potential. Surgical resection may be recommended, but the timing varies from center to center. Prognosis is excellent following surgical resection. However, type 0, with bilateral cysts, is typically lethal. Other types of CCAM have a variable prognosis. These patients should be carefully followed. Some will improve, may become asymptomatic, and not have subsequent infection or respiratory compromise.

Diagnosis

Ultrasound and chest X-ray may indicate that a congenital thoracic malformation exists. A chest CT with contrast to identify blood supply will help distinguish CCAM from a pulmonary sequestration. This may be done at one month of age in the asymptomatic patient. A definitive diagnosis of CCAM can only be made by pathology following complete excision of the malformation. Diagnostic biopsy is not usually performed as lesions may be heterogeneous.

Management

Prenatally, conservative management includes serial fetal ultrasounds. If hydrops or polyhydramnios is detected, then in utero intervention may be attempted. If there is respiratory distress at birth, the patient is stabilized. Surgical resection may be performed if the patient's respiratory status is compromised. Otherwise, if asymptomatic, the patient may be followed as an outpatient. Some centers may prefer to plan for surgical resection in the first six months of life as there is a risk of super infection and/or malignant transformation of a CCAM.

Medications: Antibiotics are used to treat interval infections of the lesion.

Surgery: If indicated, in utero surgical therapy using thoracentesis which involves insertion of a shunt, or resection of the lesion is possible. Surgical resection (lobectomy) in the first year of life is considered a definitive therapy and postponing of this procedure until a patient is symptomatic will lead to increased morbidity. In some cases, CCAM have recurred after resection.

Therapy: Chest physiotherapy and respiratory treatments are temporizing therapies, and they are not therapeutic except during interval infections.

Monitoring: Before school age, patients are monitored by pulse oximetry and blood gases at clinic visits every 2–6 months. When children reach school age, pulmonary function testing provides the most objective measure of lung function and growth. Older children who are doing well may only require pulmonary visits every 6–12 months.

Pearls and Precautions

Surgical resection is a definitive treatment, but the optimal timing of the procedure is unknown.

Malformations found prenatally have the potential to regress spontaneously. Chest X-ray and/or ultrasound performed at birth or near birth will demonstrate if the lesion persists. If the initial imaging is normal, a CT may be required to ensure that the lesion has completely regressed and does not require further intervention.

If not resected, there is the possibility of super infection and malignant transformation in CCAM types 1 and 4.

References

Langston, C. New concepts in the pathology of congenital lung malformations. Sem Pediatr Surg, 12: 17–37, 2003.

Lakhoo K. and Dinh-Suan A. Management of congenital cystic adenomatous malformations of the lung. Arch Dis Child Fetal Neonatal Ed, 94: F73–F76, 2009.

Cystic Fibrosis (CF)

Roberta M. Kato, Thomas G. Keens

This is a genetic disorder of the chloride channel in exocrine cells leading to thickened secretions in the lungs, intestines, pancreas, and liver, and increased sweat chloride. In the pulmonary system, this causes an obstructive lung disease associated with mucopurulent endobronchitis and progressive lung damage. CF is also associated with pancreatic insufficiency, liver dysfunction, diabetes, and absence of the vas deferens.

Etiology

CF is an autosomal recessive genetic disorder due to mutations in the Cystic Fibrosis Transmembrane Conductance Regulator (CFTR) gene, which is responsible for chloride transport across the cell membrane. Several hundred mutations have been identified, but the most common one affecting Caucasians is the ΔF508 deletion. Disease severity is associated with specific mutations as well as disease modifier genes such as alpha 1 antitrypsin. Viscous secretions due to abnormal transmembrane chloride transport result in obstruction of airways, pancreatic ducts and biliary drainage.

Clinical Presentation and Prognosis

Age of onset: CF may present at birth to adulthood. Signs and symptoms of this disease most commonly present during infancy to early childhood. Many states now have newborn screening for CF, so infants are now diagnosed before they are symptomatic. However, patients with mild disease may not present until adulthood.

Presenting signs and symptoms: Neonates may present with meconium ileus or intestinal atresia. More commonly patients will initially present with malnutrition and poor growth, while later may present with abdominal pain with meals, and abdominal distention and foul smelling stools that are indicative of malabsorption and pancreatic insufficiency. A majority of patients are pancreatic insufficient by 12-months of age. Cough and wheeze may occur, though may be difficult to discriminate from normal childhood respiratory illnesses. Some infants and young children present with recurrent pneumonia.

Clinical course: Patients have lifelong mucopurulent endobronchitis. Pulmonary exacerbations are common, and they require either enteral or parenteral antibiotics to manage episodes of recurrent pneumonia. Pulmonary function declines gradually over time leading to respiratory failure. Pancreatic insufficiency is life-long and diabetes requiring insulin management may develop as early as childhood. Patients are at risk for acute episodes of pancreatitis and CF related liver disease may develop in childhood. It can usually be medically managed, but may result in liver failure. Constipation is common and may result in distal intestinal obstruction syndrome (DIOS). DIOS is constipation due to dehydration of intestinal mucous. It often requires hospitalization for aggressive stool disimpaction.

Prognosis: When CF was first described in 1938, most patients died in the first year of life. Median life expectancy is now approximately 40 years of age, due primarily to daily airway maintenance therapy and pancreatic enzyme therapy. Recurrent infections, significant obstructive lung disease, and bronchiectasis result in progressive lung damage leading to respiratory failure, the most common cause of death. Liver failure is another life threatening complication.

Diagnosis

A sweat chloride concentration of greater than 60 mEq/L is diagnostic of CF. The measurement is best performed by a Cystic Fibrosis Foundation Center as the technique requires expertise, and errors can lead to false results. CFTR genetic testing provides additional diagnostic information. Testing facilities may perform initial screens for the ΔF508 mutation, followed by panels of common genetic mutations. CFTR whole gene sequencing is possible if CF is highly suspected. This is especially important in Hispanic, African-American, or Asian populations, where the most common CFTR mutations differ from those seen most commonly in Caucasians. The detection of two novel CFTR mutations, with a normal sweat chloride, should be interpreted with caution. Newborn screening, now performed in many states, has detected infants with two CFTR mutations who may not have CF disease. Further research is required to better understand this. Pancreatic insufficiency is determined by testing stool for a low fecal elastase value. Fecal fat testing is the gold standard, but due to logistical and technical problems with stool collection, this testing is rarely performed.

Management

Nutrition: The nutritional goal of a body mass index (BMI) of >50th percentile needs to be met to obtain optimal pulmonary function.

Medications: Aerosolized respiratory medications including short-acting beta-2 agonists improve airway obstruction and mucociliary function. DNase (2.5 mg aerosolized once a day) reduces the viscosity of airway secretions and has been demonstrated to reduce hospital days in CF patients. Hypertonic saline (4 ml of 7% solution aerosolized three times a day) is thought to rehydrate the fluid layer above bronchial cells, and reduce the viscosity of airways secretions. Inhaled antibiotics such as Tobramycin (TOBI), are used to eradicate and/or treat Pseudomonas aeruginosa. For those children who first show Pseudomonas, TOBI is used to attempt to eradicate the organism (300 mg per aerosol b.i.d. for 1–2 months. There is no consensus on the optimal regimen). If the organism has not been eradicated, it is used for 28-days, alternating with 28-days off as long as the patient grows Psuedomonas from sputum. Respiratory medications are given in conjunction with airway clearance techniques such as chest physiotherapy (CPT) or other vibratory extrinsic devices to improve expectoration of secretions (i.e., high frequency chest compression [HFCC] vest). Enteral and parenteral antibiotics are used intermittently for pulmonary exacerbations. Pancreatic enzymes are used on a daily basis prior to each meal to treat malabsorption (microsphere preparations are preferred, dose is 500–1000 units/kg of lipase per meal, titrated up by growth, stool frequency and type, and abdominal pain. Maximal dose is ~2,500 units/kg of lipase). Ursodiol is used in CF related liver disease (10–25 mg/kg/day in 1–2 divided doses). Anti-inflammatory medications such as ibuprofen and azithromycin improve pulmonary function. Laxatives are important in the therapy of chronic constipation such as polyethylene glycol used on an as needed or daily basis (4.25 g for toddlers, 8.5 g for preschoolers and 17 g for children 5 years or older).

Surgery: CF is not generally amenable to surgical treatment. In the event of significant hemoptysis (>100–200 mL/day), a late complication of bronchiectasis, embolization of the bronchial artery in the area of bleeding is effective. A gastrostomy tube may be indicated in patients with inadequate nutritional status as caloric demands are great in patients with CF. Lung transplantation is an option for patients with an FEV_1 <30% predicted.

Therapy: Chest physical therapy is encouraged routinely and during episodes of pneumonia. Chest physical therapy is an adjunct to parenteral antibiotics during hospitalization. Generally, patients should use chest physiotherapy for 30–60 minutes per day.

Psychiatry: Psychotherapy is used on a case-by-case basis. As with other life-threatening chronic diseases, depression is fairly common in patients with advanced disease, and psychosocial support and/or psychiatric treatment is helpful.

Social support: Social work intervention is provided with routine outpatient care. Social networking through the internet is common in patients with CF. Infection control measures have limited large gatherings such as summer camps. The Cystic Fibrosis Foundation provides information for families and holds fundraisers that bring families together, such as the CF Strides walks. See www.cff.org.

Pearls and Precautions

School/education: No special school needs. However, if the patient requires frequent hospitalizations, the school must be contacted to ensure appropriate continuation of academic studies in the hospital.

Medical devices: HFCC vest or vibratory respiratory device, nebulizer and as indicated oxygen, bilevel non-invasive mechanical ventilation, and feeding pump.

Miscellaneous: Daily airways clearance is necessary to decrease the rate of decline in pulmonary function.
CF requires a team approach to optimize a patient's care.

References

Farrell RM, Rosenstein BJ, White TB, et al. Guidelines for diagnosis of cystic fibrosis in neonates through older adults: Cystic Fibrosis Foundation consensus report. J Pediatr, 153: S4–S14, 2008.
Rowe SM, Miller S, Sorcher EJ. Cystic fibrosis. N Eng J Med, 352: 1920–2001, 2005.
Accurso FJ. Update in cystic fibrosis 2006. Am J Respir Crit Care Med, 175: 754–757, 2007.

Obstructive Sleep Apnea (OSA)

Roberta M. Kato, Thomas G. Keens

Obstructive sleep apnea is caused by increased upper airway resistance that restricts or prevents adequate gas exchange during sleep. OSA is in the spectrum of sleep related breathing disorders.

Etiology

OSA is due to a small upper airway and/or decreased upper airway skeletal muscle tone. A small upper airway is most commonly due to adeno-tonsillar hypertrophy in children age 4–8 years. In infants, OSA is almost always due to craniofacial abnormalities, such as Pierre Robin Sequence, palatal defects or macroglossia. In adolescents and older children, OSA is increasingly seen with obesity. Decreased upper airway skeletal muscle tone can be seen in children with neuromuscular disorders or cerebral palsy.

Clinical Presentation and Prognosis

Age of onset: Clinical presentation varies from birth to adulthood depending upon the etiology as described above.

Presenting signs and symptoms: Snoring is almost always present in OSA in children over one-year of age. However, some children may snore without having OSA. Parents sometimes describe obstructive apneas as loud snoring, followed by silence but struggling to breathe, which ends with an agitated arousal. These children are often restless sleepers. There are multiple associated signs and symptoms which include, but are not limited to, snoring, poor feeding, restless sleep, daytime fatigue or sleepiness, nighttime enuresis and poor school performance. Longstanding severe obstructive sleep apnea can result in pulmonary hypertension and cor pulmonale.

Clinical course and prognosis: These vary with the etiology. Adeno-tonsillar hypertrophy responds well to surgical intervention, which usually causes complete resolution of OSA. Craniofacial abnormalities may improve if surgical treatment successfully increases the size of the upper airway (i.e., mandibular distraction in Pierre Robin sequence). Sometimes a tracheostomy is required. When associated with obesity and neurologic disorders, symptoms and severity of OSA will progress without appropriate interventions. In certain scenarios, appropriate medical or surgical therapy provides a good prognosis.

Diagnosis

There are screening questionnaires that help identify children with OSA, but the specificity and sensitivity of these measures are inadequate for diagnosis. A visual inspection of the airway can be useful in identifying tonsillar hypertrophy or mandibular hypoplasia. A lateral neck X-ray will allow for assessment of obstructing lymphoid tissue. A CT of the head may be indicated in certain craniofacial abnormalities. The most important tool in the diagnosis of OSA is an overnight attended polysomnogram (PSG). A PSG will evaluate the frequency of obstructive events, hypoxia, and hypercapnia. A frequency of greater than 1.5 obstructive events per hour (apnea-hypopnea index (AHI)) is abnormal, but intervention may not be indicated until the AHI is greater than 5 events per hour, and/or hypoxia and hypercapnia are present. The PSG can also be used to assess the progression of OSA or in response to an intervention. A transthoracic echocardiogram may be performed to screen for evidence of pulmonary hypertension. This is generally required only in children with severe OSAs defined by polysomnography or patients with clinically suspected cor pulmonale.

Management

Surgery is the primary treatment for OSA in children who may tolerate this procedure. If surgical options are not available then noninvasive positive pressure ventilation with continuous or bi-level positive airway pressure—CPAP and BiPAP respectively—is used. CPAP and BiPAP can be used to temporize symptoms until surgical intervention is scheduled or during the post-operative period. Initiating CPAP or BiPAP requires an experienced respiratory therapist and assistance from the family to make the experience successful. Ideally, initiation of therapy will occur in the sleep laboratory to ensure accurate titration of pressures and adjustment of the interface. For patients with severe OSA, emergency hospitalization and inpatient initiation of CPAP or BiPAP may be required. The goal of therapy is to normalize oxygenation and ventilation, normalize the AHI, normalize the sleep pattern, and reduce or eliminate daytime symptoms.

Medications: Intranasal steroids may be used to improve the patency of the upper airway in children with severe allergic rhinitis. Otherwise, there is a minimal role for pharmaceuticals in the treatment of OSA.

Surgery: Adeno-tonsillectomy is the most common initial surgical intervention. Lingual tonsils may also require removal if they are obstructing the airway. In the cases of craniofacial abnormalities, plastic surgery can be useful in reconstructing the airway using midface advancements or mandibular distraction. If the upper airway is refractory to the above interventions, an airway may be established by tracheostomy.

Therapy: Physical therapy for weight loss is extremely important in the case of obesity.

Psychiatry: Feedback from the school with regards to social interactions and school performance provides important information regarding the significance of OSA symptoms and response to interventions.

Social support: Due to the varied etiologies, there is no one particular social support. Family support is extremely important if non-invasive ventilation is required, as the therapy will require partnership with family to ensure appropriate use especially with small children.

Monitoring: Overnight polysomnograms are performed every 6–12 months to ensure adequate ventilator support; or, sooner if symptoms indicate a possible increase in severity of OSA.

Pearls and Precautions

- A polysomnogram is required to accurately diagnose OSA.
- OSA is associated with a variety of common symptoms and should not be overlooked.
- Untreated, severe OSA can lead to cor pulmonale and be life threatening.

Medical devices: CPAP, BiPAP, and supplemental oxygen.

References

Guilleminault C. Pediatric Obstructive Sleep Apnea. Arch Pediatr Adolesc. Med, 159: 775–785. 2005.

Perez IA, Davidson Ward SL. The Snoring Child. Pediatric Annals 37: 465–470, 2008.

Primary Ciliary Dyskinesia (PCD)

Roberta M. Kato, Thomas G. Keens

Absence of coordinated movement of cilia of the respiratory epithelium results in recurrent respiratory tract infections including sinusitis, bronchitis and otitis media. PCD also involves the reproductive tract.

Etiology

PCD is a rare recessive disorder of the dynein arm genes that code for components of cilia. There are multiple dynein genes including DNAI1, DNAH5, DNAH11 and RPGR, that are each located on a different chromosome and known to be involved in PCD. RPGR is located on the X-chromosome and may be associated with retinitis pigmentosa. Though greater than 20 mutations have been identified, it is likely that there are other unidentified disease associated mutations.

Clinical Presentation and Prognosis

Age of onset: There are frequent episodes of respiratory tract infections in infancy or early childhood. Many children may continue to have recurrent respiratory infections of unknown cause until infertility occurs in adult life, prompting the correct diagnosis.

Presenting signs and symptoms: Infants may be tachypneic and will have chronic rhinitis and productive cough. In some children with chronic cough, a chest radiograph will show situs inversus (Kartagener's syndrome), suggesting the diagnosis of PCD. However, relatively few children with PCD have situs inversus.

Clinical course: Patients with PCD will have recurrent respiratory tract infections throughout life requiring intermittent therapy with enteral or parenteral antibiotics. Bronchiectasis—dilatation of bronchial airways—may develop as early as in childhood and result in decreased pulmonary function.

Prognosis: Patients require lifelong daily therapy to decrease the frequency of respiratory tract infections. There is a decline in pulmonary function over the patient's lifetime. For some patients, daily chest physiotherapy and bronchodilators will maintain normal lung function. Other patients continue to have problems with this therapy. Therefore, the prognosis for individual patients is variable.

Diagnosis

The patient may be mildly tachypneic and found to have crackles and rhinitis. There will be radiologic evidence of bronchitis, pneumonia and sinusitis. The presenting symptoms are similar to cystic fibrosis, asthma, gastro-esophageal reflux disease and other common obstructive pulmonary disorders that must first be excluded. There is a commercially available PCD mutation panel available through Ambry Genetics (866-262-7943) that will screen for mutations of DNAH5 and DNAI1. A cilia biopsy should be performed and appropriately prepared for electron microscopy to evaluate the anatomy of the dynein arms. However, normal dynein anatomy does not ensure normal function. Functional tests of cilia motion are difficult and have not been standardized. Pulmonary function tests are used to monitor the extent of airway obstruction, and they can also be used to determine the need for interval antibiotic therapy and response to interventions.

Management

The goal of management is to improve clearance of pulmonary secretions, and treat interval infections rapidly and thoroughly.

Medications: Bronchodilators are used on a daily basis to improve clearance of secretions in conjunction with manual chest physiotherapy or mechanical vibratory airway clearance techniques. Antibiotics are utilized as needed. The organisms found in PCD are similar to the respiratory flora of children of similar age. If resistance develops, sputum cultures with antibiotic susceptibility testing will guide therapy.

Surgery: Sinus surgery and placement of pressure equalizing tubes by an otolaryngologist may be indicated.

Social support: Family support is important as in any chronic illness that requires daily interventions.

Monitoring: The extent of lung disease may be monitored by pulmonary function testing and chest radiographs.

Pearls and Precautions

Immunization: Routine immunizations including annual influenza vaccination are indicated.

Medical devices: HFCC vest or other vibratory respiratory device such as acapella

Likely complications: Patients will have recurrent upper airway infections and develop bronchiectasis.

Miscellaneous: The diagnosis of PCD is based on clinical suspicion and may be supported by genetic testing or pathology.

Daily airway clearance therapy is required to maximize pulmonary function.

Respiratory tract infections must be diagnosed rapidly and treated appropriately to minimize chronic lung disease.

Reference

Storm van's Gravesandre K and Omran H. Primary ciliary dyskinesia: Clinical presentation, diagnosis and genetics. Ann Med, 37: 439–449. 2005.

Noone PC, Leigh MW, Sannuti A, Minnix, SL, Carson JL, Hazucha M, Zariwala MA, Knowles MR. Primary ciliary dyskinesia: diagnostic and phenotypic features. Amer J. Respir Crit Care Med., 169: 459–467, 2004.

Idiopathic Pulmonary Hemosiderosis (IPH)

Roberta M. Kato, Thomas G. Keens

IPH involves recurrent diffuse alveolar hemorrhage resulting in pulmonary fibrosis.

Etiology

The etiology of IPH is unknown.

Clinical Presentation and Prognosis

Age of onset: Presentation may be anytime during infancy, childhood or adulthood.

Presenting signs and symptoms: The first symptoms of alveolar hemorrhage are nonspecific and include mild tachypnea, cough and dyspnea. There may be hypoxemia, hemoptysis and fever. In infants and children, the diagnosis requires a high clinical suspicion as the classic IPH triad of signs and symptoms does not exist. The classic triad includes iron deficient anemia; radiographic evidence of diffuse pulmonary infiltrates; and, pulmonary symptoms. There may not be overt hemoptysis.

Clinical course: Patients may have recurrent episodes of pulmonary hemorrhage that require hospitalization for intravenous corticosteroids, and which can be life-threatening. Outpatient immunosuppression can lead to periods of remission. Over time, there is progressive pulmonary fibrosis resulting in decreased pulmonary function.

Prognosis: The five-year survival rate was 86% at a single center. Death is most commonly related to acute and massive pulmonary hemorrhage.

Diagnosis: The diagnosis is based on evidence of hemosiderin-laden macrophages either from bronchoalveolar lavage, gastric lavage or lung biopsy. A reticulocystosis is an indicator of acute or chronic pulmonary hemorrhage. A decrease in hemoglobin concentration with changes on X-ray, hypoxemia and respiratory distress indicates massive pulmonary hemorrhage and requires rapid intervention. However, the diagnosis of IPH can only be confirmed by open lung biopsy. This is necessary to be sure of the diagnosis because IPH requires life-long immunosuppressant therapy.

Management

Medical management with immunosuppressants is the primary therapy.

Medications: Acute episodes of pulmonary hemorrhage require the use of intravenous corticosteroids with methylprednisolone ~4 mg/kg/day divided every 6 hours until symptoms are improved. Oral immunosuppressants should be started as soon as possible to allow for tapering of corticosteroids to reduce the associated adverse effects. Oral immunosuppressants include steroids in combination with azathioprine (initially 3 mg/kg/day) or hydroxychloraquine (200 mg once daily). In some patients, a steroid free immunosuppressant regimen may be adequate.

Surgery: A surgical lung biopsy will provide tissue for diagnosis.

Therapy: Physical therapy is important if long term steroid use is required. Long term steroids will result in significant weight gain and can result in steroid induced myopathy.

Social: No specific social resources are available.

Pearls and Precautions

A high level of suspicion is required to make the diagnosis of IPH in an infant or child.

With a history of IPH, new respiratory symptoms or radiographic changes must be presumed to be signs of active pulmonary hemorrhage.

Patients with IPH are at risk for acute and life threatening pulmonary hemorrhage.

References

Godfrey S. Pulmonary Hemorrhage/Hemoptysis in Children. Pediatr Pulmonol. 37: 476–484. 2004.

Susarla SC, Fan L. Diffuse alveolar hemorrhage syndromes in children. Current Opinion in Pediatrics, 19: 314–320, 2007.

Saeed, M.M., M.S. Woo, E.F. MacLaughlin, M.F. Margetis, and T.G. Keens. Prognosis in pediatric idiopathic pulmonary hemosiderosis. Chest, 116: 721–725, 1999.

Luo, X. et al. Maintenance therapy with dose-adjusted 6-mercaptopurine in idiopathic pulmonary hemosiderosis. Pediatr Pulmonol. 43: 1067–1071. 2008.

Tracheomalacia and Bronchomalacia (Tracheobronchomalacia)

Roberta M. Kato, Thomas G. Keens

Tracheobronchomalacia is defined as collapsibility of the trachea and/or bronchi resulting in airway obstruction and impaired airway clearance.

Etiology

Specific genetic associations are not known, though studies focus on the genes involved in the formation of cartilaginous rings such as sonic hedgehog (Shh). Extrinsic compression from vascular anomalies, congenital heart disease, and masses can cause tracheobronchomalacia in some cases. Tracheomalacia is also found in congenital airway anomalies, such as tracheoesophageal fistulas, even after repair.

Clinical Presentation and Prognosis

Age of onset: If congenital etiology, presentation will be noted in infancy. If related to extrinsic compression, the presentation will vary, but it still most frequently presents in infancy.

Presenting signs and symptoms: There may be respiratory distress, chronic "honking" cough, stridor, wheeze, recurrent pneumonias, and recurrent or persistent atelectasis of a lobe.

Clinical course: Malacia can improve over time, especially if the etiology is identified and there is a therapeutic option such as surgical repair of an aberrant vessel. There are cases where severity increases with time.

Prognosis: Prognosis may be good to poor depending on the particular lesion.

Diagnosis

Diagnosis requires direct visualization by bronchoscopy. Ideally, the patient should breathe spontaneously during the procedure, as positive pressure ventilation may reduce the appearance of malacia. CT of the chest may be indicated if there is concern for an extrinsic mass or CT with contrast for evaluation of a vascular malformation.

Management

Management varies depending on the etiology and severity of the malacia.

Medications: Bronchodilators such as Albuteral are frequently used.

Surgery: Airway stents are infrequently used in growing children because they do not increase as the child grows. Because of endothelialization, stents cannot usually be removed. Therefore, one can create a progressive airway obstruction. A tracheostomy may be placed to reduce upper airway resistance or to allow for mechanical positive pressure ventilation if the lesion results in respiratory failure. Resection of short lengths of severe malacia have been performed.

Therapy: The normal cough mechanism is impaired as there is increased airway collapse with the increased intrathoracic pressure generated during a cough. Therefore, airways clearance techniques such as chest physiotherapy (CPT), are an important part of pulmonary care with tracheomalacia and/or bronchomalacia.

Psych: There are no specific psychological or psychiatric interventions recommended.

Social: There are no specific social interventions recommended.

Pearls and Precautions

Diet: A swallowing evaluation is necessary to ensure adequate and safe intake. If a primary surgical repair is not possible or complicated, a gastrostomy tube may be necessary.

Medical devices: HFCC vest, CPAP.

Likely complications: Recurrent infections and atelectasis is common.

Miscellaneous: Bronchoscopy is required to diagnose tracheobronchomalacia.

Tracheobronchomalacia should be considered in any patient that does not response to conventional pulmonary therapies.

Severe cases of tracheobronchomalacia may be life threatening.

Reference:

Masters IB. Congenital airway lesions and lung disease. Pediatr Clin N Amer, 56: 227–242, 2009.

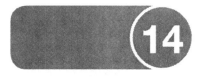

14 Rheumatolgic Disorders

Table of Contents

Behçets Disease

James N. Jarvis

Behçets disease is a multiorgan complex disease that typically involves the eyes, mucocutaneous, and genital area.

Etiology

Behçets disease in an illness of unknown etiology. While there are known human leukocyte antigen (HLA) associations suggesting links to adaptive immunity, abnormalities in neutrophil function, and the prominence of neutrophils in affected tissues, suggests complex interactions between innate and adaptive immunity.

Clinical Presentation and Prognosis

Demographics: Behçets disease is most commonly seen in children of Asian (especially Japanese), Middle Eastern, or eastern Mediterranean descent. Several series on Behçets disease in children have been published, with a mean age of onset between 7–15 years. Unlike adults, where males are more commonly affected, the ratio of boys to girls in children appears to be about 1:1 and, some series have even shown a slight female preponderance.

Presenting signs and symptoms: The most common presentation is recurrent, severe, painful oral and genital ulcers. Typical episodes last 3–10 days. Oral ulcers typically involve the lips, tongue, and palate and can usually be distinguished from benign aphthous ulcers by their severity.

Clinical course: At initial presentation, the diagnosis may not be considered as the full clinical features required for diagnosis (see below) typically evolve over time. In addition to the oral and genital ulcers, children typically develop a severe uveitis (anterior and posterior) and oligoarthritis. Central nervous system disease ranging from benign pseudotumor cerebri with headache to severe encephalomyelitis and organic brain disease (e.g., psychosis) occurs in 5–15% of children. Severe cutaneous vasculitis and/or thromboses occur in 5–15% of children.

Prognosis: The most severe complications of Behçets disease (uveitis, central nervous system disease) have traditionally been challenging to treat. Thus, long-term prognosis remains uncertain for most children. However, the emergence of newer therapies (including tumor necrosis factor (TNF) alpha inhibitors. See Medications section below) provides some hope that long-term prognosis will improve. Uveitis and central nervous system disease cause the most morbidity. Complicating the assessment of therapies is the remitting and relapsing course that many patients with Behçet's follow.

Diagnosis

There are no diagnostic tests that will establish the diagnosis of Behçets disease. Several clinical criteria have been established, and all include recurrent oral ulceration, genital ulceration, skin disease (e.g., erythema nodusm, papulopustular lesions, overt skin ulceration), and ocular involvement as major criteria. As noted, these clinical features are rarely observed at presentation and usually evolve over a period of months to years. Pathergy—the development of skin lesions with minor skin trauma—is a specific, but not sensitive sign.

Management

Medications: Treatment of Behçets disease remains largely empiric, and predicting which patients will respond to which agents has been problematic. Colchicine has been shown to reduce the severity and frequency of mucocutaneous manifestations in some patients, but is largely ineffective in ocular disease. Methotrexate, cyclosporine, tacrolimus, and thalidomide have all shown some utility in the different manifestation of Behçets. Corticosteroids, given orally, intravenously, and even as inhaled betamethasone (for oral lesions) can be effective in some patients in interrupting disease flares.

More recently, there has been considerable interest in the use of TNF inhibitors particularly in ocular disease that has not responded to topical corticosteroids. Mycophenylate mofetil has also shown some promise.

Surgery: Severe involvement of the skin or vulvae or vaginal muscosa may sometimes require debridment or skin grafting. Surgical resection of aneurysms may be required.

Consultations: Surgery, ophthalmology, dentistry, neurology, and dermatology may need to be consulted at times to treat the affected organs or systems.

Psychiatry: As with all children with chronic illness, individual psychotherapy and/or family therapy may be useful for some patients.

Monitoring: Central nervous system disease occurs in at least one fourth of patients with Behçets disease. On regular follow-up visits, attention should be paid to any neurologic symptoms, including relatively subtle changes such as alterations in personality.

Pearls and Precautions

Immunization: These patients should not receive live vaccines (measles-mumps-rubella (MMR), Varicella, Rotavirus or Inhaled Influenza Vaccine) while treated with immunosuppressant drugs.

Medications/situations that need to be avoided: Children on methotrexate should not be given other folic acid inhibitors (e.g., trimethoprim-sulfamethoxazol) as such drugs may synergize methotrexate bone marrow and hepatic toxicity.

Skin and dental care: Moderate dose topical steroids may be useful in helping to treat skin lesions. However, skin, mouth and GI tract lesions require systemic therapy for optimal control.

Likely complications: Central nervous system involvement is the most significant complication of Behçets disease. A variety of symptoms can be seen, and vascular aneurysms and stroke can be complications if the disease is poorly controlled. In addition, complications resulting from the immunosuppressive medications can be significant, particularly if steroids are required over time. The risk of infection from immunosuppression can be significant, and cushingoid features will result from prolonged steroid use. Reactivation of tuberculosis can occur with TNF inhibitors.

References

Ohno S, Nakamura S, Hori S, et al., Efficacy, safety, and pharmacokinetics of multiple administration of infliximab in Behçets disease with refractory uveoretinitis. J Rheumatol. 2004;31:1362–1368.

Kilmartin DJ, Forrester JV, Dick AD. Rescue therapy with mycophenolate mofetil in refractory uveitis. Lancet 1998;352:35–6

Juvenile Dermatomyositis (JDM)

James N. Jarvis

Juvenile dermatomyositis (JDM) refers to a chronic inflammatory vasculitis/myopathy that, in typical cases, is characterized by rash and progressive muscular weakness.

Etiology

JDM is a chronic inflammatory disease characterized by inflammation in blood vessels and peri-vascular areas of skeletal muscle and skin. The etiology of the disease is unknown. Genetic factors, both within the promoter region of the TNFA gene and HLA class II polymorphisms are both are associated with disease severity, but strong genetic links to disease pathogenesis have not been unequivocally demonstrated.

Clinical Presentation and Prognosis

Demographics: The disease is seen in all age groups and in children of all ethnic backgrounds. It is somewhat rare in adolescents.

Presenting signs and symptoms: Presenting symptoms generally occur as a constellation of features that include:

- Progressive weakness: The weakness may be quite subtle in pre-school children and manifest as simply a decrease in activity level. Parents of older children may observe difficulties going up steps (stairs or the school bus) or sometimes in activities of daily living (e.g., getting dressed).
- Rash. Four different cutaneous manifestation may be noted. These include:
    1. Heliotrope (purplish discoloration of the eyelids).
    2. Hyper-keratotic rash on the elbows and knees as well as extensor surfaces. This rash is sometimes mistaken for eczema or other forms of atopic dermatitis.
    3. Gotron's papules. These are erythematous, raised, sometimes hyperkeratotoc lesions that are prominent over the MCP, proximal interphalangeal joints (PIP), and, occasionally, distal interphalangeal joints (DIP) joints. They are highly characteristic of the disease.

4. Periungual erythema. This is often an overlooked clue into the diagnosis. When examined under microscopy (e.g., with an otoscope), these areas reveal marked capillary telangectasia and areas of capillary loss, consistent with the suspected underlying vascular nature of the disease.

Clinical course: Prior to the availability of potent anti-inflammatory therapy, JDM was progressively lethal in about 2/3 of the cases and resulted in severe disability (from muscle atrophy or calcinosis) in another third. Most deaths occurred from respiratory failure, although many deaths were also due to bowel perforation from uncontrolled vasculitis of the gastrointestinal tract. By the mid-1980s, children could be classified as likely to pursue three clinical courses: (1) monocyclic (i.e., a single disease episode responsive to treatment with no recurrences); (2) polycyclic (multiple recurrences but with good response to therapy); and (3) chronic-relapsing (poor disease control and disease exacerbations even on therapy). Whether these same disease patterns will emerge in children treated with more aggressive treatment approaches is unclear (see Medications section).

Prognosis: As noted, in the untreated child, this disease is progressive and frequently lethal. However, more aggressive management strategies have been associated with improved patient outcomes, and recurrences of JDM in adulthood are rare.

Diagnosis

In the majority of cases, diagnosis should be straightforward. Children with progressive muscle weakness and/or loss of typical activity levels who present with one or more of the characteristic rashes will commonly have elevations of one or more muscle enzymes:

- Creatine phosphokinase (CPK).
- Aldolase.
- Lactic dehydrogenase.

Elevations in serum AST/ALT levels can often distract the diagnostic work-up toward hepatic disease, particularly in children presenting with low-grade fever. A small number of children will present with rash, sometimes both typical and very prominent, with little other clinical evidence of muscle involvement. Such children usually develop typical alterations in muscle enzymes over time. MRI imaging of affected muscles may provide evidence for an inflammatory process when other clinical parameters are absent or ambiguous. Muscle biopsies may be useful in some clinical settings.

Management

Medications: The combination of methotrexate plus high-dose steroids has become the standard management for children with JDM. Weekly high-dose intravenous methylprednisolone has been shown to reduce long-term daily steroid exposure and is commonly used in addition to—or instead of—daily oral prednisone. Oral hydroxychloroquine has been shown to be effective in improving cutaneous manifestations of the disease. The roles of other immunosuppressive / anti-inflammatory drugs (TNF blockers, mycophenolate mofetil, azathiaprine, cyclophosphamide) in children who have failed methotrexate and steroids have not been studied in a sufficiently systematic way to allow general recommendations about when and where they might be helpful.

Surgery: In children in whom calcinosis is sufficiently severe to limit activity or function, surgical removal of calcinotic tissues can sometimes be beneficial.

Therapy: Physical therapy is commonly used to begin to restore muscle strength in children with lingering deficits.

Psych: Psychological issues faced by children with JDM are those generally common to children and families with a chronic, life-threatening disease. It is also useful to point out that the rash can be quite disfiguring and be accompanied by the predictable problems with peer relationships and self-esteem.

Social: The Myositis Association (www.myositis.org) and Cure JM (www.cureJM.com)are family focused organizations with resources for supporting parents and children with JDM.

Pearls and Precautions

Likely complications: Intramuscular calcinoses continue to be a major clinical challenge, particularly in children with difficult-to-control or chronic, smoldering disease.

Medications/situations/herbs that need to be avoided: Children on methotrexate should not be given other folic acid inhibitors (e.g., trimethoprim-sulfamethoxazol) as such drugs may synergize methotrexate bone marrow and hepatic toxicity.

Immunization: Children on immunosuppressive medications (e.g., methotrexate, chronic steroids, mycophenolate mofetil) should not receive live viral vaccines MMR, Varicella, Rotavirus or Inhaled Influenza Vaccine.

School: Aggressive therapy normally restores function quite quickly. School accommodations may need to be made for children who cannot easily climb stairs. Such accommodations are usually needed only temporarily.

Reference:

Banker BQ, Victor M, Dermatomyositis (systemic angiopathy)of childhood. Medicine (Baltimore) 1966; 45: 261–289.

Familial Mediterranean Fever (FMF)

James N. Jarvis

Familial mediterranean fever is an inherited, autoinflammatory condition that is characterized by periodic fever and may include polyserositis, peritonitis, and joint pain.

Etiology

FMF is a autosomal recessive genetic disease caused by defects in a gene denoted *MEFV1* or *pyrin*. The defects lead to inappropriate assembly of a protein complex called the inflammasome, with subsequent uncontrolled release of interleukin 1 and other pro-inflammatory cytokines.

Clinical Presentation and Prognosis

Demographics: FMF typically begins between the ages of 5–15 years. It is most common in children of eastern Mediterranean descent and quite rare in northern European populations.

Presenting signs and symptoms: Children typically present with recurrent episodes of fever and, quite commonly, abdominal pain from sterile peritonitis. Polyserositis (pleuritis, pericarditis, sterile peritontitis) also occurs. Typical episodes last 24–72 hours and can be quite painful. Arthralgia is common and a painful monoarthritis can occur in as many as 70% of children.

Clinical course and prognoses: Untreated, FMF pursues an unrelenting course with gradual onset of renal failure due to the deposition of amyloid proteins in the kidney. Treatment with colchicine (see Medications) ameliorates the clinical episodes and prevents or retards the development of amyloid-induced renal disease. Typically, the disease continues unabated throughout life and does not worsen or improve except with therapy.

Prognosis: For most, FMF may be easily controlled with colchicine therapy which also prevents the amyloidosis. Colchicine must be continued life-long.

Diagnosis

The diagnosis of FMF should be suspected in children with recurrent, episodic fever and abdominal pain, particularly children within high-prevalence demographics. Prior to the availability of genetic testing, diagnosis was based on the presence of specific major and minor clinical criteria that included recurrent fever, presence of amyloidosis, and response to colchicine. Genetic testing for the common MEFV1 disease-associated alleles is now widely available.

Management

Medications: Colchicine, given at doses of 1–2 mg/day (0.6 mg bid-qid) regardless of weight or age, is the most commonly used medication to prevent attacks. Those who still develop attacks despite this regimen may need to increase their dosage to 0.6 mg three or even four times daily.

Up to 5% of patients may not respond to colchicine. These patients require other therapies such as anti-IL-1 agents (anakinra) or steroid for attacks. Prolonged fever and myalgia can be treated with 1 mg/kg of prednisone for up to 6 weeks.

Consultations: In addition to rheumatology, patients who have proteinuria and amyloidosis need to be managed by a nephrologist. Patients who have renal failure also need to receive dialysis. A pain management specialist can significantly mitigate or avert the symptoms of secondary pain amplification syndrome.

Social: Education of teenagers and their parents may help with compliance.

Monitoring: Patients should be seen regularly and receive a urinalysis (urine dip may suffice) in the office to look for any proteinuria (marks non-compliance and amyloidosis) or hematuria (may mark the onset of polyarteritis nodosa).

Pearls and Precautions

Children with FMF usually feel and look vigorous and healthy between episodes. This appearance belies the intrusive, debilitating nature of the disease.

Nutrition/diet: Diet does not worsen or contribute to this disease. However, some children may develop lactose intolerance and require lactose free diet.

Likely complications: Colchicine may cause severe watery diarrhea in some children. Renal failure as a result of amyloidosis may require dialysis or renal transplant. Some patients may have coexisting diseases such as fibromyalgia, spondyloarthropathy, Henoch-Schonlein purpura, Behcet disease, and polyarteritis nodosa.

Reference

Calligaris L, Marchetti F, Tommasini A, Ventura A, The efficacy of anakinra in an adolescent with colchicine-resistant familial Mediterranean fever. Eur J Pediatr 2008; 167: 695–696.

Juvenile Idiopathic Arthritis (JIA): Pauciarticular Subtype

James N. Jarvis

Pauciarticular JIA (or oligoarticular JIA) is a term used to describe a distinct phenotype of chronic arthritis that occurs almost exclusively in children of European descent (see Demographics). By definition, such children have synovitis in 4 or fewer joints at presentation (1–2 is most typical) and maintain that phenotype for at least 5 months.

Etiology

The etiology of pauciarticular-onset juvenile idiopathic arthritis is unknown. The disease is characterized by overgrowth and invasiveness of the synovial membranes—typically of large joints (knees, ankles). Histological resemblance to the synovial pathology seen in adult rheumatoid arthritis suggests common mechanisms, although these similarities may simply reflect "final common pathway" events. Specific alleles within the HLA class II region appear to confer risk in patients of European descent, but these same alleles do not convey risk in other populations.

Clinical Presentation and Prognosis

Demographics: Pauciarticular JIA is typically a disease of pre-school girls, although boys can also be affected. This subtype of JIA is quite rare in children on the Indian subcontinent and in African American and indigenous American children living in North America. Among children of European descent, however, it is the single most common rheumatic disease and represents about 60% of children with chronic arthritis.

Presenting signs and symptoms: Joint swelling and gait disturbance are the most common presenting complaints in children with pauciarticular JIA. Children with pauciarticular JIA rarely verbalize pain, and if severe pain (e.g., that awakens a child at night) is a prominent complaint, then other diagnoses (e.g., acute lymphocytic leukemia) should be considered. The gait disturbance is often the first symptom, appearing in many cases several days or weeks before the joint swelling is visible to the child's caretaker. The symptoms are usually worse in the morning or periods of inactivity (e.g., after an afternoon nap) and improve with activity. Indeed, the constellation of relatively painless knee swelling in a European-descended child with gait disturbance, that is worse with rest and better with activity, is virtually pathognomonic of pauciarticular JIA.

Clinical course: Untreated, pauciarticular-onset JIA invariably leads to joint contracture, bony overgrowth due to hyperemia of the surrounding structures, and irreversible joint destruction occurring over the course of months (rarely) or years. Blindness from iridocyclitis is also alarmingly common in children who do not receive proper screening and treatment.

In the treated state, children with pauciarticular JIA do well. Most children are off therapy 5 years after diagnosis. However, disease recurrences in later childhood, adolescence, and/or adulthood are more common than was previously believed, although recurrences tend to respond well to therapy.

A considerable number of children with pauciarticular onset JIA will evolve—over the course of months or years—to more extensive joint involvement including the small joints of the hands, wrists, etc., and become phenotypically indistinguishable from children with polyarticular-onset disease. The disease process in these children tends to be more aggressive and typically remits only with more aggressive therapies.

Prognosis: From the standpoint of the joint disease, the prognosis for children with pauciarticular-onset JIA is excellent and most children are able to maintain or regain full function (including participation in vigorous athletic activities) throughout the disease course. The prognosis for chronic uveitis in pauciarticular JIA is good, but some loss of visual acuity is still quite common even in children who are appropriately screened and treated.

Diagnosis

The diagnosis of pauciarticular-onset JIA is entirely based on the history and physical examination. On examination, one or two (typically lower extremity) joints will feel warm with extra, "doughy" tissue surrounding them. This doughy tissue represents proliferative synovium. This finding in the setting of a child with gait disturbance that is most prominent after periods of rest, is virtually pathognomic of pauciarticular JIA. A complete blood count and differential should be performed in children with severe pain to exclude leukemia. *Neither ANA nor rheumatoid factor test have any diagnostic utility in this setting and should not be ordered for diagnostic purposes.*

Management

Medications: Non-steroidal anti-inflammatory drugs at anti-inflammatory doses (e.g., naproxen 10 mg/kg/dose given two times a day) and intra-articular steroid injections have become the treatment of choice for this disease. In rare cases, disease control is only achieved with the more potent anti-inflammatory/immunosuppressive therapy (e.g., methotrexate).

Uveitis is typically treated with topical steroids. Intractable cases usually respond to methotrexate given orally or subcutaneously. Children whose uveitis does not respond to methotrexate frequently respond to anti-TNF therapies (e.g., intravenous infliximab).

Surgery: Not typically needed. Synovial biopsy may be indicated in cases where the diagnosis is still in question.

Consultations: All children with pauciarticular JIA need regular slit lamp examinations, preferably by an ophthalmologist, to screen for chronic uveitis. Children who are ANA+ and present before the age of 5 years are at highest risk for developing this complication.

Therapy: In children with joint contractures, passive range of motion exercises may assist in restoring function as the inflammatory process begins to abate.

Psychiatric: Most children and families adjust well to this diagnosis. Need for mental health services usually reflects pre-existing family stressors.

Social: The Arthritis Foundation has many services for families provided at the local (Chapter) level: www.arthritis.org

Monitoring: Children on nonsteroidal anti-inflammatory medications should have electrolytes drawn at least twice a year. A urinalysis should be performed 2–4 times per year. Children on methotrexate should have a complete blood count and differential and comprehensive metabolic profile drawn every 3–4 months.

Pearls and Precautions

Medications that need to be avoided: Children on methotrexate should not be given other folic acid inhibitors (e.g., trimethoprim-sulfamethoxazol), as such drugs may synergize methotrexate bone marrow and hepatic toxicity.

Immunization: Children on methotrexate should not receive live viral vaccines (MMR, Varicella, Rotavirus or Inhaled Influenza Vaccine).

School/education: There is no reason to interdict ANY activity in children with arthritis. They should be allowed to do any physical activity that they feel well enough to do.

Miscellaneous: Rheumatoid factor tests are probably among the most commonly mis-used tests in pediatrics. Most children with chronic arthritis do not have positive rheumatoid factor tests, and most children with positive rheumatoid factor tests don't have chronic arthritis. Therefore, the poor positive and negative predictive values of this test make it utterly useless in evaluating children with musculoskeletal complaints.

Reference

Jarvis JN, Cleland SY, Rheumatic disease in Native American children. Curr Rheumatol Reports 2003; 5: 471–476.

Jarvis JN, Ordering laboratory tests for suspected rheumatic disease. Pediatr Rheumatol 2008; 6:19.★

Juvenile Idiopathic Arthritis: Polyarticular Subtype

James N. Jarvis

Polyarticular JIA is a term used to describe a distinct phenotype of chronic arthritis characterized by synovitis in 5 or more joints at presentation.

Etiology

The etiology of polyarticular-onset juvenile idiopathic arthritis (JIA) is unknown. The disease is characterized by overgrowth and invasiveness of the synovial membranes, including large joints (knees, ankles) and small joints (hands, fingers, feet). Histological resemblance to the synovial pathology seen in adult rheumatoid arthritis suggests common mechanisms, although these similarities may simply reflect "final common pathway" events. Children who are rheumatoid factor positive (usually adolescents) have an illness that is clinically, pathologically, and immunogenetically indistinguishable from adult rheumatoid arthritis.

Clinical Presentation and Prognosis

Demographics: This form of JIA occurs in all age groups and ethnicities encountered in a typical North American practice. It is the most common form of chronic arthritis in African American and American Indian children.

Presenting signs and symptoms: As with the pauciarticular-onset form of the disease, joint swelling and gait disturbance—not pain—is the usual presenting complaint. Patients will commonly speak of being "stiff," and the stiffness will be most prominent in the morning and improve with activity. The patient may also complain of swelling of the metacarpal-phalangeal or proximal inter-phalangeal joints. Preschoolers may present with difficulty walking or regression of gross motor milestones.

Clinical course: Untreated, polyarticular-onset JIA invariably leads to joint contracture, and irreversible joint destruction occurring over the course of months (rarely) or years. Blindness from iridocyclitis may also occur in children whose disease begins in their preschool years, particularly in children who have not had appropriate screening and therapy.

In the treated state, children with polyarticular JIA do well. However, only a small minority of these children have achieved remission (off all therapy without disease activity for ≥12 months) within 5 years of diagnosis. Furthermore, even in children who achieve remission, disease recurrences in later childhood, adolescence, and/or adulthood are more common than was previously believed. Many pediatric rheumatologists no longer reassure parents of children with polyarticular disease that their child will "outgrow" the disease process.

Prognosis: Provided adequate therapy is given in a timely fashion, the vast majority of children with polyarticular JIA will be able to lead normal lives, including the ability to engage in vigorous athletic activities. Like children with pauciarticular JIA, children with polyarticular JIA who develop uveitis commonly have some loss of visual acuity.

Diagnosis

The diagnosis of polyarticular-onset JIA is entirely based on the history and physical examination. On examination, multiple joints will feel warm with extra "doughy" tissue surrounding them. This doughy tissue represents proliferative synovium. In polyarticular JIA, it may be detected most easily in the wrists, where the synovial proliferation will obscure the extensor tendons (normally easily palpable) as they cross the carpus. Finding multiple swollen joints in a child with gait disturbance that is most prominent after periods of rest, is a classic presentation for polyarticular JIA. A complete blood count and differential should be performed in children with severe pain to exclude leukemia, for example, in a child with extremely painful swelling of both ankles and both knees. *Neither ANA nor rheumatoid factor test have any diagnostic utility in this setting and should not be ordered for diagnostic purposes.*

Management

The management of polyarticular JIA has radically changed over the past 10 years. The aggressive use of methotrexate with or without biological therapies is becoming the standard of care for most patients in most centers.

Medications: Methotrexate, 0.5 mg/kg or 20 mg/m^2 is rapidly becoming the "standard" agent for polyarticular JIA, particularly in children who are rheumatoid factor positive (as these children have a worse prognosis). Non-steroidal anti-inflammatory drugs are largely adjunctive, but are typically provided as their use may improve function sooner. Short courses of oral prednisone (1 mg/kg/day and tapering over 10–14 days) may rapidly improve function in children who are missing school or hampered in other activities of daily living. Pulse methylprednisolone (500 mg/m^2) is sometimes used for the same purpose. Children who do not achieve an inactive disease state (absence of joint swelling and normal laboratory tests) are typically placed on biological therapies. Anti-TNF therapies (etanercept, infliximab, adilumimab) are the most common, although anti-IL1 (anakinra) and T cell (abatacept) therapies are also used. Anti-IL6 therapies are in development, but currently are being used only in clinical trials in children with systemic disease.

Uveitis, which typically occurs in children whose disease starts before age 5 (but can occur in any age group) is usually treated with topical steroids. Intractable cases usually respond to methotrexate given orally or subcutaneously. Children whose uveitis does not respond to methotrexate frequently respond to anti-TNF therapies (e.g., intravenous infliximab).

Surgery: Surgery is becoming quite rare in children with polyarticular JIA. Hip and knee replacement surgeries are occasionally of benefit to children who have had severe, intractable disease and irreversible joint destruction.

Therapy: In children with joint contractures, passive range of motion exercises may assist in restoring function as the inflammatory process begins to abate.

Psychiatric: Children and families differ considerably in their adjustments to this diagnosis. Restoring normal function as quickly as possible generally obviates psychological stress. In small children, daily or weekly injections (etanercept, methotrexate, e.g.) can be a source of anxiety and stress.

Social: The Arthritis Foundation has many services for families provided at the local (Chapter) level: www. arthritis.org.

Consultations: Children with polyarticular JIA need routine slit lamp examinations as described for children with pauciarticular disease.

Monitoring: See "Pauciarticular JIA." Children on anti-TNF therapies should be monitored in the same way as children on methotrexate.

Pearls and Precautions

School/education: Early in the disease course, before the inactive disease state is achieved, children may have considerable difficulty in school, either with fine motor tasks (from synovitis in the hands or wrists) or gross motor tasks (getting from one class to another after being seated for 45–50 min). Schools are typically able to accommodate to the simple (and usually time-limited) needs of such children.

Although children with JIA were once discouraged from engaging in high-impact sports (e.g., football, ice hockey, basketball), there is no evidence to suggest that these activities are harmful. Alternatively, there is good evidence that, in general, activity is beneficial in children with all forms of arthritis. Children with polyarticular JIA who have cervical spine involvement represent an exception to this rule, and decisions for such children must be made on a case-by-case basis.

Immunization: Children on methotrexate or biologic therapies (TNF or IL-1 inhibitors) should not receive live viral vaccines MMR, Varicella, Rotavirus or Inhaled Influenza Vaccine).

Oral health: Involvement of the temporo-mandibular joints is common in polyarticular JIA and can lead to micrognathia. Good health care and habits are critical elements in preventing complications from micrognathia.

Medications that need to be avoided: Children on methotrexate should not be given other folic acid inhibitors (e.g., trimethoprim-sulfamethoxazol), as such drugs may synergize methotrexate bone marrow and hepatic toxicity.

Reference

Jarvis JN, Cleland SY, Rheumatic disease in Native American children. Curr Rheumatol Reports 2003; 5: 471–476.

Jarvis JN, Ordering laboratory tests for suspected rheumatic disease. Pediatr Rheumatol 2008; 6:19.*

Systemic Onset Juvenile Idiopathic Arthritis (SoJIA)

James N. Jarvis

Systemic-onset JIA is a disease characterized by persistent fever and rash, elevated acute phase reactants, and the insidious onset of chronic synovitis. It is a diagnosis of exclusion.

Etiology

The etiology of systemic-onset juvenile idiopathic arthritis (SoJIA) is unknown. Its strong resemblance to many auto-inflammatory syndromes and the association of the illness with elevated levels of IL-1 and IL-6 have led to speculation that this is more an illness of innate rather than adaptive immunity. The term "autoimmune" is probably inappropriate for this illness.

Clinical Presentation and Prognosis

Demographics: This illness occurs in all age groups and affects boys and girls equally. The most challenging cases tend to occur in pre-school and early school age children.

Presenting signs and symptoms: The most striking characteristic of systemic-onset JIA is the (typically abrupt) onset of high spiking fevers and rash. Fever typically occurs in a once-or-twice a day pattern, occurs daily and unrelentingly, and commonly is associated with rash. Joint swelling, which like other forms of JIA, represents proliferative synovium, may not occur until weeks, months, or even years after the onset of systemic symptoms.

Clinical course: The fever, once established, is usually unrelenting until appropriate therapy is started, and even then may be intractable. The synovitis, once established, can be very challenging to treat and typically evolves into a polyarticular pattern virtually indistinguishable from polyarticular JIA. The arthritis frequently persists years after the systemic symptoms have abated.

In severe cases, systemic disease may be associated with polyserositis (pericarditis, pleuritis), hepatic dysfunction, or myocarditis. In rare cases, the latter may be lethal. SoJIA is, in fact, the only form of JIA that has a measurable mortality rate.

Some fatalities may occur due to so-called macrophage activation syndrome (MAS). Although MAS may also be seen in polyarticular JIA and other chronic inflammatory diseases, it is most commonly associated with SoJIA. MAS should be suspected in any child with sudden onset of pancytopenia, hepatic dysfunction, and cerebral dysfunction.

Recurrences of SoJIA in adolescence or adulthood are well-described. Recurrences may include either systemic, or joint disease, or both.

Prognosis: Except in rare cases, the systemic features of the disease can either be controlled or gradually abate. The arthritis can be aggressive, progressive, and refractory to even aggressive anti-inflammatory / immuno-suppressive management approaches. The prognosis for having the disease resolve without some loss of joint integrity or function must be considered guardedly.

Diagnosis

As with the other rheumatic diseases of childhood, there is no "test" that establishes or excludes the diagnosis of SoJIA. The diagnosis is generally made only after other causes of persistent fever have been excluded. However, several clinical clues help the practitioner make the diagnosis with added confidence:

- In typical cases, the white blood cell count is above 20,000 / cu mm and the platelet count is above 500,000/cu mm. White blood cell counts of less than 10,000 / cu mm are rare.
- The fever occurs daily. Other diagnoses should be pursued in a child with intermittent fever (e.g., occurring 2–3 days per week).
- The fever can be monotonously regular in its appearance, and parents typically tell the physician that the fever occurs at specific times of the day and lasts 3–4 hours.
- When the fever is present, the child may appear quite ill. During those periods of the day when the fever is absent, the child may appear vigorous and playful.
- A salmon-colored, evanescent, maculpapular rash may appear or be more visible when the fever is present.

Management:

Medications: Until recently, corticosteroids (orally or given as intravenous "pulses") were the standard agents for controlling the systemic features of SoJIA. There is growing interest in biologics, particularly anti-IL1 agents (e.g., anakinra). Because of the important role of IL-6 in animal models of SoJIA, clinical trials of IL-6 inhibition are under way in the United States and other parts of the world. Treatment approaches for the arthritis generally parallel the approach taken for polyarticular disease.

MAS should be considered a life-threatening medical emergency, and pulse methylpredniosolone (500 mg/m2) x 3–5 daily doses should be administered as soon as the diagnosis is made. Cyclosporine may be useful in controlling disease not fully responsive to pulse steroids.

Surgery: Same as for polyarticular JIA.

Therapy: Same as for pauci- and polyarticular JIA.

Psychiatry: See polyarticular JIA.

Social : See polyarticular JIA.

Monitoring: Same as polyarticular JIA

Consultations: Same as polyarticular JIA.

Pearls and Precautions

Likely complications: While not a "likely" complication, MAS is a known and potentially lethal complication that occurs most frequently in systemic-onset JIA. MAS is usually heralded by malaise, irritability, and often low-grade fever that does not follow the double-quotidian pattern of active systemic disease. It is characterized by bone marrow, hepatic, endothelial, and cerebral dysfunction. Children typically have suddent decreases in hematocrit, white blood cell and platelet counts often found on routine monitoring for medication toxicity. MAS should be considered a medical emergency and children with this complication should be transferred immediately to a facility experienced in caring for children with this problem.

Immunizations: See polyarticular JIA.

School/Education: See polyarticular JIA.

Medications that need to be avoided: See polyarticular JIA.

Reference

Adams A. Lehman TJ, Update on the pathogenesis and treatment of systemic onset juvenile rheumatoid arthritis. [see comment]. [Review] Current Opinion in Rheumatology. 17(5):612–6, 2005 Sep.

Jarvis JN, Juvenile rheumatoid arthritis: a guide for pediatricians. Pediatr Ann 2002. 31: 437–446.

Spondyloarthropathy

(Enthesitis-Associated Arthritis in the current international nomenclature)

James N. Jarvis

Spondyloarthropathy refers to a distinct family of arthritidis characterized by (1) predominance of male patients; (2) axial skeletal involvement; and (3) extra-articular musculoskeletal involvement (bursae, tendon insertions).

Etiology

Several clues cast light on the etiology of this form of arthritis: (1) Their strong association with the HLA class I antigen B27; (2) an animal model that closely mimics the human disease-HLA B27 transgenic rodents; and (3) the failure of the transgenic rodents to develop arthritis if they are raised in a germ-free environment. These clues have led some investigators to speculate that spondyloarthropathies are diseases of abnormal antigen processing or presentation, possibly in the gut-associated lymphoid tissue. The appearance of this form of arthritis in HLA-B27+ patients with inflammatory bowel disease supports that hypothesis.

Clinical Presentation and Prognosis

Demographics: In most populations, this form of arthritis occurs predominantly in males. However, in some American Indian tribes, females may be affected as commonly as males. This may be the most common form of arthritis in children living on the Indian subcontinent and in American Indian tribes in the southwestern United States and western Canada. The arthritis is seldom seen before age 5 years and becomes more frequent in the adolescent age group.

Presenting signs and symptoms: In the pre-school or early school years, this illness can be indistinguishable from pauciarticular JIA, presenting in an identical fashion: Gait disturbance and lower extremity joint swelling. The gait disturbance will typically be more prominent after periods of rest and improve with activity. Older children or adolescents will commonly present with hip pain, and the pain shows the characteristics of other illnesses in which synovium is inflamed: The pain is worse with rest (e.g., in the morning) and better with activity. Unlike adults, sacroiliitis is seldom present at the time of diagnosis in children; therefore, low back pain is typically not a presentation of children with spondyloarthropathy.

Clinical course: Untreated, spondyloarthropathies typically result in a relentless, progressive arthritis that leads to ankylosis of the spine, destruction of the hip joints, and loss of function of other large and small joints. Acute, painful uveitis is a common and serious complication. Involvement of non-articular musculoskeletal structures (bursae, the plantar fascia, Achilles tendons, and tendonous insertions into bone [etheses]) is highly characteristic of this form of arthritis.

Prognosis: Provided that adequate care is given, the prognosis for this form of arthritis is as good as for "classic" JIA.

Diagnosis

As with other rheumatic diseases in children, the history, physical, and clinical course are the most reliable means of establishing the diagnosis. A boy presenting with lower extremity arthritis, particularly arthritis of the hip, should arouse suspicion of this diagnosis. In most cases, the erythrocyte sedimentation rate will be mild to moderately elevated (30–50 mm/hr), and the HLA-B27 antigen will be present. It is important to note that as many as 8% of the healthy Caucasian population will carry the B27 antigen; therefore, its presence is not diagnostic.

Management

Medications: Methotrexate, 0.5 mg/kg or 10 mg/m2 is rapidly becoming the "standard" agent for polyarticular JIA, particularly in children who are rheumatoid factor positive (as these children have a worse prognosis). Non-steroidal anti-inflammatory drugs are largely adjunctive but are typicaly prescribed as their use may improve function sooner. Short courses of oral prednisone (1 mg/kg/day and tapering over 10–14 days) may rapidly improve function in children who are missing school or hampered in other activities of daily living. Pulse methylprednisolone (500 mg/m2) is sometimes used for the same purpose. Children who do not achieve an inactive disease state (absence of joint swelling and normal laboratory tests) are typically placed on biological therapies. Anti-TNF therapies (etanercept, infliximab, adilumimab) are the most common, although anti-IL1 (anakinra) and T cell (abatacept) therapies are also used.

Surgery: See section on polyarticular JIA.

Therapy: See section on polyarticular JIA.

Psychiatric: See section on polyarticular JIA.

Social: See section on polyarticular JIA.

Monitoring: see polyarticular JIA.

Consult: Although the uveitis of spondyloarthropathies is typically acute and symptomatic, it is still recommended that children with spondyloarthropathies receive routine slit lamp examinations to detect indolent cases.

Pearls and Precautions

Spondyloarthropathy is one of the rare forms of chronic childhood arthritis that presents with musculoskeletal pain as a prominent complaint. However, back pain is rarely the presenting complaint. Rather, hip pain (better with activity and worse after periods of rest) is the more common complaint.

Likely complications: Extra-articular involvement of both the musculoskeletal system (tendonitis, bursitis, enthesitis [inflammation at the insertion of tendons]) and non-musculoskeletal tissues (iritis, aortitis) is common in spondyloarthropathy. Unlike the iritis of JIA, the iritis of spondyloarthropathies is usually acute and painful. Patients with this illness who develop a red, painful eye should be seen by an ophthalmologist immediately.

School/education: See section on polyarticular JIA.

Medications/situations/herbs that need to be avoided/infection control etc.: See section on polyarticular JIA.

Immunization: See polyarticular JIA

References

Aggarwal A. Misra R, Juvenile chronic arthritis in India: Is it different from that seen in western countries? *Rheumatol Int* 1994; 14: 53.

McGhee JL, Burks F, Sheckels J, Jarvis JN, Identifying children with chronic arthritis based on chief complaints: absence of predictive value for musculoskeletal pain as an indicator of rheumatic disease in children. Pediatrics 2002; 110: 354–359.

Systemic Lupus Erythematosus (SLE)

James N. Jarvis

Systemic lupus erythematosus is an archetypal autoimmune disease characterized by autoantibody formation and inflammation in multiple tissues due to immune complex deposition and complement activation.

Etiology

The etiology of systemic lupus erythematosus (SLE) is unknown. The disease is characterized pathologically by exuberant autoantibody formation and immune complex deposition and complement activation in the blood and vessel walls of numerous tissues. The strong association between SLE and genetic deficiencies of early components of the classical complement pathway (C1q, C1r, C1s, and C4) implicate defects in the processing and clearance of immune complexes and cellular debris, but no single theory of pathogenesis explains the myriad of clinical and pathological features of the disease.

Clinical Presentation and Prognosis

Demographics: Twenty percent of patients diagnosed with SLE will have onset of symptoms before age 18. That being said, SLE is rare in pre-pubertal children and even rarer in children under the age of 6 years. SLE has a nearly 1:1 female to male ratio in pre-pubertal children, but that ratio increases to 8:1 after puberty. The highest prevalence rates are reported in people of Afro-Caribbean descent, and both African Americans and American Indians appear to have higher prevalence rates than the European-descended population of North America.

Presenting signs and symptoms: Although SLE is the classic "protean" disease ("protean" from Proteos, the god who changes shapes when Odysseus grabs hold of him in order to learn how to get home in Homer's Odyssey), children and adolescents with SLE typically present with florid, unmistakable disease. Low grade fever, diffuse musculoskeletal pain (SLE is one of the few rheumatic diseases of childhood where musculoskeletal pain is a prominent complaint), malar rash (which typically is neither subtle nor evanescent); and, weight loss are commonly the constellation of symptoms that bring an adolescent with SLE to seek medical care. Only in rare cases does the illness present with asymptomatic renal disease. Thrombocytopenia and/or hemolytic anemia can be presentations of SLE, although most of these patients eventually develop systemic and/or constitutional symptoms. Isolated musculoskeletal pain, without other constitutional symptoms, is, for all intents and purposes, never the presentation of a child or adolescent with SLE.

Clinical course: The clinical course of children with SLE is highly variable and unpredictable, even in carefully monitored and managed cases. Nephritis is the most common, serious complication of SLE, but desquamating skin rashes, pancreatitis, hepatic dysfunction, strokes, pulmonary emboli and other manifestations of thrombophilia (induced or enhanced by the production of thrombophilic autoantibodies such as anti-cardiolipin antibodies), pleuritis-pericarditis, and progressive encephalopathy can all occur at any phase of the disease process.

Prognosis: Prognosis is related to the chronicity of the renal disease and the degree of immunosuppression required to maintain disease control. Even in cases where disease control is achieved, significant morbidity derives from medications used to control the disease. Corticosteroid-induced bone demineralization and growth inhibition remain frustratingly common. Immunosuppression is frequently associated with serious, life-threatening infections, and infection remains a major cause of death in childhood-onset SLE.

Diagnosis

The diagnosis of SLE is made on the basis of the signs and symptoms, pattern of end-organ involvement, and, where appropriate, biopsy of affected tissues (e.g., kidney). The vast majority of children and adolescents will have positive antinuclear antibody (ANA) tests, but it is important for the practitioner to know that positive ANA tests may be seen in as many as 30% of perfectly healthy children. Furthermore, the titer of ANA seen in healthy children overlaps that of children with SLE, and so an ANA test alone does not make the diagnosis. ANA titers of 1:3,600 are rare in healthy children, however, and can be interpreted as strong supported evidence of SLE. At the same time, titers of 1:160 or less are rare in SLE and virtually exclude that diagnosis in most cases. Children with SLE frequently have depressed levels of the complement components C3 and C4, so assays for these proteins should be included as part of the evaluation of a child or adolescent suspected of having SLE. Because of the high frequency of renal involvement, a urinalysis should also be obtained on any child suspected of having SLE. A complete blood count and differential can sometimes provide useful clues, as well. Children and adolescents with SLE often have mild leucopenia (white blood cell (WBC) 2,000–3,000/cu mm) with relative *lymphopenia.*

Management

There is no cure for SLE. Management of SLE is directed toward reduction of the inflammatory process to protect and maintain end-organ function.

Medications: Oral or intravenous corticosteroids are used to restore function and protect vital organs. Renal disease responds poorly to corticosteroids alone, and most children with renal disease are treated with steroids plus intravenous cyclophosphamide. There is growing interest in using mycophenolate mofetil as an adjunct to—or even replacement for—cyclophosphamide in select patients with lupus nephritis, but appropriately controlled studies to determine whether such an approach is as good as or better than standard therapy have not been undertaken in children. Anti-marials (most commonly, hydroxychloroquine) have been found to be efficacious in reducing the severity of some of the cutaneous manifestations of SLE and possible musculosketal symptoms. Anti-B cell antibody therapies (e.g., rituximab) have been shown to be efficacious in off-label or experimental trials, but the long-term implications for their use remains uncertain, and serious side-effects have been reported. Patients with thrombotic complications often need aggressive anti-coagulation. Pharmacokinetic factors make oral warfarin fairly cumbersome to use in this setting, and low molecular weight heparin is an increasingly attractive alternative.

Surgery: Aseptic necrosis of the hips, a complication of corticosteroid use and the underlying vasculopathy, often leads to severe pain and dysfunction in patients who have had longstanding SLE. Hip replacement surgeries have been shown to be useful even in adolescent patients with SLE whose function and quality of life have been compromised by this complication.

Psychiatric: Progressive encephalopathy, cognitive dysfunction, and thought disorders can all appear in patients with SLE as a direct result of central nervous system involvement. Establishing an etiology can often be challenging. More challenging are the depression and mood shifts that can occur as a result of medications (especially high dose steroids), the disease process itself, or the adjustment of a child or adolescent to an intrusive and often life-threatening disease.

Social: The Lupus Foundation (www.lupus.org) has excellent resources for children and adolescents with SLE.

Pearls and Precautions

Nutrition: The chronic, low-grade vasculopathy of SLE is associated with accelerated atherosclerosis, even in children and adolescents. A "heart-healthy" diet should be strongly encouraged in children and teens with SLE.

School/education: Children and adolescents with SLE confront numerous school-related issues, including most of those faced by children with polyarticular JIA. In addition, frequent school absences—because of illness or the need for monitoring and therapy—add an additional burden. Central nervous system involvement, whether manifesting as learning disabilities or emotional lability, can be particularly challenging to address.

Miscellaneous

A note on ANA testing: ANA testing has very limited utility in pediatrics. As noted in Diagnosis, as many as 30% of healthy children will have a positive ANA test. Furthermore, the titer of the positive tests seen in healthy children directly overlap the positive ANA tests seen in children with other rheumatic diseases such as juvenile idiopathic arthritis (JIA) and juvenile dermatomyositis (JDM). However, high titer ANA tests (> 1:1,080) are fairly rare in healthy children or children with other rheumatic diseases and fairly commonly seen in children with SLE. Therefore, the test does have some discriminatory ability if this is the diagnosis in question. Thus, ANA testing should be limited to attempting to answer only a *single* question in children: "Does this child have SLE?" Obviously, if that's the question, then it would be reasonable to order a complete blood count (CBC) and differential, C3, C4, and urinalysis any time one orders an ANA test on a child or adolescent.

Reference

McGhee JL, Kickingbird L, Jarvis JN, Clinical utility of ANA tests in children. BMC Pediatrics 2004; 4:13

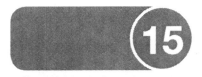

15 Medical Devices and Therapies

Table of Contents

Home Apnea Monitor

Sheila Kun

General Function and Application

Home cardiorespiratory monitor has been used for more than 30 years. The primary intent was to decrease the risk of sudden infant death syndrome (SIDS) at home. Over the years, research studies have shown that monitor use ***does not prevent*** sudden, unexpected death in all circumstances.

Indications

Recommendation per American Academy of Pediatrics: Premature infants who are at high risk of recurrent episodes of central apnea or bradycardia, after hospital discharge would benefit from its use up to 43 weeks postmenstrual age or cessation of extreme episodes.

Technology dependent infants with unstable airway or regulation of breathing, and children who are on home mechanical ventilator may benefit from this device as a back up alarm. However, there is mounting evidence that an oximeter is a much better choice for this population.

Types of Apnea

Central apnea: No breathing effort, chest movement could be related to other muscle movements, no air passing through.

Obstructive sleep apnea: No air passes through the upper airway, but the chest continues to move.

Mixed: Episodes with both central and obstructive component.

Advantages

Most apnea monitor devices are equipped with an internal memory which records episodes of apnea/bradycardia or tachycardia as long as recording parameters are set correctly. These devices allow detection of respiratory and cardiac changes for a prompt response from caregivers.

Disadvantage

Apnea monitors do not measure actual breathing or hypoxia. Therefore, as long as a patient has some chest movement, the alarms may not go off. They should not be used as a monitor for prevention of apnea or sudden infant death. Hence, the goal of monitoring needs to be clear with the caregiver. The timing of the monitor's discontinuation should also be addressed at the initiation of monitoring to prevent the parents' emotional dependence on them as an indispensable device.

Apnea monitors do not detect obstructive sleep apnea or mixed apneas.

They could provide a "false sense of security" when the goal is not well understood.

Types of Apnea Monitors

All monitors must be able to detect apnea and slow/fast heart rate. Desirable features of a monitoring device include battery back up lasting at least eight hours, and audio and visual alarms. Distinctly different alarms warn parents of equipment malfunction vs. physiological changes in the child. An optional feature is the remote unit that allows monitoring from a different room. Caution applies to allow good response time.

Memory and download capability is important to capture adverse events for subsequent analysis and help distinguish the false alarms from the real life-threatening events.

Power loss alarm is another desirable feature, which denotes low battery power.

Troubleshooting of Common Problems With the Apnea Monitor

Loose leads are the most common cause of false alarms. Ensure proper adherence of chest leads, proper placement and connections of the apnea monitor.

Another problem is the bradycardia alarm. If it is set too high, it will give false alarm. The bradycardia alarm is set at 70 beats per minute, and may drop down to 50 for infants older than 6 months.

Another false alarm is from shallow breathing. Apnea monitors will miss capturing some hypopnea/apnea.

Proper placement of the electrodes and operation of the monitor will help ensure its proper function.

Skin irritation occurs from using leads 24/7. Do allow non-monitoring times and removal of the leads to allow the skin "to breathe." Slightly position the leads at different spots to prevent chronic irritation to the same area. Hypoallergenic leads are also available.

Routine Use and Tips

The initial months of using apnea monitoring could be very stressful for the parents who have not been adequately trained on the appropriate response to the alarms. Most parents typically err on "over-reacting," rather than calmly assessing the source of the alarm. Thus, parents rapidly correct the alarms without a proper assessment of its etiology. This will lead to a series of nervous moments that provide no clues for a corrective action (e.g., lead position, assessing the patients breathing, etc.) To make apnea monitoring manageable, parents should rehearse the procedure until their response is almost "automatic."

To assure the proper function of these devices during the monitoring hours, parents should minimize any interference from other devices by keeping the monitor at least one foot away from electrical appliances, remote phones, televisions, etc. Households close to fire stations with radio signals might have interferences.

Special Considerations

For short term monitoring of life threatening central apnea or bradycardia, a rental unit is desirable so that monthly maintenance and download services are available. For clinics or medical offices, this is not a medical device that should be loaned out for obvious liability reasons.

When used as a back up alarm device for technologically dependent children, this author suggests the use of a pulse oximeter that provides more clinical data to the caregiver and functions very similarly in capturing changes in breathing and heart rate, and is also available with internal memory. However, for very young infants, the security of the pulse oximeter on the finger/toe must be considered.

Tips for The User

- Learn all the features of the apnea monitor.
- Understand when to use and when not to.
- Understand the importance of compliance.
- Rehearse and practice appropriate responses.
- Keep emergency numbers on hand.
- Stay calm and assess the reason for the alarms.
- Treat the equipment as a safety device, not a panic button.
- Follow all the cleaning and maintenance recommendations.
- For SIDS parents, practice the essential tips for the possible prevention of sudden death by, for example, keeping the infant in a supine sleeping position.

Replacement and Maintenance

- Belts and accessories are adjusted according to growth.
- Electrodes are replaced as needed and may last 2–3 days.
- Keep liquids away from the device.
- In case of a power failure, the monitor will continue to work on internal battery.
- Pack all accessories in a bag, close to the monitor. Plan ahead when traveling.
- Apnea monitoring for non- technologically dependent infant is confined usually to a few months.

Insurance and Financial Considerations

For infants with a life-threatening event outside the hospital setting or when health professionals do not directly observe the event, an apnea monitor is not easily approved. Children with a tenuous airway or on home ventilator support, approval is more readily done. Some payers require an abnormal pneumogram. Documentation of events directly observed, or polysomonogram is essential for insurance approval. The length of monitoring will determine if rental or purchase is the best recommendation. For short term monitoring of at risk infants, do include the monthly download to minimize extra written order. The vendor needs this order to get reimbursement when download service is rendered.

Dialysis

Katherine Wesseling Perry

General Function and Application

Children with acute and chronic renal failure are successfully treated with dialysis. Dialysis is either a bridge to recovery of kidney function (acute renal failure) or to kidney transplantation (chronic kidney disease). Indications for dialysis in the acute setting are: (1) Poisoning with dialyzable toxin; (2) volume overload; (3) hyperkalemia; (4) intractable acidosis; and (5) uremia. Indications for initiating dialysis in patients with chronic kidney disease include the indications listed above in addition to uremic symptoms such as: (1) Poor school performance; (2) poor appetite/nausea/vomiting; and (3) decreased energy level. Typically, dialysis is initiated when the glomerular filtration rate falls below 15 ml/min/1.73 m^2.

Peritoneal dialysis (PD) is the most common form of dialysis in pediatric patients and involves the diffusion of molecules from capillaries in the peritoneal membrane to the dialysate located in the peritoneal cavity. Fluid is removed down an osmotic gradient, generated by different concentrations of dextrose. This form of dialysis is performed at home, typically overnight.

Hemodialysis (HD) involves thrice weekly in-center purification of blood in patients with end-stage renal disease. This procedure is typically performed thrice weekly through an atrioventricular (AV) fistula (preferred), graft, or catheter (least preferable). Hemodialysis is the treatment of choice in pediatrics for conditions such as oxalosis and for the acute treatment of some inborn errors of metabolism.

Management

Electrolyte abnormalities: Severe hyperkalemia and acidosis are managed by emergent dialysis. Medical management (calcium, sodium bicarbonate therapy) is often required as an adjunct while awaiting the set up of the dialysis.

Anemia: Anemia is controlled with the use of iron and erythropoietin therapy. Iron therapy is adjusted based on iron stores (determined by iron saturation and ferritin levels); erythropoietin therapy is adjusted based on hematocrit.

Hypertension: Volume overload (salt and water retention) is by far the most common cause of hypertension in dialyzed patients. Aggressive dialysis to increase fluid removal as well as salt restriction typically controls high blood pressure. Antihypertensives are used when these measures fail. A minority of patients may have hypertension stemming from renin-release from native kidneys or from vasculitis (i.e. patients with autoimmune diseases).

Renal osteodystrophy and vascular disease: Hyperphosphatemia is controlled by phosphate binders (calcium salts, sevelamer hydrochloride, lanthanum carbonate, or, on rare occasions, aluminum hydroxide). Since progressive vascular calcification is associated with cardiac disease—the leading cause of death in both adults and children with renal failure—non-calcium containing phosphate binders (sevelamer hydrochloride) are preferred over calcium-containing compounds. Lanthanum is approved for use in adults, but not in children, while aluminum is associated with encephalopathy and osteomalacia of bone when used for extended periods of time. Serum parathyroid hormone (PTH) levels are suppressed by active vitamin D sterols (calcitriol, doxercalciferol, or paricalcitol) and/or calcimimetic (cinacalcet) agents.

Diet: A low phosphate, low potassium, low sodium diet is indicated. Adequate nutrition, particularly adequate protein (1 g/kg/d in older children and adults, more in infants. See KDOQI guidelines in Reference section for specifics) is imperative. A low protein diet is CONTRAINDICATED in pediatric CKD patients.

Consultations: A nephrologist should be the primary physician for every dialysis patient.

Surgery should be consulted for dialysis access placement (HD or PD catheter), G-tubes as necessary to maintain nutrition (particularly in young infants), and broviac catheter placement (for frequent blood draws in young infants). If possible, all three surgical procedures (catheter, G-tube, and broviac) should be placed during the same trip to the operating room. Surgery should also be consulted for repair of hernias.

Therapy: Renal osteodystrophy, chronic illness, and often multiple hospitalizations make all children with chronic kidney disease physically and emotionally at high risk for disability. Physical therapy is warranted in all children in whom gross or fine motor delay or muscle weakness is noted either on history or physical exam. Occupational therapy should be considered, particularly in infants and younger children, when an abnormal feeding and/or swallowing history are obtained.

Psychiatry: All children with chronic kidney disease are at high risk for emotional problems. Short stature, chronic illness, and repeated hospitalizations tend to isolate these children from their peers. Many uremic children have trouble learning and, when combined with multiple school absences related to their illness, school success is often limited. Thus, a psychosocial assessment is warranted for EVERY child with chronic kidney disease, including those on dialysis.

Monitoring: All children on dialysis should have a physical examination along with electrolytes, BUN, creatinine, calcium, phosphorus, and hematocrit, performed monthly. Formal dialysis adequacy tests are performed monthly in HD patients and every 3–6 months in PD patients. Growth parameters should be monitored routinely. Echocardiography (to evaluate for LVH) and a renal ultrasound (to evaluate for cysts formation) should be performed yearly.

Pearls and Precautions

Complications: Complications associated with end-stage renal disease fall into two categories: Those due to end-stage renal disease itself (including electrolyte abnormalities, anemia, hypertension, renal osteodystrophy, and vascular disease) and complications associated with the dialysis procedure (access-related infections and malfunctions).

Hemodialysis: Bacteremia is presumed present until cultures are negative in any patient with an in-dwelling catheter. Since both vancomycin (15 mg/kg) and gentamicin (2 mg/kg) are renally cleared, a single dose of each will cover gram positive and gram negative bacteria until the next session of hemodialysis.

Peritoneal dialysis: Infections are a common complication of peritoneal dialysis. Abdominal pain and cloudy effluent signify peritonitis. This condition may, at times, be managed at home. Severe abdominal pain must be managed in the hospital. Peritoneal fluid should be sent to the laboratory for cell count, gram stain, and culture. Empiric therapy for peritonitis consists of intraperitoneal (IP) ancef and ceftazidime. Antibiotic therapy should be tailored once the organism is identified and sensitivities obtained. Typically, IP therapy continues for 2 weeks. Staph aureus and Pseudomonas require 3 weeks of therapy. In the event of fungal infection, bacterial infection that does not rapidly resolve with therapy, or recurrent peritonitis, the PD catheter should be removed. Exit site infections should also be treated promptly; recurrent staph aureus or pseudomonal exit site infections may necessitate catheter removal. Catheter removal is imperative in the event of tunnel infection. A tunnel infection is recognized by the appearance of a tender "sausage" along the tunneled catheter on physical exam. Leakage of fluid at the catheter site may occur in when PD catheters are used soon after placement. The treatment of choice is to stop PD and prescribe antibiotics until the site is healed.

Hernias may develop at the umbilicus, at previous abdominal incision sites, and at the inguinal canals in patients on PD. If large, they may hinder the effectiveness of dialysis and require surgical repair.

References

KDOQI practice guidelines: http://www.kidney.org/professionals/KDOQI/.
KDIGO practice guidelines: http://www.kdigo.org/.

Feeding Pumps

Laura J. Wozniak

General Function and Application

Feeding pumps, or enteral infusion pumps, are electronic devices used to deliver nutritional solutions and other liquids to the gastrointestinal tract via feeding tubes. They are designed to deliver a continuous flow at a constant rate. Most can provide low delivery rates (<5 mL per hour) with an accuracy of +/-10%. They operate either by a rotary peristaltic mechanism or a volumetric cassette.

Indications for Use

Feeding pumps are used for patients who cannot tolerate bolus gastric feedings due to gastrointestinal and/or neurological diseases. This includes patients with short bowel syndrome, gastroparesis, gastroesophageal reflux, and/or other dysmotility problems, as well as children with severe neurodevelopmental delay and/or seizure disorders. Infusions are delivered via feeding tubes (see feeding tubes).

Advantages and Disadvantages

If deemed to be safe, bolus gastric feeds are preferred over continuous pump feeds for several reasons. Not only are bolus gastric feeds more physiologic; they are also more convenient, less expensive, and overall easier to deliver because they do not require a feeding pump.

There are many different feeding pumps, varying in complexity, flow rate ability, and cost. Pumps can be rented from suppliers of medical equipment or, more often, purchased for long-term use. When deciding which type of pump to use, there are various considerations including availability, cost, and accuracy. Prices range from approximately $500 to $1,500 depending on the pump features. Accuracy is especially important for patients who receive enteral feeds at a low flow rate, as not all pumps have the same minimum flow rate.

Types of Devices

Standard feeding pumps are designed for non-ambulatory patients. They are relatively simple to use and come with a clear set of instructions from the manufacturer. They can be programmed to run at a constant rate, but also have the ability to automatically advance in small increments over time. They are usually plugged in to an electrical outlet and mounted on an IV pole.

Portable pumps are available for patients who have an active lifestyle. These pumps are more compact, lighter (under 1–2 pounds), and come with a carrying case that can be worn as a backpack or "fanny pack." They run on batteries that have a long life and can be recharged. They operate in any orientation and therefore do not have to be maintained in an upright position.

Routine Use and Care

Guidelines for all aspects of enteral nutrition practices including ordering, preparation, delivery, and monitoring have been established by a task force of the American Society of Parenteral and Enteral Nutrition (ASPEN). This task force reviewed the available literature and published their Enteral Nutrition Practice Recommendations in the Journal of Parenteral and Enteral Nutrition in 2009. The guidelines are also available online through the ASPEN website (www.nutritioncare.org).

All feeding pumps need to be cleaned at least once daily, and also after feedings and any spills. When cleaning, pumps should be unplugged and turned off. The pumps should not be entirely immersed in water, but may be cleaned with warm soapy water (mild dish soap is fine) and a non-abrasive sponge or soft cloth. A cotton swab can be used to clean the smaller parts.

Nutrition solutions and other liquids are delivered via the feeding pump from feeding containers, most often 500 mL or 1200 mL bags. The content of these bags is individualized for each patient and may include any combination of formula, water, medications, other liquids, or blenderized solutions. Almost all feeding bags are designed to be disposable. If they need to be reused, they should be cleaned after each use with hot soapy water and rinsed thoroughly to remove any residue. The extension tubing also needs to be washed and rinsed after each use. It is important that the bags and tubing are allowed to completely dry in between uses to avoid bacterial contamination. The bags and tubing should be replaced whenever they look cloudy or unclean.

In addition to keeping the feeding pump and supplies clean, other precautions should be taken to avoid contamination. Parents should always wash their hands prior to preparing enteral solutions. Formulas that require reconstitution, dilution, or additives are at the greatest risk for contamination. Therefore, sterile, ready-to-feed products should be used whenever possible. Non-sterile solutions should have a maximum hang-time of 4 hours. Sterile solutions in an open system should have a maximum hang-time of 8–12 hours, whereas sterile solutions in a closed solution should have a maximum hang-time of 24 hours.

Troubleshooting

When patients are started on continuous feeds via feeding pumps, the parents are taught how to use the pumps by hospital staff and/or home-health companies. Most pumps are digital, with intuitive touch-panel interfaces. They are usually programmed in advance but can easily be adjusted based on patients' needs. To avoid confusion, all parents should be given a clear list of their child's feeding protocol, including:

- Type of formula (with specific mixing instructions if indicated).
- Total volume of formula (per day and per feed).
- Pump rate and duration (__ mL per hour for a total of __ hours).
- Feeding schedule (including start and stop times).

Feeding pumps are designed to alarm when they malfunction, and the instructions from the manufacturers describe how to respond to each cause of alarm. Common alarms include empty feeding container, occluded tubing, low battery, or pump motor malfunction. Depending on the manufacturer, most feeding pumps have 1–2 year warranties. In addition, they need to be periodically serviced to assure proper functioning and safety. The recommended service interval varies for different pumps, but is usually every 6–12 months.

Insurance and Financial Considerations

Reimbursement for feeding pumps and supplies varies depending on the patient's insurance plan.

Feeding Tubes

Laura J. Wozniak

General Function and Application:

Feeding tubes are used to provide nutrition and/or medications to patients who cannot tolerate them orally. This applies to patients with anatomic problems (such as esophageal atresia and short bowel syndrome), oromotor dysfunction secondary to neurologic problems, or oral aversion (as can be seen in Down syndrome, failure to thrive, or seizure disorders).

Nasogastric (NG) and nasojejunal (NJ) tubes are inserted through the nares and terminate in the stomach and jejunum, respectively. Gastrostomy tubes (G tubes) and jejunostomy tubes (J tubes) pass through the skin and abdominal wall directly into the stomach and jejunum, respectively. Gastrojejunostomy tubes (GJ tubes) have two ports, both of which enter the stomach through the same tract. The gastric port terminates in the stomach, while the jejunal port courses through the duodenum and terminates in the jejunum.

Indications/Contraindications for Use

Feeding tubes that terminate in the stomach (NG or G tubes) are good choices for patients without any history of feeding intolerance. Feeding tubes that terminate in the jejunum (NJ, J, or GJ) are more practical for patients who have gastroesophageal reflux and/or delayed gastric emptying. However, if these patients undergo a Nissen fundoplication and/or a pyloroplasty, G tubes may be safely used.

NG/NJ Tubes versus G, J, and GJ Tubes

NG and NJ tubes are ideal for patients who only require a relatively short-term temporary feeding tube (i.e., less than 3 months). NG tubes are easily inserted and removed. In fact, parents and patients can be trained to safely place NG tubes independently. NJ tubes, on the other hand, are usually positioned by interventional radiologists and require radiologic confirmation of placement. NG and NJ tubes are secured in place with tape, which can cause irritation to the skin. Active children can easily remove the tape and pull the tube out of its appropriate position.

Placement of NG and NJ tubes may lead to complications such as epistaxis and sore throat. Occasionally, more serious problems occur, including perforation of the esophagus or stomach and aspiration or pneumothorax due to incorrect placement of the tube in the trachea or lung. Long-term use of NG and NJ feeding tubes can be complicated by sinusitis, mucosal erosion, and skin breakdown. Therefore, when a tube is replaced, its position should alternate between both of the patient's nostrils. There are multiple different types of feeding tubes, each of which has its own manufacturer recommendations about how frequently the tube should be changed. Some need to be changed on a weekly basis, but those made of stiffer or more biocompatible materials (such as silastic) can remain in place for as long as 4–6 weeks.

GJ and J tubes are placed surgically via an open or laparascopic procedure. G tubes however may be placed surgically or via a percutaneous endoscopic procedure (referred to as a percutaneous endoscopic gastrostomy (PEG) tube). Compared to NG and NJ tubes, these are harder for active children to remove. They are also more cosmetically appealing because they are covered under the clothing. They can easily be removed, but will leave a scar on the abdomen and may occasionally form an enterocutaneous fistula.

Types of Devices

There are many different types and sizes of feeding tubes. Most G, J, and GJ tubes are secured in place with a balloon that sits in the lumen of the stomach or jejunum and a bolster that sits externally at the level of the skin. Some tubes have coin- or mushroom-shaped disks instead of balloons.

Skin-level or low-profile tubes, often referred to as "buttons," are also available. These tubes come in a variety of different lengths. Patients need to have their stoma length measured to determine which size tube is appropriate. The size of the tube may need to be altered with changes in the patient's abdominal circumference.

Routine Use and Care

When a G, J, or GJ tube is first placed, it may be secured in place with a suture. The tract between the skin and stomach/jejunum heals over a period of 3-4 weeks. If the tube is inadvertently removed during this time period, it needs to be replaced by a physician. A tubogram, or radiographic study using a small amount (5–10cc) of water-soluble contrast, should then be ordered to ensure that the tube is in the tract and that there is no extravasation of contrast.

Once the tract is appropriately healed, G and J tubes can be replaced by a parent, patient, nurse, or physician. Most tubes need to be changed at a minimum of every 3–6 months. In order to change a tube:

1. The new tube's balloon should be tested to be sure it is intact.
2. The end of the tube should then be lubricated.
3. The indwelling tube's balloon should be completely deflated.
4. The indwelling tube should then be withdrawn.
5. After cleaning any leakage from the skin, the new tube should be introduced into the stoma. (The easiest way to do this is when the patient is calm and the abdominal muscles are relaxed.)
6. Once the tube is advanced through the stoma, the balloon should be inflated to the appropriate volume.
7. Gentle traction should then be applied to bring the balloon up to the wall of the lumen. The external bolster should then be tightened to the level of the skin.
8. Appropriate placement can be confirmed by aspiration of enteral contents from the tube.

A small amount of clear drainage from tube stoma sites is normal. As a result, G, J, and GJ tube sites need to be cleaned at least once daily with soap and water. Use of hydrogen peroxide for cleaning should be avoided, except in the rare occasion when secretions have formed a hard crust. In this case, a half water and half hydrogen peroxide solution can be used to loosen the crust. Soap and water can then be used to clean the underlying skin. The tube should be rotated 90 degrees daily to help keep the stoma round and patent and to minimize pressure sores or skin breakdown at the stoma site. Although every attempt should be made by the care-takers to wipe and keep the site dry, avoid dressing the site by placing any gauze or dressings between the skin and external bolster.

All types of feeding tubes need to be flushed after every feeding and after all medications. This helps to prevent build-up that may clog the tube. Depending on the size of the child and the tube, a volume of 5–30cc of warm, clean tap water should be used for each flush. If the feeding tube becomes clogged, flushing warm water into the tube may help unclog it. When a feeding tube is not being used, it may be closed (clamped) or open (vented, or to gravity). Venting the tube allows for escape of gas. Leaving the tube to gravity allows for drainage of enteral contents.

Troubleshooting

Moisture or friction at the stoma site of a G, J, or GJ tube may lead to the formation of a granuloma which is moist, red, raised granulation tissue. Silver nitrate may be used to cauterize the tissue which will temporarily cause it to involute. It is important to keep the stoma site dry and to minimize friction of the tube by keeping the bolster snug against the skin. If a granuloma becomes a persistent problem, it may help to change to a skin-level or low-profile tube because these tubes cannot slide in and out of the stoma.

Occasionally the skin surrounding the stoma site can become irritated or infected. If needed, stoma powders and pastes can be used as a barrier. Petrolatum based ointments with or without zinc oxide work especially well as a moisture barrier. Antibacterial (i.e., bacitracin, mupirocin) and/or antifungal (i.e., miconazole, nystatin) powders, creams, and ointments may be needed for mild, superficial infections. If a true cellulitis develops, it should be treated with a one-week course of an enteral antibiotic that covers skin flora (such as cephalexin).

Leakage of gastric secretions from a poorly fitting tube may lead to skin breakdown. In this case, temporary use of an H2 blocker or proton pump inhibitor can help neutralize gastric acid, allowing the skin to heal. A goal gastric pH of 5–7 can be used in the short term. However, patients with feeding tubes do not need to remain on acid-blocking medications indefinitely unless they have other indications for such therapy.

If the stoma site drainage is increased from baseline, the volume of water in the inner balloon should be checked. With time, this balloon can lose water and may need to be re-filled. Occasionally, this balloon can develop a perforation, which would require replacement of the entire tube. It is also important to check that the bolster is appropriately positioned by applying gentle traction (to bring the balloon up to the wall of the lumen) and tightening the external bolster snug to the level of the skin.

Patients with feeding tubes should be instructed to always keep a spare tube at home and at school. If a tube is removed and there is no replacement readily available or the new tube cannot be easily replaced, a foley catheter can be inserted to keep the tract patent. Tubes should be replaced as soon as possible because some tracts can shrink or close within 1–2 hours, making tube replacement more difficult.

When a G, J, or GJ tube is no longer needed, it may be removed. The stoma can be covered with a 4x4 gauze with petroleum jelly on it. The stoma site will usually heal over the course of 4–6 weeks. If the site remains patent after this time period, the patient should be referred to a pediatric surgeon for possible surgical closure of the enterocutaneous fistula. Usually this involves placement of an external suture, but occasionally may involve a more invasive surgical closure.

Equipment Associated with Feeding Tubes

For all feeding tubes, extension tubing and adapters are needed to attach feeding pumps for slow bolus or continuous feeds. Bolus or gavage feeds can be given by gravity over 5–10 minutes. A large syringe with the plunger removed is the best way to administer these feeds. The rate of flow can be controlled by changing the height of the syringe (Formula will flow faster if the syringe is raised higher). Syringes can also be used to administer medications. Liquid medications are preferred, but crushed pills dissolved in water can also be given.

Venting prior to feeds to allow the escape of excess gas and/or fluids is performed by attaching a large syringe with the plunger removed or by gently aspirating air and/or fluid directly from the stomach. Drainage devices such as mucous traps or bags are available for more long-term venting. All extension tubing and other accessories should be washed in hot soapy water after use and allowed to air dry.

Other Considerations

Children with feeding tubes can participate in almost all normal activities. They can attend regular school and play sports as long as the tube is appropriately secured. When the tube is clamped, patients can bathe or go swimming. Even children who receive continuous feeds can carry on with a normal lifestyle by wearing a small backpack to keep their feeding pump with them at all times.

Insurance and Financial Considerations

Reimbursement for feeding tubes and necessary supplies varies depending on the patient's insurance plan. Medical/CCS will usually cover replacement of a standard G tube every 3 months and a skin-level G tube every 6 months.

Home Oxygen Therapy

Sheila Kun

General Function and Application

Oxygen is a necessary element to sustain life. Normal oxygen concentration is 21% at sea level. Children with low oxygen level require supplemental oxygen.

Indications

Home oxygen therapy is prescribed for children with infantile chronic lung disease and any pulmonary condition which causes hypoxemia. It can also be used as a secondary treatment for children with ventilatory muscle weakness, obstructive sleep apnea, asthma, interstitial lung disease, chronic respiratory failure and cystic fibrosis. The minimum needed flow starts with 1/8 liter per minute, and the duration of use may vary from continuous to as needed, or during certain activities such as feeding or sleeping only.

Advantages

Home oxygen therapy is considered an appropriate and relatively safe option for children with chronic respiratory problems. For young children, the most rapid lung growth is during the first two years of life. Chronic hypoxemia interferes with growth, pre-disposes patients to heart failure and possible anoxic injury. Home oxygen therapy promotes normal growth and development without restriction. The portable unit further enhances the quality of life by allowing children to go to school and have activities away from home.

Types of Oxygen

There are three main types of oxygen:

1. Compressed oxygen cylinder.
2. Oxygen concentrators.
3. Liquid oxygen system.

Compressed oxygen cylinder: Green tanks, usually large tanks or "H tanks," must be secured in a safe corner of a room. Portable smaller units called "E" or "D" tanks are mounted on a stroller stand for mobility. The gauges at the top indicate the amount of oxygen available and regulate the oxygen flow. A key is required to turn the tank on and off. Smaller carry on units are most suitable for patients on a small amount of oxygen. Normally an E-tank could last up to **7–8** hours if the patient is on 1 liter per minute of oxygen. Replacement is needed when empty.

Oxygen concentrator: These devices concentrate oxygen from the air. When connected to the wall electricity, oxygen is available without replenishing from another unit. The convenience of the concentrator is obvious as the portable units are refilled from the main unit. The portable unit can be carried with a shoulder strap or cart. A gas tank is often ordered as a back up when oxygen concentrator is used. In case of an electric black out, oxygen therapy will not be interrupted by using the gas back up system.

Liquid oxygen: Liquid oxygen is made by super-cooling oxygen gas into a liquid form. When stored, it takes up less space and provides more hours of use. The portable unit is refilled from the main unit. However, it evaporates easily. If the liquid system is not positioned properly, it could tilt and spill, gusting gas out. Try to use within a 24-hour period.

Oxygen conserving devices: Oxygen conserving devices make the delivery of oxygen more efficient and allow longer use by providing oxygen flow upon inspiration only. However, some young children require continuous flow and would not be an appropriate candidate for this system, as they may not be able to get in sync with the inspiratory cycle.

Facial interface and tubing: For most children, nasal cannula is the most popular option. Facial mask is appropriate for high liter flow such as 5 liters or more of oxygen flow. Oxygen extension tubing is also available. However, for small children on small amounts of oxygen, it is recommended that no more than 14 feet of extension tubing be used.

Troubleshooting of Common Problems with Oxygen Therapy

Running out of oxygen

To prevent running out of oxygen, families should learn to accurately estimate the needed amount and duration of their oxygen supply. The company should provide a schedule so that families can gauge their activities and plan for back up.

Irritation to the nose or face

The initial oxygen order should include humidification. Giving oxygen without humidification often causes nasal discomfort, and may lead to nose bleeds. If irritation to the nose occurs, check position of the nasal tubing; do not cut the end to make the nasal prongs fit, this would cause more irritation. One can use water based moisturizer if the nasal cavity is irritated. Contrary to old teaching, we have not seen babies getting burned from using oil on their face when oxygen is used.

Oxygen tubing does not stay

Secure the tubing with Tegaderm or hypoallergenic tape. Paper tape is not the most adhesive tape for oxygen therapy.

Child pulling the oxygen tubing

Parents have to believe that oxygen is therapeutic; otherwise, they cannot provide a positive experience for the child. Be consistent, there is no room for negotiation as this is a "medical treatment." Individual positive reinforcement methods apply. Promote comfort by using tapes that do not grab the skin.

Fire Safety

Oxygen by itself does not burn, therefore it is not flammable. However, it supports combustion and will cause fire—it would make it burn hotter and faster. The oxygen unit should be at least 6 feet away from open stove or heater. One word of caution: Do not offer a birthday cake with candles for a child who is on oxygen.

Bulky Gas Tanks and Hazards of Injury

Position H tanks safely and away from running children. Secure E tanks safely on the floor, under the rear car seat so that they don't bang against each other during transport. Liquid systems must be stood upright to prevent leakage.

Routine Use and Tips

Make sure the initial set up is correct; examine the regulator and make sure the liter flow could go up or down from the doctor's order.

Plan ahead: Check the amount of oxygen in the portable tank to ensure sufficient amount for the entire out of home activity. If routine delivery to the home is needed, mark on the calendar for the next delivery date.

Use distilled water in the humidifier bottle. Tap water could clog up the nebulizer bottle.

Special Considerations

For children who have a tracheostomy tube in place, it is easier to deliver oxygen by using direct flow via a tracheostomy collar, stating the liter per minute. A Venturi Device attached to the tracheostomy tubing is another way of providing oxygen. However, please note that a Venturi Device cannot be used with a concentrator. Also, by giving the exact percentage of oxygen, the liter flow requirement is invariably much higher, making outdoor activity cumbersome and difficult.

For patients on home mechanical ventilation, the oxygen adaptor needs to be used in the ventilator circuit. The site varies according to the type of ventilator. When in doubt, a T-connector close to the tracheostomy swivel adaptor can be used. This is not the ideal place to put the connector as it adds more direct weight to the tracheostomy tube.

1/8 of liter per minute of oxygen seems to be so minute that discontinuation should be an easy decision. However, our experience with polysomnogram in children has repeatedly demonstrated that 1/8 liter per minute does make a difference and prevent hypoxemia.

In School

Respiratory vendors can help orient and set up oxygen use in school. The amount of oxygen requirement and the number of school hours determine the type of oxygen use in the school setting.

While Traveling

Regulations regarding oxygen use during air travel are changing. The current status is that the FAA allows certain types of portable oxygen concentrators. Each airline has its own form or requirement for oxygen clearance from the medical order. Families are encouraged to inquire at least one month in advance to allow time to make arrangement with the airline or their vendor for oxygen use during flight. If oxygen is needed on a continuous basis, families are counseled to use the portable concentrator unit as the easiest option. Otherwise, the use of oxygen during flight usually requires advance arrangement plus a charge of around $75 each way. Airline staff is not responsible to evaluate the need for oxygen, but rather, accommodate the onboard provision of oxygen, based on the physician's recommendation, and the care provided by the family.

The U.S. Department of Transportation amended the 1986 Air Carrier Access Act with regard to "non-discrimination on the basis of disability in air travel." Effective May 13, 2009, the final rule adds accommodations for travelers who use oxygen and other respiratory assistive devices. Refer to http://airconsumer.ost.dot.gov/rules for the most updated policy.

Cleaning of Oxygen Tubing

Remove mucous and crusting with warm soapy water. Soak tubing in a solution of 1 part bleach and 50 parts of water. Use of commercial product such as Control 111 is also available.

Insurance and Financial Considerations

Most insurance would authorize any of the three devices based on cost and usage. For children, polysomnogram, and pulse oximeter reading are part of the medical justification. In practice, blood gas is not routinely done to demonstrate the need for oxygen therapy, even though insurance insists on that data. Payers usually require oxygen saturation below a certain level (usually 88%) to authorize. However, for children with good justification, payers may authorize these devices for patients with higher oxygen saturations.

The family is qualified for handicapped parking and discount from electric company on the use of oxygen concentrators. The savings on the concentrator is sizable when discount application is successful. New Medicare reimbursements applied as of January 2009. Recipients of Medicare should check with the vendor for specific rental and maintenance services.

Insulin Pump Therapy

Sheila Kun

General Function and Application

- An insulin pump is a medical device used for basal/bolus insulin therapy in the treatment of insulin-dependant diabetes mellitus. It is also known as continuous subcutaneous insulin infusion (CSII) therapy.

Indication

An insulin pump is an alternative to multiple daily injections of insulin (MDI) by an insulin syringe or an insulin pen and allows for intensive insulin therapy when used in conjunction with blood glucose monitoring and carbohydrate counting. An insulin pump allows the replacement of slow-acting insulin for basal needs with a continuous infusion of rapid-acting insulin.

The insulin pump delivers a single type of fast-acting insulin in two ways:

1. A **bolus dose** that is pumped to cover food eaten or to correct a high blood glucose level.
2. A **basal dose** that is pumped continuously at an adjustable basal rate to deliver insulin needed between meals and at night.

Advantages over Multiple Daily Insulin Injections

The main advantage of the pump is the ability to provide multiple basal rates for patients whose glycemic profile cannot be maintained by injection of 12- or 24-hour acting basal insulins. The second advantage relates to quality of life for some patients and avoiding insulin injections particularly in those who report pain on administration by syringe or pen, or whose lifestyles are greatly facilitated by the omission of the act of injection via needles.

An insulin pump user also has the ability to influence the profile of the rapid-acting insulin by shaping the bolus. While each user must experiment with bolus shapes to determine what is best for any given food, they can improve control of blood glucose by adapting the bolus shape to their needs.

The pattern for delivering **basal** insulin throughout the day can also be customized with a pattern to suit the pump user:

- A reduction of basal at night to prevent low blood sugar in infants and toddlers.
- An increase of basal at night to counteract high blood sugar levels due to growth hormone in teenagers.

- A pre-dawn increase to prevent high blood sugar due to the Dawn effect in adults and teens.
- In a proactive plan before regularly scheduled exercise times such as morning gym for elementary school children or after school basketball practice for high school children.

Types of Insulin Delivery by Pumps

In addition to **basal** rate administration based on glycemic profile as detailed above, **bolus** insulin via pumps can be given in a variety of individualized modes:

A **standard bolus** is an infusion of insulin pumped completely at the onset of the bolus. It is most similar to an injection. By pumping with a "spike" shape, the expected action is the fastest possible bolus for that type of insulin. The standard bolus is most appropriate when eating high carb low protein low fat meals because it will return blood sugar to normal levels quickly.

An **extended bolus** is a slow infusion of insulin spread out over time. By pumping with a "square wave" shape, the bolus avoids a high initial dose of insulin that may enter the blood and cause low blood sugar before digestion can facilitate sugar entering the blood. The extended bolus also extends the action of insulin well beyond that of the insulin alone. The extended bolus is appropriate when covering high fat high protein meals such as steak, which will be raising blood sugar for many hours past the onset of the bolus. The extended bolus is also useful for those with slow digestion (such as with gastroparesis or Celiac disease).

A **combination bolus** is the combination of a standard bolus spike with an extended bolus square wave. This shape provides a large dose of insulin up front, and then also extends the tail of the insulin action. The combination bolus is appropriate for high carb high fat meals such as pizza, pasta with heavy cream sauce, and chocolate cake. This type of meal is typically not recommended for patients with diabetes, but may be allowed in exceptional circumstances.

Parts and Associated Equipment

The device includes:

- The pump itself (including controls, processing module, and batteries).
- A disposable reservoir for insulin (inside the pump).
- A disposable infusion set, including a cannula for subcutaneous insertion (under the skin) and a tubing system to interface the insulin reservoir to the cannula.

Routine Use and Tips

Pump sites should be rotated and changed every 48 to 72 hours. Despite adequate correction, persistent hyperglycemia should be treated as a pump malfunction and subcutaneous insulin is to be administered swiftly via pen or syringes until technical issues are resolved to prevent ketoacidosis.

Use in School

School personnel need to be informed of the patient's use of pump and a school person is to be educated and designated for supervision of glucose monitoring and bolus administration for carbohydrate coverage and/or correction during school hours. Activities such as swimming require disconnection of some pumps.

Replacement and Maintenance

Pump devices usually have a toll-free number on the back of the device to be contacted in case of suspected or confirmed pump malfunction or to request updated versions as they arise. Multiple daily injections are to be used until technical issues are resolved.

Insurance and Financial Considerations

Most pumps are covered by insurance companies with appropriate medical justification which includes a variable glycemic profile and other individualized reasons for each patient (see advantages over MDI).

Home Nebulizer Therapy

Sheila Kun

General Function and Application

A nebulizer, together with the compressor, is used for delivery of bronchodilators, pulmonary anti-inflammatory medication, anti-biotics for pulmonary infections, and mucolytic agents. Liquid medications are changed into fine droplets and inhaled through a mask or mouthpiece, which is connected to the nebulizer cup. The compressor aerosolizes the liquid medication.

Indications

Patients with reactive airway disease, asthma, obstructive disease such as cystic fibrosis and chronic lung disease, use aerosol treatment on a regular and/or as needed basis.

Advantages vs. An Inhaler

- Better deposition of aerosol medication to the bronchus and lungs.
- Target at the upper and lower airway, not systemic and therefore less side effect.
- Easier to deliver treatment to small children or patients with cognitive delay who may not be able to coordinate their breathing with the medication delivered.
- More effective in an acute exacerbation than a meter dose inhaler.
- Portable units, which are battery powered, are available for out of home use.

Types of Nebulizers

The choice of the types of nebulizer is dependent on the ease of use, time it takes to aerosolize the medication and the type of aerosol treatment ordered.

Nebulizers work with all brands of compressors. However, for efficient delivery of aerosol treatment, one might want to consider the brand of nebulizer with two valves to maximize delivery, or one that has a fast flow (delivery of treatment in less than 8 minutes). Certain pharmaceutical companies designate a specific type of nebulizer for their product to achieve maximal result. Heed the specific medication recommendations offered by the manufacturer. Disposable units are available, which can be discarded per manufacturer's instructions.

Troubleshooting of Common Problems With The Nebulizer

The medication can clog up the Nebulizer kit and over time become ineffective. Proper cleaning/disposal of the Nebulizer kit is key for its efficient delivery.

Minimizing infection is another reason why disinfecting the nebulizer should be part of the patient's routine maintenance care.

- The nebulizer should be held in an upright position for adequate delivery of the droplets.
- When used with the ventilator circuit, ensure that any humidification moisture exchange (HME) device is removed, otherwise the medication could be trapped inside the HME.

Routine Use and Tips

Among many recommendations for cleaning and disinfection, we choose the approaches that are easy, manageable and safe according to a pamphlet entitled "Respiratory Stopping the Spread of Germs' By Catherine O'Malley, Charlotte Lemming, Judy Marciel, and Leslie Hazel published by the Cystic Fibrosis Foundation, 2003.

The key points are:

- Wipe the inside and outside of the nebulizer with a clean paper towel.
- Clean the equipment right after use to keep the debris from drying.
- Among the many ways of disinfecting the nebulizer tubing, the simplest method is to soak in a solution of 1 part of household bleach and 50 parts water for 3 minutes, then boiled for 5 minutes.
- Air dry the nebulizer using a paper towel.
- Good hand washing before and after the cleaning procedure.
- Contrary to popular belief, vinegar is not a strong disinfectant.

Special Considerations

- Special adaptor/connector has to be used with a child with a tracheostomy.
- If a moisture exchange device is used for tracheotomized or ventilator dependent patient, it needs to be removed to provide effective aerosol treatment.
- Oxygen can be given while the nebulizer is in use.
- If the compressor is not available or not working, one can use high oxygen flow > 6 liters per minute to drive the droplets in. This is a good tip for parents when the compressor malfunctions

Many respiratory aerosol treatments can be given together to save time and therefore improve adherence to therapy. Anti-inflammatory medication and bronchodilators are routinely mixed together for aerosol treatment. But, if multiple treatments are needed, the following example of how to sequence the respiratory treatment should be helpful.

1. Bronchodilator.
2. Mucolytic enzyme.
3. Chest clearance therapy.
4. Anti-biotic treatment.
5. Anti-inflammatory treatment.

In School

It is suggested that routine treatment at 8-hour intervals be given at home. Only those whose condition is not well controlled should receive nebulizer treatment as needed. If at all possible, use MDI for convenience and minimal interruption at school.

Tips for Oral Care

Make it a habit to rinse the mouth or brush the teeth after aerosol treatment to prevent dental or oral irritation.

Replacement and Maintenance

Disposable nebulizer cups are discarded per manufacturer's instructions weekly. Re-usable units can last up to 6 months depending on the frequency of their use.

Equipment Associated With The Nebulizer

The compressor is a simple device, connected to the nebulizer tubing. Turning the "ON" button allows air to propel the droplets along the nebulizer tubing. Cleaning and maintenance include wiping dust off with a wet paper towel, keeping it dry and clean. Always unplug the unit when cleaning. The machine part, which does not come into contact with the mucous membranes, needs no disinfection. Change the filter per manufacturer's guideline. Usually this is changed when the filter looks old. The foam filter can be washed gently if one chooses to use it again. The compressor could last up to 5 years or more depending on the frequency of its use.

Portable, battery operated compressor is available; its average use is one year.

The portable compressor is small and the total unit weighs less than 2 pounds with the external battery. Included are three versatile power source options-worldwide AC compatibility (100 to 240V), 12 volt automobile adapter, and rechargeable battery to be used anywhere.

Insurance and Financial Considerations

Public State insurance selects the most cost effective model. This might not include the one with the two safety valves. Medical justification includes the use of the type of medication used and its designated nebulizer which goes with it. The warranty on the compressor should be three years.

Portable units are not routinely approved except with strong medical justification that the frequency of treatment and that the exacerbations require immediate treatment.

Ostomies

Laura J. Wozniak, Linda M. Roof

General Function and Application

Ostomies are surgically-created openings in the abdomen or pelvis for access to, decompression of, and/or diversion from the gastrointestinal or genitourinary tract.

The term stoma, which means mouth, refers to the actual end of the opening that can be seen at the level of the skin. For each type of ostomy, a prefix is used to denote the location of the stoma within the body. Hence, those involving the gastrointestinal tract are referred to as enterostomies, while those involving the genitourinary tract are referred to as urostomies.

A gastrostomy is an opening directly into the stomach. A jejunostomy is an opening directly into the jejunum. Gastrostomies and jejunostomies are kept patent by indwelling tubes (see feeding tubes).

An ileostomy is located in the ileum and a colostomy in the colon. Patients who have undergone extensive bowel resection may have a duodenostomy or jejunostomy. A urostomy provides access to the urinary tract. These types of stomas usually empty into an ostomy bag or pouch, which is drained and changed as needed, allowing for easy collection of fecal or urinary output, respectively.

Indications/Contraindications for Use

Gastrostomies and jejunostomies are used to provide access to the gastrointestinal tract for administration of medications and/or feedings in patients who are unable to tolerate oral intake. This applies to patients with anatomical problems (such as esophageal atresia), oromotor dysfunction secondary to neurological problems, or oral aversion (as can be seen in Down syndrome, failure to thrive, seizure disorders, or brain tumors). Gastrostomies may also be used to decompress the stomach in patients who have abnormal gastric motility.

Ileostomies, jejunostomies, duodenostomies, and colostomies are often needed for diversion in patients with distal intestinal obstruction (for instance after necrotizing enterocolitis, gastroschisis, meconium ileus, or malrotation with volvulus) or inflammatory bowel disease. Urostomies are created to drain urine when the bladder and/or urethra are obstructed, for instance due to trauma or congenital abnormalities.

Advantages and Disadvantages

Surgically-created ostomies are used for patients who have underlying conditions requiring temporary, long-term, or permanent access to the gastrointestinal or genitourinary tract. They allow patients to lead active lifestyles and participate in sports and recreation. They do, however, require daily care and hygiene. Most are reversible but will leave a scar behind after surgical correction.

Types of Devices

There are many different types of feeding tubes used to access gastrostomies and jejunostomies (see feeding tubes). Likewise, there are also numerous ostomy bags and pouches available including disposable and reusable appliances. The type of system used depends on the location and type of stoma, characteristics of the output, and peristomal skin contours. Additionally, personal preferences and lifestyle are considered. In pediatrics, the ability of the patient and/or family to master self-care and pouch maintenance is also important.

The portion of the apparatus that adheres to the skin is called a "mounting plate" or "skin barrier wafer." These come in different sizes and can be personalized based on an individual patient's needs. Some appliances are a one-piece system, meaning the adhesive skin barrier and pouch are integrated together. Others come in two-piece arrangements in which the adhesive skin barrier and the pouch are separate.

Closed-end pouches are removed and changed after each use. Open-end pouches can be emptied and resealed (via a capped spout, plastic clip, or Velcro) multiple times before removal and disposal. Some pouches are clear whereas others are opaque. Small-sized pouches are available to use for swimming or other activities. Pouches are odor-proof and may be designed with filters to vent and deodorize flatus. Some patients choose to wear waist bands or specially designed ostomy belts to help their pouches remain low-profile and secure.

Routine Use and Care and Troubleshooting

The selection of which system and accessories are appropriate is determined by the patient's physician or certified ostomy nurse. Patients receive teaching on ostomy care prior to hospital discharge. Once patients become comfortable with ostomy care, they should be seen annually, or sooner if problems arise, for stoma and product needs reassessment.

Depending on the type of system used and the characteristics of the stoma, the adhesive skin barrier can stay in place for as long as 7 days. Occasionally the skin surrounding ostomies can become irritated or infected. This may be due to a poorly fitted pouch, leakage under the skin barrier, or sensitivity to the ostomy products. Various accessories to enhance wearing time and skin protection such as powder and sealants are also available. If a cutaneous fungal infection develops, nystatin powder is a good first-line option for treatment. Other problems, such as skin breakdown or bleeding, are best addressed on an individual basis by physicians or certified ostomy nurses.

Custom-tooled pouching systems are available should all conventional/commercial systems be unsuccessful in achieving a secure seal. Many manufacturers also have call-in centers where knowledgeable staff can assist with trouble-shooting.

Access to Supplies and Insurance/Financial Considerations

It is common practice to provide patients with supplies at the time of hospital discharge to use during the transition from in- to out-patient care. Pouching supplies and accessories are available from a number of different sources. Sample products are readily available from most manufacturers. Supplies for purchase are generally available from local and mail order medical supply companies and some large home care pharmacies.

After deciding upon the most ideal ostomy system, the physician must write an itemized prescription for all necessary supplies. During the hospital discharge planning process, the hospital staff should initiate a home health referral and provide a list of potential vendors. The choice of vendor is usually determined by the insurance carrier's supplier contracting list.

The vendor's choice of inventory can create a challenge when a required product is not carried. In that case, some negotiation may be needed or a comparable product substituted. The degree to which supply costs are covered is determined by the individual patient's insurance coverage. Generally insurance covers 80% of what is considered "reasonable and customary" once a deductible is met. Co-payments and the quantity of supplies allowed vary according to coverage.

Pediatric patients whose parents do not have insurance and/or have a low income may be eligible to receive state Medicaid. There is no mandated coverage for ostomy supplies, so Medicaid benefits vary from state to state. Most states address ostomy supplies in the context of inflammatory bowel disease, but they also usually cover the supply cost for patients with different diagnoses. Please see the United States Government Accountability Office: GAO Survey of State Medicaid Programs 2005 for more details regarding specific programs.

For adults, Medicare Part B covers ostomy supplies. As a national program, it has an extensive product formulary and predetermined allowable monthly amounts based upon the type of stoma. After the yearly deductible is met, the patient can expect to pay 29% of the amount approved by Medicare. Supplemental MediGap policies may cover the remaining amount.

The Crohn's and Colitis Foundation of America (CCFA) is a non-profit, volunteer-driven organization which serves as a resource for individuals with inflammatory bowel disease. The CCFA website (www.ccfa.org) has numerous references for support services available to patients and their families. In addition, there are also multiple links with general information about inflammatory bowel disease, some of which discuss ostomies.

Tracheostomy Tube for Children

Sheila Kun

General Function and Application

For the pediatric population, a tracheostomy tube is primarily used to bypass an upper airway obstruction. For children who are on home mechanical ventilation, it provides an access to the ventilator in lieu of oral intubation.

Indications

Tracheostomy is indicted for patients with upper airway obstruction such as subglottic stenosis, vocal cord paralysis and any severe anatomical upper airway obstruction.

Some children with chronic respiratory failure use a tracheostomy tube as an access to the ventilator.

A tracheostomy can be used for secretion management for children with chronic aspiration. For example, children with mental retardation and cerebral palsy may not be able to handle their own secretion.

Advantages

In the case of severe airway obstructions, a tracheostomy is the only option to allow adequate air flow.

For children with chronic respiratory failure such as central hypoventilation, severe chronic lung disease and neuromuscular diseases, a tracheostomy with positive ventilatory support is needed when the non-invasive mechanical ventilation fails.

Aspiration pneumonia is minimized when a tracheostomy is performed, as suctioning through a tracheostomy tube allows direct access to secretion in the lower respiratory tract.

Types of Tracheostomy Tube

The most common types of tracheostomy tube are made of polyvinylchloride or silicone. Both types of tracheostomy tube are very similar in appearance and use. The size is primarily determined by the inner diameter (ID), starting at 3 mm. It goes up to 6.5 mm ID. The length varies with the size. However, given the same ID, the pediatric tubes are longer than the neonatal ones. Therefore, attention needs to be paid to neonatal vs. pediatric size. If the length is too long, it could occlude at the carina. Conversely, if the tube is too short, it may easily decannulate.

Other features include extra length, customized length, cuffed and un-cuffed tubes.

Un-cuffed tubes are most commonly used. Cuffed tubes in pediatrics are reserved for rare cases such as children who are on home mechanical ventilation and unable to keep up with their ventilation requirement due to a large leak. When every approach is tried, a cuffed tube is the last resort as a means to provide adequate mechanical ventilation support. Normally, the otolaryngologist determines the size of the tracheostomy tube. However, in the case of children on home mechanical ventilation, the decision is jointly made with the pulmonologist as well.

The otolaryngologist does laryngoscopy and bronchoscopy to determine the right size and length. Its actual size and positioning can be visualized with a neck film.

Once the tracheostomy track is matured (usually seven days post surgery) parents are taught to do the tracheostomy tube change prior to discharge. The frequency of tracheostomy tube change varies from institution to institution; the most common recommendation is to change every week or every other week, and when necessary.

An obturator (like a guide) comes in with each tracheostomy tube and is used when one changes the tracheostomy tube.

Traditionally polyvinylchloride tubes were meant to be for a single time use. However, the latest product insert includes cannula and obturator cleaning with solutions such as household vinegar, sterile normal saline or water and mild detergent. There were no explicit instructions to re-use. Yet the American Thoracic Society's consensus statement in 1999 cited that they may be used for 3–4 months before the tubes stiffen.

Silicone tubes can withstand high heat and are meant to be re-usable. The cleaning procedure at home includes cleaning with warm soapy water, and sterilizing it by soaking it in a pot of boiled water. Parents are taught how to use and care for the tube before discharge.

Trouble-shooting of Common Problems with Tracheostomy Tube

Mucous plugging

The frequency of suctioning to clear mucous plugs varies from patient to patient. In general, younger patients need to be suctioned more often than older children. A large suction catheter should be used. The suctioning time is usually less than 5 seconds. Allow rest in between suctioning entries. Normal saline is usually used, but could be optional for some individual older patients. The suction catheter is introduced just beyond the end of the tracheostomy tube. However, for children with ventilatory muscle weakness, one might have to go down deeper. Since mucous plugs can form minutes after suctioning, there is no fixed schedule for suctioning. With time and training, parents learn about their children's baseline and need for suctioning.

Accidental decannulation

If the tube is not secured snugly, accidental decannulation could happen. Therefore, parents are asked to carry a spare tube as a back up. Re-insertion with the proper positioning of the head (hyper-extension of the head) is easy when the tracheostomy track is mature. In children, this is usually one week after the initial tracheostomy placement. Immediate replacement is recommended when accidental decannulation occurs as this might compromise the patency of the airway. For some children, the stoma could close in a fairly short time (minutes to hours).

Bleeding

Bleeding could be caused by:

- Aggressive suctioning.
- Dryness.
- Ill-fitted tube.
- Infection.
- Granulation tissue inside the trachea.

Control of bleeding is dependent on the etiology. Meanwhile, use of cold normal saline drops into the trachea could provide temporary relief. Bleeding from granulation tissue is a serious problem and should be handled by the specialist.

Infection

Tracheitis is not uncommon. The need to be suctioned more often is a universal sign of possible tracheitis. Treat tracheitis based on culture or symptoms.

Granulation tissue around the stoma

Granulation tissue can form with no predictable pattern. It can be treated with silver nitrate sticks (Tips: Use oil based lubricant around the surrounding skin to prevent skin abrasion from the silver nitrate); limit treatment to 2 times in a week. Another approach is to dress around the tracheostomy tube with Xeroform, a 4x4 dressing cut into stripes. After Betadine cleaning, Xeroform can be used 3 times a day until the granulation tissue shrinks. However, with some children, especially patients with darker skin, recurrence is quite likely. If the granulation tissue does not interfere with tracheal tube change, it can be left alone.

Routine care of the tracheal stoma at home: Instruct parents to use warm soapy water to cleanse daily. Frequent use of hydrogen peroxide might stimulate more granulation tissue growth and its diluted form (half –strength) should only be applied to the crusted lesions.

Caregivers during school hours: A trained personnel designated for the student is necessary, including during bus transportation. The physician reviews and signs the school protocol. Regardless of the frequency of suctioning, each student must have provision for routine care in school.

Insurance and Financial Considerations

Tracheostomy tubes and associated supplies are readily approved by both private and public insurances. However, the amount of supplies allowed could vary from insurance to insurance. Basically, the suctioning procedure at home is employing a clean technique; hence, catheters are re-usable for the same day. Parents are shown how to make the suction catheters as clean as possible. The main goal is to keep them free of mucous and dry. There is limited evidence-based research supporting the best approach to keeping the suction catheters germ-free. Physicians may complete a utilities application form that allows the families of children with a tracheostomy to receive discount allowance from the providing electric company. The patient is also qualified for handicapped parking.

Equipment Associated With Tracheostomy

Portable suction machine: When properly charged, the battery power lasts up to 45 minutes of continuous use. A stationary unit is needed for those who require frequent suctioning.

Humidification device: Compressor/nebulizer, could be optional for older children, and is normally used during sleep. Avoid water dripping into the trachea by accident.

Day time humidification: Varies with individual patient. Most children do not use a humidifier during the day and do not need a humidification moisture exchange (HME) unit.

Monitoring device for high risk patient: The consensus is that not all children with tracheostomy need to have monitoring device. But, it is common community practice to use pulse oximeter or apnea monitor for smaller children when they are not directly supervised. The degree of airway obstruction or dependency on the tracheostomy tube is one of the determining factors in considering monitoring need.

For school: Parents need to provide all necessary equipment and supplies for school use. Avoid contact sports or water play. For smaller children, use of HME could serve as a barrier while playing near sand boxes. For infants, use of a cotton bib over the tracheostomy tube could also serve as a protective layer.

Speaking valve: Per the specialist's direction, a speaking valve can be used for many children. However, its use should be initiated by the specialist who knows the child's airway the best. Some children with tight upper airway or severe chronic lung disease, may not be able to handle the speaking valve. The valve allows inhaled air coming through one way, but the exhaled air does not go through the speaking valve. Cleaning of the speaking valve is simple: Use warm soapy water for gentle cleaning. Avoid harsh brushing or detergents.

Removal of the trach tube: A tracheostomy tube is no longer needed if the reason for its use is rectified. The decannulation process involves downsizing the trach tube, capping it for tolerance and a final surgical assessment of the airway by the otolaryngologist. After the tube removal, the child is usually kept overnight in the hospital for observation.

Urinary Bladder Catheters

Katherine Wesseling Perry

General Function and Application

Intermittent urinary catheters are used to assist patients who are temporarily or permanently unable to void due to a variety of acute and chronic problems.

Indications and Counter Indications for Use

Intermittent self catheterization is the treatment of choice for management of neurogenic lower urinary tract dysfunction (urinary retention, leakage, and incontinence). Indwelling catheters and suprapubic catheterization may also be used, but are at higher risk of complications. Catheters should not be placed blindly (i.e., if they are placed at all, they must be placed with the help of an Urologist) in trauma patients with hematuria and in patients with penile anatomic abnormalities.

Routine Use and Care

Sterile, disposable catheters should not be reused.

Complications

Urinary tract *infection* and epidydimitis are common complications of catheterization. These complications can be minimized by increased catheterization frequency (optimally, performed between 4–6 times per day), avoidance of indwelling catheters, and sterile catheterization technique. Urinary tract infections in non-immunosuppressed individuals should be treated only if symptomatic. Asymptomatic bacterial colonization should not be treated.

Urethral complications include bleeding, strictures, fistulae, the formation of false passages and the development of iatrogenic hypospadias due to constant downward pressure of the catheter. These complications, particularly fistulae and iatrogenic hypospadias, are more frequent in patients with indwelling catheters

Bladder complications are rare, but may include perforation, the development of stones, and an increased risk of bladder cancer.

Allergies, particularly to latex, are common in patients requiring chronic catheterization.

UTIs should be treated more aggressively in immunosuppressed patients (i.e., those with renal transplants or other conditions requiring immunosuppressive agents) than in those with intact immune systems (i.e., patients with clumps of white blood cells in the urine and increased creatinine levels, despite lack of fever, should be considered to have infection rather than just bacterial colonization).

References

Kryger, J. 2008. "Nonsurgical management of the neurogenic bladder in children." *Scientific World Journal.* 81177–83.

Igawa, Y., J. J. Wyndaele, and O. Nishizawa. 2008. "Catheterization: possible complications and their prevention and treatment." *Int. J. Urol.* 15481–5.

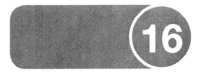 **Disease Drug Interactions**

Table of Contents

Asthma or Reactive Airway Disease

Wendy H.P. Ren, Samuel H. Wald

Absolute contraindication

Beta Blockers.

Relative contraindications

Aspirin, nonsteroidal anti-inflammatory drugs, Adenosine, high doses of H2 blocker (i.e., cimetidine).

Cautions

Morphine: Can cause histamine release, worsening bronchoconstriction and hypotension. Some intravenous preparations contain metasulphite, to which some asthmatics are sensitive.

Fentanyl: Though shorter acting with less histamine release, it can still cause bronchospasm and chest wall rigidity when given in large boluses.

Lidocaine: May prevent reflex bronchoconstriction and has little toxicity at a dose of 1–1.5 mg/kg IV, 1–3 minutes prior to intubation. Direct spraying of the airway may trigger airway reactivity so the IV route is preferable, although there have been reports of paradoxical bronchoconstriction after IV administration.

Ketamine: Produces smooth muscle relaxation and bronchodilatation both directly and via release of catecholamines. However, it should be given with an antimuscarinic or antisialagogue such as glycopyrrholate to decrease airway secretions responsible for worsening of mucus plugging.

Volatile inhalational anesthetics: Have well known bronchodilating effects. Sevoflurane is excellent for an inhalation induction having less cardiovascular effects and it does not irritate the airways as much as isoflurane or desflurane.

Neuromuscular blocking drugs: Atracurium and mivacurium are associated with histamine release. Neuromyopathy can develop after prolonged muscle relaxant drug use with an incidence of 30% in asthmatic patients. Reversal of neuromuscular blockage with neostigmine does not cause bronchospasm if atropine or glycopyrrolate are administered concurrently.

Long acting beta agonist: May increase risk of life threatening exacerbations and should be used with inhaled corticoid steroids.

Inhaled corticosteroids: Use a spacer or valved holding chambers to reduce local side effects (i.e., Thrush). Advise patients to rinse their mouths after inhalation to minimize oral bioavailability. Monitor growth charts in children. Consider calcium and vitamin D supplements.

Methylxanthines: Not recommended because it appears to provide no additional benefit to optimal short acting beta agonist and increases the frequency of adverse effects.

Chest physiotherapy: Not generally recommended; it is unknown if it is beneficial and may be unnecessarily stressful for the breathless patient.

Avoid

Exposure to environmental tobacco smoke and other respiratory irritants including smoke from wood-burning stoves and fireplaces and, if possible, substances with strong odors. Avoid exertion outdoors when levels of air pollution are high. Formaldehyde and volatile organic compounds (VOCs) have been implicated as potential risk factors for asthma and wheezing.

References

Phipps P, Garrard CS. The pulmonary physician in critical care 12: acute severe asthma in the intensive care unit. Thorax 2003 Jan;58(1):81–88

Green SM, Johnson NE: Ketamme sedation for pediatric procedures: Part 2, review and implications. Ann Emerg Med September 1990;19:1033–1046.

Expert panel Report 3: Guidelines for the Diagnosis and Management of Asthma. National Asthma Education Program. National Heart, Lung, and Blood Institute of the National Institute of Health. 2007

Chang HY, Togias A, Brown RH. The effects of systemic lidocaine on airway tone and pulmonary function in asthmatic subjects. Anesth Analg. 2007 May;104(5):1109–15

McAlpine LG, Thomson NC. Lidocaine-induced bronchoconstriction in asthmatic patients. Relation to histamine airway responsiveness and effect of preservative. Chest. 1989 Nov;96(5):1012–5

Burches BR Jr, Warner DO. Bronchospasm after intravenous lidocaine. Anesth Analg. 2008 Oct;107(4):1260–2

Burburan SM, Xisto DG, Rocco PR. Anaesthetic management in asthma. Minerva Anestesiol. 2007 Jun;73(6):357–65

Burki NK, Alam M, Lee L. The pulmonary effects of intravenous adenosine in asthmatic subjects. Respiratory Research. 2006 Nov 7:139

Leopold J.D., Hartley J.P.R., Smith, A.P. Effects of Oral H1 and H2 Receptor Antagonists in Asthma. Br. J. Clin. Pharmac. (1979), 8, 249–251

Attention Deficit Hyperactivity Disorder

Wendy H.P. Ren, Samuel H. Wald

First line treatment typically includes stimulant drugs (i.e., Ritalin, Focalin, Metadate, Methylin, Concerta, Dexedrine, Dextrostat, Adderall, Vynase, etc.).

Absolute contraindications

Advanced arteriosclerosis, symptomatic cardiovascular disease, moderate to severe hypertension, hyperthyroidism, known hypersensitivity or idiosyncrasy to the sympathomimetic amines, glaucoma, agitated states, patients with a history of drug abuse.

Relative contraindication

Do not mix stimulant drugs with monamine oxidase inhibitors (MAOI) medication (including Strattera and Dexedrine) because it can result in hypertensive crisis. The patient should be off MAOI medication for greater than 14 days before starting stimulant drugs.

Certain medicines/herbal products (e.g., cough-and-cold products, diet aids) may contain ingredients that increase heart rate or blood pressure (e.g., pseudoephedrine, phenylephrine, ephedra/ma huang).

Drugs which might increase seizure risk when combined with stimulant medications include isoniazid (INH), phenothiazines (e.g., thioridazine), theophylline, or tricyclic antidepressants (e.g., amitriptyline), among others.

Certain other drug interactions can occur with either increased, decreased, or altered effects. These include:

- Acetazolamide.
- Warfarin.
- Antihistamines such as diphenhydramine and chlorpheniramine maleate.
- Drugs classified as MAO's including the antidepressants phenelzine sulfate and tranylcypromine sulfate.
- Drugs that make the urine more acidic such as uroquid-acid No. 2.
- Glutamic acid (an amino acid related to MSG).
- High blood pressure medications such as guanethidine, hydrochlorothiazide, nifedipine, reserpine, terazosin hydrochloride, and verapamil hydrochloride.
- Lithium.
- Major tranquilizers such as chlorpromazine and haloperidol.
- Meperidine.
- Methenamine.

- Norepinephrine.
- Propoxyphene.
- Seizure medications such as ethosuximide, phenobarbital, and phenytoin sodium.
- "Tricyclic" antidepressants such as desipramine hydrochloride, imipramine hydrochloride, and protriptyline hydrochloride.
- Selective serotonin reuptake inhibitors (SSRI) antidepressants.
- Phenylbutazone, non-steroidal anti-inflammatory drugs (NSAID).
- Vitamin C, ascorbic acid.

Cautions

There is a risk of sudden death in patients with cardiac disease including structural cardiac abnormalities, cardiomyopathy, serious heart rhythm abnormalities, or other serious cardiac problems that may place them at increased vulnerability to the sympathomimetic effects of a stimulant drug. Methylphenidate in low doses lowers the heart rate and raises blood pressure.

Stimulant drugs have a risk of psychiatric side effects including hallucination. Visual disturbances such as difficulties with accommodation and blurring of vision have been reported with stimulant treatment. May also cause mood disorders, sleep disturbances, agitation, irritability, headaches and tic development.

There is some clinical evidence that stimulants may lower the convulsive threshold in patients with prior history of seizure.

Published data are inadequate to determine whether chronic use of amphetamines may cause a suppression of growth. It is recommended that growth should be monitored during treatment with stimulants and patients who are not growing or gaining weight as expected may need to have their treatment interrupted.

Decreased appetite with return of hunger, often with greater intensity, is often experienced after the drug effect has worn off.

Higher doses of methylphenidate (more than 20 mg) usually lead to children complaining of nervousness, palpitations, tremor, and/or headaches. Teenagers and adults may report mild euphoria. Experiencing euphoria is, of course, one of the features of a drug that makes it a candidate for abuse. Methylphenidate does not produce either tolerance or addiction. Methylphenidate does not accumulate in the bloodstream or elsewhere in the body, and even after years of use, no withdrawal symptoms occur when someone abruptly stops taking the drug. However, with teenagers and adults who abuse Ritalin—by taking high doses, sometimes via snorting or shooting the drug—the phenomena of tolerance, addiction, and withdrawal can occur. Generally, all stimulant drugs have the potential for tolerance, addiction, and withdrawal.

On September 30th, 2005, Eli Lilly added to its lable, a warning of the possibility that Strattera could cause suicidal thoughts in certain patients.

Be aware that one of the inactive ingredients in Dexedrine is a yellow food coloring called tartrazine (Yellow No. 5). In a few people, particularly those who are allergic to aspirin, tartrazine can cause a severe allergic reaction.

References

Daughton JM, Kratochvil CJ. Review of ADHD pharmacotherapies: advantages, disadvantages, and clinical pearls. J Am Acad Child Adolesc Psychiatry. 2009 Mar;48(3):240–8.

Mosholder AD, Gelperin K, Hammad TA, Phelan K, Johann-Liang R. Hallucinations and other psychotic symptoms associated with the use of attention-deficit/hyperactivity disorder drugs in children. Pediatrics. 2009 Feb;123(2):611–6

V A Harpin. Medication options when treating children and adolescents with ADHD: interpreting the NICE guidance 2006. Archives of Disease in Childhood – Education and Practice 2008;93:58–65

Faraone SV, Biederman J, Morley CP, Spencer TJ. Effect of stimulants on height and weight: a review of the literature. J Am Acad Child Adolesc Psychiatry. 2008 Sep;47(9):994–1009

http://www.pbs.org/wgbh/pages/frontline/shows/medicating/drugs/diller.html

http://www.coreynahman.com/strattera_atomoxetine.html

http://www.healthsquare.com/newrx/dex1129_2.htm

http://www.healthcentral.com/adhd/drug-information

http://www.healthsquare.com/newrx/add1008_2.htm

Epilepsy

Wendy H.P. Ren, Samuel H. Wald

Epilepsy is routinely treated with antiepileptic drugs in combination with other medications so attention should be taken to note possible drug interactions.

Relative contraindications

Carbamezapine: Concomitant administration with phenytoin can result in altered effects of both drugs as well as unpredictable levels. Toxicity can occur when given with lamotrigine, levetiracetam, valproate. Decrease in the effects of clonazepam, lamotrigine, oxcarbazepine, tiagabine, topiramate, valproate, zonisamide may be experienced.

Clonazepam: Its effect is decreased with phenytoin, valproate, carbamezapine and may precipitate absence status when given with valproate. When benzodiazepines are added to anti-epileptic drugs, it can result in worsening of seizures after a transient response. Withdrawing benzodiazepines must be done gradually as a sudden decrease in levels can aggravate seizures and consultation with a specialist is recommended.

Ethosuximide: Toxicity can occur when given with valproate.

Lamotrigine: Decreased effect when given with oxcarbazepine, carbamezapine or phenytoin. When given with valproate, toxicity, severe tremors, possible disseminated intravascular coagulation (DIC) and multi-organ failure can occur.

Phenytoin: Toxicity resulting in a proconvulsant effect can occur with oxcarbazepine, topiramate, and valproate; serum levels should be monitored.

Valproic acid: May increase blood ammonia leading to encephalopathy. There is also anecdotal evidence of encephalopathy with co-administration with phenobarbitone.

Cautions

Benzodiazepines: Can precipitate tonic status epilepticus in patients with Lennox-Gastaut syndrome. Although they are still the drug of choice for status epilepticus, it is important to recognize that there is the potential to worsen certain seizures in some disorders.

Carbamazepine: Can aggravate and induce absence epilepsy, juvenile myoclonic epilepsy, and other idiopathic generalized epilepsies, including Lennox-Gastaut syndrome, focal symptomatic frontal lobe epilepsy. It can cause deterioration of neuropsychological symptoms in Landau-Kleffner syndrome.

Phenytoin: Patients with Unverright-Lundborg disease may cause progressive ataxia and dementia leading to death.

Vigabatrin and Gabapentin: Have been reported to aggravate absence seizures, and myoclonic seizures.

Ketogenic diet: Avoidance of sweetened medication and intravenous solutions containing dextrose is necessary because it may lead to a fall in plasma ketones and increased risk of seizures. Monitoring of plasma acid-base balance, pH or bicarbonate (every 2–3hours), and glucose should be considered when patient is NPO to avoid severe metabolic derangements.

References

Bourgeois B. New dosages and formulations of AEDs for use in pediatric epilepsy. Neurology 2002;58(12 Suppl 7):S2–5.

Drugs for epilepsy. Treat Guidelines Med Lett 2003;1(9):57–64.

Gayatri NA, Livingston JH. Aggravation of epilepsy by anti-epileptic drugs.

Ichikawa J, Nishiyama K, Ozaki K, et al. Anesthetic management of a pediatric patient on a ketogenic diet. J Anesth 2006;20(2):135–7.

Kohrman MH. What is epilepsy? Clinical perspectives in the diagnosis and treatment. J Clin Neurophysiol 2007;24(2):87–95.

Soriano SG, Bozza P. Anesthesia for epilepsy surgery in children. Childs Nerv Syst 2006;22(8):834–43.

Valencia I, Pfeifer H, Thiele EA. General anesthesia and the ketogenic diet: clinical experience in nine patients. Epilepsia 2002;43(5):525–9.

Muscular Dystrophy

Wendy H.P. Ren, Samuel H. Wald

Absolute contraindications

Succinylcholine: Excessive potassium release from muscle cells will cause acute hyperkalemia. Succinylcholine administration to these patients will likely lead to acute rhabdomyolysis.

Relative contraindications

Inhaled volatile agents (Sevoflurane, Isoflurane, Desflurane, Halothane): Use is controversial as these may also induce acute rhabdomyolysis.

Cautions

Opioids, Benzodiazepines: Respiratory muscles will be affected and weakened which will exaggerate the respiratory depressant effects of these medications.

References

Hayes J, Duchenne muscular dystrophy: an old anesthesia problem revisited, Pediatric Anesthesia 2008;18:100-106.

Obata R, Rhabdomyolysis in association with Duchenne's muscular dystrophy, Canadian Journal of Anesthesia1999;46(6):pp 564–566.

Myotonic Dystrophy

Wendy H.P. Ren, Samuel H. Wald

Absolute contraindications

Succinylcholine: May cause prolonged muscle contractions, myotonia of the thorax and difficult ventilation.

Relative contraindications

Anticholinesterases: Unpredictable trigger episodes of myotonia in some patients.

Cautions

Opioids, Benzodiazepines: Possible exaggerated respiratory depressant effects of sedative medications.

References

Buzello W, Hazards of neostigmine in patients with neuromuscular disorders. Report of two cases. Br J Anaesth 1982;54:529.
White RJ, Myotonic dystrophy and paediatric anaesthesia, Paediatric Anaesthesia 2003;13:94–102

Pheochromocytoma

Wendy H.P. Ren, Samuel H. Wald

Absolute contraindications

Droperidol, Metoclopromide and MAO inhibitors: May produce a possible hypertensive crisis in patients with pheochromocytoma.

Relative contraindications

Glucagon: Stimulates catecholamine release, thus exaggerating symptoms.
Halothane: Increases the potential for ventricular arrhythmias.
Beta-agonist medications: Increases the likelihood of tachycardia.

Cautions

Beta Blocker: Administration of beta blockers alone in the setting of pheochromocytoma has been associated with a paradoxical increase in blood pressure due to the attenuation of beta-mediated vasodilatation in skeletal muscle. In patients known to have, or suspected of having, a pheochromocytoma, if beta-blockade is required, it should be given in combination with an alpha blocker, and only after the alpha blocker has been initiated.

References

Bitter DA. Innovar-induced hypertensive crises in patients with pheochromocytoma. Anesthesiology 1979;50:366–9

Sumikawa K, Amakata YA, The pressor effect of droperidol on a patient with pheochromosytoma, Anesthesiology 1977;46(3):359–61.

Porphyrias

Wendy H.P. Ren, Samuel H. Wald

Absolute contraindication

Barbiturates: Acute attack is most likely a consequence of a decrease in uroporphyrogen synthetase levels which interferes with heme production. Enzyme induction of increased formation of cytochrome P-450 increases levels of delta aminolevulinic acid, also precipitating an attack.

Relative contraindication

Local anesthetics: Because the porphyrias are associated with a peripheral neuropathy, the use of local anesthetics in these patients is controversial.

Cautions

Chlordiazepoxide, Chlorpropamide, Diazepam, Ergot preparations, Glutethimide, Griseofulvin, Hydantoins, Methyldopa, Meprobamate, Estrogens, Pentazocine, Progestogens and Sulfa drugs: Have all been reported to precipitate acute attacks.

Neostigmine: There is a theoretical concern for the avoidance of neostigmine in these patients for demyelination in nervous tissues, but it has thus far been used in these patients without complications.

References

Mees DE, Frederickson EL, Anesthesia and the Porphyrias, Southern Medical journal, January 1975 Vol 68, No. 1, 29–31.

Ahmed I, Childhood Porphyrias, Mayo Clin Proc. 2002;77:825–836.

Upper Respiratory Tract Infection

Wendy H.P. Ren, Samuel H. Wald

Cautions

Over the counter medications: In January 2008 the U.S. Food and Drug Administration issued an advisory strongly recommending that over-the-counter cold and cough medications not be given to infants and children under two years of age because of the risk of life-threatening side effects. Such medications may play a role in unexpected infant deaths.(1) Many cough and cold preparations are elixirs which contain up to 25% alcohol by volume. (2)

Dextromethorphan and Codeine: Neither are more effective than placebo in reduction of acute cough. Adverse reactions include obtundation, respiratory depression, somnolence, ataxia, miosis, vomiting, rash, facial swelling and pruritis.(3)(4)

Decongestants (sympathomimetics): May be associated with irritability, restlessness, lethargy, hallucination, hypertension, and dystonic reactions. Metabolism and clearance may vary with age and may be altered with concurrent use of acetaminophen.(4)(5)

Diphenhydramine: May diminish mental alertness, or in the young pediatric patient, cause excitation. Overdosage may cause hallucinations, convulsions, or death. Caution with asthmatics because may cause thickening of bronchial secretions, tightness of chest or throat and wheezing, and nasal stuffiness.(6)

Inhaled Racemic Epinephrine: Rebound edema may occur after treatment is stopped. Monitoring and observation is required for several hours after therapy. The use of steroids may reduce the need for epinephrine to manage croup.

References

(1) Rimsza, ME, Newberry, S, Unexpected Infant Deaths Associated with use of Cough and Cold Medications. Pediatrics 2008: 122:e318–e322.

(2) Drug Information for the Health care Professional (USP DI). 16th ed. Rockville, MD: United States Pharmacopeial Convention, Inc; 1996;1:1008–1104

(3) Taylor JA, Novack AH, Almquist JR, Rogers JE. Efficacy of cough suppressants in children. J Pediatrics. 1993:122:799–802

(4) Berlin, C; committee on drugs 1997. Use of Codeine and Dextromethorphan – containing cough remedies in children. Pediatrics. 1997:99:918–920

(5) Gadomski A, HortonL. The need for rational therapeutics in the use of cough and cold medicine in infants. Pediatrics. 1992,89:774–776

(6) http://www.drugs.com/pro/diphenhydramine-injection.html. accessed 4/2009

Herbal Substances' Effect on Medications

Wendy H.P. Ren, Samuel H. Wald

Anti-epileptic drugs: Borage oil and evening primrose oil contain gamolenic acid which lowers the seizure threshold.

Cyclosporin: St. John's wort may lead to graft rejection following heart, liver and renal transplantation. The mechanism is that cyclosporin blood levels drop below the therapeutic range as it is also metabolized by CYP3A.

Digoxin: Herbal laxatives may deplete potassium which increases digoxin toxicity. St. John's wort decreases digoxin levels.

Indinavir HIV medications: St. John's wort is metabolized by the same enzyme as this protease inhibitor used to treat HIV. Combination with St. John's wort may lead to lower blood levels.

Monoamine oxidase inhibitors (MAOI): Reserpine (rauwolfia alkaloid) releases and depletes norepinephrine stores. If added to a MAOI, the accumulated norepinephrine will be released.

Oral contraceptive pill: St. John's wort may cause enzyme induction via an increase in the expression of P-glycoprotein resulting in lower drug medication levels and contraceptive failure.

Selective serotonin re-uptake inhibitors: St. John's wort can potentiate serotonergic effects by duplication of action and cytochrome inhibition.

Warfarin: St. John's wort: Induction of CYP2C9 that will decrease the anticoagulant effect. Garlic may cause increase in INR.

Table 16.1: Summary of Herbal Interactions

Herbal Substance	Medication(s) Affected
Borage oil	Anti-epileptic
Evening primrose oil	Anti-epileptic
Garlic	Warfarin
Herbal laxatives	Digoxin
Reserpine (rauwolfia alkaloid)	Monoamine oxidase inhibitors (MAOI)
St. John's Wort	Cyclosporin, Digoxin, Indinavir HIV medications, Monoamine oxidase inhibitors (MAOI), Oral contraceptive pill, Selective Serotonin Re-Uptake Inhibitors, Warfarin

References

Fugh-Berman A, Ernst E, Herb-drug interactions: review and assessment of report reliability, Br J Clin Pharm 2001;52:587–95.

Izzo AA, Ernst E, Interactions between herbal medicines and prescribed drugs: a systematic review, Drugs 2001;61(15):2163–75.

Sorenson JM, Herb-drug, food-drug, nutrient-drug and drug-drug interactions: mechanisms involved and their medical implications, J Altern Complement Med 2002;8:293–308.

Williamson EM, Drug interactions between herbal and prescription medicines, Drug Safety 2003;26(15): 1075–92.

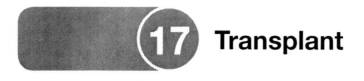

17 Transplant

Table of Contents

Cardiac Transplantation

Gary M. Satou, Thomas S. Klitzner

Although advances in the treatment of congenital and acquired heart disease have occurred in the last few decades, there remain a small number of patients for whom correction or adequate palliation cannot be performed. For this group, heart transplantation is the only remaining option. At present, artificial or other forms of heart replacement do not exist for children. Thus, human cadaveric heart replacement is the only form of cardiac transplantation. Given the scarcity of organ availability, research continues aimed at exploring artificial heart replacement options for humans of all ages.

Etiology

Heart transplantation is performed for patients with severe ventricular dysfunction. Commonly, this occurs in the setting of Dilated Cardiomyopathy and late stage congenital heart disease.

Clinical Presentation and Prognosis

Because cardiac transplantation is not a disease, but rather management, the following is applicable to either the pre-transplant heart failure patient, or the transplanted child who may present with issues such as graft rejection, infection and/or recurrent heart failure.

Age of onset: All ages. Neonates considered for transplantation usually have congenital heart disease and have undergone a surgical repair or procedure which failed. They can, however, have primary heart muscle disease such as the cardiomyopathies. Cardiomyopathy is the more common indication for heart transplantation in the older child. Cardiac transplantation for all patients is indicated when they are ill enough to be considered near-death, often in the hospital, in the intensive care unit on mechanical assistance, or when they are felt to be symptomatic with death likely within the following year or two. Thus, the age at diagnosis/presentation and the time at which myocardial failure ensues will dictate when cardiac transplantation is performed

Presenting signs/symptoms and clinical course: This depends on the etiology and timing of the heart failure. However, the general signs and symptoms of heart failure are similar irrespective of etiology. These can include systemic venous engorgement, tachypnea, tachycardia and poor tissue perfusion. There may be various types of murmurs or a gallop rhythm. There is usually hepatomegaly. There may be poor peripheral pulses and delayed capillary refill. Older patients may demonstrate lower extremity edema. Infants may be irritable with poor feeding. Older children who are able to communicate may describe nausea, vomiting, and/or abdominal pain. There may be general fatigue and shortness of breath. These symptoms occur in both the child in heart failure prior to transplantation as well as those status post cardiac transplantation with recurrent myocardial failure. The clinical course following the transplant should generally alleviate most, if not all, signs and symptoms. However, if graft rejection occurs, findings, in varying degree, may re-emerge.

Prognosis: Good, but with limitations and lifelong complexity. Though the survival of the child or the transplanted heart has improved through advances in immunosuppressive therapy, heart transplantation is not a "curative" treatment. The transplanted heart will ultimately undergo a degenerative vascular process which may include vasculitis of the coronary arteries by 7–10 years post transplant. In some patients, deterioration of the graft can occur much earlier. For all patients, lifelong immunosuppressive drug therapy is indicated.

Diagnosis

Heart failure is a clinical diagnosis as described above. Additional abnormal laboratory values and non-cardiac organ dysfunction may be present. In recent times, the serum B-type natriuretic peptide (BNP) level has been shown to trend nicely with the degree of myocardial failure. When graft rejection occurs, endomyocardial tissue biopsy, performed in the cardiac catheterization laboratory, is usually helpful in establishing the diagnosis.

Management

The pre-transplant patient will often require inpatient care prior to heart transplantation. This care can include medical management with intravenous agents including diuretics, inotropes, and afterload reducing agents. There may be a need for mechanical ventillatory support and, in some, myocardial mechanical support. The child with cardiac graft rejection will require a course of inpatient immunosuppressive therapy, along with therapy for heart failure.

Medication: While awaiting cardiac transplantation, the ill child is usually given intravenous milrinone or dobutamine for inotropic and systemic vasodilator effect. Other forms of afterload reducing agents may be used. Blood transfusions are minimized to avoid foreign antigen exposure. Lasix and other diuretic agents are administered as needed. Immunosuppression after cardiac transplantation usually includes calcineurin inhibitors such as cyclosporine or tacrolimus, as well as mycophenalate mofetil. Coticosteroids are also utilized, and, on occasion, plasmapheresis is performed with immunoglobulin infusions. Low dose aspirin therapy is used for the anti-platelet effect. Antihypertensives and other cardiac agents are used as needed. Rapamycin may be used to reduce the onset of coronary vasculopathy.

Surgery: The actual cardiac transplant operation is relatively straightforward. In short, the procedure is performed through a median sternotomy and on cardiopulmonary bypass. The recipient heart is excised and the donor heart placed, with surgical anastamoses at several sites, including the left atrium, aorta, and vena cavae. As stated above, postoperative care includes immunosuppressive drug therapy.

Therapy: Physical therapy is needed only in cases where the primary disease or systemic disorder requires such as, for example, the muscular dystrophies.

Pyscho-Social: Routine social work, psychology and psychiatry evaluations/assistance are part of the transplant evaluation and follow-process. As one may imagine, screening occurs to ensure that a family or social network for a transplant recipient is not prohibitive, given the significant time, emotional, and other requirements placed on such an individual. As well, some children will die while "listed" and waiting for a donor heart. A small number may not survive the early post-transplant period. Lifelong drug-compliance with immunosuppressives and other drugs are necessary and this can be very challenging, especially during the adolescent years.

Monitoring: Pre-transplant, the most critically ill children will usually be in the hospital. For the others, the cardiologist will be routinely visiting with them in the office to evaluate the level of heart failure symptoms, performing follow-up echocardiography and any laboratory values which may be needed, such as BNP, lactate, electrolytes and CBC. These patients generally do not have indwelling lines. Worsening clinical states will usually lead to hospitalization. Post-transplant, careful and frequent surveillance is conducted. This includes cardiac function analysis and monitoring for rejection and infections. Studies include multiple myocardial biopsies and cardiac catheterizations, angiography, echocardiography and serial blood work. Once stable after the first year post-transplant, patients are seen approximately every 3–6 months. Serial evaluation of immunosuppressive drug levels, complications of therapy and immunosuppression continue. Laboratory investigation includes electrolytes, CBC (r/o anemia), WBC (to evaluate for drug-induced neutropenia), liver function tests (LFT's), cholesterol and glucose. Renal function is assessed with serum creatine and either a nuclear glomerular filtration rate (GFR) study or creatine clearance. Occasional holter monitering and exercise (CPX) stress-testing may be performed. In general, these patients are fragile, and subtle signs or symptoms should be immediately brought to the attention of the treating pediatric cardiologist. A simple general sense of ill-being or nausea can actually be a manifestation of transplant rejection.

Pearls and Precautions

Immunizations and prophylaxis: No live attenuated vaccines are permitted as patients are chronically undergoing immunosuppression. Generally safe vaccinations include: Diphtheria, Hep A and B, Hib, HPV, Inactivated influenza, Meningococcal, Pertussis, Pneumococcal and Tetanus. Always contact your transplant center/pediatric cardiologist for any given patient. Prophylaxis is conducted for cardiac transplant patients at least for a year following transplantation and usually includes coverage for CMV (Valgancyclovir), fungus, and PCP (Bactrim).

Nutrition: Although a low fat, low salt diet is appropriate for all patients, no specific diet is demanded (unless Diabetes is present).

Dental care and procedures: Good dental hygiene is very important to reduce the risk of infective endocarditis and should be encouraged. If dental cleaning or care is performed (or other non-cardiac procedures), the cardiologist or transplant team should be contacted to discuss the patient's individual needs. Subacute bacterial endocarditis (SBE) prophylaxis is indicated for at least 6 months following the cardiac transplantation. Thereafter, it is followed on a case by case basis. The most recent guidelines for endocarditis prophylaxis can be reviewed. See References. A significant side effect of immunosuppressive therapy (calcineurin inhibitors, particularly cyclosporine) in these patients is gingival hyperplasia.

Dermatologic: Sun exposure/photosensitivity is common in cardiac transplant patients and good sun-blocking/protective therapy is important. In addition, viral warts, molluscum contagiosum, and other dermatologic abnormalities can arise and should be discussed with the cardiologist regarding evaluation and treatment.

School: Due to the new immunosuppressive regimen, children are held from re-entering school for 3 months following cardiac transplantation. Given the potential for significant amounts of time away from education both before, and possibly after transplant, additional support in the form of tutoring, home-schooling or other programs may be needed.

References

Heart transplantation in children. Denfield SW. Minerva Cardioangiol. 2008 Jun;56(3):349–59.

Pediatric heart transplantation: current clinical review. Tjang YS, Stenlund H, Tenderich G, Hornik L, Körfer R. J Card Surg. 2008 Jan–Feb;23(1):87–91

Indications for heart transplantation in pediatric heart disease: a scientific statement from the American Heart Association Council on Cardiovascular Disease in the Young; the Councils on Clinical Cardiology, Cardiovascular Nursing, and Cardiovascular Surgery and Anesthesia; and the Quality of Care and Outcomes Research Interdisciplinary Working Group. Canter CE, Shaddy RE, Bernstein D, Hsu DT, Chrisant MR, Kirklin JK, Kanter KR, Higgins RS, Blume ED, Rosenthal DN, Boucek MM, Uzark KC, Friedman AH, Young JK; American Heart Association Council on Cardiovascular Disease in the Young; American Heart Association Council on Clinical Cardiology; American Heart Association Council on Cardiovascular Nursing; American Heart Association Council on Cardiovascular Surgery and Anesthesia; Quality of Care and Outcomes Research Interdisciplinary Working Group. Circulation. 2007 Feb 6;115(5):658–76

Prevention of infective endocarditis: guidelines from the American Heart Association (multiple councils): Wilson W, Taubert KA, Gewitz M, Lockhart PB, Baddour LM, Levison M, Bolger A, Cabell CH, Takahashi M, Baltimore RS, Newburger JW, Strom BL, Tani LY, Gerber M, Bonow RO, Pallasch T, Shulman ST, Rowley AH, Burns JC, Ferrieri P, Gardner T, Goff D, Durack DT. Circulation. 2007 Oct 9; 116(15):1736–54.

End Stage Liver Disease (ESLD) & Pediatric Liver Transplantation (LTx)

Robert S. Venick

End-Stage Liver Disease (ESLD) represents a final common pathway for a number of causes of chronic liver disease. ESLD is typically marked by one or all of the following: Jaundice, ascites, encephalopathy, portal hypertension, malnutrition and liver synthetic function failure. Children with ESLD are candidates for liver transplantation (LTx).

Etiology

Extrahepatic biliary atresia (EHBA) is the leading indication for Pediatric LTx making up 40% of cases. Other forms of cholestatic liver disease [Alagille syndrome, non-syndromic paucity of bile ducts, progressive familial intrahepatic cholestasis (PFIC)] account for 15% of cases. While there are known genetic associations with Alagille syndrome and PFIC, the cause of EHBA is unknown. Fulminant hepatic failure (FHF) caused by infectious Hepatitis A Virus is the most common identifiable cause worldwide. Medication, metabolic or idiopathic causes accounts for 15% of the children requiring LTx. Other causes of LTx in children include metabolic liver disease (15%), cirrhosis (10%), and hepatablastoma (HBA) which is the most common type of pediatric liver tumors (5%).

Clinical Presentation & Prognosis

Demographics: The mean age at the time of LTx is five years old. EHBA, metabolic liver disease and HBA tend to present in infancy or the toddler years. For the most part, there are no gender or ethnic predispositions to those children who require LTx.

Presenting signs and symptoms: EHBA tends to present with jaundice and direct hyperbilirubinemia in the neonatal period and eventually with acholic stools. By definition, FHF occurs in children with no prior history of liver disease, who within eight weeks of the onset of their illness develop jaundice, coagulopathy, encephalopathy, and liver failure. HBAs most commonly present with abdominal distension or a palpable abdominal mass, failure to thrive and constitutional symptoms.

Clinical course/prognosis: Children with EHBA fail to thrive nutritionally. For those children who do not undergo hepatoportojejunostomy (Kasai procedure) or LTx by one year of age, they will almost universally succumb to malnutrition, infection or gastrointestinal bleeding due to portal hypertension. For children who develop FHF, their prognosis for spontaneous recovery is dependent on their etiology and ranges from as low as 10% to as high as 50–60%. Without hepatic recovery, death is certain in a short period of time from complications such as cerebral edema, infection or multiorgan failure.

The course of children with HBA is quite variable and depends on the time of diagnosis, size, stage and location of the tumor, particularly in relation to the vasculature and its response to chemotherapy. All of these factors go into the decision making to attempt surgical resection vs. transplantation.

Diagnosis

Lack of weight gain and vertical growth are often features of chronic congenital liver disease (i.e., EHBA). On physical exam, these children present with scleral icterus when the bilirubin is above 3 mg/dL, and will develop progressive hepatosplenomegaly, ascites and prominent superficial abdominal wall vasculature. Those children who are cholestatic for a prolonged period of time will be at risk of Vitamin D deficiency and rickets, which presents with bowing of the lower extremities, widening of the epiphyses, costochondral beading, and craniotabes (softening of the skull bones). Patients with acute hepatitis and jaundice should undergo a careful assessment of their mental status and neurologic exam including evaluation for hyperreflexia, asterixis, and focal neurologic deficits. Many HBA patients are brought to medical attention by parents who appreciate their child's abdominal distension or mass. Imaging, including CT scan or MRI, is critical in the diagnosis of HBA.

Percutaneous or surgical biopsy is the gold standard in diagnosing many forms of acute and chronic liver disease. Other modalities used in diagnosis include hepatobiliary iminodiacetic acid (HIDA) scan, intraoperative cholangiogram and genetic testing of the patient's serum.

Management

All patients with acute or chronic liver disease should be followed closely by a pediatric hepatologist, ideally one affiliated with an LTx center. Hepatic function panel, liver synthetic function (albumin, prothrombin time, fibrinogen) and fat soluble vitamins (A, D, E and K) are monitored routinely for patients with chronic cholestasis. In patients with acute liver failure Factor V and VII, ammonia levels and a host of infectious and metabolic studies will be investigated and tracked. Abdominal ultrasound is important in assessing for scarring of the liver (nodularity may be reported in cases with bridging fibrosis or cirrhosis). Ultrasound should be ordered with doppler to assess the blood flow through the portal vein and hepatic artery. While ultrasound can be used as a screening modality for a mass lesion, more detailed imaging including MRI or dual phase CT angiogram is required in such cases. For children with EHBA, early diagnosis is crucial in the first 2–3 months of life as a Kasai procedure will be performed and its success is age dependent. Following a Kasai, children are often placed on ursodeoxyxholic acid (30 mg/kg/day divided BID), and cholangitis prophylaxis (Trimethoprim/sulfamethaxszole 3–6 mg/kg/day of TMP).

Prior to LTx, children with chronic liver disease will often require supplemental nutrition which can be achieved with breast milk fortifier, calorically dense formula (i.e., 24–30 kcal/oz) polycose or MCT oil. Formulas which are high in medium chain triglyceride (i.e., pregestimil) are preferred for infants who remain cholestatic. In such circumstances, fat soluble Vitamins require monitoring and may require supplementation. Parenteral nutrition may be necessary in the pre-LTx period when children are not gaining weight appropriately and/or there is a need to fluid and sodium restrict due to ascites or respiratory compromise. Diuretics, most commonly furosemide and sprionolactone, are also employed to help manage ascites. Those children who develop portal hypertension and GI bleeding can be managed with medical therapy (ßblockers or isosorbide dinitrate- the suggested starting dose of nadolol is 1 mg/kg/d of nadolol, with titration of the drug until a 25% reduction of heart rate is achieved. Then isosorbide nitrate is added to reach a dose over the course of 1 week of 0.5 mg/kg twice a day) or serial endoscopy with sclerosis or banding of esophageal varices.

As part of the LTx evaluation, patients are seen by multi-disciplinary teams including pediatric hepatology, transplant surgery, nursing, nutrition and social work. Often times, patients may require clearance by cardiology, nephrology and dentistry. Children awaiting LTx each receive a calculated Pediatric End-Stage Liver Disease (PELD) Score which is based on their growth parameters and laboratory values. Children with acute liver failure and those with unresectable HBAs or specific disorders of metabolism may receive priority status on the waiting list (Status 1A and 1B).

Liver transplant: The options for children who receive an LTx include a cadaveric whole or segmental graft or living related donation. The latter accounts for roughly 15% of United States experience. Currently between 500–600 LTx are performed annually in the U.S. Overall, 1- and 5-year patient survival rates are 90% and 85% respectively.

Corticosteroids are typically used as part of induction immunosuppression regimens, and are generally weaned off by 6–12 months post-LTx. The vast majority of pediatric LTx recipients are managed on tacrolimus (Prograf®, FK-506) as maintenance immunosuppression. Goal trough levels of tacrolimus gradually decrease throughout the first year post-LTx. Epstein-Barr virus (EBV) and cytomegalovirus (CMV) monitoring is important in the post-LTx period and often children receive prophylaxis with ganciclovir. High risk recipients (defined as those < 12 mo. of age or an EBV negative recipient based on serologies at time of LTx) receive IV ganciclovir 5 mg/kg/q12 hours x 28 days, followed by 6 mg/kg/day IV Day 28–100 post-LTx. Low risk recipients receive 4 weeks IV ganciclovir of 6–10 mg/kg/day. Both groups then receive a total of 2 years of either acyclovir of (40 mg/kg/day divided twice a day-four times a day) or valganciclovir [dosage in mg/day= (7 x Body Surface Area x calculated Creatinine Clearance using the Schwartz Formula)] in an effort to avoid post-transplant lymphoproliferative disease (PTLD). PCP prophylaxis typically involves the use of Trimethoprim/sulfamethaxszole (TMP component 5 mg/kg/d divided q 12 Saturday and Sunday only) or Atovaquone (30 mg/kg given once daily).

Social: In the post-LTx setting, children should continue to receive any and all services which they qualify for through the Regional Center in order to maximize their development.

Monitoring: Comprehensive metabolic panel, CBC with platelets and differential, trough levels of immunosuppression are monitored regularly in the post-LTx setting. Long-term patients are screened closely for metabolic syndrome (fasting glucose, HgbA1C, fasting lipid panel).

Pearls and Precautions

Immunization: Following LTx, children should not receive live vaccines MMR, Varicella, Rotavirus or Inhaled Influenza Vaccine). All other vaccines are encouraged. For those children transplanted as infants or toddlers, it is important to check available immunization titers to make sure they have achieved a proper immune response.

Nutrition: Few dietary restrictions exist for these patients. Grapefruit is known to affect tacrolimus metabolism and should be avoided. Herbal medications are often discouraged over concern with drug interactions. The long-term sequelae of developing metabolic syndrome is particularly concerning for this cohort of patients. Healthy diet and exercise should be continually emphasized and early interventions taken whenever possible.

Skin and dental care: LTx recipients should be followed regularly by pediatric dentistry. They do not require antibiotic prophylaxis unless they have a known cardiac condition. LTx recipients on immunosuppression have an increased risk of skin cancer, therefore, sunscreen with SPF 30 or higher is important.

Toilet: Toilet training should not be much different for toddlers who have received LTx than from the general population with the exception that patients on magnesium or sodium bicarbonate supplements will tend to have more frequent and looser bowel movements which can make toilet training more challenging.

Likely complications: A frequent scenario involves a visit to the general pediatrician's office when LTx recipients develop a fever. Following a careful clinical exam, blood and urine cultures, CBC with platelets and differential, and a comprehensive metabolic panel including liver function tests should be obtained. Depending on the age, time post-LTx, presence or absence of a central venous catheter (CVC), and overall appearance of the patient, there is often a lower threshold for admission, close observation and administration of broad spectrum antibiotics. For those children with CVC, it is typical to start broad antibiotic coverage with vancomycin and a third generation cephalosporin when they present with new onset of fever above 101 Fahrenheit=38.3 celcius. For LTx recipients without a CVC, they should be carefully evaluated prior to empirically starting antibiotic therapy. The use of non-steroidal anti-inflammatory drugs (NSAID) or acetaminophen for a fever is discouraged.

School/education: Children with chronic liver disease awaiting LTx should be evaluated by the Regional Center or school district as many will qualify for physical or occupational therapy due to delays associated with chronic illness.

Medications: Common side effects of tacrolimus include neurotoxicity, hyperglycemia, hyperkalemia, hypomagnesemia, hypertension and renal insufficiency. Important drug interactions with tacrolimus include erythromycin, clarithromycin, antifungal agents, calcium channel blockers, and anticonvulsants.

Medical devices: For the first 100 days post-LTx, it is commonplace for pediatric recipients to have a CVC (to receive antiviral therapy and for lab draws). Only a small minority of the patients (typically the infants with oral aversion) will be sent home with G-tubes.

References

McDiarmid SV, Management of the Pediatric Liver Transplant Patient. Liver Transplantation 2001;Vol 7, No 11, p S77–S86.

Farmer DG, Venick RS, McDiarmid SV et al. Predictors of outcomes after pediatric liver transplantation: an analysis of more than 800 cases performed at a single institution. Journal of the American College of Surgeons 2007; 204: 904–914.

McGuire BM, Rosenthal P, Brown CC, et al. Long-term Management of the Liver Transplant Patient: Recommendations for the Primary Care Doctor. American Journal of Transplantation 2009; Vol 9, No 9:1988–2003.

Lung Transplantation

Roberta M. Kato, Thomas G. Keens

Lung transplant involves transplantation of deceased or living donor intact or partial lungs. Lung and heart transplant may be done together.

Etiology

Lung transplantation is used in patients who have such severe lung damage that death is eminent, and for which there is no medical treatment to restore lost function. The most common diseases leading to the requirement for lung transplantation are cystic fibrosis, primary pulmonary hypertension, and pulmonary fibrosis.

Clinical Presentation and Prognosis

Age of onset: Lung transplantation is most commonly performed in adolescents with advanced and incurable lung disease. However, it has been performed in infancy and in adults.

Presenting signs and symptoms: Patients with incurable lung diseases resulting in life-threatening respiratory compromise may be listed for lung transplantation if a large number of criteria are met, including the absence of complicating medical conditions which would make lung transplantation less likely to be successful, and psychosocial function and support to carry through with the considerable medical treatments required to prevent graft rejection and pneumonia.

Clinical course: Following lung transplantation, assuming that patients survive the immediate post-operative period, there is improved lung function and activity tolerance. Patients once severely debilitated and restricted will enjoy better activity tolerance and good lung function. Immunosuppression is required to prevent graft rejection. Thus, patients are carefully followed to observe for signs of acute or chronic rejection on the one hand, and infection on the other. Bronchoscopy and lung biopsies are frequently required to assess for rejection. Immunosuppressant medications are continuously monitored and adjusted, based on pulmonary function results and general health. Lung infections are typical of those seen in immunocompromised hosts. Thus, eternal vigilance is required to avoid rejection from immunosuppressant medications on the one hand, and infection on the other.

Prognosis: Relative to other solid organ transplants, lung transplantation has been more difficult to achieve good results. This may be due, in part, to the fact that the lungs are exposed to the environment, and thus more susceptible to infection than organs completely enclosed in the body. Survival of patients and transplanted lung grafts are improving with improved science and technology. Nevertheless, for the foreseeable future, lung transplantation may add years of quality life, but they are not a long-term solution for survival beyond10–20 years.

Management

Management of patients following lung transplantation is highly specialized, and it must be done by a team of physicians experienced in lung transplantation. The issues are balancing immunosuppression to prevent graft rejection on the one hand with prevention of infection on the other.

Medications: Tacrolimus, pneumocystis prophylaxis with sulfamethoxazole/trimetoprim, and prophylaxis medications as indicated including amphotericin nasal spray, fluconazole and voriconazole

Consultations: Cardiologists are routinely consulted if there is any abnormality by echocardiogram or electrocardiogram to evaluate for pulmonary hypertension. Nephrologists may be involved if there is renal insufficiency secondary to immunosuppression medication.

Surgery: Lung transplantation is a surgical procedure, but management only begins with the surgery. In pediatric patients, lung transplants are generally bilateral. Both of the child's own lungs will be removed and replaced with transplanted lungs. This is done under cardiopulmonary bypass. Simultaneous cardiothoracic transplant is less common, but may be considered if there is also severe congenital heart disease that cannot be surgically corrected.

Social: The medical treatment regimen following lung transplantation is challenging for the patient and family. Thus, a cohesive family support system and strong support of the child is important. Non-adherence with the medical regimen to prevent graft rejection remains a common cause of failure of lung transplantation.

Monitoring: Tacrolimus and creatine levels and WBC to ensure appropriate immunosuppression levels.

Pearls and Precautions

Immunization: While awaiting transplant, the patient should be fully vaccinated according to well child care guidelines. Following transplantation, no live vaccines may be given. Inactivated vaccines may be given a year following the date of transplantation.

Likely complications: Acute and chronic episodes of rejection, recurrent respiratory infections due to immunosuppression, renal insufficiency due to tacrolimus toxicity and bronchiolitis obliterans may occur.

A central catheter is placed to assist with CVP measurements to manage fluid status. A PICC line may be placed prior to discharge if long term antibiotics are required. This is necessary in patients with cystic fibrosis who will have 3–4 months of parenteral antibiotics following transplantation.

All the drugs, prescribed or not, may cause interactions which necessitates frequent drug level testing. In particular, voriconazole alters tacrolimus levels.

School/education: No specific recommendations.

Medical devices: Oxygen supplementation may be required when there are complications and daily airway care is essential as the mucociliary blanket is abnormal.

Miscellaneous

- Graft rejection starts at the time of transplant and requires close monitoring.
- New U.S. organ allocation protocols are being activated to improve allocation to children who carry the highest mortality of all lung transplant candidates.
- Immunosuppressant regimens are constantly evolving.

References

Sweet S. Pediatric Lung Transplantation. Proc Am Thorac Soc. 6: 122–127. 2009.

Woo M. Overview of Lung Transplantation. Clinic Rev Allerg Immunol. 35:154–163. 2008.

Renal Transplantation

Katherine Wesseling Perry

Indications: Renal transplantation is the treatment of choice for end-stage renal disease (ESRD) in Pediatrics.

Demographics: Since transplantation is the objective of all pediatric dialysis patients, the demographics of this population are similar to that of the pediatric CKD and dialysis populations. Renal transplantation cannot be performed in tiny infants. A minimum weight of 7–10 kg is typically required (usually over 1 year of age) for transplantation to be considered.

Management

Medications: To avoid transplant rejection, all transplant recipients are immunosuppressed which increases their risk for infection. Standard immunosuppressant therapy involves the use of steroids, calcineurin inhibitor (cyclosporine or tacrolimus) and an antimetabolite (mycophenolate mofetil or azathioprine).

Consultations: Nephrology should be consulted immediately for any transplant patient with an increased serum creatinine level.

Urology should be consulted immediately if new onset or worsening hydronephrosis is detected.

Therapy: Renal osteodystrophy, chronic illness, and often multiple hospitalizations make all children with chronic kidney disease physically and emotionally at high risk for disability. Physical therapy is warranted in all children in whom gross or fine motor delay or muscle weakness is noted either on history or physical exam. Occupational therapy should be considered, particularly in infants and younger children, when an abnormal feeding and/or swallowing history are obtained.

Psychiatry: All children with chronic kidney disease are at high risk for emotional problems. Short stature, chronic illness, and repeated hospitalizations tend to isolate these children from their peers. Many uremic children have trouble learning and when combined with multiple school absences related to their illness, school success is often limited. Thus, a psychosocial assessment is warranted for EVERY child with chronic kidney disease including those with kidney transplants.

Monitoring: Serum electrolyte and creatinine levels should be routinely measured in all transplant recipients. An unexplained increase in the serum creatinine necessitates a renal ultrasound (to evaluate for obstruction) and a kidney biopsy (to evaluate for rejection, infection, or primary disease recurrence). Electrolyte values (potassium, bicarbonate, magnesium, calcium and phosphorus) should also be followed. Calcineurin inhibition may induce a type IV RTA (acidosis and hyperkalemia) with magnesium wasting. This should be treated with bicarbonate and magnesium supplementation. Phosphate wasting is typical in the first 6 months after transplantation. Supplementation with oral phosphate and/or calcitriol should be titrated to maintain serum phosphorus levels above 2 mg/dl.

A complete blood count should be measured routinely as mycophenolate therapy may induce neutropenia. Signs of infection in the face of neutropenia must be managed aggressively.

Immunosuppressant levels (particularly of the calcineurin inhibitors—cyclosporine and tacrolimus) should be monitored regularly and used to adjust treatment dose. Certain medications including erythromycin, rifampin, verapamil, and fluconazole alter metabolism of calcineurin inhibitors. These medications should be avoided. If essential, levels of immunosuppressants should be carefully monitored and adjusted during therapy.

Blood pressure should be monitored at each clinic visit. Hypertension is common in renal allograft recipients due to medications (calcineurin inhibitors and steroids), long-term renal scarring, and renal artery stenosis. To promote renal artery dilation and improved renal blood flow, hypertension should be treated with calcium channel blockers in the immediate post-operative period. Subsequently, ACE inhibitors provide a degree of renal protection from long-term fibrosis. Cardiac function (echocardiogram) should be monitored yearly in all hypertensive patients whether blood pressure is well-controlled with anti-hypertensives or not.

Pearls and Precautions

Immunization: Live vaccines are contraindicated in all immunosuppressed patients.

Nutrition/Diet: A low salt, low sugar diet is recommended after transplantation to avoid excess weight gain and hypertension, particularly in patients treated with steroids.

Disease complications

Ureteral obstruction: Any transplant patient with an increased serum creatinine should have a renal ultrasound. Urinary tract obstruction (suggested by new or worsening hydronephrosis) should be managed by insertion of a urinary bladder catheter in combination with obtaining a Urological consult.

Rejection: Increased creatinine, fever, malaise and pain over the graft often make transplant rejection difficult to differentiate from infection. Untreated rejection leads to graft loss. Repeated bouts of rejection (from medication non-compliance or the development of donor-specific antibodies in sensitized individuals) lead to chronic allograft nephropathy and accelerated decline in renal function. Rejection is diagnosed by means of a kidney biopsy.

Infection: Common childhood illnesses are often more severe and prolonged in immuno-suppressed transplant recipients. Illnesses such as varicella, Epstein-Barr virus, and cytomegalovirus may be very severe and often require hospitalization for treatment. Bacterial infections are more likely to become disseminated in this population. Any transplant recipient—particularly in the first 3–6 months post transplant—who develops signs of infection (fever, ill-appearing) should be evaluated, cultures (including blood and urine) drawn, and antibiotic (and/or antiviral) therapy initiated quickly. Often, immunosuppressant therapy is reduced during intercurrent illness. In general, a broad spectrum of antibiotics (ceftriaxone in low risk patients, zosyn or meropenem in higher risk patients) should be initiated in febrile transplant patients in whom an organism has not been identified. Particularly in patients with indwelling lines, antibiotic therapy should include gram positive coverage.

Neoplasia: Immunosuppressed patients are at increased risk for the development of cancers. Post-transplant lymphoproliferative disease (PTLD), associated with new-onset Epstein-Barr virus disease, is the most common cancer in the pediatric age group. Signs and symptoms include a rising creatinine, fever, weight loss, and/or lympadenopathy.

Chronic allograft nephropathy (CAN) affects all transplanted kidneys in the long run. Scarring of the allograft results from repeated bouts of subclinical rejections and/or long-term therapy with nephrotoxic immunosuppressant agents. Indeed, one of the most commonly used classes of immunosuppressant medications, the calcineurin inhibitors, induce renal scarring in the vast majority of renal transplant recipients. CAN is diagnosed on renal biopsy.

Medication-induced side-effects are significant and should be monitored in all patients. Cosmetic side affects are a particular problem in adolescents as they commonly lead to problems with medication adherence. Common side effects include: Chronic renal scarring/allograft nephropathy (calcineurin inhibitors cyclosporin and tacrolimus), hirsutism (cyclosporine and minoxidil), gingival hyperplasia (cyclosporine and calcium-channel blocker anti-hypertensive agents), weight gain/obesity (steroids), diabetes (steroids, tacrolimus), osteoporosis (steroids), diarrhea and gastrointestinal upset (mycophenolate mofetil), and suppression of blood lines (particularly neutropenia) (mycophenolate mofetil).

Disease recurrence: Patients with some types of glomerular disease, including FSGS, MPGN (particularly type II), and IgA nephropathy are prone to disease recurrence post-renal transplantation. Patients with Alport's syndrome and congenital nephrotic syndrome may subsequently develop de novo anti-GBM disease post-transplantation.

References

Halloran, P. F. 2004. "Immunosuppressive drugs for kidney transplantation." *N. Engl. J. Med.* 351 2715–29.
Seikaly, M. G. 2004. "Recurrence of primary disease in children after renal transplantation: an evidence-based update." *Pediatr. Transplant.* 8 113–9.

Intestinal Failure and Intestinal Transplantation

Robert S. Venick

Intestinal failure (IF) is broadly defined as the inability of the intestinal tract to sustain life without supplemental parenteral nutrition (PN). Children with IF who do not adapt over time to achieve independence from PN are at risk of developing several complications. Intestinal Transplantation (ITx) is indicated for a subset of children with IF who develop one or more of the following life-threatening complications: Loss of central venous access (i.e., 2 or more major vessels which are thrombosed), irreversible IF associated liver disease (IFALD), severe dehydration and/or electrolyte abnormalities. In pediatrics, combined liver + intestinal transplantation is performed more commonly than isolated ITx.

Etiology

Anatomic causes of short bowel syndrome (SBS) (i.e., gastroschisis, necrotizing enterocolitis- (NEC), malrotation with midgut volvulus, and intestinal atresia) account for 2/3 of ITx in children, while disorders of motility (i.e., chronic intestinal pseudo-obstruction, Hirschsprung Disease, total aganglionosis) and congenital disorders of absorption (i.e., Tufting Enteropathy, Microvillus Inclusion Disease) make up the other 1/3.

Clinical Presentation & Prognosis

Demographics: Many of the causes of anatomic SBS are associated with pre-term labor and young maternal age. Gastroschisis and intestinal atresia will often be detected in utero. NEC and congenital disorders of absorption will typically be diagnosed in the neonatal intensive care unit, while patients with malrotation with volvulus or motility disorders may present throughout childhood. In our experience, the median age at the time of pediatric ITx is two years. There are no significant gender or racial predispositions to those children who require ITx.

Presenting signs and symptoms: Abdominal distension, feeding intolerance manifested by bilious emesis and rule-out sepsis are common presentations of SBS in neonates. Hematochezia or melena is a late-presenting sign in this group. Disorders of motility often present with delayed passage of meconium. Specifically, 95% of patients with Hirschsprung's will not pass stool in the first 24 hours of life. Congenital malabsorptive disorders typically present with failure to thrive voluminous diarrhea, dehydration and acidosis.

Clinical course and prognosis: By definition, children with IF are dependent on PN for more than 60 days. Those children who are more likely to adapt off of PN and onto full enteral feeds include patients with more than 15 centimeters of remnant small bowel, an intact ileocecal valve and full length of colon, and those with gastrointestinal continuity. The time needed to adapt can be quite variable and is the focus of ongoing multicenter studies. While the vast majority of patients on home PN tolerate it well without complications, 10–15% of those requiring long-term PN will develop IFALD, recurrent central venous catheter (CVC) infections (which may require intravenous (IV) antibiotics, removal and replacement of the line depending on the organism), metabolic bone disease or renal insufficiency. Those children who sustain such complications, and in particular those who develop IFALD manifested by persistent jaundice, abnormal liver function tests, biopsy proven cirrhosis, or portal hypertension with gastrointestinal bleeding are at especially high risk. Ideally, children with IF should be referred early to specialized centers with multidisciplinary intestinal rehabilitation and transplantation teams prior to developing such complications. Indeed infants with concomitant IF and end-stage liver disease will frequently require LTx and ITx. It is these children, due to late referrals and insufficient organ availability, who traditionally have the highest risk of waiting-list mortality of any population awaiting transplant. Currently 175–200 ITx/year are performed in the U.S. The overall 1 and 5 year patient survival rates in the modern era at experienced centers are 90% and 50–70% respectively. Infection remains the most common reason for mortality post-ITx, while rejection is the most common cause of graft loss.

Diagnosis

Prenatal ultrasound will often detect gastroschisis and intestinal atresia. NEC is a clinical diagnosis confirmed by plain films which reveal pneumatosis intestinalis and cross-table lateral X-rays which will aid in detecting the presence of free-air within the abdominal cavity. Intestinal atresia will show a paucity of distal gas on an abdominal X-ray [Kidney-Ureter-Bladder (KUB)], and can be confirmed on upper gastrointestinal with small bowel follow through (UGI+SBFT). Hirschsprung Disease is diagnosed with the following modalities: Barium enema (transition zone may be seen between aganglionic and normal bowel), anorectal manometry, rectal suction or full thickness biopsy. Chronic intestinal pseudo-obstruction is a diagnosis of exclusion in which antro-duodenal manometry may be helpful. Congenital malabsorptive disorders require upper endoscopy with small bowel biopsy, although genetic testing is now available for Microvillous inclusion disease (MVID) and Tufting Enteropathy and can be ordered in patients with a family history or high clinical index of suspicion.

Management

Intestinal failure: All children with IF (and ITx recipients) should be followed closely by a mulitidisciplinary team composed of gastroenterologists/hepatologist, pediatric and transplant surgeons, nursing, nutritionists, and social worker. Management strategies for patients with IF include medical therapy (motility agents, treatment of small bowel bacterial overgrowth, ursodeoxycholic acid, acid suppression, CVC line care teaching and antibiotic lock therapies to minimize blood stream infections); dietetic therapy (cyclic PN, PN lipid minimization to ≤ 1 g/kg/day, Omega-3 intravenous lipid preparations, specialized elemental/ semi-elemental enteral formulas high in medium chain triglycerides which are slowly advanced as tolerated, continuous vs. bolus feeds); and surgical treatments (bowel lengthening procedures, CVC placement, G-tube placement, ostomy revisions and re-establishment of GI continuity).

IF patients on chronic PN should have periodic laboratory monitoring including: Comprehensive metabolic panel, CBC with platelets and differential, coagulation studies, albumin, prealbumin, trace minerals, essential fatty acids and fat soluble vitamins.

Intestinal transplant candidates will require a number of additional infectious serologies and immune monitoring tests, assessment of vascular access using ultrasound or magnetic resonance venogram (MRVenogram), upper and lower endoscopy with biopsy, and liver biopsy. During ITx evaluation, children may require consultation by cardiology, nephrology, infectious disease, child development, physical therapy (PT), occupational therapy (OT) and dentistry. Children awaiting isolated ITx are listed as Status 1 (urgent) or 2, while those awaiting combined LTx+ITx receive a PELD Score based on their growth parameters and laboratory values.

Intestinal transplant: Induction immunosuppression typically involves IL2 Receptor Anatgonists (Daclizumab/Zenapax®, or Basiliximab/Simulect®) Anti Thymocyte Globulin (Thymoglobulin®). Maintenance immunosuppression regimens typically include tacrolimus (Prograf®, FK-506) ± Sirolimus (Rapamune®) or Mycophenolate Mofetil (CellCept®) and Steroids, which are gradually weaned at variable rates based on clinical course. Goal trough levels of tacrolimus gradually decrease the further a patient is out from ITx. Epstein-Barr virus (EBV) and cytomegalovirus (CMV) monitoring and prophylaxis is important in the post-ITx period as is PCP prophylaxis (please see ESLD & LTx Chapter for details on dosing).

In the early post-ITx period, all patients will require CVC access. PN is weaned off at a mean of 30 days post-ITx, but at many centers supplemental IV fluids and IV ganciclovir will be provided for the first 3 months post-ITx. The majority of infant ITx recipients have significant oral aversion associated with their illness and require G- or GJ-tubes for enteral nutrition and medications. In order to be able to accurately measure and monitor graft function, and survey the transplanted intestine, most pediatric ITx recipients will have ostomies in the early post-ITx period. Typically ostomy outputs <30-40 cc/kg of body weight/day are needed to maintain adequate hydration. On routine check-ups, the ostomy appearance should be assessed for color, prolapse and friability. Stoma nurse specialists are an important part of multidisciplinary teams at ITx centers. Prior to undergoing ostomy takedown, patients will need UGI+SBFT, barium enema, ileoscopy and colonoscopy with biopsies.

Consultations: Due to underlying illness and medications (aminoglycocides, diuretics, and calcineurin inhibitors), chronic renal insufficiency is prevalent in ITx recipients. Nuclear medicine glomerular filtration studies, 24-hour urine collections and nephrology follow-up are recommended. Renal dosing of medications is necessary in many ITx recipients.

Psychosocial: Due to their chronic illness and prolonged hospitalization, developmental delay is common in children with IF and ITx recipients. These children should be followed closely by child development and regional centers. Most will require physical and occupational therapy, speech therapy and feeding specialists. Social work care is crucial for these children and their families.

Monitoring: Frequent laboratory monitoring of electrolytes, LFTs, CBC with platelets and differential, nutritional markers, EBV and CMV polymerase chain reactions (PCR) and tacrolimus trough levels is the standard of care following ITx. Many centers perform surveillance endoscopy with biopsies especially in the first year post-ITx. Children with elevations or acute changes in their ostomy outputs will require a work-up for infectious enteritis including stool studies for C. Difficile, Bacterial Culture, Rotavirus, Adenovirus, Norwalk virus, viral culture and early antigen, ova and parasite, and fecal cells. If these are negative and outputs remain elevated, the child will require endoscopy to rule-out rejection.

Pearls and Precautions

Immunization: Following ITx, children should not receive live vaccines (MMR, Varicella, Rotavirus or Inhaled Influenza Vaccine). All other vaccines are encouraged. For those children transplanted as infants or toddlers, it is important to check available immunization titers to make sure they have achieved a proper immune response. A number of ITx recipients require splenectomy at the time of ITx in order to create sufficient space within their abdominal cavity. Such patients should receive 23-valent vaccine pneumococcal (Pneumovax® 23) and Pneumococcal 7-valent Conjugate Vaccine (Prevnar®) and should be on proper antibiotic prophylaxis to protect against encapsulated organisms.

Nutrition: Many centers employ elemental or semi-elemental formulas early on and avoid foods high in fat or complex carbohydrates, which are likely to be malabsorbed.

Skin and dental care: ITx recipients should be followed regularly by pediatric dentistry. At our center, these children do universally receive antibiotic prophylaxis prior to dental procedures given their highly immunocompromised state. ITx recipients on immunosuppression have an increased risk of skin cancer, therefore, sunscreen with SPF 30 or higher is important.

Toilet: The majority of these children will have ostomies for at least the first 6–12 months post-ITx. Once gastrointestinal continuity is re-established, toilet training can proceed similar to children in the general population. Challenges to toilet training include that many of these children are on continuous nighttime enteral feeds as well as magnesium and sodium bicarbonate supplements post-ITx, meaning they will tend to have more frequent and looser bowel movements.

Likely complications: Patients who present with fever, especially those early post-ITx or with a CVC, require immediate attention. Careful clinical exam and expedited work-up (blood, urine and stool cultures; CBC with platelets and differential; and a comprehensive metabolic panel) and, the prompt initiation of broad spectrum IV antibiotics. These children are amongst the most heavily immunocompromised patients in the hospital and truly require immediate, individualized attention. For those children with a CVC, it is typical to start broad antibiotic coverage with vancomycin and a third generation cephalosporin when they present with new onset of fever above 38.3 celcius. For ITx recipients without a CVC, they should be carefully evaluated prior to empirically starting antibiotic therapy. The use of NSAIDs or acetaminophen for a fever is discouraged.

School/education: Children with IF and ITx recipients should be evaluated by the Regional Center or school district as many will qualify for physical or occupational therapy due to delays associated with chronic illness.

Medications: Common side effects of tacrolimus include neurotoxicity, hyperglycemia, hyperkalemia, hypomagnesemia, hypertension and renal insufficiency. Important drug interactions with tacrolimus include erythromycin, clarithromycin, antifungal agents, calcium channel blockers, and anticonvulsants.

Medical devices: For the first 3–6 month post-ITx, it is common for pediatric recipients to have a CVC. Additionally, most of these patients will have G or GJ tubes for supplemental feeds and medications. Infants and toddlers are typically fed continuously via pumps. All children will have ostomies in the early post-ITx period.

References

Quiros-Tejeira RE, Ament ME, Reyen L, et al. Long-term parenteral nutritional support and intestinal adaptation in children with short bowel syndrome: a 25-year experience. J Pediatrics 2004;145:157–63.

Grant D, Abu-Elmagd K, Reyes J, et al. 2003 Report of the intestine transplant registry: a new era has dawned. Ann Surg 2005;241:607–13.

Fishbein TM. Intestinal transplantation. NEJM 2009; 361:998–1008

Pediatric Stem Cell Transplant (SCT)

Jerry C. Cheng, Theodore B. Moore

Currently, stem cell transplant involves the infusion of healthy pluripotent stem cells into the body to replace and carry on the function of the sick native stem cells. There are two types of SCT: Allogeneic transplant which involves infusion of stem cells from another donor; or, autologous type which involves the removal and re-infusion of the stem cells from one's own body. Allogeneic stem cells are derived from either bone marrow, stimulated peripheral blood, or umbilical cord.

Children who receive SCT should be considered immunocompromised until expert consultation with a pediatric hematologist-oncologist is available.

Etiology

Indications for pediatric SCT include two broad categories: Non-malignant and malignant diseases. Most children undergo transplant for malignant disease such as acute leukemia (primary or refractory); refractory or advanced solid tumors (Brain tumors, Ewing's sarcoma, Wilm's tumors, Neuroblastoma); or, recurrent Hodgkin lymphoma. Most malignant conditions in children involve a complex interplay between acquired genetic anomalies and poorly understood environmental factors.

Although SCT is most commonly used for the treatment of malignant conditions, it is also used to treat such non-malignant conditions as marrow failure states (aplastic anemia, fanconi's anemia); congenital immunodeficiency states (severe combined immunodeficiency); and, certain genetic/metabolic diseases (sickle cell disease, mucopolysaccharidoses, Tay-Sachs, adrenoleukodystrophy). These conditions arise as a result of specific inherited genetic mutations.

Clinical Presentation and Prognosis

Demographics: The mean age for malignant diseases varies with the specific cancer.

The vast majority of non-malignant diseases present within the first year of life. The exceptions are acquired bone marrow failure states that present after 5 years of age and adrenoleukodystrophy which can present with very subtle neurologic deficits in early childhood that progresses rapidly. There are no known racial or ethnic predilections for the aforementioned conditions. Three questions should be considered:

- Is there an ideal age for SCT?
- Is there an age when most SCT's are done?
- Is there an age when SCT's should not/aren't done?

The answer is that no, there is really no ideal age. Candidacy for transplant is an individualized decision based on clinical indications and recipient suitability.

Presenting signs and symptoms: Children who receive SCT may endure any or all of the common post-transplant complications including infection (common and opportunistic pathogens); graft-versus-host disease ((GVHD), allogeneic setting only)); endocrinopathies (thyroid, reproductive, growth failure); and medication-related end-organ damage (renal insufficiency, neurologic changes, hepatitis, and chronic hemolysis).

Infection usually presents with fever, but on occasion there may be an absence of fever if the child is on multiple immune-suppressing medications. Therefore, instability in vital signs or other signs and symptoms of septic shock may be the only presenting signs of infection and should be promptly identified. GVHD occurs in the allogeneic setting only and may present with rash (papular erythema to bullous eruption), jaundice, or diarrhea (high volume, watery to bloody). Endocrinopathies are typically detected on routine screening testing or review of systems such as fatigue in hypothyroidism. End-organ damage due to medications is common in the post-SCT setting and symptoms may include: Abdominal pain (hepatitis); alterations in mental status (posterior reversible encephalopathy syndrome); and, vomiting (hepatitis, renal insufficiency).

Clinical course and prognosis: Children who receive an autologous SCT will usually become transfusion independent by 4–6 weeks after the procedure and should have a normalizing WBC and absolute neutrophil count (ANC). Those that remain transfusion dependent or neutropenic (ANC<500) are at risk for bleeding complications and life-threatening infection. Neutropenic children may also be at ongoing risk for mucositis (from high dose conditioning chemotherapy) and secondary malnutrition. The prognosis for children who undergo autologous SCT is usually excellent (5 year survival approaches 70% for Hodgkin Lymphoma) once blood counts normalize and mucositis heals. Long term prognosis is primarily influenced by the disease state post-transplant.

The allogeneic SCT course is very different from that of the autologous setting. These children are usually immunocompromised, transfusion dependent, and at risk for significant malnutrition and end-organ damage for a much longer duration (months-years) due to the inherent need for chronic immunosuppressing medications and the aggressive conditioning therapy that is required (high dose chemotherapy, Antithymocyte Globulin (ATG), Irradiation). The duration and severity of these complications are generally influenced by two variables: Host factors and donor factors. Host factors include condition prior to transplant, serologic status for CMV, and age. Donor factors include age, gender, CMV status, ABO incompatibility and the degree of HLA mis-match (related or unrelated donor).

Complications post-allogeneic transplant usually follow a predictable timeline following the procedure as outlined in Table 17.1.

Diagnosis

A comprehensive medical history documenting the type of SCT (autologous versus allogeneic), time elapsed since SCT, active medication list, and ill contact exposures are critical. In the non-acute setting, complete review of systems and social history including Home-Education-Activity-Drugs-Sex-Suicide (HEADSS) assessment will help detect endocrinopathies and neurocognitive problems. Physical examination may reveal signs of infection (vesicular rash, lymphadenopathy, abdominal pain, erythematous or tender central line, perioral or perianal tenderness, rales); graft-versus-host disease (papular or bullous rash, jaundice, voluminous or bloody diarrhea); and medication induced toxicity (altered mental status, anemia, hemoglobinuria, renal failure).

Appropriate imaging studies such as chest X-ray, computerized tomography, or magnetic resonance imaging are indicated in helping to localize the source of infection, while the following screening labs are

Table 17.1: Post-allogeneic Transplant Complications

Days Post Transplant	Complications
1–30 (pre-engraftment phase)	1. Infection(gram negative organisms, HSV, Staph. epidermidis, Enteroccoci, fungal) 2. Mucositis 3. Veno-occlusive disease
30–100 (engraftment phase)	1. Infection (gram + and – organisms, CMV, fungal) 2. Acute graft-versus-host disease;
beyond day 100 (post-engraftment phase)	1. Infection [encapsulated bacteria, Varicella zoster virus(VZV), Pneumocystis carinii pneumonia (PCP), Epstein Barr Virus (EBV)] 2. Chronic graft-versus-host disease 3. Medication induced end organ damage 4. Endocrinopathies 5. Neurocognitive delay

generally recommended when initially evaluating an SCT recipient for an acute complaint: Complete blood count with differential; chemistry panel including calcium, magnesium, phosphorous, blood urea nitrogen (BUN), creatinine, aspartate aminotransferase (AST), alanine aminotransferase (ALT), total and direct bilirubin, and lactate dehydrogenase (LDH); urinalysis, drug levels (tacrolimus, sirolimus, cyclosporine, ormycophenolate mofetil); and, blood culture (if clinical concern for infection). If indicated, additional lab testing should include cytomegalovirus quantitative DNA polymerase chain reaction (PCR), Epstein-Barr Virus quantitative DNA (PCR), and other pathogen specific tests.

Invasive procedures that may be required for diagnosis include: Tissue biopsy of affected GVHD target organ (e.g., skin, liver, gut, or lung); or, bronchoscopy for bronchoalveolar lavage (BAL) in the setting of fever and respiratory symptoms.

Management

Children who undergo SCT are initially hospitalized for weeks to months in carefully designed isolation rooms with strict activity and dietary restrictions. In the acute outpatient setting, early expert consultation should be sought with a pediatric SCT specialist or a pediatric hematologist-oncologist. Initial triage measures should include isolation of the patient and identification of the type of complication that is present.

Infection: Blood cultures (bacterial and fungal) should be promptly drawn from central lines and/or peripherally, followed by the start of broad-spectrum antibiotics which include vancomycin (10 mg/kg/dose IV q8hours), and Ceftazidime (50 mg/kg/dose IV q8hrs). Ill appearing children should be treated with Gentamicin (4 mg/kg/dose IV q8hrs) and an antifungal of choice (voriconazole or posiconazole). Chest X-ray and pulse oximetry should be done for cough and if there is significant respiratory distress, expert consultation with a pediatric pulmonologist is recommended for a BAL. If indicated, appropriate measures to manage septic shock should be started (e.g., volume resuscitation, pressors). If there is no improvement in clinical status, consultation with an infectious disease specialist is recommended to empirically broaden anti-microbial coverage for opportunistic pathogens such as Pneumocystis jiroveci(formerly carinii).

Medication-related toxicity

- *Altered Mental Status (AMS):* Toxic elevations in commonly used calcineurin inhibitors such as tacrolimus and cyclosporine can lead to posterior reversible encephalopathy syndrome (PRES), which results in altered mental status and/or seizures. One possible cause is the recent addition of an antifungal "azole" drug. Meds should be held in this setting. Drug levels should be sent STAT and appropriate imaging with CT or MRI should be pursued. A full electrolyte panel including magnesium levels should also be drawn and any abnormalities should be corrected. Usual causes of AMS such as bleeding or mass effect should be excluded. Urgent consultation with pediatric neurology is recommended.
- *Pancytopenia:* This drop in bone marrow function may reflect underlying disease state or toxicity from immunosupressants such as cellcept or sirolimus. Cellcept is primarily myelotoxic and can lead to pancytopenia. Sirolimus is associated with thrombocytopenia and, more specifically, an aggressive variant of thrombotic thrombocytopenia purpura (elevated LDH, shistocytes, hemoglobinuria). Supportive measures in the form of transfusions of irradiated and cytomegalovirus (CMV) negative blood products are indicated. Expert consultation should be obtained before stopping immunosuppression.
- *Altered liver enzymes (AST/ALT):* Elevation of liver enzymes is very common, often due to antifungal and antiviral medications. Depending on the degree of elevation, this change in enzymes may represent liver GVHD or acute infectious hepatitis. Recommend if ALT >1000 units/Liter, sending acute infectious hepatitis panel and consider withdrawing medication. Concomitant elevation of total bilirubin above 2.0 mg/dL supports GVHD and may warrant a liver biopsy.
- *Renal insufficiency:* This is often caused by cyclosporine and less so by tacrolimus. In such cases, nephrology consultation along with prompt hydration therapy and medication adjustments may be indicated. If patient is noted to be in renal failure, emergent measures to address hyperkalemia and other electrolyte abnormalities are indicated.

GVHD: If GVHD of the skin, gut, or liver is suspected, immediate expert consultation is recommended with the appropriate specialty. This is usually coordinated with the assistance of a pediatric hematologist–oncologist. Empiric therapy to treat GVHD with steroids, immunomodulators such as daclizumab and etanercept, or other immunosuppressing medications is not appropriate without the guidance of a trained SCT specialist.

Social: Pediatric SCT recipients and families need ongoing psychosocial support. This is mostly due to the high frequency of chronic disease, developmental delay, neurocognitive delay, and adjustment disorder during adolescence. Online support groups and resources are available through the National Marrow Donor Program (www.nmdp.org).

Pearls and Precautions

Immunization: Following SCT children should not receive live vaccines (MMR, Varicella, Rotavirus or Inhaled Influenza Vaccine). All other vaccines are encouraged. For those children transplanted as infants or toddlers, it is important to check available immunization titers to make sure they have achieved a proper immune response.

Nutrition: Few dietary restrictions exist for these patients once they are no longer neutropenic. Grapefruit is known to affect tacrolimus and cyclosporine metabolism and should be avoided. Herbal medications are often discouraged over concern with drug interactions. The long-term sequelae of developing metabolic syndrome is particularly concerning for this cohort of patients. Healthy diet and exercise should be continually emphasized and early interventions taken whenever possible.

Skin and dental care: SCT recipients should be followed regularly by pediatric dentistry. They do not require antibiotic prophylaxis unless they have a known cardiac condition. SCT recipients on immunosuppression have an increased risk of skin cancer, therefore, sunscreen with SPF 30 or higher is important.

Toilet: Toilet training should not be much different for toddlers who have received SCT than from the general population with the exception that patients on magnesium or sodium bicarbonate supplements will tend to have more frequent and looser bowel movements which can make toilet training more challenging.

School/Education: Children eligible for SCT should be evaluated by the Regional Center or school district, as many will qualify for physical or occupational therapy due to delays associated with chronic illness.

Medications: Common side effects of tacrolimus include: Neurotoxicity, hyperglycemia, hyperkalemia, hypomagnesemia, hypertension and renal insufficiency. Important drug interactions with tacrolimus include erythromycin, clarithromycin, antifungal agents, calcium channel blockers, and anticonvulsants.

Medical devices: For the first 100 days post SCT, it is commonplace for pediatric recipients to have a CVC in order to receive antiviral therapy and for lab draws.

References

Blume, KG and Forman, SJ, Thomas' Hematopoetic Cell Transplantation, 4th edition, pp. 1067–1084.

Dykewicz CA, Jaffe HW, and Kaplan JE, Guidelines for Preventing Opportunistic Infections Among Hematopoietic Stem Cell Transplant Recipients, MMWR October 20, 2000 / 49(RR10);1–128.

National Marrow Donor Program Website: http://www.marrow.org/PHYSICIAN/Outcomes_Data/index.html

Pizzo, PA and Poplack, DG, Practice of Pediatric Oncology, 4th edition.

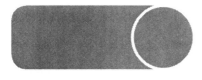

Index

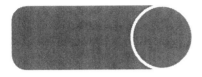

Index of Websites

LaVergne, TN USA
06 March 2011
218977LV00002B/6/P

9 781599 425351